Transition-Age Youth Mental Health Care

Vivien Chan • Jennifer Derenne
Editors

Transition-Age Youth Mental Health Care

Bridging the Gap Between Pediatric and Adult Psychiatric Care

Springer

Editors
Vivien Chan, M.D., DFAPA, DFAACAP
Student Health Center
University of California, Irvine
Irvine, CA
USA

Jennifer Derenne, M.D., DFAACAP, FAED
Department of Psychiatry
and Behavioral Sciences
Stanford University School of Medicine
Palo Alto, CA
USA

ISBN 978-3-030-62112-4 ISBN 978-3-030-62113-1 (eBook)
https://doi.org/10.1007/978-3-030-62113-1

This Springer imprint is published by the registered company Springer Nature Switzerland AG
The registered company address is: Gewerbestrasse 11, 6330 Cham, Switzerland

Preface

Transitions have the potential for amazing growth, but can also be marked by stress and anxiety. The transition from childhood to adulthood is universal and can be fraught with challenge for even the most well-adjusted individuals. Decreased parental oversight, increased responsibility, differing rates of neurobiological maturation, and the developmental challenges of separation and individuation all play a role. Young people living with a mental health condition are at high risk of worsening symptoms in the context of these stresses.

We developed this text with the goal of making a resource available to all clinicians working with transition-age youth (TAY). TAY can be wonderfully resilient, innovative, and continue to establish enduring life patterns during this critical life stage. Pediatric providers need to be aware of the potential pitfalls ahead so that they can begin to anticipate and problem solve with patients and families. Adult clinicians need to be attuned to the developmental changes and systems issues impacting TAY who are chronologically adult but maintain features consistent with the adolescent population.

We have organized the book such that the beginning part covers general, comprehensive issues of terminology and adolescent development, pithy tips for clinicians, and thoughtful considerations toward professional training issues. The second part addresses treating TAY with various mental health diagnoses. In addition to our experts' masterful contributions on mood, anxiety, adjustment/trauma, psychosis, disordered eating, attention/deficit-hyperactivity, and learning disorders, we have also called on experienced clinicians to address impulse control disorders, the obsessive-compulsive spectrum of conditions, and personality evolution. The final part of the book focuses on special populations and circumstances unique to the TAY population. We review the particular needs and resources for foster TAY, TAY who come from underprivileged and under-resourced groups including juvenile justice, LGBTQ TAY, and facets of diversity and identity wherever majority and minority groups arise. Four additional special topics, which are critical but often neglected in TAY academic writings, are included: reproductive and pregnancy issues, media use, medical leaves of absences from higher education, and, we think, a groundbreaking review of TAY disability management inclusive of visual and hearing impairments. We hope you appreciate the expertise and wisdom of leaders in our field who work with teens and young adults on both sides of the transition.

Irvine, CA, USA — Vivien Chan, M.D., DFAPA, DFAACAP
Palo Alto, CA, USA — Jennifer Derenne, M.D., DFAACAP, FAED

Acknowledgements

We wish to thank the past and current members and liaisons to the American Academy of Child and Adolescent Psychiatry's Transition Age Youth and College Student Mental Health Committee, the authors who worked so hard to contribute to this text, and the TAY that we have worked with over the years who continue to teach and inspire us.

Contents

Author Biography

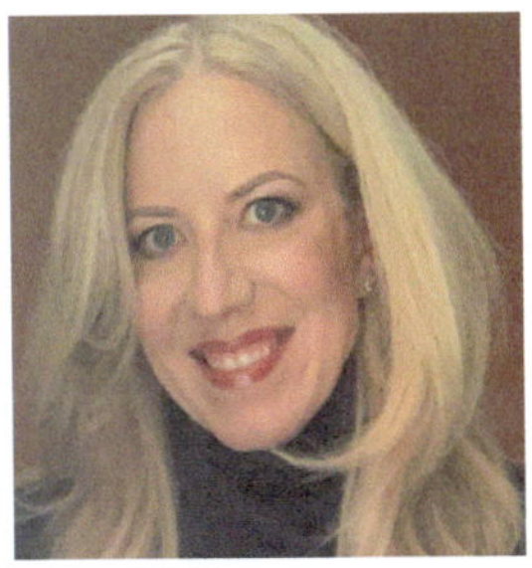

Jennifer Derenne, M.D., DFAACAP, FAED is a Clinical Professor of Psychiatry and Behavioral Sciences in the Division of Child and Adolescent Psychiatry at Stanford University School of Medicine. She graduated from the University of Wisconsin School of Medicine and Public Health and completed an internal medicine internship at Salem Hospital. She went on to pursue General Psychiatry residency and Child and Adolescent Psychiatry fellowship training at Harvard Medical School's Massachusetts General Hospital and McLean Hospital Program. She has expertise in treating anxiety, depression, and eating disorders across the lifespan, with particular interest in treating college-age students. In addition to her clinical practice, she is active in medical education and serves on the American Academy of Child and Adolescent Psychiatry College Mental Health Committee. She is currently the Psychiatric Director of the Comprehensive Care Unit for Eating Disorders at Lucile Salter Packard Children's Hospital at Stanford.

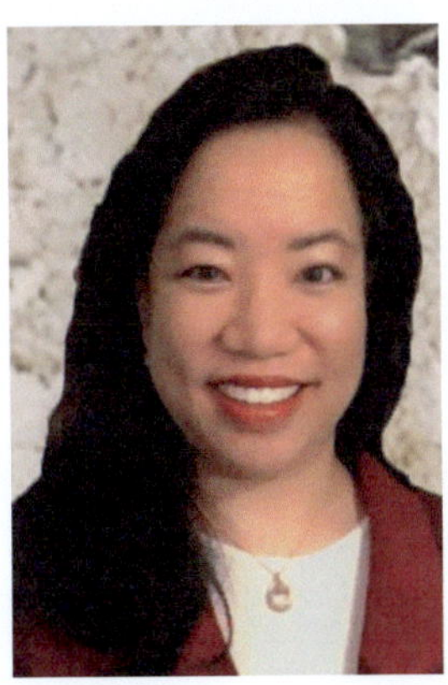

Vivien Chan, M.D., DFAPA, DFAACAP is a Distinguished Fellow of both the American Academy of Child and Adolescent Psychiatry and the American Psychiatric Association (DFAACAP/DFAPA). Nominated to Best Doctors in America and Most Distinguished Psychiatrist in Orange County by her peers, her leadership and clinical experience in the academic, public, and private mental health sectors have represented her belief in high-quality comprehensive psychiatric services for all populations, particularly in early intervention for children, adolescents, and young adults. After graduation from a 6-year accelerated, combined

BS/MD program at Northeast Ohio Medical University, she completed her general psychiatry residency and child and adolescent psychiatry fellowship at the University of California Irvine where she has been promoted to the rank of Clinical Professor in its Department of Psychiatry and Human Behavior (Volunteer Faculty Track). She is currently the Chief of Psychiatry and Mental Health Services at UCI's Student Health Center and Interim Director of Student Mental Health in the UC Virtual Care Collaborative (University of California Office of the President), and she provided psychiatric consultation in a first-episode psychosis program, Center of Resiliency, Education and Wellness (OC CREW, Orange County Health Care Agency). She also serves on the Orange County Medical Association's Physician of Excellence Committee.

Contributors

Cheryl S. Al-Mateen, MD Departments of Psychiatry and Pediatrics, Virginia Treatment Center for Children, Virginia Commonwealth University Health System, Richmond, VA, USA

Sarah H. Arshad, MD The Children's Hospital of Philadelphia, Department of Child and Adolescent Psychiatry and Behavioral Sciences, Philadelphia, PA, USA

Tracy Asamoah, MD Austin, TX, USA

Lauren P. Baker, MD Department of Psychiatry, Child and Adolescent Psychiatry, Virginia Treatment Center for Children, Virginia Commonwealth University Health System, Richmond, VA, USA

Colin W. Burke, MD Massachusetts General Hospital, Boston, MA, USA

Harvard Medical School, Boston, MA, USA

Charles Camp, MD Jacobs School of Medicine and Biomedical Sciences, University at Buffalo, Buffalo, NY, USA

Jaclyn Datar Chua, DO The Children's Hospital of Philadelphia, Department of Child and Adolescent Psychiatry and Behavioral Sciences, Philadelphia, PA, USA

Danielle Colborn, PhD Department of Child and Adolescent Psychiatry, Stanford University School of Medicine, Palo Alto, CA, USA

Shelley Co, DO State University of New York Downstate Health Sciences University/Kings County Hospital Center, Brooklyn, NY, USA

Kristin Dalope, MD UPMC Children's Hospital of Pittsburgh, Pittsburgh, PA, USA

Jana Dreyzehner, MD Life Connect Health, LLC, Nashville, TN, USA

Zhanna Elberg, MD Jacobs School of Medicine and Biomedical Sciences, University at Buffalo, Buffalo, NY, USA

Pari Faraji, MD Oregon Health & Science University, Portland, OR, USA

Elizabeth S. Firmin, BA Clinical and Research Programs in Pediatric Psychopharmacology & Adult ADHD, Massachusetts General Hospital, Boston, MA, USA

Lois Flaherty, MD Harvard University and Cambridge Health Alliance, Cambridge, MA, USA

Marcelle Friedman, MS PGSP-Stanford PsyD Consortium, Palo Alto University, Palo Alto, CA, USA

Catherine Fuchs, MD, DFAACAP Vanderbilt University Medical Center, Department of Psychiatry & Behavioral Sciences and Pediatrics, Nashville, TN, USA

Cathryn A. Galanter, MD State University of New York Downstate Health Sciences University/Kings County Hospital Center, Brooklyn, NY, USA

Anisha Garg, MD Children's Hospital of the King's Daughter, Division of Psychiatry and Psychology, Norfolk, VA, USA

Karen Goldberg, MD Life Connect Health, LLC, Nashville, TN, USA

McLeod Frampton Gwynette, MD Medical University of South Carolina, Department of Psychiatry and Behavioral Sciences, Charleston, SC, USA

Liwei L. Hua, MD, PhD Catholic Charities of Baltimore, Millersville, MD, USA

Lisa Jacobs, MD, MBA Department of Psychiatry and Behavioral Sciences, Stanford University School of Medicine, Palo Alto, CA, USA

Kristopher Kaliebe, MD USF Health Department of Psychiatry and Behavioral Neurosciences, Tampa, FL, USA

Janice Kang, PhD Department of Psychiatry and Behavioral Sciences, Stanford School of Medicine, Stanford, CA, USA

Anita R. Kishore, MD Department of Psychiatry and Behavioral Sciences, Stanford University School of Medicine, Stanford, CA, USA

Hilit Kletter, PhD Department of Psychiatry and Behavioral Sciences, Stanford School of Medicine, Stanford, CA, USA

Patricia K. Leebens, MD Department of Child and Adolescent Psychiatry, Yale Child Study Center, Yale School of Medicine, New Haven, CT, USA

Terry Lee, MD Department of Clinical Services, Community Health Plan of Washington, Seattle, WA, USA

Hope Levin, MD Counseling and Psychological Services, University of California, Los Angeles, Los Angeles, CA, USA

Natasha Marrus, MD, PhD Washington University School of Medicine, Department of Psychiatry, St. Louis, MO, USA

Adele Martel, MD, PhD Department of Psychiatry and Behavioral Sciences, Northwestern University Feinberg School of Medicine, Chicago, IL, USA

Jessica Moore, MD Department of Psychiatry, University of Texas Southwestern Medical Center, Dallas, TX, USA

Wynne Morgan, MD Department of Psychiatry, UMass Medical School, Worcester, MA, USA

Nnenna Kalaya Okereke, MD, FAPA, DFAACAP Greater Metro NYC Psychiatric, White Plains, NY, USA

Maryland Pao, MD Office of the Clinical Director, National Institute of Mental Health, National Institutes of Health, Bethesda, MD, USA

Kayla Pope, MD Winnebago Mental Health Institute, Oshkosh, WI, USA

Parna Prajapati, MD, MPH Virginia Commonwealth University, Department of Psychiatry, Division of Child & Adolescent Psychiatry, Richmond, VA, USA

Daryn Reicherter, MD Department of Psychiatry and Behavioral Sciences, Stanford School of Medicine, Stanford, CA, USA

Adelaide Robb, MD Psychiatry and Behavioral Sciences, Children's National Hospital, Washington, DC, USA

Anthony Rostain, MD, MA Cooper University Medical School of Rowan University, Camden, NJ, USA

Perelman School of Medicine, Philadelphia, PA, USA

Reem Mohamed Abdel Shafi, MD Cairns Hospital and Hinterland Service, Cairns, QLD, Australia

Vinita Shivakumar, BS Department of Psychiatry and Behavioral Sciences, Stanford University School of Medicine, Stanford, CA, USA

Stephanie Sims, MD Department of Psychiatry, University of Florida College of Medicine-Jacksonville and UF Health-Jacksonville, Jacksonville, FL, USA

Bela Sood, MD, MSHA Virginia Commonwealth University, Department of Psychiatry, Division of Child & Adolescent Psychiatry, Richmond, VA, USA

Kristen Sundin, LICSW Adolescent and Young Adult Services, Butler Hospital, Providence, RI, USA

Kevin L. Sun, MM Department of Psychiatry and Behavioral Sciences, Stanford University School of Medicine, Stanford, CA, USA

Evan Trager, MD Department of Psychiatry and Behavioral Sciences, Stanford School of Medicine, Stanford, CA, USA

Celine Turco, PHR Life Connect Health, LLC, Nashville, TN, USA

Colby Tyson, MD Psychiatry and Behavioral Sciences, Children's National Hospital, Washington, DC, USA

Erin Ursillo, LMHC Adolescent and Young Adult Services, Butler Hospital, Providence, RI, USA

Craigan Usher, MD Oregon Health & Science University, Portland, OR, USA

Timothy Van Deusen, MD Department of Psychiatry, Yale University School of Medicine, New Haven, CT, USA

Gerrit I. van Schalkwyk, MD University of Utah Department of Pediatrics, Salt Lake City, UT, USA

Roma A. Vasa, MD Kennedy Krieger Institute, Johns Hopkins University School of Medicine, Baltimore, MD, USA

Paul Weigle, MD Natchaug Hospital, Mansfield Center, CT, USA

Timothy E. Wilens, MD Harvard Medical School, Boston, MA, USA

Clinical and Research Programs in Pediatric Psychopharmacology & Adult ADHD, Massachusetts General Hospital, Boston, MA, USA

Edwin Williamson, MD Vanderbilt University Medical Center, Department of Psychiatry & Behavioral Sciences and Pediatrics, Nashville, TN, USA

Walter E. Wilson Jr, MD Vanderbilt University Medical Center, Department of Psychiatry & Behavioral Sciences and Pediatrics, Nashville, TN, USA

Margaret Wohlleber, MD Emory University School of Medicine, Atlanta, GA, USA

Amy M. Yule, MD Harvard Medical School, Boston, MA, USA

Clinical and Research Programs in Pediatric Psychopharmacology & Adult ADHD, Massachusetts General Hospital, Boston, MA, USA

Boston Medical Center, Boston, MA, USA

Boston University School of Medicine, Boston, MA, USA

Part I

An Overview of the Psychiatric Care of Transition-Age Youth

1 Transition-Age Youth: Who Are They? What Are Their Unique Developmental Needs? How Can Mental Health Practitioners Support Them?

Adele Martel

Key Points

- TAY face complex developmental challenges during a high-risk period for onset of mental illness.
- Pediatric and adult mental health providers require enhanced knowledge, skills, and attitudes to optimize treatment of TAY.
- Developmental experiences, in the context of sustained and supportive relationships, across multiple environments facilitate psychosocial development.
- Clinicians can promote post-high school success with attention to fit of activity and available supports, with TAY strengths, interests, and goals.
- Health care providers can implement health care transition in routine practice to improve TAY ability to manage illness and assume adult roles.
- Attitudes consistent with prevention, recovery, and resilience are important for working with TAY.

Introduction

The transition from adolescence to young adulthood is a unique and complex time in the life course. During this time, young people, referred to herein as transition-age youth (TAY), face significant psychosocial and maturational challenges. They make decisions about and pursue career, educational, and independent living goals and, in doing so, need to adjust to new situations and environments. They are expected to manage their own behaviors, negotiate evolving relationships with parents and other supportive adults, and be more self-reliant. TAY encounter these challenges with a brain that is not yet fully matured and in the context of less structure, decreased formal support, and less adult supervision. Though the transition from adolescence to young adulthood can be viewed as an opportunity for increased autonomy, self-exploration, and relationship building, it remains a stressful time for most young people.

TAY diagnosed with a mental health condition (MHC) during childhood or adolescence may have gaps or delays in one or more aspects of their psychosocial development, making it even more difficult for them to manage transition stresses [1]. They are at risk for symptom exacerbation, relapse, suicide, comorbid substance use disorders, and/or difficulties in social, academic, vocational, and legal realms. Among those with MHC are subgroups of young people

A. Martel (✉)
Department of Psychiatry and Behavioral Sciences, Northwestern University Feinberg School of Medicine, Chicago, IL, USA

V. Chan, J. Derenne (eds.), *Transition-Age Youth Mental Health Care*,
https://doi.org/10.1007/978-3-030-62113-1_1

with particularly high risk of not transitioning successfully into independent adulthood [2]; these include system-involved youth (special education, child welfare, mental health, and juvenile justice systems), underserved youth (racial/ethnic minority youth), and others with unique life experiences (homeless youth, immigrant youth, LGBTQ youth). TAY who enter this transition with no prior diagnoses, simply by virtue of their age [3] and developmental stage, are also at high risk for developing mental health problems and are prone to progression into substance abuse and dependency. Despite these risks, mental health services are underutilized by TAY [4, 5].

Given the potential negative impact of mental illness on young adult functional outcomes [1, 6], the mental health of TAY has become a public health priority both in the USA and abroad [2, 7, 8]. Furthermore, recognition that the brain continues to develop at least into the mid-twenties age range highlights this developmental period as an opportunity for adaptation, skill-building, prevention, and intervention, bringing increased optimism to the field. The search for strategies to engage and sustain TAY in developmentally appropriate and effective services has intensified. Child and adolescent psychiatrists (CAP) and other mental health and medical professionals working in various settings and roles can promote the mental health of TAY, enabling these young people to successfully take on adult roles as healthy workers, partners, parents, and citizens.

The purpose of this chapter is twofold: to introduce the reader to the TAY demographic cohort in the USA and to cover topics foundational for mental health practitioners to work effectively and productively with young people in transition to young adult roles and adult-oriented mental health care.

Author's Note Many of the resources listed in this chapter, and thought to be helpful for practitioners, families, and/or TAY, are shown as internet links. Typically, the links provided are from mental health or medical literature, research centers, government websites, institutions of higher education, or mental health advocacy groups and are active at the time of this writing. When commercial websites are used, they are for general informational purposes and are not an endorsement of services or products.

Terminology

Broadly defined, *transition* means "a process or period in which something or someone undergoes a change and passes from one stage, form, or activity to another" [9]. Transition, then, can refer to a period of special or unique psychosocial development and milestone achievement, an institutional transition such as graduating from high school or leaving the foster care system, or the process of moving from child-oriented mental health services to adult-oriented services. Logically, the word *transition* (also *transitional or transitioning*) is often included in the descriptive terminology used by various child-serving systems, to refer to individuals moving from adolescence to adulthood. "Youth aging out" and "young adults aging out," terms mostly used in the foster care system, and pediatric terms "children with special health care needs" and "youth/young adults with special health care needs" are exceptions.

The descriptive term *transition-age youth* and its many grammatical variants* are used by stakeholders across multiple child-serving systems. This has led to some confusion as to a consistent definition of *transition-age youth*, and whether variants of the term are system specific. Complicating matters is when a definition from a document focusing on a subset of youth from one service sector is taken out of context and makes its way into the lay literature, including online information sources. On a positive note, across service systems, the age ranges used to define *transition-age youth*, though not identical, overlap and typically include individuals pre- and post- the age of majority (18 years old [y.o.]).

***Author's Note** Grammatical variants include transition age(d) youth +/− a hyphen after the word transition; transitional age(d) youth +/− a hyphen after the word transition; transitioning youth, transitional youth, and youth in transition.

Historical Perspective

The young adult outcomes of youth involved with various child-serving systems (special education, pediatric primary care, child and adolescent mental health, child welfare, and juvenile justice) were under intense scrutiny mostly starting in the 1980s [10]. The implementation of civil rights, entitlement, and disability legislation, along with advances in the identification and treatment of chronic medical and mental health conditions, reinforced this interest. Stakeholders evaluated the availability of, access to, engagement in, and impact of services designed to support the transition to adulthood of vulnerable youth [1, 11–14]. The ages, disabilities, and circumstances of the populations studied, and the terminology used, varied somewhat given the different perspectives (Table 1.1). Transition planning became a focus across service systems, and, of relevance, the word "transition" had formally entered the lexicon of multiple child-serving systems around the same time [15–18].

In the field of child and adolescent mental health, early studies on young adult outcomes focused on youth with serious emotional disturbance (SED), the population of interest being defined as those having serious emotional or behavioral difficulties that are psychological in origin, in combination with significant functional impairment, and arise by age 18 y.o. [1, 19]. In a paper informed by a 1995 workshop sponsored by the Center for Mental Health Services [12], the term *transitional youth* was used to label this population. The terms *transition-aged youth* [20] and *youth in transition* [19] have also been used. Many youth with SED have multisystem involvement [1], possibly resulting in these terms being used for specific subpopulations of youth in child-serving systems. Multiple terms continue to be used in the mental health literature for those transitioning to adulthood [21–24]. Experts hope

Table 1.1 The need for transition services across child-serving systems

Service system	Early key documents with reference to transition services	Terminology used in early documents	Typical age range for transition planning, research, or funding
Mental health	*1986* A System of Care for Severely Emotionally Disturbed Children [15] *1996* The Transition to Adulthood among Adolescents Who Have Serious Emotional Disturbance [12]	Youngsters between 18 and 21 y.o. Transitional youth	14–16 to 24–26 y.o. (sometimes to 30 y.o.)
Education	*1983* Programming for the Transition of Youth with Disabilities: Bridges from School to Working Life [16]	Youth with disabilities	14–16 to 22 or 23 y.o. (16 y.o. mandatory)
Foster care	*1986* The Independent Living Initiative (P.L. 99–272) [18] *1999* Foster Care Independence Act[a]	Eligible youth age 16 y.o. and over Children aging-out	14–16 to 21–23 y.o.
Pediatric primary care	*1989* Surgeon General's Report: Growing Up and Getting Medical Care [17]	Children with special healthcare needs	12–14 to 18–26 y.o.

Select documents and/or legislation from various child-serving systems are listed, along with the words used to refer to the populations of interest at the time. The age ranges listed in the last column are not specific to the early documents but represent the typical ages of those individuals in transition to young adulthood addressed by stakeholders from the various systems

[a]Foster Care Independence Act of 1999, Pub. L. No. 106–169, 113 Stat. 1882 (Dec 14, 1999)

that fewer words will be used as the field of TAY mental health advances [23].

In the latter studies, youth with SED were typically 14–16 to 25 y.o. The Substance Abuse and Mental Health Services Administration (SAMHSA) refers to those aged 16–25 y.o. with the terms *youth and young adults* as well as *transitional aged youth* [25, 26]. This age range roughly corresponds to what is traditionally considered mid to late adolescence and young adulthood. Some organizations and researchers include youth as young as 12 y.o. when talking about the transition age period considering the decreasing age of puberty and/or desire to begin transition planning early. Others extend the upper age limit to 30 y.o., to capture the wide variation in the timing of the achievement of young adult milestones in the USA. In his work on the transition to adulthood, Arnett defined *emerging adults* (EA) as ages 18–25 to 29 y.o. [27]. There is obviously overlap in the age ranges of the TAY and EA cohorts. However, an important difference is that the EA group does not include youth prior to having reached the age of majority. When narrower or more broad age ranges are used, these may be dictated by guild definitions of ages served, age constraints imposed by legislation or funding agencies, bureaucratic limitations based on chronologic ages served, or even for reasons of scientific method (e.g., the availability of an already existing control group or carefully specifying a target population). In all instances, it is important to discern the rationale for the age range listed and not automatically assume the transition age period is being redefined.

To summarize, in the mental health sector, the term *transition-age youth* and its variants have long been associated with youth and young adults at high risk of poor transition outcomes secondary to complex needs, lack of a support system, and multiple challenges. There has been fluidity in the precise grammatical form of the term used, but these nuances seem to have little import in regard to the population being discussed or the service sector in which a youth "resides." Perhaps of more relevance is not the slight variant of the term used, but that the age range of study populations continues to reflect the developmental transition and the need to bridge service systems.

Evolving Terminology

The terminology in federal initiatives as well as in the literature is evolving. In its Now Is The Time Healthy Transitions grants, SAMHSA focuses not only on youth and young adults with serious mental health conditions (SMHC) but also *those at risk for developing a SMHC* and, importantly, *those in the general public* [28]. This expanded focus may be a reflection of the epidemiologic data showing that *all* youth of transition age are at risk for mental health issues, substance abuse disorders, and suicide. It also speaks to the renewed federal emphasis on wellness promotion, screening, early detection, and early intervention in mental health across all ages and in a wide range of settings [29]. Therefore, TAY is being used more often to refer to *all* individuals in an age range, regardless of presence or absence of a MHC, service system involvement, and unique life circumstances as has been done historically. Interestingly, the *transition-age youth* form of the term is being used more consistently in the literature from different child-serving systems though the definitions continue to vary [30–32]. Lastly, the term *youth and young adults* is being used more often for those between the ages of 15–16 y.o. and 26–30 y.o.

Defining Transition-Age Youth

Establishing an approximate age range and shared terminology for those in transition from adolescence to young adulthood should serve to highlight the unique developmental features of this population and help guide the creation of policies and services designed to support them. While acknowledging that there are subpopulations of TAY at significantly increased risk for poor functional outcomes, for the purposes of this chapter, the term transition-age youth refers to the population demographic spanning middle and late adolescence [33] to young adulthood [7] roughly ages 15–26 y.o. [2, 21].

Demographics

Based on the US Census [34], individuals ages 15 through 26 years numbered approximately 52 million in 2010, accounting for nearly 16% of the total US population [34]. Along with the rest of the nation, the TAY group has become increasingly diverse in regard to ethnicity and race. The racial/ethnic makeup of the adolescent and young adult population varies by region. It is projected that the nation will become minority White in 2045 with the minority tipping point coming in 2020 for youth under 18 y.o. and in 2027 for the 18–29 y.o. age group [35].

In terms of activity (Fig. 1.1), a large proportion of TAY are in the process of pursuing their education. In 2017, nearly 22 million or 57.3% of civilian, noninstitutionalized 16–24-year-olds were enrolled, either full or part-time, in educational programs leading to a high school diploma or equivalency credential, a college diploma (Associates or Bachelors), or an advanced degree [36]. Of note, the overall high school status completion rate of 18–24-year olds has trended upward across most racial/ethnic groups, with the gap between White and Black rates no longer significant in 2017 [37]. However, compared to Whites and Hispanics, Black men and women have sustained little gain in college completion rates over the past two decades [38].

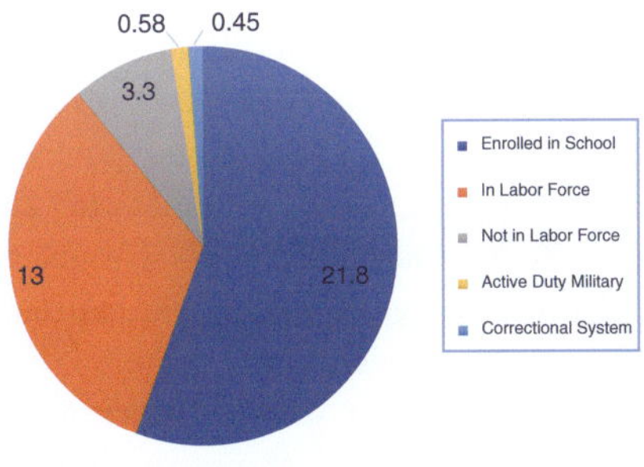

Fig. 1.1 School enrollment and other activities of U.S. 16–24 year-old in 2017. Numbers (in millions) of 16–24-year-olds involved in various activities. Of the 21.8 million enrolled in school, 12.1 million are enrolled in college. The civilian, noninstitutionalized group consists of those enrolled in school and those in and out of the labor force. Data from multiple sources was used to create this graphic; however, total numbers approximate the estimated total population of 16–24-year-olds in 2017 of 39 million [36, 42–46]

Of the 16.3 million civilian, noninstitutionalized 16–24-year-olds *not* enrolled in school, 79.5% were in the labor force in 2017. According to definitions used by the Bureau of Labor Statistics [39], those in the labor force include regular or temporary workers, working on a part- or full-time basis. Those who are unemployed but are actively pursuing gainful employment and are available to work are also considered part of the labor force. As might be predicted, labor force participation rates for both men and women were highest for those with a bachelor's degree and lowest for those with less than a high school diploma, whereas unemployment rates showed the reverse association [36]. The unemployment rate for Black youth not enrolled in school was higher than rates of other racial/ethnic groups [36].

Young people neither enrolled in school nor part of the labor force include those working toward nondegree credentials such as certifications and licenses and those involved in unpaid internship and apprenticeship programs. Others in this group are referred to as *disconnected youth*; they are neither in the labor force nor in school for a variety of reasons and include those with disabilities and those with child/family caretaking responsibilities [40]. Due to definitional and methodological differences in surveys, estimates of the number of *disconnected youth,* ages 16–24 y.o., vary, but the percentage of disconnection (11.5% in 2017) has trended down [41]. Black and Native American youth have the highest disconnection rates, and disconnected youth tend to have lower educational attainment (half of this group has a high school diploma) and live in poverty [41]. There is a concern that extended detachment from school or work may result in missed opportunities to learn new skills, gain experiences, establish networks, and build relationships with caring adults all of which can impact the transition to adulthood and, in turn, expression of mental health.

Over half a million young people under the age of 25 y.o. are active duty members of the military [42]. This group accounts for about 45% of all active duty military members. Characteristics of this group include 84% male gender, 69% White, 19% Black, and about 16% of Latino/Hispanic ethnicity. Nearly 98% of active duty members hold at least a high school diploma or its equivalent, while only just under 22% hold a bachelor's degree or higher.

The estimated number of 16–24-year-olds involved with the juvenile and adult correctional systems is about 450,000 [43–45]. The correctional system population estimate includes those in adult prisons and jails, youth detention centers, long-term secure facilities, and reception/diagnostic centers, plus those in residential treatment, group homes, and individuals on parole or probation. It is difficult to provide more precise numbers, as data sets use different or overlapping age ranges, define youth or young adults differently, and/or combine numbers from locked facilities and unlocked residential or community facilities/programs. That said, Black male and female young people are overrepresented in the correctional system [44, 46].

Pathways to Adulthood

The transition to adulthood is traditionally characterized by the achievement of markers or milestones such as completing formal education, starting and keeping a full-time job, being financially independent, living independently and away from home of origin, getting married, and starting a family [47, 48].

In its seminal report on young adults, the Institute of Medicine [7] provides a detailed description of historical and current patterns in the timing and sequencing of transition markers and a robust discussion of the societal trends (rapid changes in technology, restructuring of the economy, evolving social mores, gender role fluctuations, use of birth control, etc.) impacting the patterns. Evidence suggests that the transition to adult roles in contemporary American society has become protracted and more individualized with diversity in sequencing of markers [7, 47, 48]. "Due to the less structured pathways of this period, social support and social psychological resources are more important than ever before in facilitating youths' transition to adulthood," [49] highlighting deficits in support and creating more stress for some young people.

Many young adults focus on educational and socioeconomic attainment while delaying marriage and parenting, lengthening the time to achieve transition markers. The median age of first marriage has been increasing for decades and, in 2019, was about 28 and 30 years of age, respectively, for women and men (including same-sex married couples). Likewise, the mean age of mothers at first birth increased to 26.8 y.o. in 2017 [50]. The average age to have a baby varies with educational attainment, marital status, race/ethnicity, socioeconomic status, experience in the child-welfare system, and geographic location [50, 51].

Regarding living arrangements, more than half of 18–24-year-olds live in their parents' home [51]. They are more likely to be enrolled in school and out of the labor force compared to peers living independently or living with roommates [51]. Greater variability in the sequencing of markers is also observed. Some young adults leave home but return to live with parents, combine school and work activities or alternate between them, transfer between schools, cohabitate before marriage, and have non-marital and/or within-cohabitation children.

TAY who initiate family formation "early" (by age 21 y.o.), due to choice or circumstance, by nonmarital, unintended childbearing, or multiple partner fertility, experience young adulthood differently. They tend to have fewer opportunities and lower educational and occupational attainment and "experience greater stress, less social and economic support…and poor physical and mental health" [7]. To some extent, these findings may reflect socioeconomic and health disparities that existed before youth become parents, but they also emphasize "the cumulative advantages and disadvantages that young adults face" [52]. Unfortunately, differences within a generational cohorts' achievement of transition markers reflect ongoing inequalities in the availability of options, opportunities, and resources [47, 48].

Epidemiology

The trajectory into young adulthood, including the expression of mental wellness or mental illness, and positive or negative functional outcomes, is the result of a complex and dynamic interplay of biological, psychological, social, and cultural risk and resilience factors over the lifetime of an individual. For example, exposure to adverse events in childhood and/or adolescence are associated with negative mental health outcomes in adulthood [53]. TAY belonging to socially disadvantaged groups based on race, ethnicity, gender, sexuality, SES, nativity, and systems involvement have many risk factors for mental illness and are often overrepresented in the group of TAY with MHC. However, maintaining a life course perspective, the impact and meaning of these factors can change with ongoing maturation, environmental context, and exposure to new opportunities, experiences, and relationships [54].

Mental health and substance use disorders are major causes of disease burden in youth and young adults in the USA. Data from the 2017 global burden of disease study [55] show that over 45% of the years lived with disability (YLDs) in each of the specified age groups were caused by mental health and substance use disorders (Fig. 1.2). Statistics for neurological disorders, musculoskeletal disorders, and skin/subcutaneous disorders *in combination*, which also are main contributors of YLDs in TAY, are shown for comparison sake.

Suicide is the second leading cause of death in the 15–24-year-old age group. In 2017, the suicide rate for this age group was 14.5/100,000. For the younger members of this group (15–19 y.o.), the overall rate was 11.8/100,000, and for the older members of this group (20–24 y.o.), the overall rate was 17/100,000 [56]. In both age cohorts, males had higher suicide rates than

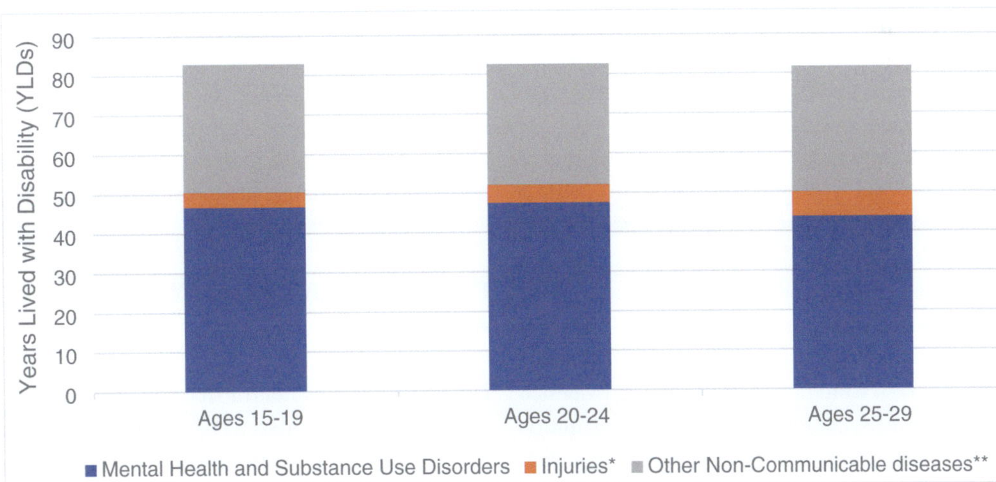

Fig. 1.2 Burden of disease in young people aged 15–29 years in the United States for 2017. Data obtained from the Global Health Data Exchange Tool for 2017 [55]. Years Lived with Disability (YLDs) are a measurement of the burden of disease. YLDs essentially represent the number of years that an individual lives with a functional impairment caused by a disease (its morbidity). *Injuries include road injuries, other unintentional injuries, and self-harm and interpersonal violence. **Three noncommunicable disease categories are *combined* – neurological disorders, musculoskeletal disorders, and skin/subcutaneous disorders

females. Among 18–24-year-olds, non-Hispanic White and American Indian or Alaska Native populations have higher rates of suicide compared to non-Hispanic Black, Hispanic, Asian, or Pacific Islander young adults [57]. College students have a lower risk of attempting suicide with a plan and a lower rate of completed suicide compared to their non-college attending peers [58, 59]. LGBTQ TAY have high rates of suicidal ideation and attempts [60]. Based on the 2018 National Survey of Drug Use and Mental Health, approximately 3.7 million young adults aged 18–25 y.o. (11.0%) had serious suicidal thoughts, the highest prevalence among adults across all age groups [61]. These data highlight the importance of suicide prevention and intervention in TAY.

Other epidemiological studies looked at the onset, prevalence, continuity across development, and sociodemographic correlates of psychiatric disorders. TAY are at an age of peak vulnerability for the new onset of psychiatric disorders. In the cross-sectional, retrospective National Comorbidity Survey Replication Study (NCSR), Kessler et al. [3] found that 50% to 75% of DSM-IV defined anxiety disorders, mood disorders, impulse control, and substance disorders emerge between the ages of 14 and 24 y.o. Schizophrenia, which has a 1% 12-month prevalence in the general population, is also diagnosed in the late teens and twenties, with the earlier age of onset biased toward males [62].

It is generally accepted that at least one in five adolescents and young adults struggles with a mental health condition. TAY experience the full range of psychiatric disorders with anxiety, depression, behavior disorders, and substance use disorders being most common [63, 64]. Comorbidity is common across the TAY age range [65–67]. Cumulative or lifetime prevalence of a range of psychiatric disorders, across multiple age groups, is graphically shown in Fig. 1.3. Gender differences in prevalence rates exist, with females having a higher overall rate of anxiety and mood disorders and males having higher rates of behavior and substance use disorders in both adolescence and young adulthood [64]. There are some racial/ethnic disparities in the rates and trajectories of substance use during adolescence and young adulthood [68]. Otherwise, when socioeconomic and other environmental risk factors are accounted for, "…ethnic and/or racial minority transitional adults do not demonstrate greater risk for diagnosed mental health conditions" [69].

Developmental Psychopathology

Having a mental health disorder in childhood or adolescence is a risk factor for having a disorder in adulthood [6, 70]. Homotypic patterns of continuity are common from adolescence to young adulthood. Two heterotypic patterns of continuity that are of interest are as follows: depression and anxiety tend to cross-predict one another, and child/adolescent oppositional defiant disorder tends to predict adult anxiety and depression [71]. Across mid to late adolescence and then into young adulthood, the prevalence rates of classes of disorders can change; for example, there is a surge of substance use disorders in late adolescence. Likewise, the prevalence rates of certain disorders within a class can also change across developmental transitions; for example, the prevalence rate of panic disorder increases from childhood to adolescence and into young adulthood while the rate for separation anxiety disorder decreases [70]. General knowledge of continuities can help with patient psychoeducation about prognosis, early intervention, and anticipatory guidance about transition planning.

Functional Outcomes in Young Adulthood

Having a mental health disorder in childhood or adolescence is also a risk factor for suboptimal outcomes [1, 72] in multiple domains of young adult functioning (health, educational, financial, social, legal), although that is not always the case. "There is a high degree of variation among young people with serious mental health disorders in terms of symptoms, causes, course of the disorder, response to treatment, mechanisms of change, and out-

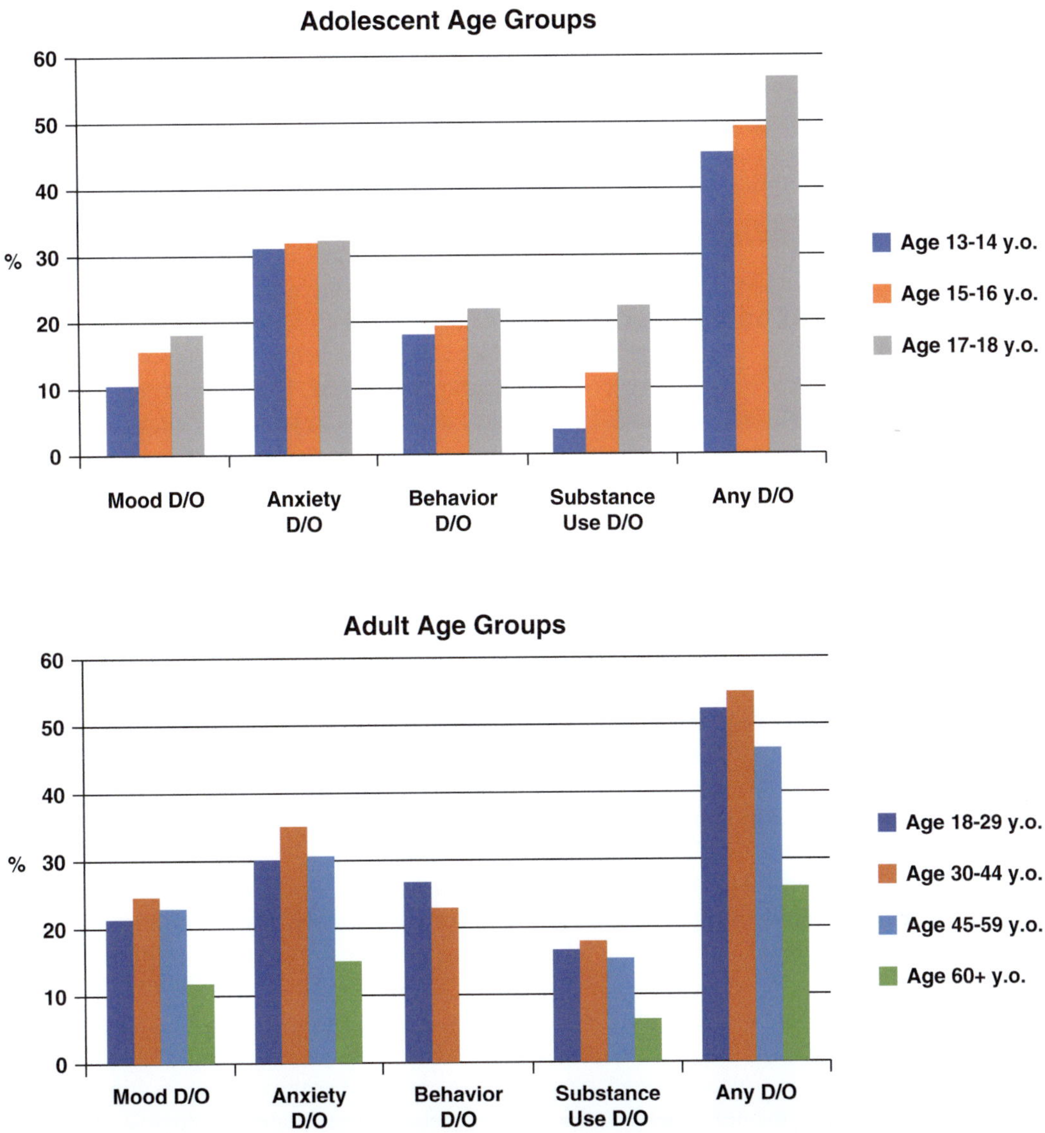

Fig. 1.3 Lifetime prevalence of DSM IV disorders. Lifetime prevalence of a broad range of mental disorders in US adolescents and adults by age groups. Top chart shows data from the cross-sectional, retrospective, National Comorbidity Survey Replication – Adolescent Supplement [64] and the bottom chart shows data from cross-sectional, retrospective National Comorbidity Survey Replication [66]

comes over time" [73]. As a group, young adults with histories of a diagnosable psychiatric disorder or even subthreshold psychiatric problems in childhood or adolescence have higher rates of adverse functional outcomes compared to non-cases, even when controlling for psychosocial hardships and adult psychiatric disorder [6, 74]. Youth with SED in the National Longitudinal Transition Study had poor social adjustment and high rates of criminal justice system involvement [75]. TAY with MHC struggle to complete college [76]. Breslau et al. [77] found that mental disorders were significantly associated with termination of schooling prior to completion at the primary, high school, and college levels and suggest that economic, social, and health difficulties may be mediated to some extent by low educational attainment. Notwithstanding the importance of prevention and early intervention in childhood and adolescence, the continuation of developmentally appropriate services and supports across the transition to adulthood should help mitigate short- and long-term functional sequelae of having a mental health condition.

Help-Seeking in TAY and Barriers to Help-Seeking

Despite the high prevalence of mental health conditions in this age group, use of mental health services is low [7]. Hower et al. [5] examined age transition effects on treatment utilization by a sample of youth with bipolar disorder, and Copeland et al. [4] used data from a longitudinal, prospective study to look at changes in service use among participants with a range of psychiatric disorders. In both studies, there was a decline in service utilization with the transition from late adolescence into young adulthood. The decline in treatment use was seen across all service sectors with a marked decrease in education sector services [4]. The latter finding is not unexpected given that aging out of or crossing over from child-serving to adult-serving systems can disrupt mental health and other support services. The use of general medical health services is low in young adults versus older adults [7]. Similarly, the percentages of young adults (19–25 y.o.) who received treatment services for any mental illness, serious mental illness, or a major depressive episode in the past year (37%, 54%, and 50%, respectively) were the lowest among all adult age groups [61]. Untreated or inadequately treated mental health conditions in TAY can serve as an obstacle to negotiation of the important demands of this developmental period such as educational completion, career establishment, and relationship building.

Identifying barriers to help-seeking for TAY can inform changes in treatment approaches, systems of care, and policy in order to better engage and maintain them in treatment [78–80]. Using a socio-ecological approach, barriers to help-seeking can be found at all levels. Community and societal level barriers exist, including public stigma against those with mental illness [81] and ongoing disparities in access to care [82]. These important and complex issues are beyond the scope of this chapter although providers working with diverse TAY need to remain mindful of the existence and impact of such issues. Barriers to help-seeking at the system level center around the multidimensional needs of TAY with MHC and the differences between adolescent and adult health systems [31, 83]; at the practitioner level, they center around provider training and competencies; at the individual level, they range from practical issues to stage-related attitudes (Fig. 1.4). An understanding of adolescent and young adult development in conjunction with improvements in comprehensive transition preparation and planning services as well as enhancing provider competence in working with TAY may address these barriers and facilitate help-seeking [2, 7].

TAY Development and Developmental Needs

The achievement of traditional milestones or markers of adulthood involves gradually working through developmental tasks intrinsic to the TAY developmental period, i.e., identity formation, separation and individuation, and achieving intimacy. In turn, these tasks require a foundation of biopsychosocial maturation in multiple aspects of development including biological, cognitive, moral, social, and emotional.

Aspects of Biopsychosocial Maturation

Throughout this discussion of typical TAY development, it is useful to keep in mind that aspects of biopsychosocial development are on different time courses within and among individuals. Maturation in one or more facets of development can be facilitated or delayed or may not progress at all given various individual characteristics, situations, or experiences [84]. Also, even when

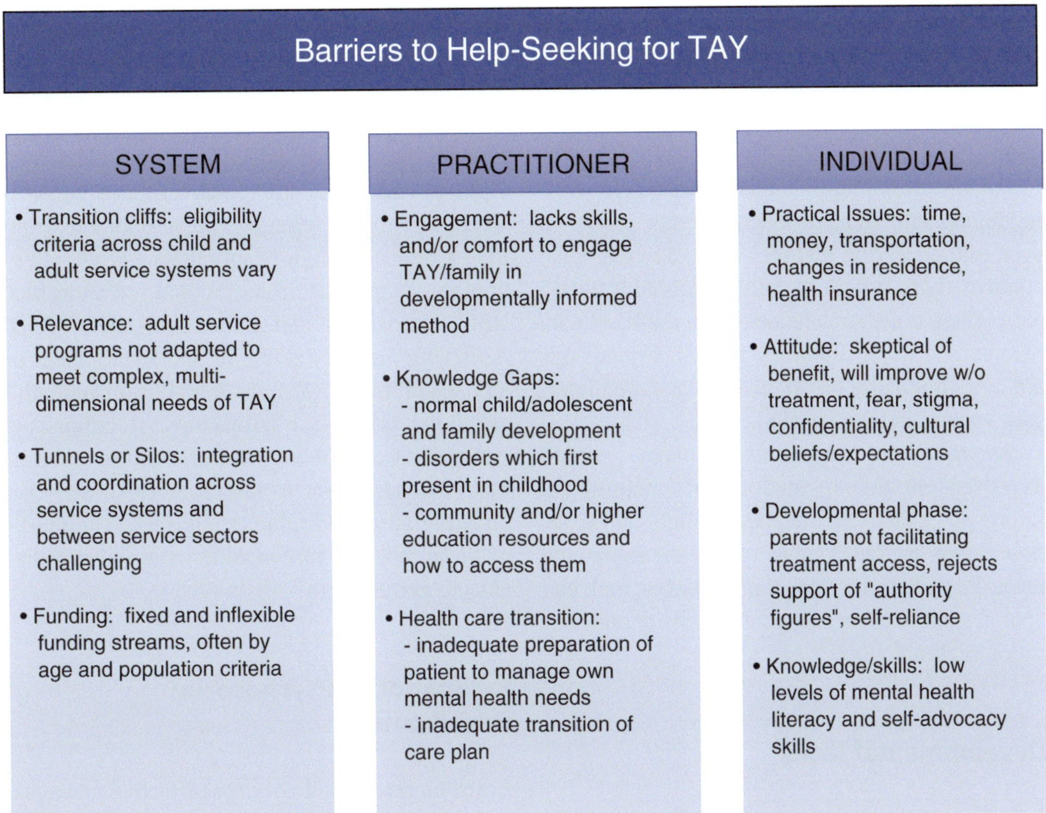

Fig. 1.4 Barriers to help seeking for TAY. Specific examples of barriers which exist at the system, practitioner, and individual levels for TAY moving from child-oriented to adult-oriented mental health care [79, 80, 83]

typical developmental gains are made, TAY are challenged to apply their new skills in novel and challenging contexts, and they may revert to less mature skills under stress [85].

The overt *biological* changes that take place in adolescence (increases in body mass and height, primary and secondary sexual characteristics, and improved coordination) are profound and are typically completed long before the age of majority. Brain development, however, continues late into the second decade of life and influences gradual maturation of other lines of development throughout that time. Brain development is asynchronous with the emotional and reward parts of the brain developing earlier than the prefrontal cortex which is associated with executive functioning [86]. Changes in the prefrontal cortex include increased myelination of nerve fibers, increased connectivity with other parts of the brain, and shifting levels/distribution of dopamine activity in prefrontal-limbic pathways. Brain development is dynamically influenced by internal factors (hormones, neurotransmitters, immune factors) and external factors (experiences, opportunities, and environmental contexts) which potentially allow for improvement in functioning and trajectory into adulthood.

TAY experience important and gradual changes in their *cognitive* abilities. With increased capacity for abstract and hypothetical thinking, they can prioritize and execute plans for the future, consider multiple ideas simultaneously, weigh the pros and cons of their actions/choices, think more creatively and use symbolic thinking, and demonstrate improved self-awareness and self-reflection [1, 84, 87].

Moral development evolves from a right/wrong framework to one in which TAY "value diversity of people and perspectives and appreciate that there may be many right answers to a problem" [84]. Over this developmental period, TAY can be more empathic and act for the greater good.

Social development is characterized by shifting relationship dynamics with parents, increased peer influence, and changes in socio-ecological contexts (high school to college, school to work, etc.). There is a natural tendency for conflicts with parents and other authority figures. Friendships are more mutuality based, involving shared interests, values, and loyalty [88].

Emotional development evolves toward improved emotion regulation. TAY acquire an improved capacity to integrate thought and emotion. They are better able to weigh immediate rewards with risks and consequences and can "put more brakes on emotional intensity and sensation seeking" [84].

Developmental Tasks

As biopsychosocial maturation proceeds, TAY are better able to negotiate three important developmental tasks [85] intrinsic to this developmental period. Working through developmental tasks supports the transition into adult roles and responsibilities.

Identity formation and consolidation is a primary developmental task of TAY. The goal is to develop a cohesive, accurate, and stable sense of self which "serves as an internal framework for making choices and provides a stable base from which one can act in the world" [89]. Identity development involves (1) integrating all aspects of one's identity, e.g., race/ethnicity, sex, gender, religion, privilege, and culture; (2) articulating realistic goals based on innate abilities, learned knowledge and skills, other life experiences, and vulnerabilities; and (3) defining and refining a personal value system. *Separation and individuation* is another developmental task that spans the adolescent years and continues into young adulthood. This task was first confronted during early childhood and is revisited. TAY become more aware of being separate from parents and others and having independent thoughts, feelings, and values. They are challenged to (and usually want to) become more autonomous and self-reliant in making/pursuing life choices, in day-to-day functioning, and in governing their behaviors. Optimal outcomes are positive sense of self-worth and "being separate and autonomous from their parents and significant others…while maintaining supportive transactional relationships with the parents and important others" [87]. *Achieving intimacy* refers to the development of and commitment to more mature and mutually satisfying intimate relationships. Relationships include those involving romantic and sexual intimacy but also refer to increasingly substantive, discriminating, and valued friendships. Hallmarks of these relationships include trust and self-disclosure and concern.

Facilitation of Psychosocial Development

Based on research, theory, and effective practices, three different groups have recently developed frameworks or standards related to the dimensions of and foundations for young adult success [89–91]. The research groups support positive youth development and resilience-focused approaches to working with TAY [92, 93]. Despite somewhat different initial aims, each framework highlights that to facilitate psychosocial development and the successful pursuit of desired young adult outcomes, TAY need opportunities for developmental experiences, in the context of sustained and supportive relationships, across multiple environments. Developmental experiences are "opportunities for action and reflection that help young people build self-regulation, knowledge and skills, values, agency and integrated identity" [89]. The benefits of such experiences are maximized within developmental relationships, those with adults and peers, which can help TAY translate experiences to promote psychosocial maturation. Features of developmental experiences [89] and developmental relationships [91, 94, 95] are shown in (Fig. 1.5). For TAY, experiences and social interactions are available in the contexts of

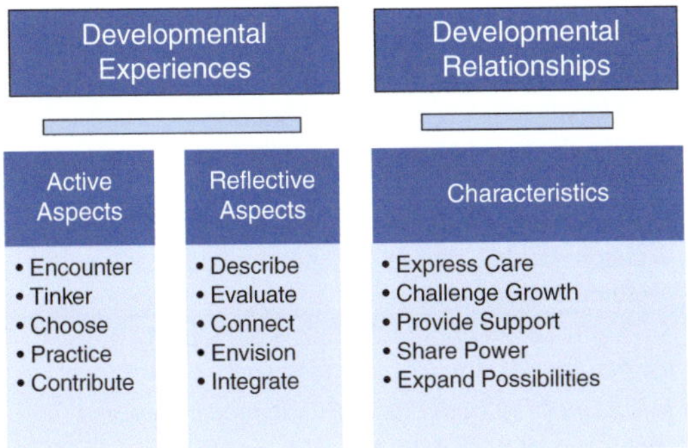

Fig. 1.5 Facilitation of psychosocial development. Features of developmental experiences [89] and developmental relationships [95] which facilitate psychosocial development

family (broadly defined), partners, peer group, school, work, and community. Though not unlike what is needed in earlier periods of development, intentional opportunities for TAY require attention to their specific needs for increasing autonomy, identity exploration, and peer interactions. Mental health providers can utilize these concepts to inform their own work with TAY and to guide others who strive to promote psychosocial maturation and a smooth transition into adulthood.

The National Collaborative on Workforce and Disability "Guideposts for Success" framework [90] describes in more detail experiences and relationships which all youth need to succeed during the transition years in the following five areas:

- School-Based Preparatory Experiences
- Career Preparation and Work-Based Learning Experiences
- Youth Development and Leadership Opportunities
- Connecting Activities (opportunities, services, and supports to become independent adults)
- "Family" Engagement and Supports

Guideposts also identify what additional supports youth with disabilities need to achieve independence in adulthood. The first iteration of Guideposts [96] was adapted to specifically address youth with mental health needs [97]. In Guideposts 2.0 [90], the School-Based Preparatory Experiences section is extended to include postsecondary education. Though initially created for the transition out of high school to the workforce, Guideposts can be applied more broadly, given the emphasis on self-determination, self-advocacy, family involvement, and transition preparation and planning, which are also important considerations for TAY who are in transition to an adult model of mental health care.

Psychosocial Development in TAY with MHC

As a group, young people with MHC have gaps or delays in one or more areas of psychosocial development [1, 88] making it even more difficult for them to navigate normal developmental tasks and to function in novel post-high school environments. Cognitive delays may interfere with educational and vocational achievement and the ability to execute plans or to change behaviors based on self-reflection. Delays in social development can make it difficult to negotiate workplace social rules, resolve conflicts with roommates, and renegotiate relationships with parents/caregivers, while delays in moral development may contribute to criminal behavior [88]. Ongoing characteristics of an illness itself (such as mood dysregulation, lethargy, inattention, impulsivity, language difficulties, episodic nature of some MHC, time management) and/or side effects of pharmacotherapy can prevent the young person from gaining the benefits of maturation-promoting experiences.

During an already complex and stressful developmental transition, TAY with MHC are expected to complete more tasks and mature undertakings than those without special challenges. They need to assume primary responsibility for their mental health care, have some understanding of how their illness might impact functioning in college, at work, and in the community, and consider what supports they need to promote success. They are expected to advocate for themselves, recognize warning signs of relapse, develop relationships with new treatment providers, and navigate new systems of care [98]. Maintaining a life course and resilience-focused perspective, TAY with MHC may benefit from scaffolds and supports which extend across the transition from late adolescence into young adulthood to hone skills, accomplish developmental tasks, achieve personal goals, and establish a supportive social network (not unlike many youth without MHC).

Implications for Mental Health Treatment

Informed by the developmental tasks and needs of TAY, their risk for mental health and substance use disorders, known barriers to help-seeking, and guided by the System of Care (SOC) concept and philosophy [15, 99], it is possible to articulate key features of developmentally appropriate treatment services for TAY (Table 1.2). For many mental health providers, items on this list may be viewed as how they routinely approach patient care across all age groups. Still, it is important to contemplate how these treatment characteristics specifically apply to TAY who [1] have a strong developmental drive to separate and establish an independent adult life, [2] experience change and new demands in all facets of their lives as they move toward adulthood, [3] have brains that are still maturing, and [4] are at risk for discontinuation of institutional supports and other services, including disruption of health care.

Table 1.2 Important Features of Behavioral Health Treatment Services for TAY

Individualization of care, respecting the personal history, developmental status, culture, and maturational process of each young person
Prioritization of TAY voice in setting goals, treatment decision-making, and the design, implementation, and evaluation of services
Strengths-based approach to promote identity formation, self-efficacy, and resilience
Involvement of family balancing independence and need for continued support
Multidimensional approach, supporting needs and goals in education, employment, relationships, health, stable housing, and community engagement
Coordination of care across service sectors to simplify access, and across systems with age limitations to avoid care disruption
TAY/age-specific settings and programs, with *peer support providers* (if applicable), to increase appeal and help reduce stigma
Attention to *natural and informal supports* across ecological contexts to help build supportive and enduring social networks
Screening for problematic *alcohol and/or substance use* with brief interventions and/or referral to treatment
Transition preparation and planning for movement to adult-oriented mental health services including psychoeducation, self-advocacy, and health management skill development
Public health approach with early identification and intervention to enhance young adult outcomes
Utilization of technology in planful, legal, and ethical fashion, to communicate with TAY and to engage them in treatment
Utilization of emerging *evidence-based practices* (EBP) for TAY and/or adaptation of existing EBP that have established effectiveness in other age groups

A TAY Version of the SOC Framework

The SOC concept and philosophy was updated in 2010 [99], acknowledging its applicability to different age groups. Figure 1.6 shows the original, child-focused SOC framework [15, 99] and a new version adapted herein for working with late adolescents and young adults, as informed by their unique needs and evidence-based or promising best practices. The traditional eight overlapping areas of needed services and supports are relevant to TAY. The framework underscores a holistic or recovery approach to mental health treatment which is preferred by young people with MHC [99, 100]. This TAY SOC framework differs from the original in a few ways. The labeling of the central circle in the figure has been modified to reflect the population of focus – TAY. Also, "other natural supports" has been added to emphasize that TAY may choose to involve family and/or individuals from outside the family, in their mental health care and life planning. The words "legal" and "adult" were added to the area labeled "juvenile justice services" given that for TAY, legal supports and services may extend into the criminal justice system and may be needed for benefits management, dis-

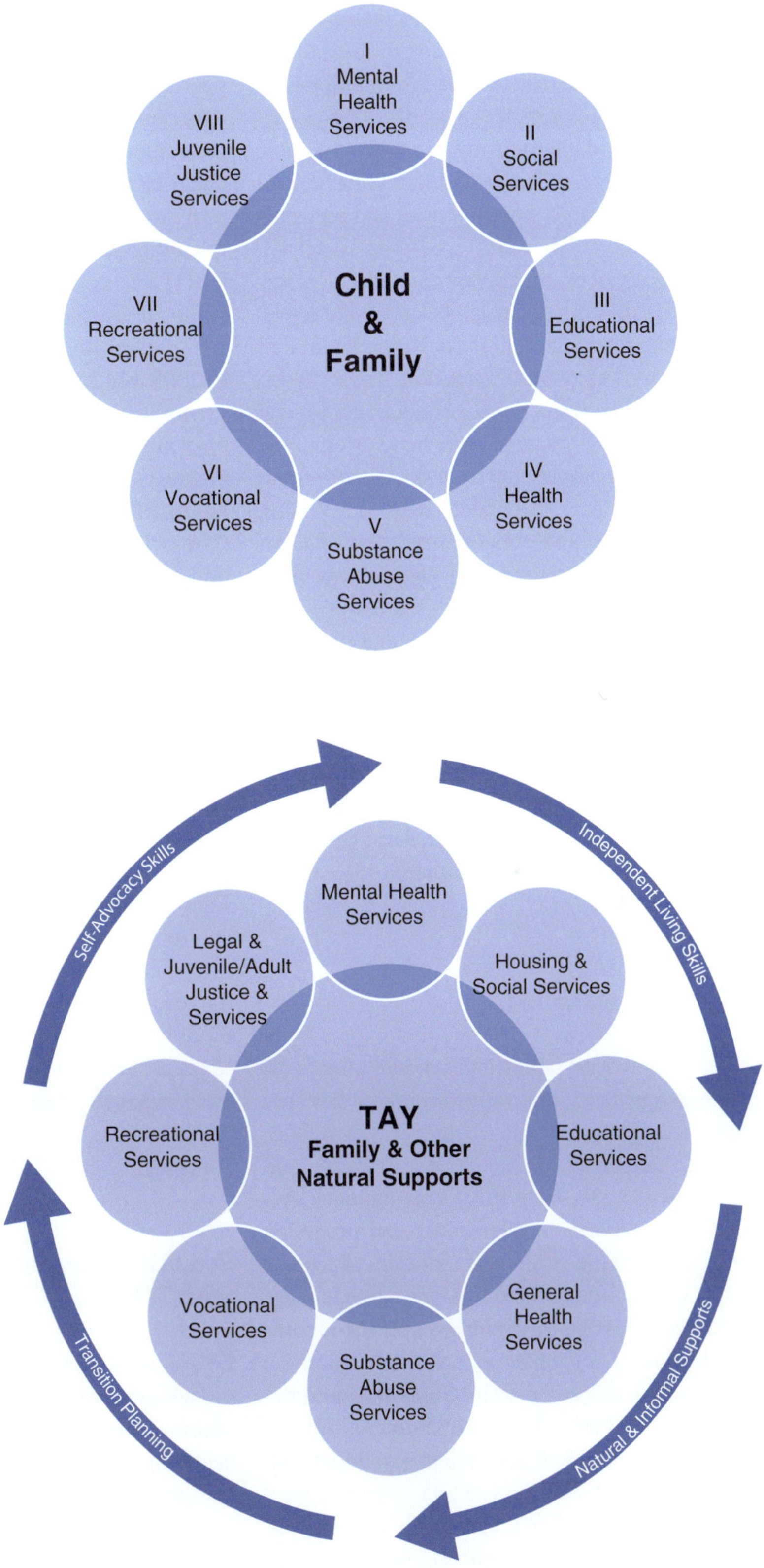

Fig. 1.6 A System of Care Framework for TAY. The top diagram shows a reproduction of the original SOC framework. (*It is included and modified with permission of the Georgetown University Center for Child & Human Development, Georgetown University Medical Center*). The bottom diagram shows a modified version as applicable to TAY. The arrows represent essential services/supports which should be part of the services array within each of the eight dimensions

ability rights and advocacy, debt restructuring, etc. "Housing" has been added to the area labeled "social" in the original framework to emphasize the heightened importance of stable, safe, accessible, and affordable housing for this vulnerable population. "Social" services include basic support services such as clothing, meal and transportation vouchers, showers, parenting supports, protective services, and foster care/adoption services [15]. Four arrows have been added to represent essential services/supports which should be available to TAY within each dimension. Given that TAY frequently change socio-ecological contexts, service areas, and service systems, the ongoing development of certain skills can smooth those transitions. TAY need help developing skills to identify and enlist natural supports. An expanded and dynamic social network not only supports the transition to adulthood but provides a safety net when TAY are not engaged in formal supports. Independent living skills build self-efficacy and may facilitate access to and use of other services. Likewise, self-advocacy skills and transition planning services (learning to anticipate the changes ahead) can help TAY guide their service plan and obtain accommodations to optimally function in new environments.

Applying System of Care Concept and Principles to TAY

Assisted by federal policy and funding initiatives, and driven by need, innovative programs that specialize in serving TAY have been developed, integrating elements of the SOC concept and principles [23, 24, 101, 102]. This includes evidence-based *coordinated specialty care* programs for young people with first episode psychosis [103] and the Transition to Independence Process (TIP) Model [104]. Also, interventions found to be efficacious in older populations, such as Individualized Placement and Support Supported Employment [105] and Clubhouse programs [106], many of which also favor individualized, coordinated, and multidimensional supports, have been tailored for the TAY age group. Researchers are evaluating the core features and efficacy of such programs. One core feature of specialized programs worth mentioning is the integration of peer support specialists, individuals with lived experience, in service delivery [107, 108]. Researchers are also developing fidelity measures and disseminating best practice guidelines for programs designed for TAY with MHC. Two rehabilitation and research training centers (RRTCs), co-funded by SAMHSA and the National Institute on Disability, Independent Living, and Rehabilitation Research (NIDILRR) in 2008 and 2014, have been instrumental in this work [24]. The websites of these RRTCs (https://www.umassmed.edu/TransitionsACR/; https://pathwaysrtc.pdx.edu/), along with a recently NIDILRR-funded cross-disability RRTC in VA (https://vcurrtc.org/), have a wealth of information and resources for policymakers, researchers, clinicians, transition specialists, special education teachers, families, and patients.

Beyond informing policy and program development, independently practicing mental health clinicians can apply SOC principles and methods to engage TAY in treatment [109]. Such providers coordinate care between service sectors by establishing regular communications with primary care providers and school personnel. They help bridge the gap between child-oriented and adult-oriented service systems by transmitting medical records and communicating with the receiving clinical team. Providers can use the modified framework to visualize the range of services a patient may need to support transition and to identify their own knowledge gaps regarding available community resources and TAY contexts.

Provider Competencies for Working with TAY

Providers working with TAY require enhanced knowledge, skills, and attitude competencies to optimize treatment of young people with mental health needs during the transition years. Core competencies for program-related transition service providers and a provider competency scale have been developed [107, 110, 111]. Though somewhat useful for individual practitioners across disciplines, more detailed knowledge and skill competencies are needed. The remainder of this chapter addresses specific areas of knowledge essential to working with TAY. A brief discussion of skills and attitudes follows as a segue to information in subsequent, diagnosis-based chapters.

Provider Knowledge: Laws, Legislation, and TAY

Whether TAY are moving on to higher education, employment, and/or independent living, it is essential for providers and other stakeholders to have a basic understanding of the protections and opportunities various civil rights laws and entitlement legislation offer to TAY with disabilities (Fig. 1.7), including those with MHC. Providers "can better advise youth and their families, work with representatives from other agencies, and develop transition plans taking advantage of these protections and opportunities" [112]. Additional resources on this topic are listed at the end of the chapter.

The Individuals with Disabilities Education Act (IDEA), a reauthorization of Public Law 94–142, ensures that students with disabilities are identified and provided with a Free Appropriate Public Education (FAPE). An Individualized Education Program (IEP) outlines specialized instruction, supports, accommodations, and qualified personnel to meet the needs of the student. Of relevance to TAY, IDEA requires the inclusion of transition services in the IEP which will be in effect when the student turns age 16 y.o. (younger in some states) to help prepare the student for post-high school endeavors. The transition plan may specifically be referred to as an Individualized Transition Plan (ITP). The transition plan includes a statement of student goals and plans for after high school and what services the school itself, and in collaboration with other agencies, is going to provide to assist the student in achieving the goals.

IDEA no longer applies after graduation from high school. IEPs and ITPs do not automatically continue to institutions of higher education (IHEs) nor to places of employment. Instead, after high school, young people with disabilities may be eligible to receive disability-related accommodations under civil rights laws. Young people may need help understanding that a MHC can be a disability when it limits one's ability to function in various environmental contexts, whether for a discrete period of time, or across the lifespan [113]. Within civil rights legislation, an individual with a disability is a person who [1] has a physical or mental impairment that substantially limits one or more major life activities, [2] has a record of such an impairment, or [3] is regarded as having such an impairment.

Section 504 of the 1973 Rehabilitation Act [114] prohibits discrimination against people with disabilities and guarantees equal access to participation in programs and services that receive federal financial assistance. The Americans with Disabilities Act (ADA) of 1990 [115] and the ADA Amendments Act of 2008 [116] extend this antidiscrimination mandate to entities that do not receive federal financial assistance. In order to receive disability-related accommodations, college students with disabilities must disclose their disability to the school's Office of Disability Services (or an office of some other title) and request specific supports in a timely manner that follows the procedures set forth by the institution. Employees who choose to disclose a disability typically go through the Human Resources Department or an Employee Assistance Program. Reasonable accommodations include changes in the classroom or work environment, modification in policies, practices or procedures, and provision of auxiliary aids and services, which enable an individual with a disability to have an equal opportunity to participate in an academic program or job. IHEs and employers are not required to eliminate or modify requirements of an academic program or essential functions of a job, nor are they required to lower performance standards.

Section 504, the ADA, the Fair Housing Act of 1968 [117] and its amendments, and other federal, state, and local laws provide protection for disabled individuals regarding housing. Additional information for disabled individuals

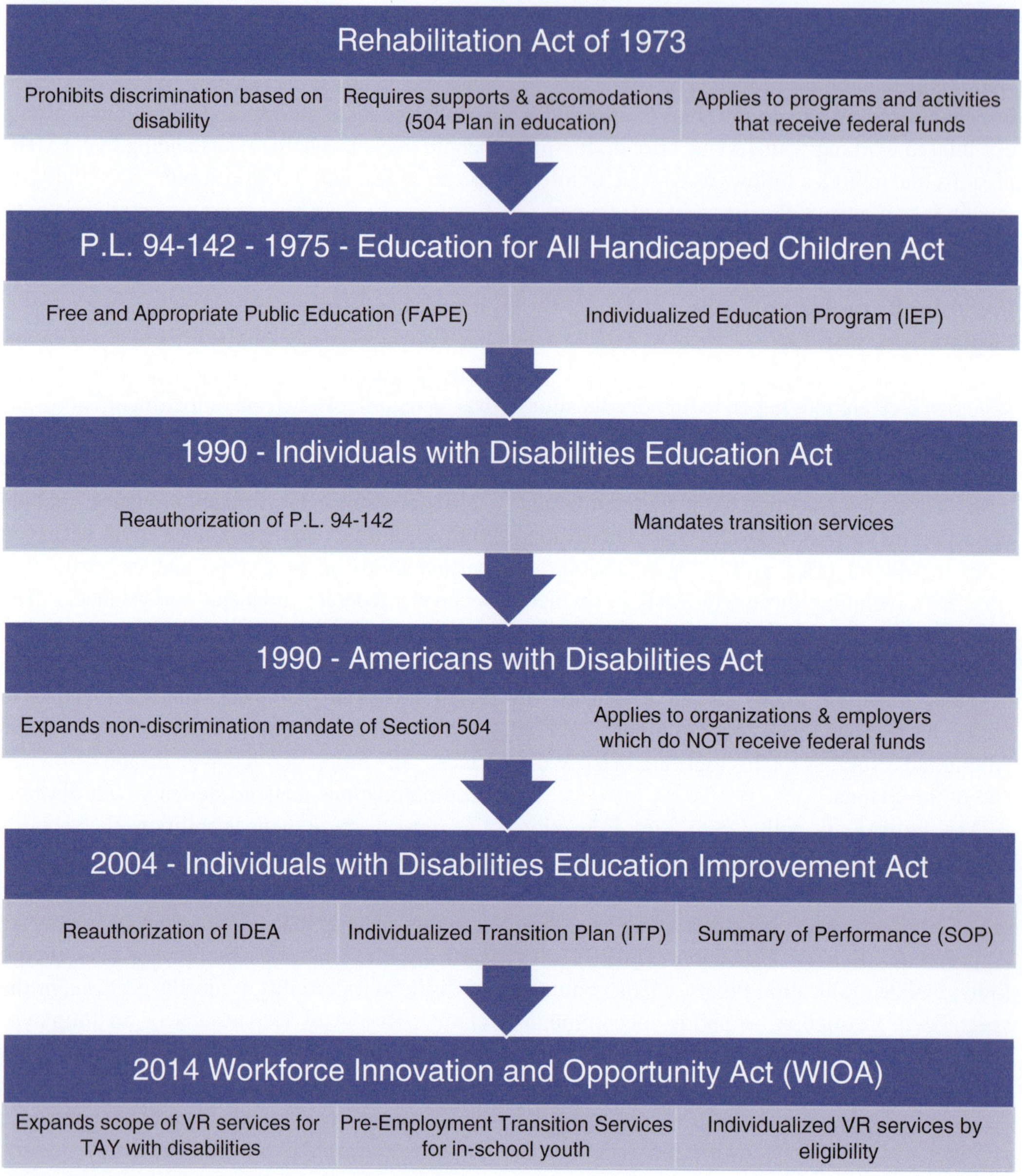

Fig. 1.7 Transition-related laws and legislation. Timeline of some important disability laws/legislation relevant to transition services and accommodations for TAY with MHC

about housing rights and responsibilities, reasonable housing accommodations, and housing options are listed at the end of the chapter.

The 2014 Workforce Innovation and Opportunity Act (WIOA) increases vocational rehabilitation (VR) services for both in-school and out-of-school youth (ages 14–24 y.o.) with disabilities (including psychiatric disabilities), who have one or more barriers to employment. The WIOA prioritizes competitive integrated employment [118].

There are other entitlement programs available to eligible TAY with MHC such as social security disability income and supplemental security income. The details of these programs are beyond the scope of this chapter, but providers are sometimes tasked with completing forms related to these benefits.

Providers are familiar with state medical record privacy laws and the federal privacy rules and protections afforded under the Health Insurance Portability and Accountability Act (HIPAA) of 1996. However, *student health records maintained at school* are protected under a different federal law, the Family Educational Rights and Privacy Act (FERPA). This law applies to all schools that receive funds under an applicable program of the US Department of Education. When a student turns 18 y.o. or attends higher education, the rights afforded under FERPA transfer from parents to the eligible student. Protection does not apply in certain circumstances, such as in a health or safety emergencies, or if there is an underage substance violation. Whether treatment records are covered by HIPAA and/or FERPA, 18-year-old patients or eligible students need to complete and sign authorization forms for information to be disclosed to parents and other third parties (for FERPA, specific authorization forms are required). The intersection of HIPAA and FERPA on campuses is nuanced and well-described by Chan et al. [119] and in an updated joint guidance [120]; consultation with compliance officers or legal advisors can be sought. After careful discussion with college-bound patients, getting release forms signed prior to matriculation which allow communication with parents and with new providers on/near campus can be helpful. Parents can call providers and the school with concerns or observations of their TAY regardless of the existence of a release.

For some TAY with MHC, additional personal, financial, and healthcare decision-making options need to be considered for when the young person turns 18 y.o. These include, but are not limited to, healthcare proxy, psychiatric advanced directive, supported decision-making, guardianship, and conservatorship. A helpful resource for youth, families, and providers is *Moving to Adult Life: A Legal guide for Parents of Youth with Mental Health Needs* [121].

Provider Knowledge: Health Insurance

Insurance-related barriers to seeking mental health care by young adults improved with the implementation of the Affordable Care Act (ACA). Between 2010 and 2018, the percentage of uninsured 19–25-year-olds declined from over 30% to 14.4% [122]. Still, it remains imperative for health care providers (HCP) to discuss with patients and families the importance of maintaining health insurance across age transitions. HCP need basic knowledge of the insurance options available to TAY and how TAY and their families might access those plans.

Medicaid and the Children's Health Insurance Program (CHIP) provide free or low-cost health coverage. *Medicaid* provides health coverage to many Americans including eligible children and adolescents, pregnant women, and people with disabilities. Some states have expanded Medicaid coverage to adults based on income criteria only. An uninsured young adult may, therefore, qualify for Medicaid in certain states. Emancipating/emancipated foster children who meet certain criteria may stay on Medicaid up to the age of 26 y.o. [123]. A disabled individual on SSI (supplemental security income) does not automatically lose Medicaid coverage when turning 19 y.o. but needs to be reevaluated regarding disability status using adult criteria. The *Children's Health Insurance Program* (CHIP) provides low-cost health coverage to children, up to age 19 y.o., in families that earn too much money to qualify for Medicaid but cannot afford private coverage. In some states, CHIP covers pregnant women. Young people and families can apply online, year-round, at https://www.healthcare.gov/medicaid-chip/. For Medicaid and CHIP, the Federal government establishes certain parameters for all states to follow, but the programs are administered by states with variable eligibility criteria and coverages nationwide. Individuals cannot simply transfer Medicaid from one state, or even county, to another, nor use benefits while temporarily out of state except under certain circumstances.

TAY may stay on a parent's health insurance plan, whether an employee-sponsored insurance (ESI) plan or a marketplace plan, up to the age of 26 y.o. The young person does not have to be claimed as a dependent by the parents or living with the parents, nor are there restrictions based on student status, employment status, or marital status. There is an annual open enrollment period, although certain life events may qualify a young person for a special enrollment window.

Other options for TAY are school-sponsored or college plans [124], ESI plans, state/federal marketplace plans (https://www.healthcare.gov/get-coverage/), and plans through trade/professional associations or membership organizations, depending on the post-high school path. College plans and ESI plans may be difficult to maintain if not attending school or working full time.

Provider Knowledge: Options for Life After High School and Available Supports

TAY with MHC can succeed in various post-high school endeavors with careful attention to available supports and the fit of a program, institution, or activity with the young person's interests and goals, strengths, and needs. Providers familiar with the broad range of post-high school options, in combination with their knowledge of developmental psychopathology, are better able to guide TAY with MHC and their families in planning for the transition to post-secondary education and training, work, and/or independent living.

Post-Secondary Education and Training (PSET) Options

PSET is characterized by diversity. Programs/institutions vary by mission, size, geographic location, selectivity, availability of formal and informal supports, types of degrees awarded, research activity, control (public or private), and whether they are operated on a nonprofit or for-profit basis. Students attend part-time, full-time, in-person, or through distance-learning options, reside in campus housing (on or near campus), or commute to school. Though most schools are coed, there are some single-gender institutions. Others may focus on special populations such as historically Black colleges, Hispanic-serving institutions, and religiously affiliated schools.

Four-year colleges or universities offer baccalaureate degrees and equip graduates with skills and knowledge for a broad range of professions. It is important for providers to remind patients and families that there are multiple pathways to complete a bachelor degree. Many young people enroll in a 4-year degree-granting institution immediately after high school while others opt to attend a two-year institution and then transfer to complete a four-year degree. Others take a gap year (a planned break from schooling) between high school and college and spend time working, traveling, and/or volunteering. Whether the gap year is self-designed or part of an established program, it provides a break from formal academic work and an opportunity for growth and personal development. It is possible to defer enrollment by choice or by recommendation of the accepting IHE to complete a gap year. For a variety of reasons, including as a possible accommodation for a mental health-related disability, some young people choose to or are encouraged to take reduced course loads or attend school part-time, understanding that they will take longer than 4 years to graduate and/or will attend school year-round. (In the case of part-time status, patients should pay careful attention to qualifications to maintain student health insurance as well as time-to-degree financial aid limits.) Some students transfer between 4-year institutions, including those seeking more robust mental health, academic, and social support services. The take-home message is that for TAY with MHC who aspire to earn a 4-year degree, there are many paths to success.

Two-year colleges (community or junior college) typically offer associate degrees, preparing students for entry-level positions in certain occupations, and/or transfer to a four-year degree-granting institution. Many community colleges also offer career and technical training programs leading to a certificate, or an associate degree, and a fast track into a career. Attendance at a local community or junior college is one way to ease into a four-year degree. It affords a young person the opportunity to explore interests, develop more academic and independent living skills, utilize familiar supports (family, peers, tutors, treatment providers), and/or stabilize after a mental health crisis. Cost tends to be lower, and many students combine part-time work and school.

Career, technical, or vocational/trade schools offer education options that focus on developing a skill set and knowledge base for a specific career or trade. At these schools, students usually earn a certificate or associates degree. Programs are available in various fields of study including health care, technology, emergency services, and skilled trades such as electricians, plumbers, and auto mechanics. Career and technical education programs may even begin in high school and continue into higher education at the 2-year college level [7]. Many programs require apprenticeships and/or internships that help students gain practical experience and fulfill licensing requirements. Programs typically last 2 years or less, focus on hands-on training, and provide more direct paths to jobs, characteristics which may be a best fit for some individuals.

Work

Going directly to the workforce after high school, whether driven by personal preference, economics, or sociocultural expectations, is another post-high school path for young people with MHC. Work not only provides money, but it is a source of structure, social interaction, and self-esteem [125]. TAY should seek jobs with opportunities for advancement and ideally, work with products and services which interest them. In best cases, a young person entering the workforce after high school will have had volunteer, internship, and/or part-time work experiences as a prelude to employment. An extended period of work may allow TAY to increase self-awareness and perhaps even reassess the need for PSET. Some employers may offer financial support for continuing education. *AmeriCorps*, a network of national service programs [126], is an option after high school which involves a work commitment with the benefits of educational monetary awards, personal development, access to health insurance, student loan forbearance, and a living allowance (depending on the program). The *Job Corps* [127] is a national, residential career training program for eligible, at-risk young people, between the ages of 16 and 24 y.o. Participants can complete their high school education, obtain career technical skills, and gain employment; some Job Corps graduates go on to higher education. For some TAY with disabilities, receipt of social security benefits is a disincentive to seeking employment, for fear of losing their benefits. These youth and families can seek benefits counseling and investigate social security work incentive programs [112] to understand how they can participate in meaningful and fulfilling work while maintaining entitlement income.

Military

Joining the military can be a good option for TAY who do well with structure and have a desire to serve their country. It offers distinct advantages for TAY in the development of leadership and teamwork skills, work ethic, and goal directedness. The military provides an opportunity to build a career in the service, move on to a civilian job, and/or qualify for financial support to attend PSET. A young person is disqualified from serving in the US military with a current diagnosis or verified past medical history of most mental health disorders [128]. Some disorders are permanently disqualifying and not eligible for medical waiver. For other disorders, including ADHD, learning disorders, depressive disorders, and certain anxiety disorders, the cumulative duration of treatment, period of time symptom- and treatment-free (including medication), need for inpatient or residential treatment, and documentation of adverse academic, occupational, or work performance are taken into consideration. TAY should work with a recruiter to learn about qualifications and waivers. Asking for a waiver does not guarantee the waiver will be granted. It will likely require more tests at the individual's expense and the provision of additional documentation. Patients who are passionate about joining the military may unilaterally decide to terminate treatment; providers should openly discuss these concerns with patients and encourage them to taper and stop medication with medical supervision. Professionals can provide verifying documentation if requested/authorized by the patient. Possible mental health sequelae of military service, difficulty reentering civilian life and adjusting to the social and academic challenges of PSE, require careful and coordinated transition planning.

"Independent Living" as a Post-High School Possibility

All TAY need to develop independent living skills whether they remain in the parental home after high school graduation or live in apartments, college dormitories, military housing, etc., with or without a roommate, partner, or spouse. However, for some TAY and their families, "independent living", *defined here as residential living arrangements separate from those in the home of the parent or guardian where the youth was raised,* may be a post-high school outcome of interest [112]. Providers may need to suggest this option to some patients and families, keeping in mind the relevance of safety and stability, community integration, and self-determination to housing options for TAY with serious MHC and other disabilities [100]. Options range from complete independence to 24/7 care, considering the level of informal and formal supports required by an individual [112, 129]. Some programs have strict eligibility criteria or may not specifically serve TAY. The availability of and funding for various residential options can vary by state and navigating the supports for independent living can be difficult. Patients and families should begin to address this goal early, by working with educational transition staff and contacting their local NAMI affiliate, Public Housing Authority, Community Mental Health Center, Vocational Rehabilitation (VR) Agency, and state departments of mental health and/or developmental disabilities services for information. If a TAY does not qualify for an out-of-home living situation and continues to live at home, respite services should be considered for parents and other caregivers to help restore the energy and commitment needed to care for youth with serious emotional disturbance [1].

Mental Health Care on or near Campus

The mental health, wellness, and disability services available on or near campuses are as diverse as the available PSET options available to youth. Home-based providers are not expected to know the details of services on each campus but can recommend that patients and families explore what is available starting with initial college tours. Patients, parents, and providers can supplement that information [130] by researching college websites and/or calling a campus health administrator to get additional details on the following [131]:

- Types of counseling services including access, session limits, fees, and wait times
- Psychiatric services including criteria to access, fees, and wait times
- Location of services on/near campus and transportation availability
- Breadth of disability services and required documentation to apply for accommodations
- Student-driven mental health support/advocacy groups
- Wellness groups
- Student health insurance and/or acceptance of family's current insurance plan
- Student of Concern Team [132]
- Availability on/off campus of:
  - Emergency/crisis services
  - Intensive level mental health services (inpatient, partial hospital program (PHP), and intensive outpatient program (IOP))
  - Specialized mental health services (substance abuse and eating disorders)

Based on the ongoing mental health needs of the transitioning student and available services, providers can attempt to guide youth and families in college selection. However, for various reasons, mental health is not always made a priority [133] increasing risk for a suboptimal transition.

Other Supports on Campus

Providers should know about other sources of enhanced support for their patients headed to college. The TRIO Programs [134] are Federal outreach and student services programs designed to identify, serve, and assist low-income individuals, first-generation college students, youth aging-out of foster care, and individuals with disabilities, to progress through the academic pipeline from middle school to post baccalaureate programs. Many of these youth also experience mental illness. TRIO grant recipients are institutions of higher education, public and private agencies, organizations including community-based organizations, or combinations of such entities, with experience in serving disadvantaged youth and secondary schools.

Summer bridge programs are designed to enhance nonacademic and/or academic readiness skills and support the overall transition to a new environment. Young people from underrepresented and vulnerable groups and those from certain diagnostic groups [135] may choose or be required to attend a summer bridge program. The content of summer bridge programs varies, but typically includes orientation to campus resources and campus life, study skills, remedial academic work, connections with advisors and mentors, and engagement with peers. Students may continue to have access to one or more of these features into the academic year depending on the program. Summer bridge programs may be funded by TRIO but not necessarily.

Supported Education (SEd) has emerged as a promising practice for supporting individuals with psychiatric disabilities in reaching their PSE goals [136–138]. SEd programs have specialized staff who coordinate campus mental health, and other supports, meet one-on-one and in groups to help with academic skills, help navigate the campus system of care, facilitate getting accommodations, improve motivation, and help students cope with mental health issues. SEd providers may also consult to the IHE about campus mental health policies and practices. Some SEd programs are campus initiatives while others are accessed through community mental health centers, university research centers, and other settings. Ringeisen et al. [138] discuss funding options for SEd services, which are often expensive.

Employment Supports

TAY with psychiatric disabilities who plan/desire to head to work may need guidance and support preparing to apply for and find a job, advancing in or maintaining employment, or integrating into the community. Mental health providers can be helpful to these TAY patients by knowing some basics about vocational rehabilitation services.

Pre-Employment Transition Services (Pre-ETS) are a specific set of services funded by state VR agencies for students with a disability who are still enrolled in school. Students must meet eligibility criteria for Pre-ETS but an application is not required. These services, offered either in a group or on an individual basis, include [112, 118]:

- Job exploration counseling
- Work-based learning experiences, which may include in-school or after-school opportunities, or experience outside the traditional school setting (including internships) provided in an integrated environment to the maximum extent possible
- Counseling on opportunities for enrollment in comprehensive transition or postsecondary educational programs at IHEs
- Workplace readiness training to develop social skills and independent living
- Instruction in self-advocacy, which may include peer mentoring

Another set of transition-related VR services is available to both in-school and out-of-school youth. These are provided in group settings and do not require an application. At the other end of the continuum are individualized transition services, which are available to all individuals who are determined to be eligible and require an application, and an approved Individualized Plan for Employment (IPE) must be developed. Collaboration with state education agencies and even IHE's may be required based on the IPE.

VR services vary to some extent by state, are limited by available funding, and target those most in need. TAY with MHC, who are disconnected, who have experience in the justice or foster care systems, and who are disadvantaged based on opportunity and healthcare disparities, would likely qualify for and benefit from VR services but need to know how to access and apply for them.

Other possible services to support the career development of TAY include the Individual Placement and Support (IPS) model of supported employment (SE) especially when it is systematically modified for young adults [102, 105], and Clubhouses [106]. HYPE (Helping Youth on the Path to Employment) is a manual-based intervention to support TAY with MHC to develop their careers [139]. It integrates the IPS model of SE with SEd and includes other enhancements; it is poised to be tested on college campuses across the country.

Provider Knowledge: Domains of Adolescent and Young Adult Functioning

To ease the stress of transition and promote mental wellness and stability, practitioners must assess, monitor, and help move patients (and families) forward in their readiness for transition in multiple domains of function relevant to post-high school success and transition to adult-oriented mental health care [131]. Critical to this task is the gradual shift of responsibility for these functions from the parent or other adult (such as tutor, mentor, special education teacher) to the TAY. The child-oriented mental health provider, often a CAP, is not solely responsible for promoting a patient's independence in multiple domains. Instead, the CAP often takes on a facilitative role in health care transition, highlighting patient needs and then engaging other members of the transition team, including a transition case manager, if available, to promote transition readiness. It is possible that a young person may not be fully competent in all domains at the time of transition, but TAY can still be successful if sufficient supports are in place where still needed [90].

Health Condition Knowledge and Skills

Health condition knowledge ranges from the basics of knowing the name and symptoms of one's condition(s) to understanding the triggers and warning signs of relapse. Health condition skills include the ability to present acute concerns to medical provider(s), get prescriptions filled, and describe a complete treatment history. Learning about health insurance is included in this domain. Progressively nuanced and complex health knowledge and skills, important for TAY with MHC to develop, are shown in the format of a readiness assessment (Fig. 1.8). Providers can discuss these topics with patients and families and engage them in assignments and activities to build youth knowledge and skills. A Health and Human Services document entitled "Teaching adolescents how to use the healthcare system" suggests sample tasks to assign adolescents to enhance readiness in this domain. There are many assistive mobile apps which may appeal to TAY which help track mood, anxiety, time management, medication compliance, etc. A young person leaving home, confident about their abilities to manage their mental health condition, should be better able to weather the stress of transition and focus on young adult pursuits.

Self-Advocacy Knowledge and Skills

Self-advocacy knowledge and skills taught in elementary, middle, and high school take on critical importance for young adults seeking accommodations in PSE, on the job, and in the community. Self-advocacy knowledge includes understanding how one's condition/disability impacts learning and/or working and what accommodations and supports will enable participation in future endeavors. Individuals with disabilities should know their rights and responsibilities and the pros and cons of disclosure in various settings. Self-advocacy skills include the ability to ask for help, effectively disclose a disability, and advocate for accommodations and supports across different settings. Clinicians, parents, education personnel, vocational rehabilitation counselors, and others should work together and encourage patients to participate in and/or lead their 504, IEP, ITP, IPE, and other individualized planning meetings, maintain a portfolio of documents related to the disability, and read results of educational, psychological, and other testing. Providers can consider role play activities so patients can practice disclosure skills. Successful post-school transitions require that adolescents assume prominent roles in their own educational and life planning. TAY can use the Summary of Performance (SOP) as a guide for self-advocacy in post-high school settings although it is not a guarantee of services and supports. The Summary of Performance (SOP) is required for some youth under the reauthorization of the IDEA of 2004 [140].

TRANSITION READINESS ASSESSMENT and ACTION PLAN *for Youth with Mental Health Conditions*

Please fill out this form to help us see what you already know about your condition and how to manage it. We can work together to address what you need to learn. If you need help with this form, please let us know.

NAME DATE OF BIRTH DATE OF ASSESSMENT	I know this or I do this	I need to learn	What can I do to practice or prepare? Who can help?
HEALTH CONDITION KNOWLEDGE			
I know the name of my condition/disability			
I know how my condition impacts my social functioning			
I know what to do in case of an emergency			
I know the triggers for and warning signs of a relapse			
I know the circumstances and conditions which trigger trouble for me (destabilization and/or relapse)			
I know how alcohol/drugs might affect my health condition			
I know how sleep (or lack of it) affects my condition			
I know how pregnancy might affect my health condition			
I know strategies and tools to help stabilize me			
I understand how my family's cultural beliefs might affect health care decisions			
I know pertinent family medical and psychiatric history			
HEALTH CONDITION SKILLS			
I can name my providers(s) and reach them			
I meet privately with my doctor for part of each office visit			
I can present acute concerns to my provider(s)			
I make and keep track of my own appointments			
I can explain my condition in a few sentences			
I can present my treatment history or have easy access to it			
I discuss short- and long-term treatment goals and needs with my provider			
I understand/complete/sign medical forms (health history, permission for treatment, release of records, HIPAA Policy)			
Once I turn 18, I will meet alone with my doctor unless I have signed consent forms			
I have decided about emergency contacts and possible parental access to providers after I turn 18 years old			
MEDICATION KNOWLEDGE			
I know if I am allergic to any medications and what happens			

Fig. 1.8 Transition readiness assessment and action plan for youth with mental health conditions. This readiness assessment is designed to assess the health condition knowledge and skills of youth with a broad range of mental health conditions. The team can record action plans to address knowledge and skills gaps

I know the names and purposes of my medication(s)			
I know my baseline eating, sleeping, elimination patterns			
I know the general side effects of my medication(s)			
I know the sexual side effects of my medication(s)			
I know the blood work needed for my condition/medications			
I know what will happen if I abruptly stop taking my med(s)			
I know to ask about possible medication interactions			
I know how substance use may affect my medication(s)			
I know to ask if my medication(s) impact family planning			
I know about abuse, misuse, and diversion of medications			
MEDICATION SKILLS			
I can read a prescription bottle			
I take my medications independently			
I keep track of and fill my prescriptions			
I store my medications in a safe location			
HEALTH INSURANCE			
I know why it is important to have health insurance			
I carry my insurance card and know about copays			
I have a plan for health insurance after the age of 18			

Fig. 1.8 (continued)

In addition to the above, patients headed to PSE need to know if their testing results are up-to-date and what documentation is required to apply for accommodations on standardized college entrance examinations and in PSE settings. It can be helpful to patients for providers to discuss the differences between high school and college as a way to increase patient interest in developing knowledge and skills in self-advocacy. Then, they can better anticipate and advocate for the supports they will need to complete PSE [141]. Additional resources on this topic are listed at the end of the chapter.

Independent Life Skills

It is never too early to learn/practice some fundamental daily life skills. Already knowing how to do laundry, cook simple meals, set and wake up to an alarm, etc., can help decrease stress and avoid relapse [131] for a young person adjusting to a new job, college life, and/or a new housing situation. Basic daily activities, such as bathing, dressing, toileting, ambulating, and eating, are often referred to as activities of daily living [142]. For TAY patients who struggle with these activities, high levels of personal support are necessary. In comparison, instrumental activities of daily living (IADLs) are activities that allow an individual to live independently in a community [143]. These activities include:

- Comfortably communicating on the phone and via computer
- Maintaining one's living environment
- Managing personal hygiene
- Planning and preparing meals
- Getting to where one needs to go by driving, hiring taxis, or ridesharing services, using public transportation
- Managing finances
- Balancing time between work, social, and leisure activities
- Managing health

It is best to build these skills over time, preferably years, using age-appropriate tasks. For TAY, the Casey Life Skills Assessment covers a range of independent life skills, and the Resources to Inspire Guide provides many examples of tasks to build skills [144]. These tools were designed for foster youth in transition but are more broadly useful, including the questions about supportive adults given the importance of developmental relationships and social networks during the transition to adulthood.

In the area of managing finances, there are specific financial terms to understand and tasks for the TAY to accomplish [145], depending on the post-high school path. For example, a young person headed to college needs to plan, along with family, how to pay for college. The Free Application for Federal Student Aid (FASFA) allows a student to apply for federal grants, work-study, and loans and allows easy comparison of the financial aid packages IHEs are offering (https://studentaid.gov/). The FAFSA requires parents' financial information if the student is considered a dependent. For TAY headed to work, it is important to understand W4 forms, employee benefits, taxation, and retirement accounts. For TAY renting a first apartment, understanding the terms of a lease, security deposit, and rights and responsibilities as a tenant is useful. The Casey Life Skills Assessment addresses these issues.

Executive Functioning (EF) Skills

Across post-high school contexts, the abilities to organize and prioritize tasks, regulate alertness and sustain attention, shift tasks, manage frustration, utilize memory, and self-regulate are important for success. For TAY with MHC, EF deficits can represent core features of a disorder or can stem from delayed psychosocial maturation, negative life experiences, and other etiologies. The treatment team should attempt to engage the young person in self-assessment of independent EF skills. It is important to be mindful of the sometimes extensive supports, in the form of a structured home setting, tutors, medications, and school accommodations which have contributed to success while at home and in high school [131]. The patient will need time to practice strategies others have been facilitating; medications may prove helpful as well (although EF deficits in psychiatric disorders may contribute to lack of treatment adherence). College and job selections should be challenging but tailored to the young persons' interests and skill strengths. Knowing what was helpful at home can help the young person advocate for similar supports in PSE and in the workplace. EF skills are usually more thoroughly assessed with neuropsychological testing.

Psychosocial Development

Facilitation of psychosocial development has been discussed earlier in the chapter. Family interactions related to opportunities to make decisions, communicate needs, express feelings, resolve conflicts, take on responsibilities, and participate in cultural traditions should be explored. The extent and quality of peer interactions, including dating, and availability of friends who are supportive should be assessed. The ability to take the perspective of others, deal with peer pressure and/or bullying, and recognize signs of an abusive relationship should be discussed. Experiences such as volunteer work, part-time employment, and extracurricular activities can expose the TAY to others and help build self-knowledge and confidence. Asking about interests, hobbies, dreams, and goals encourages identity exploration.

A somewhat related issue occurs when a young adult remains at home after high school or returns to live at home for a mental health-related reason with or without additional financial issues. This situation can be a strain for the young person in regard to self-esteem, autonomy, and decision-making and may put emotional and financial strain on parents [146]. Family assessment and intervention may be necessary, to help steer the family system toward a more normative developmental trajectory.

Anticipatory Guidance: Safety Issues and Thinking Ahead

This sixth and last domain is less about assessment and more about helping the young person envision themselves in their new environment. It is an opportunity to discuss difficult topics and to offer information and guidance to help prepare patients (and their families) for the expected changes and stresses associated with this transition. How and when to stay connected with family and friends and other informal supports should be planned out. Obstacles to treatment compliance for young adults (such as disliking new provider(s) or hoping for a "fresh start") and barriers to accessing accommodations (such as fear of being stigmatized and being deemed ineligible for services) should be openly discussed. Means to reduce stress and promote wellness which are available in the new environment should be investigated. Other topics include abuse, misuse, and diversion of medications; accessing online peer support networks; dealing with the adult legal system; internet safety, community safety, and dating safety; protection from STDs and unwanted pregnancies and date rape; and discrimination and harassment. Particularly in college, but also in the workplace and community, TAY will be exposed to new lifestyles, values, ideas, and ways of behaving which provide new choices and temptations. This can help to consolidate identity or create stress. Sometimes new choices can lead to traumatic events, addiction, unwanted pregnancies, and legal difficulties which can derail post-high school plans [131]. Lastly, it is important for the provider to express flexibility and acceptance if treatment compliance waivers or post-high school plans need to be changed or adjusted.

Provider Skills

Armed with an enhanced knowledge base, providers working with TAY should be able to:

1. Partner with and actively engage diverse TAY in treatment services and other supports. TAY have clear and strong thoughts on how providers can more effectively communicate and partner with them [147]. Logan and Mullen [148] recently summarized tips and strategies for providers to engage young adults. Practitioners should utilize approaches such as positive assessment [149], shared decision-making [150], trauma-informed care [151], cultural formulations [152], and motivational enhancement therapy [153].
2. Assess suicide risk, manage crises, and promote protective factors in TAY [154].
3. Screen for problematic substance use, provide brief interventions, and know when to refer for comprehensive services [68].
4. Integrate parents/caregivers in the care of late adolescents and young adults (if appropriate), including assessment for parental accommodation [146].
5. Collaborate across agencies and systems that support young people.
6. Facilitate transitions to young adult roles and adult-oriented mental health care by designing opportunities to gain skills and experiences in key domains of functioning.
7. Develop comprehensive transfer of care plans in collaboration with patients and others which are individualized and developmentally sound.
8. Monitor the literature for new evidence-based treatments for TAY, including those that are adaptations of treatments already shown to be effective in other age groups.

Provider Attitudes

Important attitudes for providers working with TAY have been embedded throughout this chapter. Models and concepts focused on prevention, recovery, and resilience involve hope for the future and encourage the building of bridges to support young people across environmental contexts. Maintaining a developmental mindset means valuing the pursuit of identity and the importance of self-determination. It also means appreciating TAY noncompliance from a developmental perspective and willingness to reframe setbacks and failures as learning experiences.

Health Care Transition (HCT)

To meaningfully address the multiple needs of TAY with MHC and promote their continued engagement in treatment, it is essential for mental health practitioners to address transition preparation and planning in routine clinical care. Providers must be able to identify the broad goals of HCT and explain them to patients and families. HCT should be integrated into clinical practice in a way that addresses the developmental and treatment needs of youth, supports families, and is practical and sustainable for clinicians. *HCT challenges practitioners to utilize their enhanced knowledge, skills, and attitudes to work with TAY intentionally and productively.*

Definition of Health Care Transition

Transition is defined in the health care literature as a purposeful and planned process of change that attends to the medical, psychosocial, educational, and vocational needs of adolescents, as they move from child-oriented to adult-oriented models of health care [155, 156]. The goal of transition in health care is to maximize lifelong functioning and potential, by ensuring uninterrupted, developmentally appropriate, and comprehensive health care services as adolescents move into young adulthood [157]. HCT does not necessitate a change in health care provider, but it does require the provider to shift to an adult approach to health care and to help prepare TAY to communicate about their health care needs, manage all aspects of their own care, understand privacy and consent, recognize the need for supports, and be more independent in day-to-day functioning. When referral and transfer of care to a new provider is required, it must be understood that transfer of care is only one aspect of transition preparation and planning and, in and of itself, does not address the broad focus of HCT as described.

Planned HCT for young people with special health care needs is a core component of the US Healthy People health prevention agenda [158]. Specifically, for young people with MHC, the need for transition preparation and planning is supported by professional groups whose constituents work on both sides of the transition [157, 159–164]. Advocacy groups, representing the experiences and perspectives of patients and their families, encourage transition planning and usually have transition resources on their websites [129]. Young people, themselves, have preferences and expectations about the content, process, and benefits of transition preparation and planning [165–167].

Practice-Based Health Care Transition Preparation and Planning with TAY

In 2011, the American Academy of Pediatrics, the American Academy of Family Practitioners, and the American College of Physicians developed a clinical consensus report [157] providing recommendations for HCT planning for all youth beginning in early adolescence. This report offers practical guidance, suggesting timelines and activities, to support practice-based HCT planning. Like transition guidelines for youth who receive special education services [112, 168] and those in foster care [164], the recommended practices are grounded in the knowledge of normal development and align with SOC principles. Youth participation and self-determination [111], communication and collaboration among transition team members, and appropriate parental involvement are essential components of the recommendations.

The *Six Core Elements of Health Care Transition,* published by Got Transition™ [169], essentially translates the consensus document into a structured transition process and provides associated clinical tools, to help ease the challenges of incorporating HCT into routine practice. Medical specialists are encouraged to adapt the process and tools to their populations. Regarding mental health, the clinical HCT tools have been adapted for youth with intellectual disabilities/developmental disabilities [170] and for college-bound youth headed to college with a range of mental health conditions [171]. Cleverly et al. [172] used the Six Core Elements as a framework to organize a literature review on core components and indicators of successful transition from child to adult mental health services. Encouragingly, a structured HCT process is associated with positive outcomes [173, 174]. The Six Core Elements are described below and depicted in Fig. 1.9.

A *transition policy* for the practice introduces the concept, process, and content of HCT to youth (as early as age 12 y.o. and preferably by age 14 y.o., or at the time of diagnosis) and caregiver(s). The policy typically describes how the practice intends to support a healthy transition from adolescence to young adulthood. For example, providers encourage youth to gradually take on responsibility for their own health care and other aspects of their lives and encourage caregivers to provide opportunities for skill-building. The policy also provides information on privacy and consent and any patient age or geographic limitations that exist for the practice. Many CAP naturally incorporate transition concepts into their work, but they need to be more cognizant of their HCT practices. Being transparent with patients and families about transition helps to foster teamwork, avoid misunderstandings, and engage youth.

Transition tracking and monitoring is used to track each patient's progress through the steps of transition planning. Initiating transition planning should not be dependent upon request but by established eligibility criteria such as age. The EMR may be used here to flag patients poised for transition planning.

Transition readiness involves systematic identification of youth needs in order for them to achieve independent management of their health condition. Structured readiness assessments or questionnaires can help the provider identify what the young person already knows, what tasks can be done independently, and what still needs to be learned. The provider, youth, and family can then jointly develop action plans to remediate gaps in health care knowledge and skills. For all youth, but particularly those with MHC, it is also important to track knowledge and skills in other essential domains of function (Table 1.3).

Given the nature of psychiatric practice, it is recommended that a face-to-face global review (or re-review) of a youth's current functioning, in addition to structured readiness assessments, be conducted [131]. This is an opportunity to understand the youth's post-high school goals, strengths and vulnerabilities, diagnosis and prognosis, long- and short-term treatment needs, and current level of supports.

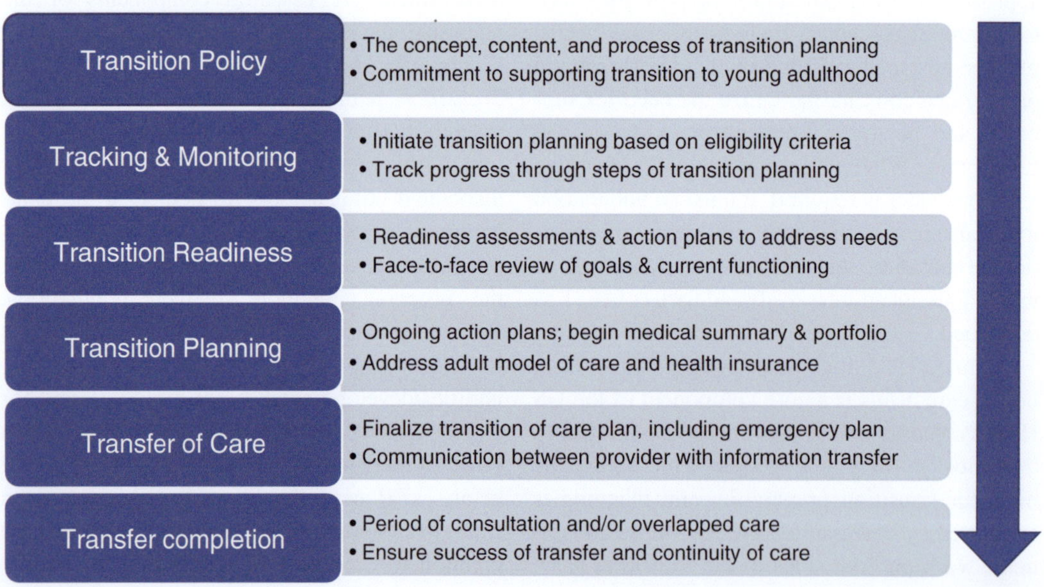

Fig. 1.9 Summary of the Six Core Elements of Health Care Transition

Table 1.3 Readiness assessment tools

General Health Care Transition Readiness Assessments
Transition Readiness Assessment for Youth/Young Adults http://www.gottransition.org/resourceGet.cfm?id=239
Transition Readiness Assessment Questionnaire TRAQ 5.0 © Wood, Sawicki, Reiss &, Livingood, 2012 http://www.hscj.ufl.edu/jaxhats/docs/traq_5.0.pdf
UNC STARx Program - STARx Questionnaire https://www.med.unc.edu/transition/transition-tools/trxansition-scale/
Independent Life Skills Assessment
Casey Life Skills Assessment and Resources to Inspire Guide | Casey Life Skills https://www.casey.org/casey-life-skills-resources/
Readiness Assessments with Focus on Youth with MHC
Specialized Transition Readiness Assessment and Action Plan for Youth Heading to College with a Mental Health Condition https://www.aacap.org/app_themes/aacap/docs/families_and_youth/Readiness_Assessment_Action_Plan_College.pdf Published as Supplemental Material in Academic Psychiatry 2015; 39(5): 549–554 Updated & Published in Promoting Safe and Effective Transitions to College with Mental Health Conditions, Springer 2018
Landmark College - A Guide to Assessing College Readiness https://www.collegechangeseverything.org/events/2018-media/Session-1I-College-Readiness-Guide.pdf Focus on academic and executive function skills
Virginia's College Guide for Students with Disabilities http://www.doe.virginia.gov/special_ed/transition_svcs/outcomes_project/college_guide.pdf

Transition planning is informed by transition readiness assessment and patient goals. Activities, discussions, and tasks are completed over time. Progress is assessed and action plans reworked. This is also a time to discuss how the model of care changes when the patient turns 18 y.o., particularly regarding health care decision-making, self-advocacy, and possible changes in insurance coverage. Whether or not the young person needs/wants to change providers and the timing of the transfer of care are both important areas of planning. The patient and provider can work together on a Mental Health and Medical Summary and a Transition Portfolio [170], both of which can serve as tools for psychoeducation. A thoughtful review of the SOC Framework modified for TAY can help identify service areas which need to be addressed in the transition care plan.

Transfer of care and *transfer completion* require detailed planning and clear and timely communication. Ideally, the young person's condition is stable at the time of care transfer. If that is not the case, post-high school plans may need to be adjusted and/or additional supports must be put in place. Once a new provider is identified, authorized communication takes place between providers to exchange patient health information and to clarify the date of transfer and roles of each provider. A transfer of care plan (or transition care plan) is the plan established for ongoing mental health treatment and other supports for the young person and should include an emergency care plan. HCT guidelines recommend that about 3 months post-transfer, the pediatric provider contacts the young adult, the family, and the adult provider to verify that transfer of care has occurred and to offer consultation assistance. Studies show that TAY appreciate a period of parallel care at the time of transfer and/or a case manager who can cross system boundaries [165]. For TAY headed to college, there are special considerations when a home-based provider and a college provider plan to share treatment responsibilities [171].

By virtue of the age range they treat, child and adolescent clinicians bear the major responsibility for transition preparation and planning

[133, 172]. Adult mental health providers, however, also need to understand and implement HCT practices in order to receive young adult patients, help them adjust to a new model of mental health care, and promote their ongoing journey to young adulthood. *Development and the need for bridging supports do not stop at the transfer of care.*

Conclusion

TAY face significant, complex and dynamic psychosocial and maturational challenges at a time which coincides with the onset of many mental health disorders. Mental health and wellness are important for young people to productively pursue post-high school goals. Concerns about the ability to engage and retain these youth and young adults in mental health treatment have prompted calls for services that are age specific and developmentally appropriate. Progress has been made over the past two decades, with much of the work grounded in the SOC concept and philosophy as relevant to TAY. There remains room for expanding the evidence-based outcomes literature. Mental health practitioners working on both sides of the transition need to fully appreciate the developmental stage. They have a shared responsibility in promoting patient psychosocial maturation and independent management of their mental health and other daily living needs, as they support patients in their transition to adulthood. Developing a mental health workforce trained to work with this population [175] should be a priority across disciplines.

Appendix

Helpful Resources

Transition-Related Laws

- Laws and Guidance Overview https://www2.ed.gov/policy/landing.jhtml?src=pn
- Disability Overview https://www.hud.gov/program_offices/fair_housing_equal_opp/disability_overview
- The Fair Housing Act https://www.justice.gov/crt/fair-housing-act-1#disability
- WIOA: New Law Helps Youth & Young Adults Get Jobs – What Families Need to Know https://escholarship.umassmed.edu/cgi/viewcontent.cgi?article=1127&context=pib

Reasonable Accommodations at School and at Work

- Getting Accommodations at College: Tools for School https://escholarship.umassmed.edu/cgi/viewcontent.cgi?article=1066&context=pib
- Academic Accommodations for Students with Psychiatric Disabilities https://www.washington.edu/doit/academic-accommodations-students-psychiatric-disabilities
- Higher Education Supports Tool Kit: Assisting Students with Psychiatric Disabilities https://cpr.bu.edu/app/uploads/2011/09/Higher-Education-Support-Toolkit.pdf
- Outside-the-Box College Accommodations Real Support for Real Students https://escholarship.umassmed.edu/cgi/viewcontent.cgi?article=1110&context=pib
- Disability Employment 101. Appendix IV. Reasonable Accommodations and the ADA https://www2.ed.gov/about/offices/list/osers/products/employmentguide/appendix-4.html
- Job Accommodation Network http://janweb.icdi.wvu.edu
- Entering the World of Work: What Youth with Mental Health Needs Should Know About Accommodations https://www.dol.gov/odep/pubs/fact/transitioning.htm

Self-Advocacy Knowledge and Skills

- The 411 on Disability Disclosure – A Workbook for Youth with Disabilities http://www.ncwd-youth.info/wp-content/uploads/2016/10/411_Disability_Disclosure_complete.pdf
- Do I Tell My Boss?: Disclosing My Mental Health Condition at Work https://escholarship.umassmed.edu/cgi/viewcontent.cgi?article=1077&context=pib

- Supporting Student Led Transition Planning for Students with Emotional Behavioral Disturbance https://www.umassmed.edu/globalassets/transitionsrtc/our-models/test/products/student-led-support-pre-pub.pdf
- Teens on IEPs: Making My "Transition" Services Work for Me https://escholarship.umassmed.edu/cgi/viewcontent.cgi?article=1067&context=pib

Transition Preparation and Planning for Life After High School

- High School and Life after High School Parenting Guides https://www.parenttoolkit.com/grade-levels/life-after-high-school https://www.parenttoolkit.com/grade-levels/high-school
- Children and Adults with Attention-Deficit/Hyperactivity Disorder (CHADD). Preparing for the road ahead: teens and the transition to adulthood. https://chadd.org/adhd-weekly/preparing-for-the-road-ahead-teens-and-the-transition-to-adulthood/
- Autism Speaks. Transition Tool Kit https://www.autismspeaks.org/tool-kit/transition-tool-kit
- Learning Disabilities Association of America. Transition. https://ldaamerica.org/?s=transition
- How Is High School Different than College https://www.smu.edu/provost/sasp/NeatStuffforNewStudents/HowIsCollegeDifferentfromHighSchool
- The differences between high school and college https://centerontransition.org/publications/download.cfm?id=71
- Planning Ahead for Your Mental Health Care as You Transition to College https://www.settogo.org/cardstack/planning-ahead-for-your-mental-health-care-as-you-transition-to-college/#card=1
- Transitioning from High School to College with a Psychiatric Illness: Preparation https://www.aacap.org/AACAP/AACAP/Families_and_Youth/Facts_for_Families/FFF-Guide/Transitioning-From-High-School-to-College-With-A-Psychiatric-Illness-Preparation-114.aspx
- Starting College with a Psychiatric Illness https://www.aacap.org/AACAP/AACAP/Families_and_Youth/Facts_for_Families/FFF-Guide/Starting-College-with-a-Psychiatric-Illness-115.aspx
- Managing a Mental Health Condition in College https://www.nami.org/Your-Journey/Teens-Young-Adults/Managing-a-Mental-Health-Condition-in-College

References

1. Davis M, Vander SA. The transition to adulthood for youth who have serious emotional disturbance: developmental transition and young adult outcomes. J Mental Health Admin. 1997;24(4):400–27.
2. Martel A, Fuchs DC, editors. Transitional age youth and mental illness: influences on young adult outcomes. Child and Adolescent Psychiatric Clinics of North America. Volume 26–2. Philadelphia: Elsevier; 2017. 410p.
3. Kessler RC, Berglund P, Demler O, Jin R, Walters EE. Lifetime prevalence and age-of-onset distributions of DSM-IV disorders in the National Comorbidity Survey Replication. Arch Gen Psychiatry. 2005;62:593–602.
4. Copeland WE, Shanahan L, Davis M, Burns BJ, Angold A, Costello EJ. Increase in untreated cases of psychiatric disorders during the transition to adulthood. Psychiatr Serv. 2015;66(4):397–403.
5. Hower H, Case BG, Hoeppner B, Yen S, Goldstein T, Goldstein B, et al. Use of mental health services in transition age youth with bipolar disorder. J Psychiatr Pract. 2013;19(6):464–76.
6. Copeland WE, Wolke D, Shanahan L, Costello EJ. Adult functional outcomes of common childhood psychiatric problems: a prospective, longitudinal study. JAMA Psychiat. 2015;72(9):892–9.
7. Institute of Medicine, National Research Council. Investing in the health and well-being of young adults. Washington, D.C.: The National Academies Press; 2015. 502 p.
8. Malla A, Iyer S, McGorry P, Cannon M, Coughlan H, Singh S, et al. From early intervention in psychosis to youth mental health reform: a review of the evolution and transformation of mental health services for young people. Soc Psychiatry Psychiatr Epidemiol. 2016;51:319–26.
9. National Collaborative on Workforce and Disability. Transition truths: an overview of transition systems.

2015. http://www.ncwd-youth.info/publications/transition-truths-an-overview-of-transition-systems/.
10. Osgood DW, Foster EM, Flanagan C, Ruth GR, editors. On your own without a net: the transition to adulthood for vulnerable populations. Chicago: Univ Chicago Press; 2005. 401 p.
11. Wagner M. Outcomes for youths with serious emotional disturbance in secondary school and early adulthood. Futur Child. 1995;5(Pt 2):90–112.
12. Davis M, Vander SA. The transition to adulthood among adolescents who have serious emotional disturbance. Center for Mental Health Services: Rockville; 1996. https://eric.ed.gov/?id=ED418526.
13. Clark H, Unger K, Stewart E. Transition of youth and young adults with emotional/behavior disorders into employment, education and independent living. Community Alternatives. 1993;5(2):19–46.
14. Altschuler DM. Policy and program perspectives on the transition to adulthood for adolescents in the juvenile justice system. In: Osgood DW, Foster EM, Flanagan C, Ruth GR, editors. On your own without a net: the transition to adulthood for vulnerable populations. Chicago: Univ Chicago Press; 2005. p. 92–113.
15. Stroul BA, Friedman RM. A system of care for severely emotionally disturbed children and youth. 1986. https://www.ncjrs.gov/pdffiles1/Digitization/125081NCJRS.pdf.
16. Will M. OSERS programming for the transition of youth with disabilities: bridges from school to working life. Washington, D.C.: Office of Special Education and Rehabilitative Services; 1983. https://files.eric.ed.gov/fulltext/ED256132.pdf.
17. Magrab PR, Millar, HEC, editors. Growing up and getting medical care: youth with special health care needs. Summary of conference proceedings; 1989 Mar 13–15; Jekyl Island, GA. Washington DC: National Center for Networking Community Based Services. Georgetown University Child Development Center; 1989. https://collections.nlm.nih.gov/ext/document/101584932X870/PDF/101584932X870.pdf.
18. U.S. Department of Health and Human Services. Administration for Children, Youth and Families. Independent Living Initiative Title IV-E. 1987. https://www.acf.hhs.gov/sites/default/files/cb/pi8701.pdf.
19. Davis M. Addressing the needs of youth in transition to adulthood. Admin Pol Ment Health. 2003;30(6):495–509.
20. Vander Stoep A, Taub J, Holcomb L. Follow-up of adolescents with severe psychiatric impairment into young adulthood. In: Liberton C, Kutash K, Friedman R, editors. A system of care for children's mental health: expanding the research base. 6th Annual Research Conference Proceedings; 1993 Mar 1–3. Tampa: Research and Training Center for Children's Mental Health, University of South Florida. p. 373–80.
21. Wilens TE, Rosenbaum JF. Transitional aged youth: a new frontier in child and adolescent psychiatry. J Am Acad Child Adolesc Psychiatry. 2013;52(9):887–90.
22. Manteuffel B, Stephens RL, Sondheimer DL, Fisher SK. Characteristics, service experiences, and outcomes of transition-aged youth in systems of care: programmatic and policy implications. J Behav Health Serv Res. 2008;35:469–87.
23. Davis M, Koroloff N, Ellison ML. Between adolescence and adulthood: rehabilitation research to improve services for youth and young adults. Psychiatr Rehabil J. 2012;35(3):167–70.
24. Davis M, Munson MR. Youth and young adult mental health: interventions, services, systems, and rehabilitation. Psychiatr Rehabil J. 2018;41(4):253–7.
25. Substance Abuse and Mental Health Services Administration. Healthy transitions: improving life trajectories for youth and young adults with serious mental disorders program. 2018. https://www.samhsa.gov/grants/grant-announcements/sm-18-010.
26. Substance Abuse and Mental Health Services Administration. Enhancement and expansion of treatment and recovery services for adolescents, transitional aged youth, and their families. 2018. https://www.samhsa.gov/grants/grant-announcements/ti-18-010.
27. Arnett JJ. Emerging adulthood: a theory of development from the late teens through the twenties. Am Psychol. 2000;55(5):469–80.
28. Substance Abuse and Mental Health Services Administration. "Now is the time" healthy transitions (HT): improving the life trajectories for youth and young adults with, or at risk for, serious mental health conditions. 2014. https://www.samhsa.gov/grants/grant-announcements/sm-14-017.
29. Interdepartmental Serious Mental Illness Coordinating Committee. The way forward: federal action for a system that works for all people living with SMI and SED and their families and caregivers. 2017. https://store.samhsa.gov/product/The-Way-Forward-Federal-Action-for-a-System-That-Works-for-All-People-Living-With-SMI-and-SED-and-Their-Families-and-Caregivers-Full-Report/PEP17-ISMICC-RTC.
30. Vincent GM, Drawbridge D, Davis M. The validity of risk assessment instruments for transition-age youth. J Consulting Clin Psychol. 2019;87(2):171–83.
31. Davis M, Koroloff N, Sabella K, Sarkis M. Crossing the age divide: cross-age collaboration between programs serving transition-age youth. J Behavior Health Services Res. 2018;45(3):356–69.
32. Packard Tucker L, Dworsky A, Van Drunen M. Alameda County's youth transitions partnership program – a promising model for supporting transition-age youth in foster care. Chicago: Chapin Hall at the University of Chicago; 2020.
33. Hardin AP, Hackell JM, AAP Committee on Practice and Ambulatory Medicine. Age limit of pediatrics. Pediatrics. 2017;140(3):e20172151.

34. United States Census Bureau. National population by characteristics: 2010–2019. https://www.census.gov/data/tables/time-series/demo/popest/2010s-national-detail.html. Accessed 1 June 2020.
35. Frey WH. The U.S. will become minority white in 2045, census projects. Updated Sept. 2018. https://www.brookings.edu/blog/the-avenue/2018/03/14/the-us-will-become-minority-white-in-2045-census-projects/ be36.
36. U.S Bureau of Labor Statistics. College enrollment and work activity of recent high school and college graduates – 2017. Released Apr 26, 2018. https://www.bls.gov/news.release/archives/hsgec_04262018.htm.
37. National Center for Educational Statistics. Trends in high school dropout and completion rates in the United States. https://nces.ed.gov/programs/dropout/ind_03.asp. Accessed 1 June 2020.
38. National Center for Educational Statistics. Digest of education statistics - table 326.10. https://nces.ed.gov/programs/digest/d18/tables/dt18_326.10.asp. Accessed 1 June 2020.
39. U.S. Bureau of Labor Statistics. Labor force statistics from the current population survey concepts and definitions. Updated June 2020. https://www.bls.gov/cps/definitions.htm.
40. Fernandes-Alcantara AL. Disconnected youth: a look at 16 to 24 year olds who are not working or in school. Congressional Research Service; 2015. https://fas.org/sgp/crs/misc/R40535.pdf.
41. Lewis K. Making the connection: transportation and youth disconnection. New York: Measure of America, Social Science Research Council; 2019. https://ssrc-static.s3.amazonaws.com/moa/Making%20the%20Connection.pdf
42. Department of Defense. 2017 Demographics. Profile of the military community. https://download.militaryonesource.mil/12038/MOS/Reports/2017-demographics-report.pdf. Accessed 1 June 2020.
43. National Center for Juvenile Justice. Easy access to the census of juveniles in residential placement: 1997–2017. https://www.ojjdp.gov/ojstatbb/ezacjrp/asp/Age_Sex.asp. Accessed 1 June 2020.
44. Sawyer W. Youth confinement: the whole pie 2019. Prison policy initiative. https://www.prisonpolicy.org/reports/youth2019.html. Accessed 1 June 2020.
45. Bronson J, Carson EA. U.S. Department of Justice. Prisoners in 2017 https://www.bjs.gov/content/pub/pdf/p17.pdf. Accessed 1 June 2020.
46. Sawyer W, Wagner P. Mass Incarceration: the whole pie. Prison Policy Initiative. 2019. https://wwwprisonpolicyorg/reports/pie2019html Accessed 1 June 2020.
47. Shanahan MJ. Pathways to adulthood in changing societies: variability and mechanisms in life course perspective. Ann Rev Sociol. 2000;261(1):667–92.
48. Oesterle S. Background Paper: Pathways to Young Adulthood and Preventive Interventions Targeting Young Adults. Board on Children, Youth, and Families; Institute of Medicine; National Research Council. Improving the health, safety, and well-being of young adults: workshop summary. Washington, D.C.: National Academies Press (US); 2013. https://www.ncbi.nlm.nih.gov/books/NBK202209/.
49. Benson JE, Elder GH. Young adult identities and their pathways: a developmental and life course model. Dev Psychol. 2011;47(6):1646–57.
50. Martin JA, Hamilton BE, Osterman MJK, Driscoll AK, Drake P. Births: final data for 2017. Natl Vital Stat Rep. 2018;67(8):50p. https://www.cdc.gov/nchs/data/nvsr/nvsr67/nvsr67_08-508.pdf.
51. Vespa J. The changing economics and demographics of young adulthood: 1975–2016. Current Population Reports. April 2017. 23 p. https://www.census.gov/library/publications/2017/demo/p20-579.html
52. Frech A. Pathways to adulthood and changes in health-promoting behaviors. Adv Life Course Res. 2014;19:40–9.
53. Hughes K, Bellis MA, Hardcastle KA, Sethi D, Butchart A, Mikton C, et al. The effect of multiple adverse childhood experiences on health: a systematic review and meta-analysis. Lancet Public Health. 2017;2:e356–66.
54. Leebens PK, Williamson ED. Developmental psychopathology: risk and resilience in the transition to young adulthood. Child Adolesc Psychiatr Clin North Am. 2017;26(2):143–56.
55. Global Health Data Exchange. GBD results tool for 2017. Seattle: Institute for Health Metrics – University of Washington; 2020. http://ghdx.healthdata.org/gbd-results-tool. Accessed 1 June 2020.
56. Miron O, Yu K-H, Wilf-Miron R, Kohane IS. Suicide rates among adolescents and young adults in the United States, 2000–2017. JAMA. 2019;321(23):2362–4.
57. Jiang C, Mitran A, Miniño A, Ni, H. Racial and gender disparities in suicide among young adults aged 18–24: United States, 2009–2013. National Center for Health Statistics Health E-Stat. Sept 2015. https://www.cdc.gov/nchs/data/hestat/suicide/racial_and_gender_2009_2013.pdf.
58. Drum DJ, Brownson C, Burton Denmark A, Smith SE. New data on the nature of suicidal crises in college students: shifting the paradigm. Prof Psychol Res Pract. 2009;40(3):213–22.
59. Han B, Compton WM, Eisenberg D, Milazzo-Sayre L, McKeon R, Hughes A. Prevalence and mental health treatment of suicidal ideation and behavior among college students aged 18–25 years and their non–college-attending peers in the United States. J Clin Psychiatry. 2016;77(6):815–24.
60. Rodgers SM. Transitional age lesbian, gay, bisexual, transgender, and questioning youth: issues of diversity, integrated identities, and mental health. Child Adolesc Psychiatr Clin N Am. 2017;26(2):297–309.
61. Substance Abuse and Mental Health Services Administration. Key substance use and mental health indicators in the United States: Results from the 2018 national survey on drug use and health (HHS Publication No. PEP19–5068, NSDUH Series

H-54). Rockville: Center for Behavioral Health Statistics and Quality, Substance Abuse and Mental Health Services Administration; 2019. Retrieved from https://www.samhsa.gov/data/.

62. Chan V. Schizophrenia and psychosis: diagnosis, current research trends, and model treatment approaches with implications for transitional age youth. Child Adolesc Psychiatr Clin N Am. 2017;26(2):341–66.
63. Blanco C, Okuda M, Wright C, Hasin D, Grant B, Liu S-M, et al. Mental health of college students and their non-college-attending peers. Arch Gen Psychiatry. 2008;65:1429–37.
64. Merikangas KR, He J-P, Burstein M, Swanson SA, Avenevoli S, Cui L, et al. Lifetime prevalence of mental disorders in U.S. adolescents: results from the national comorbidity survey replication-adolescent supplement (NCS-A). J Am Acad Child Adolesc Psychiatry. 2010;49(10):980–9.
65. Kessler RC, Avenevoli S, Costello J, Green JG, Gruber MJ, Mclaughlin KA, et al. Severity of 12-month DSM-IV disorders in the National Comorbidity Survey Replication Adolescent Supplement. Arch Gen Psychiatry. 2012;69(4):381–9. B.
66. Kessler RC, Chiu WT, Demler O, Walters EE. Prevalence, severity, and comorbidity of 12-month DSM-IV disorders in the National Comorbidity Survey Replication. Arch Gen Psychiatry. 2005;62:617–27.
67. Kessler RC, Avenevoli S, Costello EJ, Georgiades K, Green JG, Gruber MJ, et al. Prevalence, persistence, and sociodemographic correlates of DSM-IV disorders in the National Comorbidity Survey Replication Adolescent Supplement. Arch Gen Psychiatry. 2012;69(4):372–80. A.
68. Bukstein OG. Challenges and gaps in understanding substance use problems in transitional age youth. Child Adolesc Psychiatr Clin N Am. 2017;26(2):253–69.
69. Rivas-Drake D, Stein GL. Multicultural developmental experiences: implications for resilience in transitional age youth. Child Adolesc Psychiatr Clin N Am. 2017;26(2):271–81.
70. Costello EJ, Copeland W, Angold A. Trends in psychopathology across the adolescent years: what changes when children become adolescents, and when adolescents become adults? J Child Psychol Psychiatry. 2011;52(10):1015–25.
71. Copeland WE, Adair CE, Smetanin P, Stiff D, Briante C, Colman I, et al. Diagnostic transitions from childhood to adolescence to early adulthood. J Child Psychol Psychiatry. 2013;54(7):791–9.
72. Vander Stoep A, Beresford SAA, Weiss NS, McKnight B, Cauce AM, Cohen P. Community-based study of the transition to adulthood for adolescents with psychiatric disorder. Am J Epidemiol. 2000;152(4):352–62.
73. Gralinski-Baker JH, Hauser ST, Billings RL, Allen JP. Risks along the road to adulthood: challenges faced by youth with serious mental health disorders. In: Osgood DW, Foster EM, Flanagan C, Ruth GR, editors. On your own without a net: the transition to adulthood for vulnerable populations. Chicago: Univ Chicago Press; 2005. p. 272–303.
74. Costello EJ, Copeland W, Angold A. The Great Smoky Mountains Study: developmental epidemiology in the southeastern United States. Soc Psychiatry Psychiatr Epidemiol. 2016;51:639–46.
75. Wagner M, Newman L. Longitudinal transition outcomes of youth with emotional disturbances. Psychiatr Rehabil J. 2012;35(3):199–208.
76. Mojtabai R, Stuart E, Hwang I, Eaton W, Sampson N, Kessler R. Long-term effects of mental disorders on educational attainment in the National Comorbidity Survey ten-year follow-up. Soc Psychiatry Psychiatr Epidemiol. 2015;50(10):1577–91.
77. Breslau J, Lane M, Sampson N, Kessler RC. Mental disorders and subsequent educational attainment in a US national sample. J Psychiatr Res. 2008;42(9):708–16.
78. Hunt J, Eisenberg D. Mental health problems and help-seeking behavior among college students. J Adolesc Health. 2010;46(1):3–10.
79. Gilmer TP, Ojeda VD, Fawley-King K, Larson B, Garcia P. Change in mental health service use after offering youth-specific versus adult programs to transition-age youths. Psychiatr Serv. 2012;63(6):592–6.
80. Broad KL, Sandhu VK, Sunderji N, Charach A. Youth experiences of transition from child mental health services to adult mental health services: a qualitative thematic synthesis. BMC Psychiatry. 2017;17(1):1–11.
81. Thornicroft G, Mehta N, Clement S, Evans-Lacko S, Doherty M, Rose D, et al. Evidence for effective interventions to reduce mental-health-related stigma and discrimination. Lancet. 2016;(10023):387, 1123–1332.
82. Lê Cook B, Trinh N-H, Li Z, Hou SS-Y, Progovac AM. Trends in racial-ethnic disparities in access to mental health care, 2004–2012. Psychiatr Serv. 2017;68(1):9–16.
83. Skehan B, Davis M. Aligning mental health treatments with the developmental stage and needs of late adolescents and young adults. Child Adolesc Psychiatr Clin N Am. 2017;26(2):177–90.
84. Simpson AR. Young adult development project. Boston: Massachusetts Institute of Technology; 2018. https://hr.mit.edu/static/worklife/youngadult/individual.html.
85. Grayson P. Overview. In: Grayson P, Meilman P, editors. College mental health practice. New York: Routledge; 2006. p. 1–20.
86. Chung WW, Hudziak JJ. The transitional age brain: "the best of times and the worst of times". Child Adolesc Psychiatr Clin N Am. 2017;26(2):157–75.
87. Gemelli R. Normal child and adolescent development. Washington, D.C.: American Psychiatric Press, Inc; 1996. 582 p.

88. Davis M, Sabella K, Smith LM, Costa A. Becoming an adult: challenges for those with mental health conditions. Research Brief 3. Worcester: University of Massachusetts Medical School, Department of Psychiatry, Systems and Psychosocial Advances Research Center (SPARC), Transitions Research and Training Center; 2011. https://escholarship.umassmed.edu/cgi/viewcontent.cgi?article=1064&context=pib.
89. Nagaoka J, Farrington CA, Ehrlich SB, Heath RD. Foundations for young adult success: a developmental framework. Chicago: The University of Chicago Consortium on Chicago School Research; 2015. https://consortium.uchicago.edu/sites/default/files/2018-10/Foundations%20for%20Young%20Adult-Jun2015-Consortium.pdf.
90. Larson M, Bolton A, Williams T. Guideposts for success 2.0: a framework for successful youth transition to adulthood. Washington, D.C.: Institute for Educational Leadership, National Collaborative on Workforce Development for Youth; 2019. https://files.eric.ed.gov/fulltext/ED598433.pdf.
91. Scales PC, Benson PL, Oesterle S, Hill KG, Hawkins JD, Pashak TJ. The dimensions of successful young adult development: a conceptual and measurement framework. Appl Dev Sci: Positive Youth Development Interventions: Advancing Evaluation Theory and Practice. 2016;20(3):150–74.
92. Kim-Cohen J. Resilience and developmental psychopathology. Child Adolesc Psychiatr Clin N Am. 2007;16(2):271–83.
93. Guerra NG, Bradshaw CP. Linking the prevention of problem behaviors and positive youth development: Core competencies for positive youth development and risk prevention. In NG Guerra and CP Bradhsaw (eds), Core competencies to prevent problem behaviors and promote positive youth development. 2008. New Dir Child Adolesc Dev. 2008;122:1–17.
94. Li J, Julian MM. Developmental relationships as the active ingredient: a unifying working hypothesis of 'what works' across intervention settings. Am J Orthopsychiatry. 2012;82(2):157–66.
95. Search Institute. The developmental relationships framework. Search Institute: Minneapolis; 2018. https://www.search-institute.org/wp-content/uploads/2018/05/Developmental-Relationships-Framework_English.pdf.
96. National Collaborative on Workforce and Disability for Youth. Guideposts for success. Washington, D.C.: Institute for Educational Leadership; 2005. http://www.ncwd-youth.info/wp-content/uploads/2018/03/Guideposts-for-Success-English-Print-Quality-1.pdf.
97. Podmostko M. Tunnels and cliffs: a guide for workforce development practitioners and policymakers serving youth with mental health needs. Washington, D.C.: National Collaborative on Workforce and Disability for Youth, Institute for Educational Leadership; 2007. http://www.ncwd-youth.info/wp--content/uploads/2017/10/Mental_Health_Guide_complete.pdf.
98. Martel A. The practice gap in health care transition: focus on young people heading to college with a mental health condition. In: Martel A, Derenne J, Leebens PK, editors. Promoting safe and effective transitions to college for youth with mental health conditions: a case based guide. Switzerland: Springer International; 2018. p. 3–9.
99. Stroul B, Blau G, Friedman R. Updating the system of care concept and philosophy. Washington, D.C.: Georgetown University Center for Child and Human Development, National Technical Assistance Center for Children's Mental Health; 2010. https://gucchdtacenter.georgetown.edu/resources/Call%20Docs/2010Calls/SOC_Brief2010.pdf.
100. Friesen B, Koroloff N. Housing and transition: meeting the needs of young adults with mental health conditions. Portland: Research and Training Center for Pathways to Positive Futures, Portland State University; 2018. https://pathwaysrtc.pdx.edu/pdf/proj-4-SPAC-housing-transition.pdf.
101. Ojeda VD, Hiller SP, Hurst S, Jones N, McMenamin S, Burgdorf J, et al. Implementation of age-specific services for transition-age youths in California. Psychiatr Serv. 2016;67(9):970–6.
102. Ellison M, Huckabee SS, Stone RA, Sabella K, Mullen MG. Career services for young adults with serious mental health conditions: innovations in the field. J Behav Health Serv Res. 2019;46(1):1–14.
103. Nossel I, Wall MM, Scodes J, Marino LA, Zilkha S, Bello I, et al. Results of a coordinated specialty care program for early psychosis and predictors of outcomes. Psychiatric Serv. 2018;69(8):863–70.
104. Clark HB, Hart K. Navigating the obstacle course: An evidence-supported community transition system. In: Clark HB, Unruh DK, editors. Transition of youth and young adults with emotional or behavioral difficulties: an evidence-supported handbook. Baltimore: Brookes; 2009. p. 47–94.
105. Bond GR, Drake RE, K. Effectiveness of individual placement and support supported employment for young adults. Early Interv Psychiatry. 2016;10(4):300–7.
106. Mckay CE, Osterman R, Shaffer J, Sawyer E, Gerrard E, Olivera N. Adapting services to engage young adults in ICCD clubhouses. Psychiatr Rehabil J. 2012;35(3):181–8.
107. Jivanjee P, Grover L, Thorp K, Masselli B, Bergan J, Brennan EM. Training needs of peer and non-peer transition service providers: results of a national survey. J Behav Health Serv Res. 2020;47(1):4–20.
108. Delman J, Klodnick V. Effectively employing young adult peer providers: a toolkit. Worcester: Transitions to adulthood center for research. https://www.umassmed.edu/globalassets/transitionsrtc/publications/effectivleyemployingyoungadultpeerproviders_a_toolkit.pdf. Accessed 18 July 2020.
109. Winters NC, Pumariega A. Practice parameter on child and adolescent mental health care in community systems of care. J Am Acad Child Adolesc Psychiatry. 2007;46(2):284–99.

110. Sellmaier C, Jivanjee P, Brennan EM, Grover L. Development and psychometric testing of the transition service provider competency scale. J Behav Health Serv Res. 2019;46(2):353–62.
111. Jivanjee P, Brennan EM, Grover L, Sellmaier C, Roser E, Pathways Transition Training Collaborative, Youth M.O.V.E. National, Pathways Transition Training Partners. Transition mental health service provider core competencies. Portland: Research and Training Center for Pathways to Positive Futures, Portland State University; 2018. https://www.pathwaysrtc.pdx.edu/pdf/projPTTP-core-competencies-2018.pdf.
112. Morgan RL, Riesen T. Promoting successful transition to adulthood for students with disabilities. New York: Guilford; 2016. 296 p.
113. Gruttardaro D, Crudo D. College students speak: a survey report on mental health. National Alliance on Mental Illness: Arlington; 2012. https://www.nami.org/getattachment/About-NAMI/Publications-Reports/Survey-Reports/College-Students-Speak_A-Survey-Report-on-Mental-Health-NAMI-2012.pdf.
114. Office of the Assistant Secretary for Administration and Management. Section 504, Rehabilitation Act of 1973. Washington, D.C.: U.S. Department of Labor. https://www.dol.gov/agencies/oasam/centers-offices/civil-rights-center/statutes/section-504-rehabilitation-act-of-1973. Accessed 1 June 2020.
115. Americans with Disabilities Act of 1990, Pub. L. No. 101–336, 104 Stat. 327 (July 26, 1990). https://www.govinfo.gov/content/pkg/STATUTE-104/pdf/STATUTE-104-Pg327.pdf.
116. Americans with Disabilities Amendments Act of 2008, Pub. L. No. 110–325, 122 Stat. 3553 (Sept. 25, 2008). https://www.congress.gov/110/plaws/publ325/PLAW-110publ325.pdf.
117. An act to prescribe penalties for certain acts of violence or intimidation, and for other purposes. Pub. L. No. 90–284, 82 Stat. 73 (April 11, 1968). https://catalog.archives.gov/id/12199297.
118. Logan D, Golden L, Osmani K. Family advisory Board of the Transitions ACR. WIOA: new law helps youth & young adults get jobs – what families need to know. Worcester: University of Massachusetts Medical School, Department of Psychiatry, Transitions to Adulthood Center for Research; 2019.
119. Chan V, Rasminsky S, Viesselman JO. A primer for working in campus mental health: a system of care. Acad Psychiatry. 2015;39:533–40.
120. U.S. Department of Education, U.S. Department of Health and Human Services. Joint Guidance on the Application of the Family Educational Rights and Privacy Act (FERPA) and the Health Insurance Portability and Accountability Act of 1996 (HIPAA) To Student Health Records. December 2019 update. https://studentprivacy.ed.gov/resources/joint-guidance-application-ferpa-and-hipaa-student-health-records. Accessed 1 June 2020.
121. Allison J, Childs J, Lambert L, Silver A. Moving to adult life: a legal guide for parents of youth with mental health needs. Boston: Parent/Professional Advocacy League; 2015. https://ppal.net/wp--content/uploads/2011/01/Legal-guide-single-page-all-for-web.pdf.
122. Cohen RA, Terlizzi EP, Martinez ME. Health insurance coverage: early release of estimates from the national health interview survey, 2018. Washington, D.C.: National Center for Health Statistics; 2019. https://www.cdc.gov/nchs/data/nhis/earlyrelease/insur201905.pdf
123. Fernandes-Alcantara AL, Baumrucker EP. Medicaid coverage for former foster youth up to age 26. Washington, D.C.: Congressional Research Service; 2018. https://fas.org/sgp/crs/misc/IF11010.pdf
124. American College Health Association. ACHA guidelines standards for student health insurance/benefits coverage. Maryland: American College Health Association; 2017. https://www.acha.org/documents/resources/guidelines/ACHA_Standards_SHI_Benefits_Programs_Nov2017.pdf
125. Torres Stone RA, Sabella K, Lidz CW, McKay C, Smith LM. The meaning of work for young adults diagnosed with serious mental health conditions. Psychiatr Rehabil J. 2018;41(4):290–8.
126. Corporation for National and Community Service. Be the greater good: Americorps. Washington, D.C.: Corporation for National and Community Service. https://www.nationalservice.gov/programs/americorps/join-americorps. Accessed 1 June 2020.
127. U.S. Department of Labor. What is job corps? Washington, D.C.: U.S. Department of Labor; Updated 3/2020. https://www.doleta.gov/job_corps/.
128. Office of the Under Secretary of Defense for Personnel and Readiness. Medical standards for appointment, enlistment, or induction into the military services. Arlington: Department of Defense; 2018. https://www.esd.whs.mil/Portals/54/Documents/DD/issuances/dodi/613003p.pdf
129. National Alliance on Mental Illness (NAMI). Transitions: supporting a young adult with a mental illness. https://2a392k31wksy2wkejf1y03dp--wpengine.netdna-ssl.com/wp-content/uploads/sites/188/2019/10/NAMI-Transitions2019.pdf. Accessed 15 July 2020.
130. Chan V. Understanding campus mental health services and the campus system of care. In: Martel A, Derenne J, Leebens PK, editors. Promoting safe and effective transitions to college for youth with mental health conditions: a case-based guide. Switzerland: Springer International; 2018. p. 37–42.
131. Leebens PK. Essential domains in transition planning and the roles of various constituents. In: Martel A, Derenne J, Leebens PK, editors. Promoting safe and effective transitions to college for youth with mental health conditions: a case-based guide. Switzerland: Springer International; 2018. p. 11–27.
132. Higher Education Mental Health Alliance (HEMHA). Balancing safety and support on cam-

pus: a guide for campus teams. 2012. http://hemha.org/wp-content/uploads/2019/01/campus-teams-balancing-safety-support-campus-jed-guide.pdf.
133. Martel A, Derenne J, Leebens PK. Helping patients and families navigate the transition to college: common themes, lessons learned, and best practices. In: Martel A, Derenne J, Leebens PK, editors. Promoting safe and effective transitions to college for youth with mental health conditions: a case-based guide. Switzerland: Springer International; 2018. p. 271–7.
134. U.S. Department of Education – Office of Postsecondary Education. Federal TRIO programs. Updated 5/2020. https://www2.ed.gov/about/offices/list/ope/trio/index.html.
135. Nelson V. What is a summer college bridge program? College Parent Central. https://www.collegeparentcentral.com/2011/05/what-is-a-college-summer-bridge-program/. Accessed 1 June 2020.
136. Eisenberg D, Lipson S, Posselt J. Promoting resilience, retention, and mental health. New Dir Stud Serv. 2016;156:87–95.
137. Biebel K, Mizrahi R, Ringeisen H. Postsecondary students with psychiatric disabilities identify core services and key ingredients to supporting education goals. Psychiatr Rehabil J. 2018;41(4):299–301.
138. Ringeisen H, Langer Ellison M, Ryder-Burge A, Biebel K, Alikhan S, Jones E. Supported education for individuals with psychiatric disabilities: state of the practice and policy implications. Psychiatr Rehabil J. 2017;40(2):197–206.
139. Stone R, Ellison M, Huckabee S, Mullen M. Innovative practices to support careers of young adults with mental health conditions. Worcester: University of Massachusetts Medical School, Department of Psychiatry, Systems and Psychosocial Advances Research Center (SPARC), Transitions Research and Training Center; 2017. https://www.umassmed.edu/contentassets/7fad776e301747ff8adbae8fd4999944/booklet_final_2.pdf.
140. U.S. Department of Education. Additional requirements for evaluations and reevaluations Sec. 300.305 Individuals with Disabilities Education Act. https://sites.ed.gov/idea/regs/b/d/300.305. Accessed 1 June 2020.
141. Fowler CH, Getzel EE, Lombardi A. Facilitating college supports to ensure student success. New Direct Adult Contin Educ. 2018;2018(160):101–12.
142. Katz S, Ford AB, Moskowitz RW, Jackson BA, Jaffe MW. Studies of illness in the aged. The index of ADL: a standardized measure of biological and psychosocial function. JAMA. 1963;185(12):914–9.
143. Guo HJ, Sapra A. Instrumental activity of daily living (IADL). StatPearls [Internet] Publishing LLC; 2020. Bookshelf ID: NBK553126. PMID: 31985920. https://www.ncbi.nlm.nih.gov/books/NBK553126/.
144. Lee T, Morgan W. Transitioning to adulthood from foster care. In: Martel A, Fuchs DC, editors. Child Adolesc Psychiatr Clin N Am. 2017;26(2):283–96.
145. Lieber R. A financial checklist for your newly minted high school graduate. The New York Times. 2019 May 31.; https://www.nytimes.com/2019/05/31/your-money/teenager-financial-preparation.html.
146. Livesey CMW, Rostain AL. Involving parents/family in treatment during the transition from late adolescence to young adulthood. Child Adolesc Psychiatr Clin N Am. 2017;26(2):199–216.
147. American Academy of Child and Adolescent Psychiatry (AACAP). Youth voice tip sheet. Communication between child and adolescent psychiatrist & youth. 10 tips to improve the conversation. Washington, D.C.: AACAP; 2012. https://www.aacap.org/App_Themes/AACAP/docs/youth_resources/misc/Youth_Voice_Tip_Sheet_2012.pdf.
148. Logan D, Mullen M. Strategies for engaging young adults. Shrewsbury: University of Massachusetts, Systems and Psychosocial Advances Research Center (SPARC); 2018. https://escholarship.umassmed.edu/cgi/viewcontent.cgi?article=1132&context=pib#:~:text=If%20technology%20is%20available%20to,to%20connect%20with%20young%20adults.
149. Schlechter AD, O'Brien KH, Stewart C. The positive assessment: a model for integrating well-being and strengths-based approaches into the child and adolescent psychiatry clinical evaluation. Child Adolesc Psychiatr Clin N Am. 2019;28(2):157–69.
150. Elwyn G, Frosch D, Thomson R, Joseph-Williams N, Lloyd A, Kinnersley P, et al. Shared decision making: a model for clinical practice. J Gen Intern Med. 2012;27(10):1361–7.
151. The National Child Traumatic Stress Network. Trauma-informed care. Los Angeles: National Center for Child Traumatic Stress, University of California; https://www.nctsn.org/trauma-informed-care. Accessed 1 June 2020.
152. Pumariega AJ, Rothe E, Mian A, Carlisle L, Toppelberg C, Harris T, et al. Practice parameter for cultural competence in child and adolescent psychiatric practice. J Am Acad Child Adolesc Psychiatry. 2013;52(10):1101–15.
153. Mistler LA, Sheidow AJ, Davis M. Transdiagnostic motivational enhancement therapy to reduce treatment attrition: use in emerging adults. Cogn Behav Pract. 2016;23(3):368–84.
154. Sood AB, Linker J. Proximal influences on the trajectory of suicidal behaviors and suicide during the transition from adolescence to young adulthood. Child Adolesc Psychiatr Clin N Am. 2017;26(2):235–51.
155. Blum RW, Garell D, Hodgman CH, Jorissen TW, Okinow NA, Orr DP, et al. Transition from child-centered to adult health-care systems for adolescents with chronic conditions: a position paper of the Society for Adolescent Medicine. J Adolesc Health. 1993;14(7):570–6.
156. Paul M, Ford T, Kramer T, Islam Z, Harley K, Singh SP. Transfers and transitions between child and adult mental health services. Br J Psychiatry Suppl. 2013;54:s36–40.
157. American Academy of Pediatrics, American Academy of Family Physicians, and American

College of Physicians, Transitions Clinical Report Authoring Group. Supporting the health care transition from adolescence to adulthood in the medical home. Pediatrics. 2011;128(1):182–202.

158. Office of Disease Prevention and Health Promotion. Healthy people. Washington, D.C.: U.S. Department of Health and Human Services; https://www.healthypeople.gov/. Accessed 1 June 2020.
159. AACAP. Moving into adulthood resource center. Washington, D.C.: AACAP; 2019 update. https://www.aacap.org/AACAP/Families_and_Youth/Resource_Centers/Moving_Into_Adulthood_Resource_Center/Home.aspx.
160. Soe K, Babajide A, Gibbs T. Council on children, adolescents, and their families. Position statement on transitional aged youth. Washington, D.C.: American Psychiatric Association; 2019. https://www.psychiatry.org/home/policy-finder?k=transitional%20aged%20youth
161. American Psychological Association. Services for transition age youth fellowship. https://www.apa.org/pi/mfp/psychology/stay/.
162. Young CC, Calloway SJ. Transition planning for the college bound adolescent with a mental health disorder. J Pediatr Nurs. 2015;30(5):e173–82.
163. Collins G, Wolter JA. Facilitating postsecondary transition and promoting academic success through language/literacy-based self-determination strategies. Lang Speech Hear Serv Sch. 2018;49(2):176–88.
164. Child Welfare Information Gateway. Core/Foundation Training for Caseworkers: transition to adulthood and independent living. Washington, D.C.: Children's Bureau, Administration for children and Families, U.S. Department of Health and Human Services; https://www.childwelfare.gov/topics/management/training/curricula/caseworkers/core/outofhomecare/transition-living/. Accessed 1 June 2020.
165. Hovish K, Weaver T, Islam Z, Paul M, Singh SP. Transition experiences of mental health service users, parents, and professionals in the United Kingdom: a qualitative study. Psychiatr Rehabil J. 2012;35(3):251–7.
166. Dunn V. Young people, mental health practitioners and researchers co-produce a transition preparation programme to improve outcomes and experience for young people leaving Child and Adolescent Mental Health Services (CAMHS). BMC Health Serv Res. 2017;17(1):293–304.
167. Syverson EP, McCarter R, He J, D'Angelo L, Tuchman LK. Adolescents' perceptions of transition importance, readiness, and likelihood of future success: the role of anticipatory guidance. Clin Pediatr. 2016;55(11):1020–5.
168. Koroloff NM. Moving out: transition policies for youth with serious emotional disabilities. J Mental Health Admin. 1990;17(1):78–86.
169. Got Transition. Six core elements of healthcare transition™. Washington, D.C.: The National Alliance to Advance Adolescent Health; 2020. https://www.gottransition.org/six-core-elements/.
170. American College of Physicians (ACP). Condition-specific tools. Intellectual disabilities/developmental disabilities (ID/DD). Philadelphia: ACP; 2016. https://www.acponline.org/system/files/documents/clinical_information/high_value_care/clinician_resources/pediatric_adult_care_transitions/gim_dd/idd_transitions_tools.pdf.
171. Martel A. Adaptation of pediatric health care transition guidelines for use with youth headed to college with mental illness: building a toolkit. In: Martel A, Derenne J, Leebens PK, editors. Promoting safe and effective transitions to college for youth with mental health conditions: a case-based guide. Switzerland: Springer International; 2018. p. 43–70.
172. Cleverly K, Rowland E, Bennett K, Jeffs L, Gore D. Identifying core components and indicators of successful transitions from child to adult mental health services: a scoping review. Eur Child Adolesc Psychiatry. 2020;29:107–21.
173. Schmidt A, Ilango SM, McManus MA, Rogers KK, White PH. Outcomes of pediatric to adult health care transition interventions: an updated systematic review. J Pediatr Nurs. 2020;51:92–107.
174. White PH, Cooley WC, Transitions Clinical Report Authoring Group; American Academy of Pediatrics; American Academy of Family Physicians; American College of Physicians. Supporting the health care transition from adolescence to adulthood in the medical home. Pediatrics. 2018;142(5):e20182587. https://doi.org/10.1542/peds.2018-2587.
175. Derenne J, Martel A. A model CSMH curriculum for child and adolescent psychiatry training programs. Acad Psychiatry. 2015;39:512–6.

2 Tips for Child and Adolescent Psychiatry Providers

Patricia K. Leebens

There is no constant but change.
–Buddha

Key Points

- It is important that children and adolescents begin practicing strategies to cope with change early and throughout childhood and adolescence.
- Pediatric clinicians should periodically review a youth's diagnoses and treatment needs with the parents and teen to inform decisions about post-high school plans.
- Clinicians who work with youth and families should help parents establish opportunities for the teen to practice increased self-care and independence.
- The pediatric provider must work with families to develop a mental health treatment plan and new supports in the post-high school environment.
- It is important for the pediatric clinician to continue to collaborate with new providers throughout the handoff and transition process.

Introduction

Homo sapiens, like all living species, are dynamic, ever-changing, and constantly interacting with their multiple settings and environments. Change, expected or unexpected, can lead to healthy growth and adaptation—with increased skills to cope with challenges—or can overwhelm the individual and lead to short-term dysregulation or long-term disability. The recent COVID-19 pandemic, with broad and varying rates of morbidity and mortality worldwide, has revealed how individual vulnerability along with environmental and cultural differences can interact, producing a wide variety of outcomes.

Human development from childhood to adulthood requires negotiating many changes and transitions. Successful coping is influenced by the individual child's strengths, as well as the effective support from parents in addition to other significant individuals and systems in the child's life. Pediatricians and family practice providers, as well as child and adolescent psychiatrists (CAP), play important roles in identifying a child's strengths and vulnerabilities. They identify and treat medical and/or mental health conditions, encourage opportunities for activities and experiences to increase independence in the youth, and assess the effectiveness of the child's home, school, and community environments.

P. K. Leebens (✉)
Department of Child and Adolescent Psychiatry, Yale Child Study Center, Yale School of Medicine, New Haven, CT, USA

V. Chan, J. Derenne (eds.), *Transition-Age Youth Mental Health Care*,
https://doi.org/10.1007/978-3-030-62113-1_2

The evolution of adolescents into adults can be a particularly challenging transition. Because of variations in emotional and cognitive maturity, levels of individual and parental psychopathology, differences in environmental stresses or supports, and possible risk factors for the worsening or onset of psychiatric or substance abuse disorders, the transition age youth (TAY) is particularly vulnerable in the initial steps into adulthood (1). This chapter focuses on practical suggestions for the child and adolescent psychiatrist to assist youths and their parents in the preparation and execution of post-high school plans.

Assessing Response to Change as Part of Routine Evaluation

Understanding a child's biopsychosocial development becomes an important part of the initial and ongoing psychiatric or mental health evaluation. That assessment involves evaluating home, school, and community environments for their ability to support healthy growth, including coping with expected and unexpected changes. How does the youth cope with routine change (e.g., starting a new school year, change of seasons, arrival of a new sibling, the move to a new home, changes in schedule on the weekend)? How does the family cope with unexpected changes (e.g., prolonged illness in a family member, severe damage or loss of home due to a natural disaster, sudden death of a grandparent, exposure to violence or trauma)?

If the assessment of the child and family reveals areas of concern that might benefit from ongoing therapeutic interventions, the CAP can help nurture the family throughout the process. This provides important support for managing symptoms, optimizing functioning, and improving parent-child interactions. Promoting a positive response to therapeutic interventions includes the following:

- Provide a warm and accepting therapeutic environment.
- Model effective communication with the child/youth.
- Employ motivational interviewing strategies to engage the youth in future planning and to improve independence and self-esteem.
- Demonstrate the importance of collaborating with the school and other members of the child's support team.
- Describe diagnoses in developmentally appropriate terms.
- Explain the reasons for therapy and medication recommendations at initiation of interventions and when adjustments are made.
- Help manage parent-child conflicts to decrease ineffective and possibly abusive interactions.
- Help parents provide positive opportunities to improve the youth's self-esteem, coping skills, and resilience.

Guiding Parents to Encourage Healthy Responses

Following the initial assessment and feedback in appropriate developmental terms, the goals of treatment should be established with the cooperation of the youth and the parents. This will help them anticipate changes and transitions that may lie ahead in the child's life and in the therapeutic process. If possible, goals should be described in ways so that progress can be identified in behavioral terms. Goals of treatment should be adjusted to respond to upcoming changes in the family's life (e.g. transition to middle school, coping with exposure to drugs and alcohol, driving a car responsibly, using electronics reasonably). Treatment goals should also include increasing the youth's independence through family chores, overnights with "best buddies," learning to seek help at school and from other significant adults, sleep-away camp, and managing personal hygiene (e.g., showering, brushing teeth, wearing deodorant, picking out appropriate clothing).

Parent guidance meetings with the CAP or other mental health providers can assist the parents in understanding and anticipating normal child and adolescent development or variations in development that may be a result of the child's learning or psychiatric difficulties. Routine transitions in the child's life can be discussed with the parents in advance so that they may help the youth anticipate upcoming changes and develop strategies to deal with them. Such parent guidance meetings with the CAP can also provide parents with a safe, nonjudgmental setting to express their frustration, sadness, and anger with the challenges of parenting a child with special needs. Such meetings can also help parents learn to work as a co-parenting team, so they are not giving their child mixed messages or opportunities to "split" the parents around expectations and rules (2).

The CAP can coach parents to support their child to grow and develop healthy responses to normal developmental changes (i.e., understanding and coping with bodily changes, getting to know new teachers and classmates in a new school year, locating and meeting helping personnel in a new school). Parent-child meetings with the CAP can help demonstrate that problems and concerns can be brought up and discussed in healthy, nonpunitive ways. The CAP can also encourage the youth's participation in annual reviews of the individualized educational plan (IEP) and in establishing educational goals for post-secondary transitions.

The CAP can encourage steps toward independence in the adolescent by increasing the time spent alone with the youth during the therapeutic appointments and by reviewing the child's diagnoses and medications with them in developmental terms. When age appropriate, the youth can be encouraged to set up appointments with the CAP, to contact the CAP if there are questions about medications or concerns about side effects, and to notify the CAP when medication renewals are needed. The CAP can assist the child and parents in identifying changes that may represent a re-emergence of symptoms of the disorder or condition (e.g., decreased sleep, difficulty concentrating, low mood, increased substance use, isolating from family and friends) and to devise plans to cope with possible decompensations.

Post-High School Planning

Establishing an Empathic and Effective Working Relationship

The CAP can help begin post-high school planning early, by helping the young teen become aware of talents, interests, and future goals. Using OARS techniques from Motivational Interviewing (**O**pen Ended Questions, **A**ffirmation, **R**eflective Listening, and **S**ummarize and recap plans for forward movement) helps the CAP establish an empathic working relationship with a youth who may be unsure, insecure, or actively resistant to making and clarifying future plans (3, 4).

For example, through initial open-ended questions, a CAP may learn that a 14-year-old teen with attention deficit hyperactivity disorder (ADHD) has a dream to become a physician like his mother, but he is afraid to admit that because he does not think he is smart enough or a good enough student. The CAP can encourage the teen to talk more about how he became interested in medicine, what kind of aspects of medicine he finds most interesting, and what the teen understands about what kind of schooling is needed to become a physician. Nonjudgmental questions by the CAP can help the teen think about the pros and cons of such a career choice, and the CAP can encourage the teen to plan opportunities to learn more about the role of physician (e.g., doing volunteer work in a hospital, participating in summer internships at medical schools, talking to his mother, and, if possible, shadowing her on a typical work day). The CAP can play an important role in affirming the youth's interests and process of exploration, even if the youth changes directions often in the course of exploring their dreams.

Discussing the teen's thoughts and feelings about these "practice" opportunities to learn more about medicine may reveal that the teen is more interested in becoming a physical therapist or a full-time bench researcher, thus leading to an adjustment of the post-high school plans as well as changes in current activities (e.g., seek out chances to be an internship with a researcher, or interviewing and shadowing a physical therapist friend of his mother).

Work with the parents could include helping them support the teen to try opportunities to learn about his career interests, even if the parents think the choice may be too hard for a child with ADHD. They may be worried about the expense of supporting their child for the entirety of medical training. Both parents and teens may be hesitant to look at "nontraditional" post-high school interventions such as a gap year, Job Corps, a post-high school transitional living program, getting a part-time job while living at home, or the military. The CAP can help the teen and parents assess the youth's readiness for the demands of college by encouraging the youth to attend post-high school planning meetings at school and by reviewing necessary skills needed for college as listed in readiness assessments (see resources, Casey Foundation). A variety of resources are available to assist the youth and their parents in exploring post-high school options and in preparing for a successful transition (see resources).

Even if the CAP begins therapeutic work with the teen well into their high school career, a review of the youth's interests, talents, and dreams can help focus the transition process. Using the young person's interests and dreams as a springboard for discussion can help with motivation and can also stimulate their awareness of skills and abilities that might need to be nurtured and developed to be able to accomplish designated goals.

If an initial assessment was done years earlier by the CAP, an updated feedback session with the teen and their parents should be done to review: (1) strengths and vulnerabilities of the child and the family, (2) DSM-5 diagnoses, (3) reasons for current therapeutic interventions (i.e., therapy, in-home services, medications, special supports at school or after school), and (4) beginning discussion about what interventions and supports may be needed in the new, post-high school setting. If multiple options are being considered, the teen and parents should be encouraged to consider the range of supports that might be needed depending upon which path is chosen. A one- or two-page summary of the feedback meeting can serve as a roadmap for preparing for possible post-high school options and the interventions needed for a successful transition (see Appendix 1).

Throughout middle and high school, parents can encourage the adolescent to explore interests through extracurricular and volunteer activities. Experiences like day and sleep-over camp, family outings and vacations, and independent reading can highlight. Parents can encourage increased independence and self-confidence in their teens by encouraging them to participate in after-school activities such as music lessons, art, sports and part-time jobs. Transition plans should take into account the youth's maturity level, educational, medical, and psychiatric needs, as well as current interests and future plans. When thinking about post-high school plans, families should include a variety of educational options (e.g., two- or four-year colleges, vocational or trade schools, apprenticeships) as well as alternative plans (e.g., work, military, gap year, independent living programs).

The CAP, coordinating with the school and other therapeutic providers, can assist the TAY and parents in focusing on realistic plans. Both parents and teens may require support and honest discussion, by taking into account the youth's strengths and need for appropriate, but not overly intrusive, support. The CAP may have to address a parent's need to hold tightly to their child, who they may view as fragile and unprepared for adult responsibilities. Or, the CAP may have to encourage the teen to accept support (e.g., academic or work accommodations, tutors, mentors, job coach) from their new environment. A parent guidance meeting may aid the CAP in reviewing the TAY's psychiatric and educational needs in a frank and direct way. This meeting may be a reminder to a parent—one depleted by years of coordinating care for offspring with special needs—of the need for continued support. As part of the process of formulating post-high school plans, the CAP can help the youth and parents outline the pros and cons of various options, taking into account the youth's needs and access to services (see Fig. 2.1).

TRANSITION OPTIONS	QUICK TIPS OF PROVIDER DISCUSSION POINTS
Learning About Post High School Options	• use office computer to tour important websites together related to post high school plan (e.g., college, military, GAP year options, Job Corps, etc.)
	• with teen alone and/or with parents
Turning Age 18 years old	• if still your care, prepare releases of information ready at the first appointment after 18th birthday • frame as "privilege" (rather than "responsibility") of signing documents to help coordinate care • reassure youth about disclosure notifications, unless emergency. • Include releases when possible for: parents, school, current treaters, future treaters if known, other support persons in current and new setting
College/University as Plan	• review process of applying for accommodations and see what documentation needs to be submitted and by whom. • assist youth and parents to check out educational and mental health services (on campus/off campus; fees; need to buy the college health insurance?) when visiting campuses or perusing websites of potential college choices • plan to contact youth and new providers 3 weeks into first semester and at midterm to see if current supports are adequate
College Chosen	• consolidate information into a Transfer of Care plan, including emergency plans.
Non - College Plan	• identify what is the goal of non-college choice? (e.g., earn money; gain work experience to help focus choices when going to college; experience living away from home; improve maturity and responsibility; get military to help with education costs; live in another country or culture). • try to estimate cost and duration of non-college plan
Non - College Plan Chosen	• review expectations are about the non-college choice with TAY, parents, and supports • consolidate youth information into a Transfer of Care plan, if needed

Fig. 2.1 Quick tips transition guide provider discussion points

It can be helpful to subscribe to the "Tarzan" theory of transition, in which, like the literary character, Tarzan, one needs to get a firm grasp on the new vine before letting go of the old one. Success in a new environment may require gathering and using information about the new setting, along with practicing skills in order to improve one's chance for success. Getting information about a new setting is not simply compiling information, but getting comprehensive details about the new environment. Understanding how services and access to supports may differ in the two communities (e.g., one outpatient psychiatric clinic has cognitive behavioral therapy, but not in another; the youth's insurance pays for services at the home city, but not in the college community) may be the difference between success and a suboptimal transition.

Empowering the TAY to develop independent living skills prior to graduation from high school will help ease the stress of coping with a new setting. Below are some of the skills which may transfer to the new environment:

- Driving a car responsibly, including basic auto maintenance
- Doing laundry, household cleaning, and basic healthy cooking
- Earning money, budgeting, and managing credit or debit card
- Managing class schedules, assignment deadlines, and appointments
- Appropriately seeking help from others, including professors, tutors, academic advisers, medical providers, and therapists
- Maintaining good medication compliance, including getting medications renewed in a timely fashion
- Understanding the possible dangers that can result from excessive drug and alcohol use
- Knowing the signs and symptoms of worsening illness and what to do if that occurs

Becoming familiar with the physical layout of the new environment can also help ease disorientation during the transition period. Visiting the new campus or worksite and locating significant services or buildings (e.g., personnel office, work location, library, dining hall, dormitory, health service, Dean's office, financial aid, disability services, etc.) can help the youth feel more comfortable and prepared.

Choosing Educational, Occupational, and Mental Health Supports

Once post-secondary plans are selected, psychiatric treatment options should be identified in the new setting. This could include an outpatient clinic provider, solo practitioner, college counseling services, or continuing with the current provider. Once plans are consolidated, the following tasks should be undertaken:

- Providers should obtain releases of information allowing the current and newly identified psychiatric provider to exchange information. These should be signed by the youth if age 18 years or by the parents if under age 18 years.
- Discuss the process for setting up an intake appointment and arranging transportation between the TAY's housing and the new provider(s).
- If the youth chooses college as a post-high school plan and struggles with learning disabilities or psychiatric conditions that disrupt functioning in completing academic tasks, the CAP should review the process of obtaining educational accommodations through the campus Office of Disability. Copies of recent (within the last 3 years, usually) psychoeducational testing may be required to obtain accommodations for ADHD or other learning disabilities. The CAP may be required to submit documentation of psychiatric conditions which would indicate a teen's eligibility for academic accommodations. Examples include extended time to complete tasks, flexibility with deadlines, and the option to complete tests in a smaller room with a limited number of students present. Required forms or letters of support should be submitted by the current provider.
- Complete a "transfer of care plan" which describes the youth's DSM-5 diagnoses, concurrent medication regimen, any allergies or concurrent medical conditions, and signs of the youth's reemergent symptoms. It should also detail an emergency plan, and names and contact information of current and new providers and services.
- Review the new provider's website(s) to determine whether an agency or center provides any additional supportive services. CAP should create a brief summary of the youth's current and past treatments, as well as any follow-up needed.
- CAP, youth, and parents should review signs that the youth is more symptomatic and may need urgent or emergent care. The TAY should know how and where to seek help in the new environment. It may also help for them to store important emergency numbers in their cell phone. If appropriate, the CAP should encourage the family to discuss issues such as finances, health habits, and expected communication with parents.

- Accountability issues should also be discussed. For example, given the high cost of college or special post-high school programs, does the parent expect to see copies of the youth's grades or performance evaluations? Do the parents have a limit to the amount of financial support that they can extend to the TAY for tuition or living expenses?
- The youth, parents, and CAP should discuss possible alternative contingency plans as well as more challenging plans if things go better than anticipated. They may need to transfer to a college in their hometown in order to get more family support or take a semester off to focus on treatment. If things are going well, they may be able to transition to living in a residence hall on campus instead of living at home or may be able to make the jump to attending college after a successful gap year of working and living independently.

Conclusion

Growing up is challenging at best and can be overwhelming when coping with psychiatric or educational disabilities. A youth's self-esteem and plans for the future can be eroded with educational delays or failure. Parents can despair for their child and become overly protective or neglectful if they themselves are overwhelmed. A youth with special needs may need multiple educational and psychiatric supports, including help in the home. Medical monitoring and multiple medications may be needed to help them function, and planning for the future may be daunting. A child and adolescent psychiatrist has specialized training to help the child and family with these complex issues. The transition can showcase successful support from home, school, and therapeutic supports. Or, the transition can be a poorly planned and fragmented journey that leads to regression, discouragement and disappointment, as well as possible disability for the young adult.

A healthy and successful transition to adulthood requires careful planning, long-standing opportunities to practice new life skills and independent learning, as well as a carefully choreographed transition of support services and therapeutic providers. The CAP has a key role as conductor of this complicated orchestra. Nothing is sweeter nor builds self-esteem and self-confidence more than real success.

> Growth has not only rewards and pleasures but also many intrinsic pains and always will have. Each step forward is a step into the unfamiliar and is possibly dangerous. It also means giving up something familiar and good and satisfying. It frequently means a parting and a separation with consequent nostalgia, loneliness, and mourning. It also often means giving up a simpler and easier and less effortful life in exchange for a more demanding, more difficult life. Growth forward is in spite of losses and therefore requires courage and strength in the individual, as well as protection, permission, and encouragement from the environment. –Abraham Maslow, Motivation and Personality (1954)

Appendix 1: Post-High School Feedback and Planning Meeting

Suzy, 16 Years Old

Strengths	Vulnerabilities
Good student; hard working	Susceptible to mood swings/anxiety
Supportive parents	Depression with suicidal thoughts
Persistent	History of abuse and trauma
Bilingual	Difficulty trusting others
Willing to seek help	Straddling two cultures
In treatment; has insurance	Self-esteem issues
Has friends; good with kids	Difficulty with intimacy

Possible Post-High School Plans (1) 4-year college in hometown; (2) gap year working with kids; (3) 4-year college away from home

DSM-5 Diagnostic Summary

- Bipolar II Disorder (F31.81), current episode Depressed
- Persistent Dysphoric Disorder (Dysthymia) (F34.1)
- Generalized Anxiety Disorder (F41.1)
- r/o Posttraumatic Stress Disorder, Chronic (F43.12)

- Overweight; h/o iron deficiency anemia; family history diabetes and hypertension
- History of trauma and abuse; parent-child conflicts; developmental stresses

Response to Treatment Current medication regimen (lithium 600 mg/900 mg; fluoxetine 10 mg) has provided stability for the last 18 months, along with weekly participation in CBT-informed psychotherapy with Dr. B. Six months of an intensive outpatient treatment program at age 14 helped improve parent-child functioning and peer relationships. Parent guidance meetings every 3 months have been very helpful.

Recommendations

1. Follow up on medical issues: (a) EKG; (b) lithium level, thyroid function tests, vitamin D, folate, and vitamin B12, CBC, ferritin, reticulocyte count, fasting glucose, HgbA1c; (c) pelvic exam.
2. Review current IEP with school; bring along school advocate to request increased accommodations for more time on tests because of severe anxiety. Plan for Suzy to attend IEP meetings at school.
3. Treat underlying medical issues if emerge following above medical evaluations.
4. Begin regular exercise routine for improved health and mood; monitor weight.
5. Continue TF-CBT work with Dr. B.
6. Consider addition of antipsychotic medication (i.e., low-dose aripiprazole or ziprasidone) to augment mood stabilizers and to help with cognitive distortions and overreactions when triggered by trauma reminders.
7. Consider judicious use of antidepressant medication if depressed mood persists beyond addition of antipsychotic medication.
8. Consider volunteer activities, hobbies, art classes, singing in a choir for structure, enjoyment, and mastery.
9. Work on Transition Plan for college:
   (a) Self-advocacy (practice asking for help with teachers/counselors at school).
   (b) Health management and relapse prevention (know names and doses of meds and side effects).
   (c) Investigate on campus supports and college-friendly environments for bipolar disorder (internet browsing).
   (d) Update educational assessments to obtain accommodations.
   (e) Consider gap year or other post-high school plans to improve confidence in new settings and to work on advocacy and independent living skills.
   (f) Work on getting driver's license, doing own laundry, getting part-time job working with kids, opening checking account.

Resources

- https://www.casey.org/casey-life-skills-resources/. Readiness assessment
- https://www.parentcenterhub.org/whatiscpir/. *Collection of information and products created for Parent Centers around the US serving families of children with disabilities. Useful info about many post-high school options. In English and Spanish.*
- https://dbhdid.ky.gov/dbh/documents/ksaods/2015/Golden.pdf. Motivational Interviewing with Adolescents, Department for Behavioral Health, Developmental and Intellectual Disabilities, State of Kentucky.
- https://www.gottransition.org/. A website to improve transition from pediatric to adult health care through the use of new and innovative strategies for health professionals and youth.
- https://www.settogo.org/. A Jed Foundation Program which provides information, tools and guidance to help teens decide whether to go to college or straight to a career. Helpful information for parents as well.
- https://staff.aacap.org/AACAP/Families_and_Youth/Resource_Centers/Moving_Into_Adulthood_Resource_Center/Home.aspx. Helpful resources for child and adolescent psychiatrists working with teens with special needs transitioning into adulthood.

- https://sites.ed.gov/idea/files/postsecondary-transition-guide-may-2017.pdf. A helpful transition guide to postsecondary education and employment for youths with disabilities.

References

1. Leebens PK, Williamson ED. Developmental psychopathology: risk and resilience in the transition to young adulthood. Child Adolesc Psychiatr Clin N Am. 2017;26(2):143–56.
2. Martel A, Derenne J, Leebens PK, editors. Promoting safe and effective transitions to college for youth with mental health conditions: a case-based guide to best practices. New York: Springer International Publishing; 2018.
3. Miller W, Rollnick S. Motivational interviewing. 3rd ed. New York: Guilford Press; 2013.
4. Naar-King S. Motivational interviewing in adolescent treatment. Can J Psychiatr. 2011;56(11):651–7.

15 Going on 26: Tips for Working with Transitional-Age Youth

3

Maryland Pao

Key Points

- Some of the challenges in bridging the transition from pediatric to adult mental health care may arise from the conceptual differences imparted in adult and child and adolescent psychiatric training.
- All providers are challenged to keep TAY, who are unpredictable and evolving, engaged during evaluation and treatment of potentially emerging mental disorders.
- When interviewing TAY, clinicians should not make any assumptions about the person's level of experience around sexuality, substance use and abuse, or other "outrageous" behaviors but rather take a comprehensive biopsychosocial approach to appropriately interpret findings.
- It may be helpful for adult psychiatrists who treat TAY to incorporate developmental domains (informed by Piaget and Erikson) into their clinical interviewing and treatment formulations.
- Given uneven developmental trajectories in emotion, social cognition and intellect, clinicians may need to facilitate TAY participation in shared medical decision-making with their families.
- TAY development crosses systems of care from school to employment, from family to an individual focus, even differing psychiatric diagnostic disorders, all of which has implications for the adult and child and adolescent psychiatrists caring for them.

M. Pao (✉)
Office of the Clinical Director, National Institute of Mental Health, National Institutes of Health, Bethesda, MD, USA
e-mail: paom@mail.nih.gov

Introduction

Adult psychiatrists are fundamentally interested in where people and their trajectory stories intersect with mental illness; child and adolescent psychiatrists (CAPs) and adult psychiatrists may differ in how they conceptualize their patients and their goals. CAP view their patients including transitional age youth (TAY), defined here as 15 years through 26 years [1], through the multifaceted prism of ongoing development and focus on facilitating coping and adaptation for optimal development rather than concentrating primarily on identifying psychopathology to initiate treatment. A significant challenge for all clinicians working with TAY is keeping them engaged in

V. Chan, J. Derenne (eds.), *Transition-Age Youth Mental Health Care*,
https://doi.org/10.1007/978-3-030-62113-1_3

evaluation and treatment at this critical time when they are not fully independent but are at significant risk for onset of mental disorders and developing substance use disorders [2]. When interviewing TAY, clinicians should not make any assumptions about the person's cognitive level, verbal abilities, or psychosocial experiences, including level of experience around sexuality, substance use and abuse, or other "outrageous" behaviors without a comprehensive biopsychosocial assessment. Recalling aspects of developmental theories can enhance psychological and psychiatric understanding when working with TAY.

Concept of Development

"The developmental perspective emphasizes maturation of the brain in the context of social experience, the environmental interface" [3]. The concept of development is complex and requires an understanding of many biological concepts including sensitive periods, monitoring separate streams of development (physical growth, motor development, language, cognitive, emotional, attachment, social, and sexual) and their trajectories, and awareness of the continuity and discontinuity of human characteristics and symptoms [3]. Eisenberg noted, "The point to be stressed is that the developmental process begins with the information encoded in the genome but its phenotypic expression is continuously modulated by sequential interactions with environmental variables at each stage of development, not excepting circulatory, nutritional and toxic factors during intrauterine life and the obstetrical characteristics of the birth process itself" [4]. He further stated, "What is crucial is an understanding of the interactions between the two [nature vs nurture], interactions that determine the trajectory of development [4].

It is clear that "Early life exposure to adverse childhood experiences (ACE), like trauma, abuse or maltreatment in childhood has been linked to alteration of the brain structure and the neurobiological stress-response systems which have consequences for health and emotional well-being [5]" and demonstrate enduring effects [6]. While negative experiences such as loss are virtually unavoidable, experiencing a major loss, as an example that of a parent in early childhood, may have a greater, more pervasive impact on the person's outcome, illustrating the concept of sensitive periods and critical windows in childhood development [3].

The term transitional age youth (TAY) typically refers to the demographic spanning older adolescence (15–16 years) to young adulthood (24–26 years) [1]. The lack of preciseness in part reflects that this cohort is characterized by uneven brain development [7, 8] and puberty as well as psychosocial transitions that are not uniformly accomplished by a specific age and may be highly influenced by culture [9]. However, there do appear to be some universal culturally determined tasks of achieving adulthood and self-sufficiency related to educational attainment, employment, contribution to a household, role in relationships and parenting, and positive community contributions [10].

Two Useful Developmental Theories

Two key theories of development that may be useful to adult psychiatrists include that of Jean Piaget regarding a child's development of cognitive understanding of the world around them and how they categorize experiences and that of Erik Erikson who proposed a theory of psychosocial developmental tasks humans face as they mature.

Piaget and Cognitive Development

In the early twentieth century, Piaget, a Swiss developmental psychologist, proposed a developmental stage theory based on his observations of how children acquired knowledge using mathematical, physical, and logical practices [11, 12]. Piaget believed the brain matured biologically along with environmental experiences to develop cognitive understanding of the world through language and reasoning. He proposed four stages

Table 3.1 Piaget's Cognitive Stages of Development [12]

Cognitive stage	Age	Main task	Perspectives
Sensorimotor	0–24 months	Uses senses to explore world; concept of object permanence begins	Focus on self
Preoperational	2–7 years	Repetitive actions; symbols and mental images are sustained; begins mastery of logic and language	Focus on self
Concrete operational	7–11 years	Classification of objects; reasoning and inference occur with trial and error; concept of conservation	Focus on self Begins to understand perspective taking of others
Formal operational	12–adulthood	Hypothesis testing Abstract thinking-reversibility and propositional operations	Taking perspective of others is more developed

of cognitive development that all humans pass through sequentially, though not always achieving all four stages fully. This has relevance for adult psychiatrists when evaluating a patient's ability for abstract thinking related to illness, illness causality, and treatment. The stages are sensorimotor (0–2 years), preoperational (2–7 years), concrete operational (7–11 years), and formal operational (12 years to adulthood) [12]. See Table 3.1 for a summary of Piaget's Cognitive Stages.

Piaget did not focus on social cognition and his theory does not emphasize the role of social adaptation or cultural influences which are critical factors. Nevertheless, it is crucial that adult psychiatrists consider a TAY's chronologic age and consider what cognitive stage they have achieved. Not all TAY have fully matured in formal operational thinking, and this can impact understanding or, more aptly, misunderstanding of medical information and unfulfilled expectations by clinicians as to what they believe the TAY should be doing in self-care or treatment. For example, it may be difficult for a TAY to be willing to take a prophylactic medication (i.e., antibiotic) for a condition when they feel well and the medication is likely to cause side effects; it is difficult for them to appreciate long-term benefit as they are focused on the here and now. They may also believe they are immortal and do not believe nonadherence to treatment regimens will seriously impact them. Medical decision-making today requires an ability to comprehend and manipulate large quantities of information and options. Clinicians working with TAY need to make a conscious assessment of the TAY's decision-making capacity at the time of the evaluation [13] as well as consider how to work with families in these decisions which may need to be shared to improve outcomes [14].

Erikson and the Stages of Psychosocial Development

Erik Erikson, a psychoanalyst, described in the mid-twentieth century, a theory of eight developmental stages of psychosocial development that all humans confront in the life cycle [15]. According to Erikson, the primary developmental tasks for TAY are separation-individuation, identity formation, and achieving intimacy. Additional stages in the later adult life include concerns with career consolidation, generativity, and being a keeper of meaning and integrity [15].

Overall, TAY are trying to develop their own identity and value systems basically around what is the balance between "being" and "doing" in their sociocultural contexts. They tend to view others' stances as black or white and, perhaps due to not fully formed brain circuits and lack of experiences, have a low tolerance for hypocrisy. Acquiring the ability to understand nuance and see shades of gray generally expands as young adults mature. Expanding the gray areas in situations is a potential focus for practicing cognitive behavioral therapy in TAY (see Table 3.2 for a summary of Erikson's Psychosocial Developmental Stages).

Table 3.2 Erikson's Stages of Psychosocial Development [15]

Stages	Approximate ages (years)	Psychosocial crisis/ developmental task	Favorable outcome	Unfavorable outcome
Childhood				
1	0–1	Trust vs mistrust	Hope and trust in environment and future	Suspicion in environment and fear of future
2	1–3	Autonomy vs shame/doubt	Sense of adequacy and self-control	Sense of shame and self-doubt
3	3–6	Initiative vs guilt	Ability to initiate one's own activities with purpose	Sense of guilt and inadequacy to be on one's own
4	6–12	Industry vs inferiority	Ability to learn, organize, and feel competent	Feeling inferior at learning and organizing
Transition				
5	Adolescence	Identity vs confusion	Seeing oneself as unique and an integrated self	Confusion over who and what self really is
Adulthood				
6	Early	Intimacy vs isolation	Able to commit to others; to love	Unable to form sustained meaningful or affectionate relationships
7	Middle	Generativity vs stagnation	Concern for family and society in general	Concern only for self and one's own well-being and prosperity
8	Late	Integrity vs despair	Sense of integrity and fulfillment; able to face death without major regrets	Dissatisfaction with life; despair in facing death with many regrets

Differences in Adult and Child and Adolescent Psychiatry

All CAPs have received 2 years of training in adult psychiatry, and all adult psychiatrists have had exposure to child and adolescent psychiatry, so what is the gap that needs to be bridged? All psychiatric professionals are concerned with the well-being of the patient and restoring them to the best mental health and functioning possible. However, given cognitive, emotional, and social development do not proceed in lock step and adults are not suddenly fully mature at age 18 years, there is considerable overlap of in the provision of psychiatric care in patients 18–26 years old. In addition to some notably different presentations of childhood psychiatric disorders such as attention deficit hyperactivity disorder or autism spectrum disorders, there are major differences in the systems in which the person is operating. (See Table 3.3 for summary of differences between child and adult psychiatric care.) There are differences in who identifies the problem for a child versus an adult, what parties are involved in the assessment and treatment, and the consequences of failure of treatment may have different legal and social outcomes. Working with TAY requires going back and forth across these different systems and approaches. CAPs are especially sensitive to the variability in developmental trajectories of TAY, especially in cognitive and emotional development. They appreciate the essential role of the family in adaptation. CAPs try to ameliorate adversity whether it is due to chronic or serious medical or psychiatric illness, natural disasters, trauma, or abuse. They attempt to facilitate optimum child development (which may include helping parents) and hope to prevent mental illness.

Some Helpful Key Questions for Adult Psychiatrists to Remember

1. **Does the TAY have a past psychiatric history?** Many mental disorders start in adolescence [2, 5].

   Ask: *Have you ever seen a school counselor, therapist, or psychiatrist before, even as a child? How did those experiences go? (This may identify positive or negative response to suggesting*

Table 3.3 Differences between child and adult psychiatric care

	Child	Adult
Who identifies the problem?	Parent/other-school/self	Self
How do the problems present?	Problematic behaviors for others Problematic behaviors for self	Problematic behaviors for self Problematic behaviors for others
Who seeks the solutions?	Family/school/self	Self
Assessment	Youth/parent/other-school	Adult/(outside informant)
Provider's treatment approach	Individual focus Family focus	Individual focus
Who makes treatment decisions?	Paternalistic/shared decision-making	Autonomy/shared decision-making
Target of treatment	Specifically focused on health/pathology Psychosocial developmental aspects considered	Specifically focused on pathology/health
Preferred treatment modality	Non-pharmacologic	Pharmacologic
Provider role in treatment adherence	Helps with regimen	Accepts refusal
Provider role in care coordination	Communication with school/other services more reliable	Coordination with other services may be variable
Legal	Minor until 18 years; no decision-making authority (some exceptions by state for certain decisions	Legally responsible as an adult for all actions

psychiatric treatments.) Have you ever been on psychiatric medications before ever?

2. **Take a detailed school history**. This information may indicate signs of early trouble in cognitive, social, or emotional domains; school, like job stability for adults, is a place for a youth to demonstrate persistence, self-mastery, and signs of early resilience. How difficulties in school are managed also gives clues to parental and environmental responses.

   Ask: *How far did you go in school? Ever repeat or skip a grade? Did you need any extra help in school? What were your grades like? What was hard in school? What was easy? Is school or home better?*

Specific Approaches to Working with TAY

Setting Up the Interview

- Working with TAY requires more time during the evaluation period in order to get a detailed clinical history for two main reasons: First, it takes more questions to get answers from TAY. Second, it requires additional information gathering, including from the parent/s or caregivers and other sources such as teachers.

History Taking

- If a parent/s accompany/ies the TAY, start by asking the TAY if they would like to be interviewed first, or if it would be okay to start with the parent/s present. This allows an immediate assessment of the family relationship regarding how comfortable they are speaking in front of one another and builds trust through respecting the TAY as an independent voice. After asking the TAY questions around history of the present illness, they may be curious to listen to the parental version. Information regarding childhood milestones is generally provided by parent/s which the TAY may find interesting. If the TAY declines to have parent/s in the initial interview, then indicate you will meet with each of them separately starting with the TAY in order to gain the trust of the TAY. Most parent/s will honor this request unless the TAY is on the younger end of the age spectrum or has cognitive difficulties.

- TAY are generally more accurate when describing internalizing symptoms such as mood, anxiety, and sleep, while parent/s may be more accurate regarding externalizing symptoms such as inattentiveness, hyperactivity, aggressive, or disruptive behaviors. While both perspectives are helpful, the clinician may need to seek additional information, with parental and TAY permission, from school personnel.
- It is important to ask about early milestones (e.g., social, motor, language) and details about school history that may indicate delayed neurologic development or other early vulnerabilities.
- It is critical to ask TAY by themselves about risk behaviors around sexuality, substance use and abuse, or social media use. It's a faster-paced world today. While TAY still benefit from having boundaries to push up against to understand the limits of their emotions and behaviors, experimentation, risk taking, and limit testing are a normal and expected part of development, and they may not wish to share everything in front of parent/s.
- It is also necessary to meet with parent/s alone, at least briefly, for observations on the struggling TAY and to provide additional context of which the TAY may not be aware (e.g., parents suffer from their own mental health problems or have serious work or financial problems, family history of suicide or psychotic illness, or other "family secrets"). Parent/s may also provide strategies/treatments they have tried using to assist the TAY or may reveal serious parenting problems.

Mental Status Exam

- Don't be fooled by good verbal and social skills which may mask uneven cognitive skills such as lack of ability to think abstractly or follow multiple directions. By the same token, do not assume poor speech skills are equivalent to intellectual disability.
- Be prepared for responses that range from regressive and basic to sophisticated and mature, "15 or 26 years" or anything in between. This is the fun and the challenge of working with TAY.
- Confidentiality is tricky when working with TAY. Be sure to be explicit to the TAY about what will or will not be shared with other adults. Talk with your colleagues about best practices and be aware of local legal policies regarding working with youth under age 18 years [16]. If they are over 18 years, depending on state policies, obtain releases of information to share information with parents and other providers.

Assessment/Formulation

- Consider predisposing (e.g., genetics, family history, lead poisoning, h/o ADHD), perpetuating (e.g., abusive environment, marital conflict), and precipitating factors (e.g., relocation, new medical illness, bullying) in formulation. Determine physical, emotional, and social developmental levels and decision-making capacity and remember these developmental trajectories may not all be in sync.
- Consider what psychosocial developmental tasks are salient and create a treatment plan that facilitates growth in those areas.
- Think about developmental discrepancies and how one might tailor treatments to the variability, e.g., adding a case manager or school counselor as part of the needed treatment to decrease anxiety in college may be more appropriate than adding an anxiolytic medication.

Treatment Planning

- Working with TAY on treatment issues requires flexibility, persistence, authenticity, and patience.
- On engagement, "Moreover, adult psychiatrists may require additional education to understand and treat mental health disorders that may persist from childhood (e.g., autism, ADHD) or emerge during the TAY years (substance abuse) and acquire the capacity to work with systems and families, negotiate reim-

bursement, and navigate boundaries and confidentiality" [1].

- Goals for treatment should be realistic, made explicit, and may require some negotiation to reach agreement. Tasks should be broken down into achievable parts and be specific. Prepare TAY and family for difficult tasks that may require behavioral plans be put in place over time. For example, fostering further independence may be the act of assisting the TAY to locating a phone number and having them make a medical appointment for themselves.

Conclusion

Working with TAY in mental health care requires a psychiatrist to be flexible, persistent, and authentic and have patience given their responses can range from immature to age appropriate to maturely sophisticated just within one patient. This is the fun and the challenge of working with TAY. Awareness of cognitive and psychosocial developmental theories is useful. Adult psychiatrists may be more effective by keeping a developmental perspective in mind along with their usual diagnostic and treatment approaches when working with TAY.

Acknowledgments This research was supported by the Intramural Research Program of the NIMH (Annual Report Number ZIAMH002922).

References

1. Wilens TE, Rosenbaum JF. Transitional aged youth: a new frontier in child and adolescent psychiatry. J Am Acad Child Adolesc Psychiatry. 2013;52(9):887–90.
2. Merikangas KR, He JP, Burstein M, Swanson SA, Avenevoli S, Cui L, et al. Lifetime prevalence of mental disorders in U.S. adolescents: results from the National Comorbidity Survey Replication--Adolescent Supplement (NCS-A). J Am Acad Child Adolesc Psychiatry. 2010;49(10):980–9.
3. Harris JC. Developmental neuropsychiatry, vol. 1. New York: Oxford University Press; 1998. p. 167–8.
4. Eisenberg L. Development as a unifying concept in psychiatry. Br J Psychiat. 1977;131:225–37.
5. Michelle K-I, et al. ACEs and all cause mortality. Eur J Epidemiol. 2013;28:721–34.
6. Anda RF, Felitti VJ, Bremner JD, et al. The enduring effects of abuse and related adverse experiences in childhood. A convergence of evidence from neurobiology and epidemiology. Eur Arch Psychiatry Clin Neurosci. 2006;256(3):174–86.
7. Giedd JN. The teen brain: insights from neuroimaging. J Adolesc Health. 2008;42:335–43.
8. Casey BJ, Heller AS, Gee DG, Cohen AO. Development of the emotional brain. Neurosci Lett. 2019;693:29–34.
9. Oesterle S. Background paper: pathways to young adulthood and preventive interventions targeting young adults. In: IOM (Institute of Medicine) and NRC (National Research Council), editor. Improving the health, safety, and well-being of young adults: workshop summary. Washington, DC: The National Academies Press; 2013. p. 147–76.
10. Pao M. Conceptualization of success in young adulthood in child Adolesc Psychiatr Clin N Am. Martel A, Fuchs C (eds.) 2017;26(2):191–8.
11. Gardner H. Frames of mind: the theory of multiple intelligences. New York: Basic Books; 2011.
12. Piaget J. The stages of the intellectual development of the child. Bull Menn Clin. 1962;26:120–8.
13. Skehan B, Davis M. Aligning mental health treatments with the developmental stage and needs of late adolescents and young adults. Child Adolesc Psychiatr Clin N Am. 2017;26(2):177–90.
14. Ruggeri A, Gummerum M, Hanoch Y. Braving difficult choices alone: children's and adolescents' medical decision making. PLoS One. 2014;9(8):e103287.
15. Erikson E. Childhood and society. New York: Norton; 1950.
16. https://www.aafp.org/about/policies/all/adolescent-confidentiality.html. Accessed 2/16/2020.

4 Developing a Physician Workforce to Bridge the Gap Between Pediatric and Adult Psychiatric Care

Jessica Moore

Key Points

- It is crucial to train the emerging physician workforce on issues of transition from pediatric to adult care.
- All psychiatrists should be prepared to help youth move through the various pathways of transition by being cognizant of childhood development, means for effective transfer, and diverse systems of care.
- Early exposure for medical students to child and adolescent psychiatry helps to build their knowledge base in development and issues of transition.
- A model transitional age youth fellowship incorporates college mental health, community TAY clinics, integrative didactics, and focused training in development.
- Interorganizational collaboration allows for optimal use of resources, innovative training experiences, and improved advocacy for youth in transition.

Transition has long been discussed in medical training, initially in the context of the need for appropriate handoff of patient information between colleagues. Since the 1990s, the term transition has come to be applied to population-based health relative to systems of care. Discussions in transition have evolved to consider the developmental biopsychosocial changes that take place during late adolescence and young adulthood. Despite this broadening of the scope, medical schools and residency training programs continue to struggle with how to educate future physicians on issues of transition. This is in part, because of existing myths about this transitional age youth (TAY). Physicians may falsely believe that development is no longer clinically relevant after adolescence. They may think that TAY are developmentally similar to either adolescents or persons in late adulthood and would consider adjustments in assessment, treatment, or management. Some may also assume that academic achievements are indicative of well-being and therefore mental health needs of this population are low. In other words, a student who is academically talented enough to matriculate to college no longer needs care. In fact, an understanding of development across the life span is critical: TAY have developmental challenges that set them apart from adolescents and from those in older adulthood. The literature has repeatedly emphasized that transition is not a discrete event to be com-

J. Moore (✉)
Department of Psychiatry, University of Texas Southwestern Medical Center, Dallas, TX, USA
e-mail: Jessica.Moore@utsouthwestern.edu

V. Chan, J. Derenne (eds.), *Transition-Age Youth Mental Health Care*,
https://doi.org/10.1007/978-3-030-62113-1_4

pleted in one clinic visit [19, 27, 28]. Rather, transition describes a process that occurs in stages over time. The term transfer better describes the handoff from pediatric to adult provider [20, 27]. Youth face multifactorial vulnerabilities and may fall through the cracks as they attempt to navigate this transitional period. It is vital that adult psychiatrists and child and adolescent psychiatrists are educated on how to address these cracks in order to promote the well-being of these patients. This chapter will explore ways to bridge the gap between pediatric and adult care from an educational standpoint at the individual, institutional, and systematic level. (1) It will discuss the essential knowledge for individual trainees to know, as well as (2) institutional interventions for general psychiatry and child and adolescent programs to implement, and (3) ways to improve considerations of transition at a systemic level.

Individual-Level Interventions: What Every Psychiatrist Should Know About Transitional Age Youth

Foundational to treating the TAY group is understanding distinct neurobiological changes of transitional age youth. There is a discrepancy between early, well-formed subcortical systems (amygdala, nucleus accumbens) responsible for emotion, reward, and pleasure and the late-developing cortical systems (prefrontal cortex) that are responsible for inhibition and regulation. This discrepancy contributes to the risk taking and impulsivity for which TAY are so well known [12]. This is a critical period from a neurodevelopmental standpoint, as it is the time that the pruning of prefrontal cortex takes place. As this occurs TAY are more able to implement planning and problem solving. These core brain changes guide necessary treatment interventions, especially the need for consistent environmental structure to support youth as they learn to regulate their emotions, which is important for trainees to understand [14]. Neurobiology relevant to TAY can be taught in didactic lectures, in clinic case conferences, in journal clubs, and on clinical wards [13, 17, 39].

General psychiatry trainees should be educated on disorders that often present in childhood and persist into adulthood. It is important to be able to discern between childhood and adult presentations of specific disorders and how psychopathology might evolve over time. In particular, understanding presentation, prognosis, and treatment of various psychiatric disorders is key. For example, 50% of childhood attention-deficit/hyperactivity disorder (ADHD) cases persist into adulthood, often as inattentive type, with intelligence quotient (IQ) and comorbid psychiatric disorders as predictors of severity [25]. When considering autism spectrum disorders (ASD), an adult provider might anticipate that disorder communication improves over time, while difficulty with social functioning and restricted interests endures. While certainly there are increasing numbers of those with ASD attending college, a significant portion of patients will have poor outcomes related to independent living, academic pursuits, or occupational goals [47]. And finally, eating disorders are well known to have a peak during adolescence, with predominant symptoms of disordered eating. However, in young adults distorted thoughts about weight and body image may continue but with fewer episodes of disordered eating [44]. Many patients may have their first episode of psychosis or mania during this transitional age youth period, and, as such, psychiatrists must provide accurate assessment, diagnosis, and treatment of these disorders while being keenly aware of the biopsychosocial issues that may impact the course. As noted previously, TAY are particularly vulnerable to substance use disorders due to incomplete neurobiological development, changes in peer influences, and decreases in environmental structure. It is necessary for psychiatrists to be able to navigate these changes in order to provide optimal care.

The path to transition to adulthood varies between cultures. Whereas some cultures may value quick movement towards independence, others may continue to hold community and family at its core. For some young adults, moving out of the home and being financially independent in college may be typical, and, for others, continuing to live in the home and staying connected to family until marriage may be more common. As the nation becomes more diverse, youth may face issues of acculturation when their own personal values of community and independence may not look the same as their peers. If trainees are to avoid pathologizing culturally relevant behavior during an individual's development, they should be able to appreciate these cultural factors. Trainees might find the American Psychiatric Association's (APA) Cultural Formulation Interview and the American Academic and Child and Adolescent Psychiatry (AACAP) Practice Parameter for Cultural Competence in Child and Adolescent Psychiatry of particular use [27, 38].

As the number of people attending college, in general, has increased across the nation, so has the number of youth with psychiatric disorders attending college [23, 25]. A well-informed psychiatrist should be aware of educational challenges, such as obtaining a 504 Plan or an Individualized Education Plan (IEP), and how these accommodations are impacted upon the completion of high school. Psychiatrists should be able to help their patients who have learning disabilities gain access to a college's office of disabilities. Being aware of essential legal statutes, including section 504 of the 1973 Rehabilitation Act and the Individuals with Disabilities Education Act (IDEA), allows psychiatrists to better advocate for their patients [10, 33]. Pursuing college directly after high school is not the path for all TAY: some may go on to work towards full-time employment and independent living; others may take a gap year before college, and still others may need ongoing structured support from caregivers. Psychiatrists ought to be aware of all of these pathways and of ways to best support TAY and their families through each of these avenues (Table 4.1).

Table 4.1 Managing varied pathways to transition

Pathways to transition	Considerations for psychiatrist
High school directly to college	Family and personal expectations for college Family/support network communication plan HIPPA/FERPA Navigating social and peer groups Skills for independent living Academic readiness Transfer of high school accommodations Preparedness to navigate adult healthcare systems/health knowledge Transition of care: on campus/off campus or continuing care from a distance
Employment and independent living	Job readiness and career planning Managing household chores Preparedness to navigate adult healthcare systems/health knowledge Issues of confidentiality Transportation Financial supports Emergency plan Insurance changes Retention in psychiatric services
Consideration of a gap year (taking time off after high school and before college)	Interventions to maintain structure Consideration of employment Financial supports Social/peer functioning Academic readiness Opportunities to build resilience Plans for transition to college
Need for ongoing structured support (chronic medical conditions, intellectual disabilities, autism spectrum disorders, etc.)	Discussions of guardianship and/or medical power of attorney Applications for disability Long-term plans for housing Respite care and caregiver support Case management needs Emergency care plan Financial supports

As youth age out of pediatric care, only 38.4% of those with mental illness received mental health care in the last year [45]. The reasons for this underutilization of services are multifactorial. One reason may be that there is a dearth of resources that might appropriately serve patients in this stage of development. Therefore, it is important for psychiatrists to be familiar with community and state resources for these youth in order to best get them connected to care. In particular, having adequate resources for those aging out of foster care, youth with autism, and those with intellectual disabilities is key. To improve treatment continuity and service utilization, it remains prudent for psychiatry residents to know how to transition a patient from pediatric to adult care. This involves being knowledgeable about the timing for when to start conversations about transition, in the appropriate time for transition, and helping patients and families prepare for transition. Child and adolescent psychiatrists must learn methods to teach pediatric patients about their diagnosis, indications for their medications, ways to schedule appointments, and tools for navigating the mental health system. For the providers that are receiving adult patients, they should be aware of how to help a pediatric patient transition to adulthood. This consists of helping patients balance autonomy in medical decision making with maintaining parental support when needed, teaching patients to advocate for themselves, and helping them manage insurance issues. Providers to adult patients need to develop skills for having conversations with parents about guardianship and addressing requests for disability. There are structured tools that psychiatrists can utilize to assess and facilitate transition. Child and adolescent psychiatrists might employ the Transition Readiness Assessment Questionnaire (TRAQ) to help determine areas of strength and weakness during transition [50]. Individuals working with these populations should be aware of the American Academy of Pediatrics (AAP), American Academic of Family Physicians (AAFP)/American College of Physicians (ACP) joint guidelines on transition, discussed further below [8]. Also, the website Got Transition.org has developed a toolkit consisting of "six core elements," describing optimal healthcare transition [20, 29].

Institutional Interventions: Changing How Medical Schools and Residency Programs Approach Transition

The importance of addressing transition at the institutional level has been recognized across the field of medicine. The 2011 joint AAP/AAFP/ACP statement describes a specific algorithm for improving transition to adulthood [8]. Similarly, a 2015 report by the Institute of Medicine (IOM) and the National Research Council of the National Academies details the needs unique to young adults and makes recommendations for systemic-, institutional-, and individual-level interventions [34]. What is noted in each of these reports is in the need for changes in the healthcare workforce. In particular, both primary care physicians and specialists need to have training in transitioning youth to adult care and in clinical exposure to adult manifestations of childhood diseases [8, 34]. Despite these clear guidelines, residency programs struggle to educate and train residents on issues of transfer and transition. In many specialties, the focus is on transfer of care rather than biopsychosocial needs of transition. This is best expressed through a closer look at the Accreditation Council for Graduate Medical Education (ACGME) requirements for residency programs (Table 4.2). All residency and fellowships discuss the need for trainees to be able to transfer care to another provider, though this is not specific to transfer from pediatric to adult care. Despite these requirements, very few (3%) pediatric trainees felt "fully competent" in discussing issues of transfer with patients, and many (25–54%) pediatric trainees reporting having no training or exposure to communicating about transfer with another provider [21, 33, 41]. There is even less training with topics of transition, with the majority of pediatric residents (75%) reporting not having specific exposure in issues of transition to adulthood [33]. This lack of exposure is not related to lack of interest, as most residents

Table 4.2 (ACGME) Program requirements for medical specialties and subspecialties and mention of TAY, transition, or transfer

Program	ACGME mention of TAY or transition
Residency and Fellowship Common Program requirements [1, 2]	**Transitions of care:** "clinical assignments to optimize transitions in patient care, including their safety, frequency, and structure"
Pediatrics [6]	**Program definition:** "Pediatrics encompasses the study and practice of physical and mental health promotion, disease prevention, diagnosis, care, and treatment of infants, children, adolescents and young adults"
Adolescent Medicine [3]	**Resources**: "An adequate number and variety of adolescent medicine patients ranging in age from approximately 10 years through young adulthood" **Patient care**: "provide direct and consultative care to adolescents and young adults" **Medical knowledge:** "transition to adult providers"
Child and Adolescent Psychiatry [4]	No mention of young adulthood or transitional age youth
Psychiatry [7]	**Resources**: "There should be patients of different ages and genders from across the life cycle" **Medical knowledge:** "psychological development throughout the life cycle"
Internal Medicine-Pediatrics [5]	**Program definition** "The combined training allows development of a physician knowledgeable in the full spectrum of human development, from newborns to the age"

(70%) want more curriculum on transition and transfer [30, 32].

Given these educational challenges, combined residency programs often provide improved training for working with TAY. The development of the combined internal medicine-pediatrics program has been an initiative to for physicians to treat patients with chronic illnesses across the life span. While not a combined program, the subspecialty of adolescent medicine seeks to uniquely consider those patients who exist between childhood and adulthood [3]. In 2020 the American Society of Adolescent Psychiatry offered psychiatrists an opportunity to further develop their skills in working with TAY by offering a non-American Board of Psychiatry and Neurology (ABPN) certification in adolescent and young adult psychiatry. Innovative combined programs in pediatrics, psychiatry, and child and adolescent psychiatry (otherwise known as the "Triple Board") were developed as a pathway to those interested in both medical pediatrics and child psychiatry. However, most combined-program graduates spend most of their practice in child and adolescent psychiatry, and there is no adolescent medicine equivalent to connect the divide between pediatric and adult psychiatric care [21].

Clearly more intervention is needed across all fields of medicine to educate trainees on TAY, starting at the medical student level. Medical students can be taught early on in training about transition. For example, these topics can be incorporated into the didactic curriculum when they are learning about development across the life span. Additionally, efforts focused on increasing interest in child and adolescent psychiatry allows further training in issues of development, regardless of the specialty students ultimately choose. While general psychiatry training has become more popular, child and adolescent psychiatry has not reaped these same gains (Fig. 4.1).

Early exposure to child and adolescent psychiatry through didactics, increasing contact with child and adolescent fellows, increasing the number of child and adolescent faculty in medical school leadership, and developing engaging clinical rotations may increase interest in the field. Conversely, lack of exposure to child and psychiatry early in training is a significant factor deterring students from pursuing the specialty [49]. Even with this knowledge, child and adolescent psychiatry is generally underrepresented in medical student curriculum, with only 27% of schools requiring rotations and only 23% of students on average participating in rotations [17]. For those medical schools who do not have access to clinical rotations, providing online modules

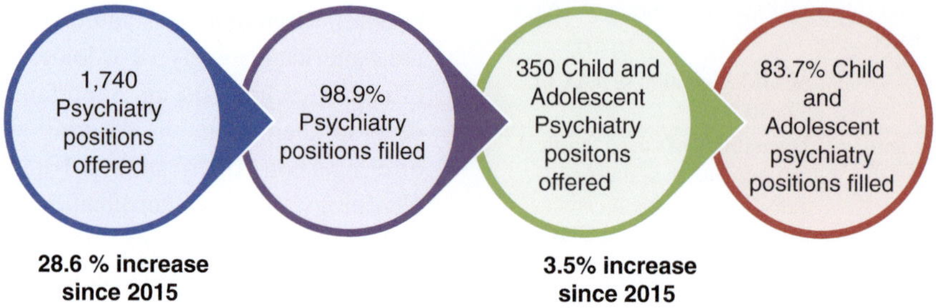

Fig. 4.1 2019 National Resident Match Program (NRMP) data for offered and filled positions in Psychiatry and Child and Adolescent Psychiatry [35, 36]

illustrating common child psychiatric diagnoses can be a useful alternative. Implementing medical student-run clinics that are available to even first-year students can serve as opportunity for early exposure to both pediatric and adult psychiatry. Students participating in student-run free clinics are more comfortable with mental illness and have increased interest in pursuing psychiatry [32].

At the resident level, general psychiatry programs and subspecialty programs have also struggled to adequately integrate transition into didactic and clinical rotations. While ACGME Psychiatry requirements indicate that residents should be knowledgeable about development across the life span, only 2 months of organized clinic experience in child and adolescent psychiatry are required [4]. Disappointingly, child and adolescent psychiatry ACGME requirements have left transitional age youth unaddressed [7] (Table 4.2). Comparable to adolescent medicine, it would be beneficial for pediatric and adult psychiatry ACGME requirements to incorporate education on both young adulthood and transition of care from pediatric to adult care.

Considering that residents report clinical rotations are the ideal method to learn about transition and transitional age youth, residency programs need to be prepared to provide well-developed rotations in this area [30]. Rotations that serve this population may exist on college campuses, inpatient settings, primary care clinics, or psychiatry outpatient clinics. Rotations that focus on transitional age youth can be learning opportunities for both residents and fellows. As such, it is quite necessary to have effective collaboration between general psychiatry and psychiatry subspecialty departments. Program directors may need to collaborate on scheduling, funding, and adequate supervision. While it may be advantageous, supervisors for these rotations do not have to be child and adolescent psychiatry-trained. However, it is essential that they have training and experience in caring for young adults as well as robust background in development, childhood-onset diagnoses, learning disorders, ADHD, and adolescent substance abuse [23]. Supervisors should also be well-versed in navigating systems of care, such as college campuses and foster care.

College student mental health rotations may serve as a training site for child and adolescent psychiatry fellows and for general psychiatry residents. Child and adolescent psychiatrists may transition care to college counseling centers or may opt to continue to see their college-aged patients from a distance. However, they are often unaware of the challenges that their patients face accessing care on campus or how to appropriately manage care from afar. Conversely, general psychiatry-trained providers caring for these patients may not be cognizant of the developmental challenges these students faced prior to their arrival to college. Since college is also a time that many students have first episodes of various psychiatric conditions, institutions of higher education (IHEs) are faced with how to serve and ensure the safety of these students. Unfortunately, college counseling centers and health centers are often understaffed and under resourced to manage the increasing demands. Data from the most recent Association for University and College Counseling Center Directors (AUCCCD) survey indicate that more than half (53.4%) of college counseling centers don't have any psychiatrists, and for those that do, the average full-time equivalent (FTE) is 0.61 [26]. Additionally, 57% report needing an increased number of psychiatrists and nearly half (47%) report needing those psychiatrists to work more hours [26]. It is also the case that smaller IHEs have less access to psychiatrists and fewer community resources [22]. Psychiatry training programs can collaborate with local universities and colleges to help fill this service gap and to provide unique rotation opportunities. These collaborations should not just be relegated to connections to other large, resource-rich institutions. For example, psychiatry trainees can be well utilized at community colleges and minority serving institutions, which are likely to serve underrepresented minorities who may have equivalent psychiatric needs but less access to care [31, 32].

College mental health rotations give residents the opportunity to see comparatively high functioning patients for therapy and medication management, in addition to those in the academic center-partnered community clinics that serve primarily the seriously mentally ill [14, 24]. Trainees able to provide both medication management and psychotherapy services may be of particular use in smaller college clinics in which available therapy services might be sparse. College mental health rotations also allow trainees to provide interventions outside the clinical setting, such as providing psychoeducation in campus outreach programs which promote awareness and reduce stigma [31]. As the conundrum of suicide on college campus continues, resident physicians can both learn about and implement prevention, intervention, and postvention strategies. For example, residents might learn what suicide prevention strategies are evidence-based and then work with a multidisciplinary team to operationalize them on campus.

Residents rotating at college counseling centers can become skilled in providing developmentally appropriate care and learning the psychological challenges that that transitional age youth might face, including exploring their sense of identity, living away from parents, navigating new interpersonal relationships, and learning to manage their own health care. Residents should also be taught how to obtain a detailed developmental history so that they learn to differentiate between variations in normal development and psychopathology. In creating a college mental health rotation, it is vital to provide adequate, onsite when possible, supervision to trainees. College students are seen on average for 3.8 visits at college counseling centers, typically over the course of several months [26]. In turn, trainees should participate in the rotation at least for 6 months and ideally for a year in order to see a student for a full course of treatment. Having upper-level trainees (PGY3 and PGY4 or subspecialty fellows) allows trainees to best employ their knowledge of crisis management, consultation, and inpatient psychiatry. Upper-level trainees may utilize these rotations sites for scholarly research and to implement quality improvement projects that may enhance smaller clinics. While possible, having trainees on rotation early in training would require increased supervision, especially for crisis management. College mental health rotations often get positive feedback from residents [14]. Nevertheless, there may be challenges in developing a collaborative college mental health rotation. For instance, legal implications of ownership of medical records and privacy laws may limit trainee participation. Financial barriers, such as cost of resident or supervisor salary and cost of an electronic medical record, may be particularly challenging for smaller institutions. Other challenges might include travel distance to rural IHEs, call coverage or availability of after-hours services, and appropriate space for trainees to provide clinical services [22]. With proper planning and support, these barriers can be overcome.

While many TAY with psychiatric conditions attend college, this may not be the trajectory to everyone. Some TAY may opt to take a gap year with a subsequent planned transition to college. For others, navigating independent living may be the next milestone. Consequently, trainees should be prepared to help patients and families traverse a variety of routes to adulthood. Residents and fellows would benefit from participating in psychiatry rotations supporting transitional age youth who are not necessarily college students. These rotations include programs that support transition out of foster care, clinics in the juvenile justice system, early psychosis programs, young adult eating disorder programs, and young adult services at community mental health centers. Services for young adults with autism spectrum or intellectual disabilities tend to be limited but in high demand. Subsequently, patients may end up being treated in pediatric clinics long beyond what would be considered usual and appropriate [43, 46]. Rotations in these clinics fill a service gap and also give residents exposure to a unique population [24]. Providing adequate exposure to childhood onset disorders, like intellectual disabilities, allows residents to feel more comfortable in working with these disorders, even when they are treating adult populations [20, 30].

At the core of treating TAY in the community is the ability to work on a multidisciplinary team that may comprise social workers, case managers, psychologists, nutritionists, and other medical providers. This is a skill that can be modeled for trainees in inpatient hospital settings and in outpatient clinics [46]. Working on these teams calls for an approach that not just values managing a patient's symptoms but also incorporates their personal, family, and community strengths. Psychiatry trainees may also find it useful to rotate in an adolescent/young adult medicine clinic in order to gain experience in working with chronically medically ill adolescents. This population may have psychiatric comorbidities that put them at risk for prolonged and suboptimal transition [9]. Resident dyad transition clinics, in which internal medicine, pediatrics, and internal medicine-pediatrics residents work together to address biopsychosocial issues of transition, can serve as an opportunity for psychiatry residents to provide consultation [11].

Formal didactic instruction is at the core of any residency or fellowship program. Yet, many child and adolescent psychiatry programs do not address fundamental topics of transition during didactic lectures [16]. General psychiatry residents need high-quality training in human development, incorporating adequate time to discuss the challenges and changes that occur in late adolescence and young adulthood. Curricula need to also include robust diagnosis-specific teaching on topics such as learning disorders, ADHD, and developmental disabilities, which are often covered only superficially in general psychiatry training. Establishing an integrative didactic experience for both general psychiatry residents and child and adolescent fellows is a good method to learn about issues of transition [42]. Integrative didactics allow for increased collaboration between divisions within departments that may be siloed. General psychiatry residents can get a developmental perspective from their child and adolescent counterparts, while child and adolescent fellows may also get a refresher on some of the challenges of general psychiatry that they may have long forgotten. Curricula on transitional age youth can include a range of topics from transfer of care to the neurobiology of development to college mental health systems of care (Table 4.3). While instructors for this cur-

Table 4.3 Sample topics for a didactics series on transitional age youth

Sample transitional age youth didactic topics
Introduction to college mental health and systems of care
Unique developmental needs of transitional age youth
Neurobiological features of transitional age youth
Optimal transition of youth with mental health conditions from pediatric to adult care
Addressing suicide on college campus: prevention, intervention, postvention
College mental health and the law
Supporting students who struggle w/ transition to adulthood
Unique needs for minority and first-generation students in higher education
Addressing learning disorders and developmental disabilities in transitional age youth
Substance use in transitional age youth and college students
Diagnosing and managing ADHD in young adults

riculum need not only be child and adolescent psychiatrists, they should be adequately trained in topics of development and transition. Creating didactics that are taught throughout the course of residency rather than limited to a specific post-graduate year is preferable and allows for repetition and improved integration with clinical knowledge [30]. Didactic instructors need not be limited to lecture format but should also consider case-based discussion, journal club, online modules, and flipped-classroom teaching.

Clinical experiences in college student mental health and TAY-serving community clinics combined with well-thought-out didactics are valuable. Connecting these elements to build a comprehensive one-year transitional age youth fellowship would provide immense benefit to resident education, community partnerships, and college counseling centers. Trainees in a transitional age youth fellowship would be experts in biopsychosocial transition, college health systems, and young adult development. There are only a few established psychiatry student mental health fellowships across the nation, including those at Stanford, University of Chicago, and the Ohio State University [16]. These fellowships consist of rotations in college student mental health clinics, didactics, and independent scholarly pursuits. A transitional age youth fellowship expands upon already innovative student mental health fellowships to include all TAY, not just those in college. For instance, trainees in a public psychiatry fellowship have been able to integrate both college mental health and TAY clinic into an already established fellowship [40]. Ideally, transitional age youth fellows would rotate in multiple college mental health clinics that vary in size and classification (private versus public, and two-year versus four-year) and that serve diverse populations (predominately white institutions, historically black college/universities, and Hispanic-serving institutions). Fellows might also serve a more active administrative role in clinic development, implementation of campus screening tools for depression, and campus-wide mental health promotion. Fellows may work on leadership skills and gain multidisciplinary team experience by attending behavioral intervention team meetings (also called CARE, student at-risk response teams, or Students of Concern Committee) which operate to identify students of concern on college campus. An ideal TAY fellowship would collaborate with child and adolescent fellowships to create a developmentally focused program. Having adequate training in child and adolescent psychiatry that encompasses both outpatient and inpatient experiences as well as exposure to eating disorders, learning disorders, suicide risk assessment, and substance abuse is important. A well-rounded transitional age youth fellowship would consist of experience in child and adolescent rotations, dedicated training in community TAY clinics, college mental health clinics along with comprehensive integrative didactics (Table 4.3), and pursuit of scholarly work.

Early career psychiatrists (ECPs) who are interested in both child and adolescent psychiatry and general psychiatry may find themselves pressured to choose one path over the other. It is crucial that ECPs stay connected to supportive colleagues and mentors. This could be for career development, emotional support, or clinical consultation. Practically, this means staying connected to other college student mental health psychiatrists, pediatricians, and internists interested in transition, and psychologists at campus counseling centers. Listservs that operate by means of email is a good way to get support and garner ideas on ways to handle administrative issues, clinic practice habits, and systems of care. The field of college student mental health and transitional age youth is ever evolving; ECPs must remain up to date on systems of care, legal implications, and best practices. Attending conferences, which may hold in-depth workshops on how to care for transitional age patients, allows ECPs to earn continuing medical education credits (CME), maintain current medical knowledge, and access professional mentorship [28]. Even as they learn to navigate practicing independently, ECPs can also become leaders in this growing field. One way to do this is by serving as faculty for academic medical centers. As previously noted, in order to maintain well-executed rotations and didactics, experienced TAY faculty are needed. ECPs can help fill this gap. Finally, ECPs are able to be role models or mentors, which has been noted to be a significant factor for medical students choosing to go into child and adolescent psychiatry and general psychiatry [48].

Systemic Interventions: Improving Pathways to Adulthood Through Organized Medicine and Systems of Care

While individual- and institutional-level changes are important, systemic changes need to take place in the field of psychiatry to better bridge the gap between pediatric and adult care. The literature has indicated that child and adolescent psychiatrists are uniquely skilled to provide care for TAY [49]. AACAP's Transitional Age Youth and College Student Mental Health (TAY-CSMH) committee has investigated the unique needs of this vulnerable population [15]. It is notable that significant reasons for advocating for focus on this population are to allow for improved clinical training, interorganizational collaboration, and advocacy [15]. National psychiatric organizations like AACAP, APA, the American Association of Directors of Psychiatric Residency Training (AADPRT), and the Association of Directors of Medical Student Education in Psychiatry (ADMSEP) have been created in order to connect psychiatrists, provide resources, develop best practice guidelines, and propel the field forward through advocacy. While these organizations have been successful in achieving these goals, they often operate independently and without consultation with each other. Having interorganizational collaboration would readily allow pooling of relevant resources and skilled leaders. For example, the Higher Education Mental Health Alliance (HEMHA) is a partnership between a number of relevant organizations, including AACAP, APA, AUCCCD, and the American College Health Association (ACHA), to systemically further mental health initiatives on college campuses. Similarly, in 2010 the ADMSEP Task Force on Child and Adolescent Psychiatry in Medical Education (CAPME) was developed as a collaboration between members of APA, AACAP, AAP, and AADPRT to address much-needed improvements in child and adolescent psychiatry medical student education [18]. This collaboration allowed for development of online learning modules, standardization of learning objectives, and improvement in child and adolescent psychiatry rotations for medical students. Both APA and AACAP have demonstrated interest in TAY through the development of committees focused on this population: the Council on College Mental Health and the aforementioned TAY-CSMH Committee, respectively. Ongoing collaboration between these committees allows for further development of strategies to help this population, increases possibilities for academic publications targeting this population, and connects organizations to trainees. For medical students and residents who travel to annual conferences, committee meetings might be their first in-depth introduction to organized psychiatry. Committees are a way for trainees to hone their advocacy skills, improve collaboration between academic institutions, and provide a chance to learn more about TAY that may not be traditionally taught during training.

Finally, discrepancies in age restrictions between federal, state, and local agencies do a disservice to patients trying to progress to adult care [24, 37]. TAY are often unable to transition out of pediatric care all at once, as they attempt to find a new therapist, psychiatrist, primary care provider, social worker, and work program who may each have different criteria for appropriate transition. Improved interagency communication and consistency would increase service utilization for young adults.

Conclusion

Navigating the divide between pediatric and adult care is a valuable skill that deserves more focus during training. There are distinct developmental challenges that all psychiatrists must be able to manage in order to support ideal transition. For medical students, early exposure to development across the life span and improving resident/fellow clinical and didactic experiences are essential to building a workforce trained to work with transitional age youth. It is also vital for systemic changes to be in place to better allow for interorganizational and interagency collaboration to bridge the gap. Once individual, institutional, and systemic interventions are in place, TAY can better utilize services, effectively get connected to adult providers, and make progress in achieving developmental milestones.

References

1. Accreditation Council for Graduate Medical Education. ACGME Common Program Requirements (Fellowship). https://www.acgme.org/Portals/0/PFAssets/ProgramRequirements/CPRFellowship2019.pdf. Retrieved 25 Nov 2019.
2. Accreditation Council for Graduate Medical Education. ACGME Common Program Requirements (Residency) https://www.acgme.org/Portals/0/PFAssets/ProgramRequirements/CPRResidency2019.pdf. Retrieved 25 Nov 2019.
3. Accreditation Council for Graduate Medical Education. ACGME Program Requirements for Graduate Medical Education in Adolescent Medicine (Subspecialty of Pediatrics). https://www.acgme.org/Portals/0/PFAssets/ProgramRequirements/321_AdolescentMedicine_2019.pdf?ver=2019-08-01-123255-437. Retrieved 25 Nov 2019.
4. Accreditation Council for Graduate Medical Education. ACGME Program Requirements for Graduate Medical Education in Child and Adolescent Psychiatry (Subspecialty of Psychiatry). https://www.acgme.org/Portals/0/PFAssets/ProgramRequirements/405_ChildAdolescentPsychiatry_2019.pdf?ver=2019-06-19-091518-287. Retrieved 25 Nov 2019.
5. Accreditation Council for Graduate Medical Education. ACGME Program Requirements for Graduate Medical Education in Combined Internal Medicine – Pediatrics. https://www.acgme.org/Portals/0/PFAssets/ProgramRequirements/700_InternalMedicinePediatrics_2019.pdf?ver=2019-06-18-144517-517. Retrieved 25 Nov 2019.
6. Accreditation Council for Graduate Medical Education. ACGME Program Requirements for Graduate Medical Education in Pediatrics. https://www.acgme.org/Portals/0/PFAssets/ProgramRequirements/320_Pediatrics_2019.pdf?ver=2019-06-18-155134-967. Retrieved 25 Nov 2019.
7. Accreditation Council for Graduate Medical Education. ACGME Program Requirements for Graduate Medical Education in Psychiatry. https://www.acgme.org/Portals/0/PFAssets/ProgramRequirements/400_Psychiatry_2019_TCC.pdf?ver=2019-03-27-090422-550. Retrieved 25 Nov 2019.
8. American Academy of Pediatrics, American Academy of Family Physicians, and Report Authoring Group. Supporting the health care transition from adolescence to adulthood in the medical home. Pediatrics. 2011;128:181–202.
9. Bloom SR, Kuhlthau K, Van Cleave J, Knapp AA, Newacheck P, Perrin JM. Health care transition for youth with special health care needs. J Adolesc Health. 2012;51(3):213–9.
10. Chan V. Special needs: scholastic disability accommodations from K-12 and transitions to higher education. Curr Psychiatry Rep. 2016;18:21.
11. Chung RJ, Jasien J, Maslow GR. Resident dyads providing transition care to adolescents and young adults with chronic illnesses and neurodevelopmental disabilities. J Grad Med Educ. 2017:222–7.
12. Chung WW, Hudziak JJ. The transitional age brain: "the best of times and the worst of times". Child Adolesc Psychiatr Clin N Am. 2017;26:157–75.
13. Coverdale J, Balonm R, Beresin EV, Louie AK, Glendon RT, Goldsmith M, Roberts LW. Teaching clinical neuroscience to psychiatry residents: model curricula. Acad Psychiatry. 2014;38:111–5.
14. DeMaria PA, Matthew J, Kay J, Schwartz V, Steinhouse R, DiMino J. Psychiatry resident rotations in university and college counseling centers: a pilot study of rotation types and challenges. J Coll Stud Psychother. 2013;27:4, 337–44.
15. Derenne J, Chan V, Martel A, Sondheimer A. The case for expanding AACAP's age of purview from 18 to 26 years of age. Am Acad Child Adolesc Psychiatry News. 2016;47:68–9.
16. Derenne J, Martel A. A model CSMH curriculum for child and adolescent psychiatry training programs. Acad Psychiatry. 2015;39:512–6.
17. Dingle AD. Child psychiatry: what are we teaching medical students? Acad Psychiatry. 2010;34:75–182.
18. Fox GS, Stock S, Briscoe GW, Beck GL, Horton R, Hunt J, et al. Improving child and adolescent psychiatry education for medical students: an inter-organizational collaborative action plan. Acad Psychiatry. 2012;36:461–4.
19. Gleason MM, Fritz G. Innovative training in pediatrics, general psychiatry, and child psychiatry: background, outcomes, and experiences. Acad Psychiatry. 2009;33:99–104.
20. Hart L, Maslow G. The medical transition from pediatric to adult-oriented care: considerations for child and adolescent psychiatrists. Child Adolesc Psychiatr Clin N Am. 2018;27:125–32.
21. Hart L, Van Deusen R, Gonzaga AM. Pediatric residents' attitudes and practice patterns regarding tran-

sition to adult-oriented care. J Community Healthc. 2017;10:149–55.
22. Kay J, Schwartz V, editors. Mental health care in the college community. Hoboken, NJ: Wiley-Blackwell. 2010.
23. Kirsch DJ, Domakonda M, Doerfler LA, Ahn MS. An elective in college mental health for training adult psychiatry residents in young adult psychiatry. Acad Psychiatry. 2015;39:544–8.
24. Lamb C, Murphy M. The divide between child and adult mental health services: points for debate. Br J Psychiatry. 2013;202:S41–4.
25. Leebens PK, Williamson ED. Developmental psychopathology risk and resilience in the transition to young adulthood. Child Adolesc Psychiatr Clin N Am. 2017;26:143–56.
26. LeViness P, Bershad C, Gorman K. (2017).The Association for University and College Counseling Centers Directors Annual Survey Reporting period: July 1, 2016 through June 30, 2017. Association for University and College Counseling Centers. Available at https://www.aucccd.org/assets/documents/Governance/2017%20aucccd%20survey-public-apr26.pdf. Accessed 20 July 2019.
27. Lewis-Fernández R, Aggarwal NK, Hinton L, Hinton DE, Kirmayer LJ, editors. DSM-5® handbook on the cultural formulation interview. Arlington, VA: American Psychiatric Publishing, Inc. 2016.
28. Martel A, Derenne J, Chan V. Teaching a systematic approach for transitioning patients to college: an interactive continuing medical education program. Acad Psychiatry. 2015;39:549–54.
29. McManus M, White P. Transition to adult health care services for young adults with chronic medical illness and psychiatric comorbidity. Child Adolesc Psychiatr Clin N Am. 2017;26:367–80.
30. Menito S. Resident preferences for a curriculum in healthcare transitions for young adults. South Med J. 2012;105:462–6.
31. Moore J, Pollio D, Hong B, Valencia C, Sorrell M, North C. Pilot design and implementation of a mental health and wellness clinic at a Historically Black College/University. Community Ment Health J. 2018;54:371–5.
32. Murzl CA, Durns TA, Mowrey LT, Tubbs AS, Boeve SA. A medical student-run child and adolescent psychiatry clinic: one institution's experience. Acad Psychiatry. 2017;41:582–6.
33. Nazarian BL, Glader L, Choueiri R, Shipman DL, Sadof M. Identifying what pediatric residents are taught about children and youth with special health care needs and the medical home. Pediatrics. 2010:S183–9.
34. National Research Council. Investing in the health and Well-being of young adults. Washington, DC: The National Academies Press; 2015.
35. National Resident Matching Program, Results and Data: 2019 Main Residency Match®. National Resident Matching Program, Washington, DC. 2019. Retrieved from https://mk0nrmp3oyqui6wqfm.kinstacdn.com/wp-content/uploads/2019/04/NRMP-Results-and-Data-2019_04112019_final.pdf. 15 Nov 2019.
36. National Resident Matching Program. Results and data: specialties matching service 2019 appointment year. Washington, DC: National Resident Matching Program; 2019. Retrived from https://mk0nrmp3oyqui6wqfm.kinstacdn.com/wp-content/uploads/2019/02/Results-and-Data-SMS-2019.pdf. 15 Nov 2019.
37. Osgood DW, Foster EM, Courtney ME. Vulnerable populations and the transition to adulthood. Futur Child. 2010;20:209–28.
38. Pumariega AJ, Rothe E, Mian A, Carlisle L, et al. Practice parameter for cultural competence in child and adolescent psychiatry. J Am Acad Child Adolesc Psychiatry. 2013;52:1101–15.
39. Roffman JL, Simon AB, Prasad KM, Truman CJ, Morrison J, Ernst CL. Neuroscience in psychiatry training: how much do residents need to know? Am J Psychiatr. 2006;163:919–26.
40. Romero M, Munir F, Runnels P. Integrating a college mental health track into a public psychiatry fellowship. Acad Psychiatry. 2015;39:555–7.
41. Sadun RE, Chung RC, Polloc MD, Maslow GR. Lost in transition: resident and fellow training and experience caring for young adults with chronic conditions in a large United States' academic medical center. Med Educ Online. 2019;24:1–7.
42. Sexson SB, Thomas CR, Pope K. Models of integrated training in psychiatry and child and adolescent psychiatry. Acad Psychiatry. 2008;32:377–85.
43. Soe K. The wicked problem of transitional care for youth with autism. Am Acad Child Adolesc Psychiatry News. 2019;50:198–9.
44. Slane J, Klump KL, McGue M, Iacono WG. Developmental trajectories of disorder eating from early adolescence to young adulthood: a longitudinal study. Int J Eat Disord. 2014;47:793–801.
45. Substance Abuse and Mental Health Services Administration. Key substance use and mental health indicators in the United States: results from the 2017 National Survey on Drug Use and Health (HHS publication no. SMA 18-5068, NSDUH series H-53). Rockville: Center for Behavioral Health Statistics and Quality, Substance Abuse and Mental Health Services Administration; 2018. Retrieved from https://www.samhsa.gov/data/. 30 Nov 2019
46. Van Deusen TC. Child and adolescent psychiatrists are experts in transitional aged youth, aren't we? J Am Acad Child Adolesc Psychiatry. 2014;53:446–7.
47. Volkmar F, Wolff J. When children with autism become adults. World Psychiatry. 2013;12:79–80.
48. Volpe T, Boydell KM, Pignatiello P. Choosing child and adolescent psychiatry: factors influencing medical students. J Canad Acad Child Adolesc Psychiatry. 2013;22:260–7.
49. Wilens TE, Rosenbaum JF. Transitional aged youth: a new frontier in child and adolescent psychiatry. J Am Acad Child Adolesc Psychiatry. 2013;52:887–90.
50. Wood DL, Sawicki GS, Miller MD, Smotherman C, Lukens-Bull K, Livingood WC, et al. The transition readiness assessment questionnaire (TRAQ): its factor structure, reliability, and validity. Acad Pediatr. 2014;14:415–22.

Part II

Clinical Topics

Unexpected Peaks and Valleys: Navigating the Path to Adulthood with a Mood Disorder

5

Colby Tyson and Adelaide Robb

Key Points

- TAY are a vulnerable population that have the worst access to mental health care across the life span, are at high risk for new-onset psychiatric illness, and are at risk of falling in-between gaps during provider transition.
- TAY are navigating a developmental period marked by milestones that revolve around formation of identity, independence, and formation of relationships, which can all be significantly affected by a mood disorder. These challenges may also make advocating for oneself in treatment more difficult.
- TAY with mood disorders are at high risk for adverse adult outcomes as related to education, employment, health, and social functioning.
- While recovery rates of MDD in TAY are high, so are recurrence rates into the second and third decades of life. Compared to adult-onset MDD, TAY have longer episode duration and increased rate of bipolar switching.
- Risk factors for bipolar switching in TAY diagnosed with MDD include family history of depression or bipolar disorder, mania or hypomania precipitated by medications, and history of psychotic depression.
- Bipolar spectrum illness in TAY can initially present with depressive episodes that are not identified as part of the bipolar course until a later manic or hypomanic episode.
- A TAY presenting with new-onset psychosis should be screened carefully for underlying mood disorders with psychotic features to avoid inappropriate management.
- Chronic irritability alone is not a diagnostic indicator for bipolar disorder (BP). The clinician should assess the pattern of irritability, associated mood disorder criteria, and identifiable triggers to irritability prior to giving a diagnosis of bipolar disorder.
- Childhood-onset bipolar disorder is associated with a more severe course of illness compared to adult-onset bipolar disorder, including more polarity switches, longer periods of subthreshold symptoms, more depressive and mixed symptoms, and increased suicidal behaviors.

C. Tyson (✉) · A. Robb
Psychiatry and Behavioral Sciences, Children's National Hospital, Washington, DC, USA
e-mail: ctyson@childrensnational.org; arobb@childrensnational.org

V. Chan, J. Derenne (eds.), *Transition-Age Youth Mental Health Care*,
https://doi.org/10.1007/978-3-030-62113-1_5

- Bipolar disorder not otherwise specified (NOS) carries high rates of conversion to BP I and BP II, and subthreshold symptoms are associated with increased morbidity when compared to controls.
- Medication management of MDD in youth has focused on the use of selective serotonin reuptake inhibitors (SSRIs), serotonin-norepinephrine reuptake inhibitors (SNRIs), and tricyclic antidepressants (TCAs). TCAs are not commonly used due to side-effect profile, lethal risk in overdose, as well as lack of efficacy in placebo-controlled trials in youth.
- Second-generation antipsychotics effectively treat TAY with bipolar spectrum disorders; however, youth may be more sensitive to metabolic side effects.
- Anti-epileptic mood stabilizers in TAY are less efficacious in youth than in adults. However, lithium has been proven effective in the treatment of bipolar disorder in TAY.
- Treatment of comorbid attention-deficit/hyperactivity disorder (ADHD) with stimulants is safe and efficacious but should be done in the context of a mood stabilizer.
- Successful transition into adulthood for TAY with mood disorders includes interventions that span family, educational, occupational, and health care systems.
- Special considerations should be taken when working with TAY in foster care, those who are ethnic and racial minorities, and those who identify as part of the lesbian, gay, bisexual, transgender, and queer (LGBTQ) community.

Case History

Savannah is a 17-year-old girl with bipolar I disorder, generalized anxiety disorder (GAD), and alcohol use disorder in remission. She is currently in 12th grade at a local public high school with a 504 plan that gives her accommodations related to her anxiety and mood difficulties. Savannah lives with her two siblings and mother during the school year and spends the summer with her father, who lives in another state. Her family history is significant for her maternal grandmother having what mother describes as "manic depressive disorder," requiring hospitalizations and with a history of suicide attempts. Savannah's father has a history of alcohol use disorder, in sustained remission.

Developmentally, Savannah met all milestones appropriately; however, her mother describes her as having been a "difficult" baby who had trouble self-soothing and had sleep difficulties. She was described as "slow to warm up" to peers but otherwise could engage socially once familiar with people and her surroundings. As Savannah entered elementary school, she began refusing to go to school, had several somatic complaints with frequent visits to the nursing office, and was often noted by teachers to be distracted in class. Neuropsychological testing confirmed severe anxiety and ruled out a comorbid learning disorder. At that time, she was diagnosed with generalized anxiety disorder, started cognitive behavioral therapy (CBT), and was trialed on various serotonin selective reuptake inhibitors (SSRIs). Medication management was limited by side effects, primarily activation. Ultimately, her engagement in CBT was effective in reducing her anxiety, and she was able to remain in class and somatic complaints decreased.

In eighth grade, Savannah gradually pulled away from her friend group. Her grades fell, she quit the track team, and she was noted to have an increase in irritability. She also described a lack of energy, decreased appetite, trouble sleeping, passive suicidal thoughts, and had outbursts that led to destruction of property at home. She was reevaluated by a child and adolescent psychiatrist (CAP) given concerns for depression. On evaluation, in addition to depressive symptoms, her parents and Savannah described brief periods (4–5 days) of time that she had trouble sleeping and would stay up all night doing school work, reorganizing her room, and cleaning. Savannah would seem fine the next day without fatigue and continued to attend school. They also noted a slight increase in the rate of her speech, and Savannah described her thoughts as "racing." Savannah described stealing random small items and sneaking alcohol from her parents' cabinets. She started smoking marijuana as she reported that it helped her feel calmer and get to sleep. It was at this time that her CAP identified these episodes as hypomania and diagnosed her with bipolar II disorder. She was started on aripiprazole to target her mood and restarted weekly therapy.

Savannah appeared to be doing well. She rejoined her extracurricular activities, her mood stabilized, and her school functioning improved. However, in the beginning of 11th grade, Savannah started going to more parties and was breaking curfew. Her grades declined, she was sleeping more, and her parents found empty bottles of alcohol under her bed. Savannah eventually reported to her CAP that she had started drinking for social purposes to fit in with her friends. She noticed that drinking alcohol was helpful with her anxiety and had begun drinking heavily, sometimes at home alone and before bedtime to help her sleep at night. She had been worried about alcohol interfering with her medication, so she was intermittently taking her aripiprazole. Savannah was also concerned about her rapid decline and agreed to substance treatment. She stopped using alcohol and marijuana as part of her program and reported improvement in her mood with motivation to continue with her sobriety. However, her parents soon noted that she was speaking quickly, pacing around her room at night talking out loud to herself, and appeared energetic despite little sleep in the past week. Savannah's mood became more labile; she started making paranoid comments and referring to herself in third person. She was found to be manic with psychotic features and was hospitalized, where she was diagnosed with bipolar I disorder. Her aripiprazole was switched to risperidone, and she was started on lithium with resulting rapid stabilization in her mood and resolution of her psychosis.

Following her hospitalization, Savannah was transitioned into a partial hospitalization program for ongoing adjustments of her medications and assistance with transitioning back to school. Her 504 plan was modified to include accommodations to assist with managing side effects from her medications. Accommodations included access to water throughout the day; extended time for tests and assignments, given her slowed cognition; and counseling support in school. The summer after 11th grade, she did not go to visit her father and, instead, remained near home to continue her treatment. She took on a part-time job at a hair salon shampooing hair and assisting with tasks around the salon.

Savannah engaged with a tutor over the summer and has not had an episode of mania, hypomania, or depression in 8 months and is now starting 12th grade. Savannah has also started playing more of an active role in her treatment (i.e., *scheduling her own appointments and managing her medications). While she is not refusing parental involvement, she is hesitant about including her parents in her care at this time, as she feels she wants to be independent and learn to manage on her own.*

In her therapy sessions, Savannah is reflecting on her goals and expresses concern about college and what having bipolar disorder would mean for her going away to her dream school. She asks her clinician, "Does this seem like a realistic option for me?"

Savannah is entering a critical time in development as she transitions into adulthood, and she shows good insight to question her level of readiness. Given all that has taken place in her life related to her mental health needs, answering her question is not straightforward. It is important for the clinician to have proper understanding of her diagnosis and risks, assess how the diagnosis may interfere with this developmental stage, and know what planning and treatment options need to be considered before we can answer her question of whether she can head away to her dream school in the next few months.

Background on Mood Disorders in TAY

While there is some variability in what is defined as transitional age youth (TAY), typically we are referring to older adolescents (15–16 years old) spanning to young adulthood (24–26 years old) [55, 92]. This age group encounters many challenges and is highly vulnerable for several reasons:

1. Young people between 12 and 25 years old have the worst levels of access to mental health across a whole life span [57].
2. This is a high-risk time for new onset of psychiatric illness. Per the National Comorbidity Replication Study, 50–75% of anxiety, disorders, mood disorders, impulse control disorders, and substance use disorders emerge between the ages of 14 and 24 years [43, 55].
3. Those TAY who are receiving mental health care services risk falling into the gap of aging out from pediatric specialists but having limited access to clinicians comfortable with this age group.
4. This developmental period is marked by milestones that revolve around formation of identity, independence, and formation of relationships, which can all be significantly affected by the stability of one's mental health.

Overall, there is a strong movement to assess the needs and the use of developmentally informed interventions for TAY related to their mental health care needs. There has been significant work focusing on early interventions for first-episode psychosis (which tends to present in TAY) and looking at the use of comprehensive, multidisciplinary, and team-based treatment approaches [64]. Studies so far have shown the benefit of such an approach to improve prognosis in first-episode psychosis. Similar models and practice guidelines would likely benefit TAY also dealing with other mental health illnesses, such as mood disorders [57], and we will give suggestions on this later in this chapter.

Adult Outcomes

Mental health has a tremendous effect on adult outcomes. The Great Smoky Mountains Study is a longitudinal epidemiological study of children of ages 9–13 years in 11 rural counties in North Carolina that looked at psychiatric diagnoses, correlates, and risk factors. Annual assessments were completed until age 16 and then again at 19, 21, and 25 years of age. These assessments were looking for adverse outcomes related to health, the legal system, personal finances (high school dropout, inability to keep a job, and residential instability), and social functioning. Common childhood disorders assessed included anxiety disorders, mood disorders, conduct, oppositional defiant disorder (ODD), attention-deficit/hyperactivity disorder (ADHD), and substance use disorders. Compared to those with no history of psychiatric problems, participants with a childhood disorder had six times higher odds (OR, 5.9 (95% CI, 3.6–9.7)) of at least one adverse adult outcome and nine times higher odds (OR, 8.7 (95% CI, 4.3–17.8)) of having two or more adverse adult outcomes [23]. Findings also demonstrated that even if the symptoms were subthreshold or did not persist into adulthood, these disorders were still associated with adverse adult outcomes.

Specifically when it comes to mood disorders, data indicate that a mood disorder in childhood increases risk for a mood disorder in both adolescence and adulthood [92]. Regarding bipolar disorder, compared to adult onset, early- and TAY-onset cases have data that suggest that they are more complicated when these youth become adults, with a higher risk for other neuropsychiatric disorders, comorbidity, and mixed presentations [92]. These factors would undoubtedly have a negative effect on adult outcomes.

One group looked at a subset of 367 youth with bipolar disorder from the Course and Outcome of Bipolar Illness in Youth (COBY) study and divided them into groups of mood trajectories: predominantly euthymic, moderately euthymic, ill with improving course, and predominantly ill. School, employment, and disability status were assessed over a median of 11.5 years of follow-up and demonstrated the following findings [41]:

- Predominantly euthymic youth were more likely to be in school or employed.
- Persistently ill youth were more likely to be on disability.
- About 44% of predominantly euthymic and 93% of ill with improving course youth continued to experience psychosocial impairment, indicating that despite resolution or improvement in symptoms, impairment can persist.
- Predictors of poor psychosocial functioning included early onset, low socioeconomic status (SES) and current comorbidity.
- Low SES and current comorbidity predicted not being enrolled in school and unemployment.

Having a mood disorder also influences academic achievement. Analysis of the 2001–2002 National Epidemiologic Survey on Alcohol and Related Conditions (NESARC) data led to several findings related to college achievement and completion. A subset included 2188 college students and 2904 not attending college in a group of 19–25-year-olds and compared rates of psychiatric conditions. There was no difference found in overall rates of psychiatric illness between those attending college and those not attending, and almost half reported a psychiatric disorder in the past year. In addition, bipolar disorder was less common among individuals in college [13]. Also, using the NESARC data set, researchers looked at a subset of 15,800 adults aged 22 years and older who at least entered college and evaluated associations between specific psychiatric disorders and postsecondary educational achievement. Findings showed that five disorders were associated with failure to graduate college: bipolar I disorder, marijuana use disorder, amphetamine use disorder, cocaine use disorder, and antisocial personality disorder [42]. The National Comorbidity Survey in 1990–1992 and the follow-up in 2001–2003 examined a total of 5001 people aged 15–54 years in a two-wave panel survey and noted that those with bipolar disorder at the initial wave were less likely to graduate from high school. In addition, students were less likely to graduate from college if they developed bipolar disorder after the initial survey [62].

Adolescent depression is associated with impairment in future social functioning, employment, academic achievement, and verbal intellectual performance [31, 44, 45]. The National Population Health Survey (NPHS) followed a subset of 1027 adolescents (aged 16–17 years initially) with MDD every 2 years over a 10 -year course and assessed adult outcomes. Negative outcomes identified included depression recurrence, higher severity of symptoms, migraine headaches, poor self-rated health, low levels of social support, and heavy drinking [67]. It also appears that functional outcomes are worse for very early-onset depression compared to later-onset depression. A subgroup of 4041 participants from the Sequenced Treatment Alternatives to Relieve Depression (STAR*D) study were grouped based on age at onset. Early age at onset was associated with never being married, more impaired social and occupational functioning, poorer quality of life, greater medical and psychiatric comorbidity, more lifetime depressive episodes and suicide attempts, and greater symptom severity and suicidal ideation in the index episode [45, 96]. Some data suggest that this effect on psychosocial functioning in adulthood is primarily due to a frequent recurrent course as opposed to early onset [94]. Regardless, data highlight the need to consider age at the onset and recurrence of depressive episodes when assessing the risk for impaired psychosocial functioning in adulthood.

As we think about Savannah, she is at significant risk related to her educational achievement and future adult functioning. Even if she were to go to college, her diagnosis of bipolar I disorder puts her at higher risk of not graduating. Her risks do not indicate telling her not to pursue her dream but, instead, signifies to the clinician the need for proper planning, guidance, and treatment to ensure her successful transition into adulthood and the need for continued treatment as an adult.

Diagnosing Depression in TAY

Epidemiology

The 12-month prevalence of depression is approximately 2% in childhood and increases to a cumulative prevalence of approximately 20% by age 18 years [7, 8, 25, 32, 83]. Data from the National Survey on Drug Use and Health (NSDUH) for 2005–2014 showed an increase in prevalence rates. In adolescents (aged 12–17 years), the 12-month prevalence of major depressive episodes increased from 8.7% to 11.3%. For young adults (aged 18–25 years), prevalence increased from 8.8% to 9.6% [63]. Females appear to have higher rates of MDD compared to males [3, 63]. Increase in depression throughout this age group is thought to be associated with postpubertal changes that include an alteration in hormone levels, increased capacity for self-awareness and social understanding, increased stress due to developmental transitions, increased cognitive maturity allowing for rumination, and changes in parent and peer dynamics [32, 83]. The rates above do not incorporate children and adolescents with subthreshold symptoms who are also at risk for progression to full diagnosis and associated morbidity. It is thought that approximately 5–10% of children and adolescents fit into this category [7, 8].

Criteria

Major depressive disorder is characterized by the presence of five or more specific criteria (Box 5.1) for at least two consecutive weeks with at least one of the symptoms being (1) depressed mood or (2) loss of pleasure or interest. Symptoms should be a change from baseline with impairment in functioning. Specific specifiers exist to distinguish various subtypes. Specifiers include the following: with anxious distress, mixed features, melancholic features, atypical features, mood congruent psychotic features, mood incongruent psychotic features, catatonia, peripartum onset, and seasonal pattern [27]. The specifiers *with psychotic features* and *with mixed features* are thought to confer increased risk for bipolar disorder [7].

Box 6.1 Diagnostic Symptoms for Major Depressive Disorder

1. Depressed mood (can be irritable mood in children and adolescents)
2. Anhedonia
3. Decrease or increase in appetite
4. Insomnia or hypersomnia
5. Psychomotor agitation or retardation
6. Decrease in energy
7. Increase in guilt or feelings of worthlessness
8. Poor concentration
9. Suicidal ideation or behavior

Considerations Specific to TAY

While much of the overall diagnostic criteria for MDD are similar between TAY and adults, there are important factors to consider and recognize when working with TAY. An observational study spanning two decades looked at youth initially aged 8–13 years with MDD. Assessments measured recovery and recurrence rates of a depressive episode and looked at possible psychosocial and clinical predictors of outcomes. Recovery rates ranged from 96% to 100% across MDD episodes, while length of episodes ranged from 6 to 7 months. Up to 72% of those who recovered from a first episode of MDD had a further episode with a median interepisode interval of 3–5 years [45]. There was no single variable that consistently predicted recurrence or recovery. Overall, the study showed that early-onset MDD has risks of depression into second and third decades of life, which cover the developmental time span of TAY. In a separate study looking at cortisol levels and levels of social support as predictive and protective factors in youth aged 13–18 years, it was noted that higher cortisol levels were associated with longer time to recovery, while a higher level of social support was protective [72].

When comparing the abovementioned longitudinal study in youth to the National Institute of Mental Health (NIMH) Collaborative Depression Study conducted in adults, clear similarities and

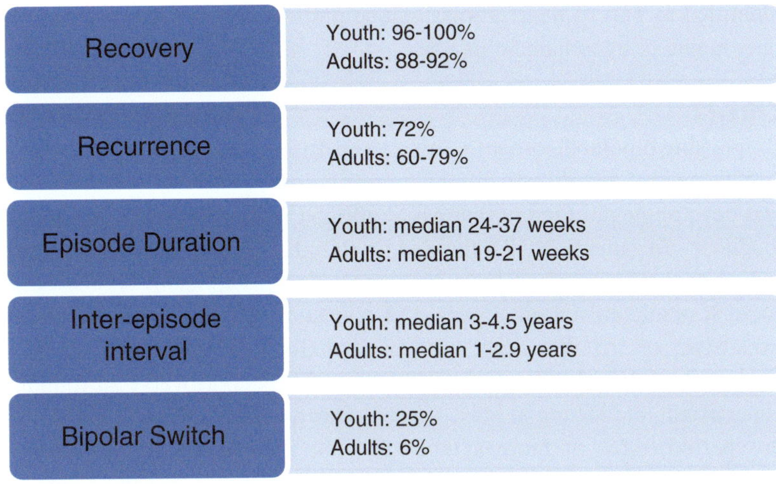

Fig. 5.1 Comparison of NIMH Depression Collaborative Study in adults and longitudinal observational study from childhood to young adulthood

differences between adult-onset and child-onset depression course were observed (Fig. 5.1) [45, 78, 79].

It is important to be aware of the risk of bipolar switching as approximately 20–40% of youth initially diagnosed with MDD go on to be diagnosed with bipolar disorder [7, 9]. At the same time, not every youth with depression will later be diagnosed with bipolar disorder. Factors that should be assessed that point to a higher risk include psychotic symptoms, mania or hypomania precipitated by medication, and family history of depression or bipolar disorder [7, 9]. In the Collaborative Depression Study of adults, predictors of conversion from MDD to bipolar disorder included family history, number of manic symptoms at baseline, psychosis, and age of onset [4].

Overall, change in polarity appears to be more frequent in early-onset depression when compared to adult onset, which we see highlighted in Savannah's case. Her initial symptoms led to a diagnosis of MDD with later episodes of hypomania and mania, changing her diagnosis to bipolar I disorder.

Diagnosing Bipolar Spectrum Illness in TAY

Epidemiology

Savannah's course of illness highlights the need to conceptualize bipolar disorder on a spectrum, especially when discussing TAY. Bipolar spectrum disorders include bipolar I disorder (BP I), bipolar II disorder (BP II), cyclothymic disorder (CyD), bipolar disorder not otherwise specified (BP NOS), and other specified bipolar and related disorders (OS-BRD) and can all present in the child and adolescent population [37]. Rates of lifetime mania in teens vary from 0.1% to 1.7%, and rates of bipolar spectrum disorders are as high as 6.7% [19, 58, 82]. In one cross-sectional survey, comparison of those aged 13–14 years with the TAY aged 17–18 years demonstrated a nearly twofold increase in rates of mania in the older group [58]. Specifically related to TAY, a population-based survey assessed the lifetime prevalence of bipolar disorder in subjects aged 15–24 years. Weighted lifetime prevalence was 2.1% in individuals aged 15–18 and 3.8% in those aged 19–24 years [47]. Metaanalysis of epidemiological studies show that pediatric bipolar disorder is overall more common than autism or schizophrenia and less common than depression and ADHD [37]. Similarly to pediatric depression, bipolar spectrum disorders appear to have higher rates post-puberty compared to prepuberty. This may be confounded by a few factors: (1) there is lack of data looking at prepubertal patients; (2) in early-onset bipolar disorder, retrospectively there may have been minimization of initial hypomanic symptoms; and (3) the child may have presented with depressive episodes initially that were not identified as part of their bipolar course until a later manic or hypomanic episode.

Criteria

Diagnosing bipolar disorder in TAY can be difficult because of variation in clinical presentation and developmental factors that can confound a diagnosis. In general, BP I is defined by an individual presenting with at least one manic episode. A manic episode is a period of elevated, expansive, or irritable mood and abnormally increased goal-directed activity or energy that is persistent and lasting at least 1 week. During this period, three or more symptoms (four if mood is irritable) from Box 5.2 are present. Some individuals may have had depressive or hypomanic episodes; however, this is not required for a diagnosis of BP I. BP II is defined by episode(s) of hypomania (similar criteria to mania symptoms in Box 5.2 but with shorter duration of at least 4 days and less impairment) in addition to current or past episodes of major depression. Cyclothymic disorder is defined by multiple periods of hypomanic and depressive symptoms lasting for at least 2 years in adults and 1 year in children and adolescents. These symptoms do not meet the criteria for a hypomanic episode or a depressive episode. BP NOS and OS-BRD are diagnosed when an individual experiences alternating manic, hypomanic, and depressive symptoms but the symptoms do not meet the criteria for BP I or BP II [27]. Overall, each diagnosis is based on specific changes in mood and behavior that are atypical and exceed normal expected development, persist for a specific duration, and have varying impact on functioning based on where one falls on the spectrum [37].

Box 6.2 Symptoms of Mania and Hypomania

1. Increased self-esteem or grandiosity
2. Decreased need for sleep
3. Increased rate in speech or pressured speech
4. Flight of ideas or racing thoughts
5. Distractibility
6. Increased goal-directed activity
7. Excessive risk-taking behaviors or impulsive behaviors

Considerations Specific to TAY

Clinicians should be aware of special considerations related to the diagnosis and illness course of bipolar spectrum disorders. There is a historical controversy surrounding whether chronic severe irritability in the pediatric population is part of the bipolar spectrum. As of 2017, there has been an increasing agreement that chronic irritability is not sufficient enough to diagnose pediatric bipolar disorder [18, 37]. Severe irritability in youth can be seen with several psychiatric disorders. For example, an anxious child may have repeated outbursts and aggression when exposed to anxiety-provoking stimuli. This behavior can be inadvertently reinforced by accommodating factors in the environment and can lead to the perception of chronic irritability. Longitudinal data demonstrate that nonepisodic irritability in youth is more likely to be associated with generalized anxiety disorder and unipolar depression in adulthood and does not predict bipolar disorder [50, 81]. If the irritability has an episodic quality and is associated with other symptoms of bipolar disorder without an identifiable trigger, then this may indicate that the chronic irritability is part of the symptom profile of a TAY with bipolar spectrum illness [37].

Identification of comorbid illness is extremely important as it is associated with a worse course and clinical outcome in pediatric bipolar disorder. This can be difficult to do as symptoms of a bipolar spectrum illness may overlap with other diagnoses. One suggestion to help delineate comorbid illness is to assess what symptoms persist in the setting of euthymia [37]. *For example, with Savannah, once her mood was stable, her generalized anxiety persisted. Her anxiety contributed to her deciding to stay up all night studying, her urge to use alcohol and drugs, and her avoidance of situations that lead to isolation. This places her at risk for exacerbating her mood symptoms.*

In Savannah's case, while bipolar I disorder is her primary diagnosis, identifying and treating her GAD and alcohol use disorder have been just as important. Savannah's comorbid alcohol use disorder is consistent with data associating adolescent-onset bipolar disorder with high risk for substance use disorder [93]. Data from a subset of 5673 participants aged 15–24 years from the Canadian Community Health Survey (CCHS) demonstrated high rates of comorbidity with anxiety disorders, substance use, and suicidality [47]. TAY with mood disorders can also present with psychosis and are at risk of being misdiagnosed with a primary psychotic disorder. This misdiagnosis can lead to inappropriate medication management, protracted illness course, and stigmatization throughout medical treatment.

When reviewing the clinical course of bipolar spectrum illness in youth, there are specific risks associated with this population. Multiple studies of these youth have shown [11, 37]:

- High recurrence rates of depression, hypomania, or mania.
- Patterns of comorbidity similar to those seen in adult bipolar disorder.
- Childhood onset is associated with a more severe course of illness compared to adult-onset bipolar disorder, including more polarity switches, longer period of subthreshold symptoms, more depressive and mixed symptoms, and increased suicidal behaviors [6, 69–71].

The major COBY study, in which 413 youth aged 7–17 years with bipolar I, bipolar II, and bipolar NOS were assessed longitudinally over an initial 4-year period, had the following pertinent findings [11]:

- The polarity of the index episode predicted the polarity of subsequent episodes.
- Twenty-five percent of youth with BP II converted to BP I.
- Thirty-eight percent of BP NOS converted to BP I or BP II.
- Poorer outcomes were associated with early-onset, comorbid disorders; diagnosis of BP NOS; long duration of illness; low socioeconomic status; and family history of mood disorders.
- Youth with BP I and BP NOS spent more follow-up time with subsyndromal compared to syndromal symptoms.
- While experiencing syndromal symptoms, all groups spent more time in depression and with mixed/cycling symptoms compared to mania or hypomania.
- After 2.5 years, 81.5% of participants had full recovery after the onset of the initial episode:
  - BP I rates of recovery were greater than those of BP NOS.
  - BP I and BP II had a shorter time of recovery compared to BP NOS.
  - One and a half years following recovery, 62.5% had syndromal recurrence.

While significant attention has focused on BP I and BP II, there is also an increased focus on pediatric subthreshold bipolar disorder (BP NOS, OS-BRD). The prevalence of subthreshold bipolar disorder in adolescents ranges from 1.2% to 13.3%. As seen in the COBY study, youth with subthreshold bipolar disorder are at risk for progression to bipolar I and bipolar II. A 10-year prospective longitudinal and family study that assessed 2210 youth aged 14–24 years indicated that those with a history of MDD and subthreshold bipolar disorder at baseline converted more often to BP I when compared to their counterparts with a history of MDD only (7.2% vs. 1.7%, respectively) [4, 95]. It is unclear exactly what factors contribute to the conversion from subthreshold bipolar disorder to BP I or II. However, one study looked at 140 children and adolescents meeting the COBY criteria for BP NOS and assessed them longitudinally with a mean duration of follow-up being 5 years. Conversion to BP I or BP II occurred in 63 subjects (45%), with the strongest predictor being a first- or second-degree family history of mania or hypomania [4]. There is also evidence looking at psychiatric diagnoses of parents and association with subthreshold bipolar symptoms that indicate that children of parents with bipolar disorder have 13 times higher odds of meeting the criteria for BP NOS. In addition, parents with bipolar disorder were more likely to have offspring diagnosed with BP NOS (7.2%) compared to receiving a diagnosis of BP I (2.1%) or BP II (1.3%) [4, 11].

Not only is there raising awareness of pediatric patients with subthreshold bipolar disorder, there are also data supporting increased morbidity compared with youth without a bipolar spectrum illness. A recent meta-analysis looked at morbidity for this population as it relates to functional impairment, severity of mood disorders, psychiatric comorbidities, suicidal ideation and behaviors, and mental health treatment between two paired groups: subthreshold pediatric bipolar disorder vs. controls and subthreshold pediatric bipolar disorder vs. pediatric BP I. The meta-analysis indicated the following [86]:

1. Youth with BP I disorder were more impaired than those with a subthreshold diagnosis, were more likely to have suicidal ideation or attempts, and were more likely to utilize mental health services.
2. Youth with subthreshold bipolar disorder and BP I disorder did not demonstrate differences related to degree of depressive symptoms or rates of comorbid disruptive behavior, mood, anxiety, and substance use disorders.
3. Compared to controls, subthreshold bipolar disorder patients did have greater functional impairment, greater severity of mood symptomatology, higher rates of suicidality, and higher rates of psychiatric comorbidities, such as disruptive behavior and substance use.

These data support the idea of viewing bipolar disorder as a spectrum of illness. TAY who present with subthreshold symptoms and may not initially meet the criteria for BP I or BP II are at significant risk for conversion and impairment as they transition into adulthood. *Savannah initially presented with anxiety and depressive episodes with prominent irritability. She then experienced hypomanic episodes with mixed features, culminating in her first manic episode at age 17 years in which she converted from bipolar II to bipolar I disorder. Her course of illness falls in line with what we know about bipolar spectrum illness in pediatrics, especially TAY. Savannah has a family history of bipolar disorder, has comorbid illness, and experienced early onset of symptoms. These factors put her at a higher risk of impaired adult functioning, ongoing depressive and mixed symptoms, and relapse of substance use as she navigates her transitional years. Savannah is also demonstrating good insight and is expressing motivation to take on managing her mood disorder. With proper planning and treatment, these risks can be mitigated.*

Transition Planning

What Is a Successful Transition?

Savannah is questioning her ability to meet her previously established goals in the context of intermittent exacerbations of her mood disorder. It is important for her clinician to help her establish what a successful transition would look like for her and then start the collaborative planning process to guide her along the way.

There is no exact template for a successful transition into adulthood. The clinician and patient need to consider cultural aspects, personal interests, core values, and the social determinants of health and how they connect to goal setting. However, there are core concepts to a successful transition that can serve as guidance when evaluating if someone is proceeding in the right direction.

The transition from adolescence into adulthood consists of meeting milestones related to formation of identity, obtaining self-sufficiency, separation-individuation, and establishing intimacy [30, 55]. To meet these milestones, a youth needs to be successful at several tasks. Tasks include taking care of their mental and physical health, avoiding risky behaviors with negative life-altering consequences, educational attainment, employment, avoiding or ceasing illegal behaviors, developing and maintaining a social support network [23, 55], and accepting responsibility for decision-making. In addition, this is a time of continued neuronal pruning which affects executive functioning, decision-making, and emotional maturity [21].

These tasks as a TAY can be overwhelming and challenging to successfully obtain without guidance and support. Any chronic illness such as a mood disorder that has presented throughout childhood and adolescence can cause deviation in normal development. With each exacerbation of mood symptoms requiring stabilization, a developmental pause button is pushed. The presence of ongoing subthreshold symptoms can then lead to detour signs along the path of development. By the time a teen with a chronic illness reaches the transitional age period, they are likely no longer on a normal developmental trajectory yet expected by society to traverse the transition into adulthood as if they were. Unfortunately, this leaves them at higher risk of a disrupted transition.

For example, a TAY with MDD who is isolating, no longer motivated, and has anhedonia will have a limited social network, a lack of identifiable interests, and trouble with future-oriented thinking. This youth will have trouble with planning for adulthood and identity formation and may have a limited skill set when applying for college or employment. A TAY with bipolar disorder who is experiencing mood lability and is engaging in risk-taking behaviors will have difficulty with relationships, will have lack of consolidation of a sense of self, and may have made impulsive decisions that lead to long-term health and financial burden.

Overall, mood disorders in TAY can lead to increasing reliance on caregiver or social supports secondary to the effect on development. *We see this in Savannah's case. She does not have much in her academic portfolio to apply to college as she spent a large portion of her high school years stabilizing her mental health. She now needs more support than her peers in determining what the next appropriate step is for her after high school.*

Risk Factors for Impaired Transitions

Savannah's case demonstrates several risk factors for an impaired transition into adulthood. Up until recently, her mother managed her mental health needs, kept track of her symptoms, and administered her medications, leaving Savannah to play a minimal role in her own health care. Savannah also presents with several psychiatric comorbidities with a history of intermittent sobriety. While she is motivated for treatment, she is ambivalent regarding her mother remaining involved in her treatment planning during her transition. Lastly, she has several accommodations through her 504 plan that will not automatically transfer to college or to a place of potential employment.

Risk factors for impaired transitions are as follows [74]:

- Limited previous opportunities to practice independent life skills
- School accommodations that cannot easily be translated to employment or college setting
- Lacking ability to self-advocate
- Psychiatric comorbidities
- Lack of understanding of diagnosis and treatment
- Poor organizational skills
- Lack of transitional support systems
- Ambivalence regarding ongoing treatment
- Reluctance to engage in lifestyle modifications to support maintaining mood stabilization
- Recent clinical destabilization

Identification of risk factors for impaired transition allows for planning and incorporation of targeted interventions to mitigate these risks.

Predictors of Successful Transition

It is equally important to identify predictors of a successful transition in order to use these factors to propel a TAY forward.

Predictors of a successful transition include the following [74]:

- Insight into the need for scaffolding and support during transition
- Understanding of diagnosis and treatment planning

- Extended period of mood stability
- Help seeking and self-advocates
- Engagement in healthy lifestyle choices (sleep, nutrition, exercise, etc.)
- History of ability to be away from home
- Previous positive work experience
- Engagement in and compliance with mental health treatment

Savannah demonstrates insight into her need for treatment and is now taking an active role in her care. She is scheduling and attending her appointments and is seeking support from her providers. During periods of stability, Savannah has a history of attending overnight camp successfully and working at a beauty salon. These data points demonstrate that with proper support and management of her mood, Savannah has the ability to function with some level of independence. While this does not mean that she is ready to transition to college thousands of miles away, it does allow for a better assessment of her capabilities and possible next steps in her planning.

Planning is essential in helping Savannah and any TAY transition into adulthood. This process should include a strategy that addresses identification of early warning signs of decompensation, interventions to maintain stabilization, supports available, and plans of what to do in a crisis, especially if the patient is impaired and has limited capacity to participate in treatment decisions. One intervention to facilitate management during a crisis is the creation of a psychiatric advanced directive (PAD). A PAD allows an individual to communicate their mental health treatment preferences and designate others to make decisions on their behalf in future situations in which they may be unable to participate in their treatment planning [80]. A university study recruited 40 students with serious mental health illness and assessed the use of PADs. Positive aspects included allowing students to have control over their treatment and negatives included breach of privacy and stigmatizing those with mental illness [76]. There is limited data regarding outcomes related to the use of such tool in transitional age youth; however, it is one that could be considered when helping TAY, especially in the context of chronic episodic mood disorders.

Treatment Considerations

Psychopharmacology

Medication management is one of many components in the treatment of mood disorders. While many of the same medications are used in the adult and adolescent populations, there are differences in FDA approval, risk related to side effects, and response rates. Here, we will give a general overview of the medication options for the treatment of mood disorders with details specific to TAY.

Depression

A clinician should first assess the severity of MDD, which is driven by impairment of functioning, suicidality, presence of psychosis, and severity of symptoms. In a patient identified with mild severity, it is likely that supportive interventions alone (psychoeducation, brief supportive therapy, psychosocial support, etc.) may be sufficient. Randomized control trials (RCTs) have shown that up to an average of 50–60% of children and adolescents with MDD respond to placebo [7, 17] and 15–30% respond to brief nonspecific treatments [7, 73]. If a patient is identified as having moderate or severe MDD, treatments that include specific psychotherapies and medication management should be considered.

Overall, medication management of MDD in youth has focused on the use of SSRIs, SNRIs, and TCAs. TCAs are not as commonly used due to side-effect profile, lethal risk in overdose, as well as lack of efficacy when compared to placebo when treating youth with MDD [5, 39]. Paroxetine is also not typically used because of lack of demonstrated efficacy. Current US Food and Drug Administration (FDA)-approved medications for the treatment of MDD in youth include escitalopram (aged 12–17 years) and fluoxetine (aged 8–18 years). While many may start with using these two SSRIs, a clinician should assess family history use of antidepressants and response, possible drug-drug interactions, allergies, risk of noncompliance, cost, comorbid diagnosis, and symptom profile to evaluate if an alternative non-FDA-approved medication may be more suitable. For example, in a patient who is on several nonpsychotropic medications for chronic medical illness and has a family history of depression responsive to sertraline, a provider may consider sertraline. While not classified as FDA approved, in a multicenter randomized double-blind placebo controlled trial, sertraline demonstrated efficacy in the treatment of children and adolescents with depression [88]. If a patient has a partial response to monotherapy or comorbid ADHD, medications such as bupropion have been used to augment antidepressants when treating MDD [26, 85].

While dosing and side-effect profiles of SSRIs and SNRIs are similar in TAY and adults, TAY are subject to the black box warning on antidepressants. In 2004, the US Food and Drug Administration completed a meta-analysis that indicated a risk of increased spontaneously reported suicidal ideation and, to a lesser degree, suicide attempts in patients less than 25 years of age taking antidepressants; however, no completed suicide attempts were found in the study [16, 77]. This led to the announcement of a black box warning on antidepressants. There is controversy surrounding this finding as there are several studies that do not show significant worsening of suicidality in this population [14]. In addition, following the announcement of this warning, there was a decrease in the prescribing of antidepressants and a shift from generalist to psychiatrist prescribing [68]. There was also noted an increase in suicide rates in the years that followed these changes in prescribing practices. In addition, most studies indicate a positive relationship between SSRIs and reduction in adolescent and adult suicide. The overall take-home point is while there is evidence of a small increase in suicidal ideation, due to the potential benefits of antidepressant treatment, the American Academy of Child and Adolescent Psychiatry (AACAP) practice parameters still support the use of antidepressants in patients under 25 years of age with careful monitoring. Practice parameters note the recommendation that youth be seen every week for the first 4 weeks and biweekly thereafter. Assessments can be done face to face when possible but can also be briefly carried out by phone [10]. When assessing increasing suicidality in the context of medications, it is important to assess for the presence of an undertreated mood disorder, side effects that could worsen mood, whether the patient is currently disclosing suicidality that was present prior to the initiation of medications, and if suicidality can be connected with changes in psychosocial factors.

Bipolar Disorder

Medication management is a core component of treatment for bipolar spectrum illness. Prior to initiating medications, a clinician should assess the phase of illness, additional specifiers, comorbidities, family history, side-effect profile, and evidence of effectiveness in the literature for the TAY population [19].

Several antipsychotics and mood stabilizers have FDA approval in adults for bipolar spectrum illness, while only a handful have FDA approval in adolescents. For mania or mixed mania in children and adolescents, the second-generation antipsychotics that are FDA approved for ages 10–17 years include risperidone, aripiprazole, quetiapine, and asenapine. Olanzapine is FDA approved for ages 13–17 years. Atypical antipsychotics have shown larger effect size than anticonvulsant mood stabilizers when treating mania/mixed mania [19, 24]. In the Treatment of Early Age Mania (TEAM) trial, 279 medication-naïve patients aged 6–15 years with manic or mixed phase bipolar disorder were treated with risperidone, lithium, and divalproex sodium with response rates, respectively, of 68%, 35%, and 24%. Overall, it was noted that risperidone was more effective than lithium or divalproex sodium, especially for youth with ADHD [37, 87].

Lithium has FDA indication for acute and maintenance treatment of mania in patients aged 7 years and older. A randomized controlled 8-week trial in youth aged 7–17 years with BP I manic/mixed episode compared lithium to placebo. The change in Young Mania Rating Score (YMRS) was significantly larger in lithium-treated participants (5.51 (95% confidence interval: 0.51–10.50)) ($P = 0.03$), thus highlighting lithium being superior to placebo in reducing manic symptoms in pediatric patients [34, 37]. A recent review of the data from the COBY study sought to compare outcomes in participants initially aged 7–17 years at intake with a mean follow-up of 10 years who were taking lithium versus non-lithium mood stabilizers. When compared to non-lithium mood stabilizers, lithium was associated with less suicide attempts, fewer subthreshold depression symptoms, better psychosocial functioning, and less parent-reported aggression [38]. Lithium has previously been associated with decrease in suicidality in adults. A randomized, double-blind, placebo-controlled discontinuation trial examined youth aged 7–17 years with mixed or manic episode who had received 24 weeks of lithium treatment in the Collaborative Lithium Trials (COLT 1 and CoLT 2) with responders being randomized to continue lithium or be cross-titrated to placebo for up to 28 weeks. Those who continued lithium had a lower hazard ratio of recurrence compared to those who were cross-titrated to placebo. These data support using lithium as a maintenance treatment and the associated safety and tolerability [36].

While divalproex is FDA approved in adults, it has been noted to have less efficacy in trials looking at bipolar youth as noted in the TEAM trial. Given that our population of TAY spans both adolescence and adulthood, it is important to keep this factor in mind. However, divalproex remains used in adolescents, and there are positive trials that support its use [84]. An NIMH RCT compared lithium, divalproex, and placebo in youth aged 7–17 years with bipolar mania. Those treated with divalproex had a larger reduction in YMRS ($\Delta M = 8.3$) scores compared to placebo ($\Delta M = 5.3$) ($P = 0.04$) [37, 46]. Another study compared lithium to divalproex as maintenance treatment in youth aged 5–18 years and noted similar effectiveness [33]. Negative studies include a 4-week RCT in which divalproex ER was not better than placebo in the treatment of mania [37, 90]. Topiramate and oxcarbazepine have not been found to be significantly better than placebo [19, 37, 89]. In a placebo-controlled randomized withdrawal trial, adjunctive lamotrigine was compared to placebo in a group of 10–17-year-olds with bipolar I disorder receiving conventional bipolar disorder treatment. Lamotrigine did demonstrate additional benefit with delayed time to occurrence of mood episodes; however, this was only statistically significant in adolescents aged 13–17 years [35].

In adult bipolar depression, FDA- approved medications include olanzapine and fluoxetine combined, quetiapine, and lurasidone. The combination of olanzapine and fluoxetine now has an FDA indication for bipolar depression in youth aged 10–17 years [37]. As of 2018, lurasidone has been FDA approved for ages 10–17 years. There is often a significant concern regarding the use of antidepressants in bipolar depression for fear of inducing a switch into mania. Overall, the frequency of antidepressant-induced mania has been studied in several naturalistic and controlled studies, with rates ranging from 7% to 10% [56]. In addition, being on a mood stabilizer does not reliably protect from flipping into mania when an antidepressant is introduced. Guidelines recommend avoiding monotherapy with antidepressants in this population. If considering an antidepressant in a youth initially presenting with MDD, it is important to assess family history of a bipolar spectrum illness and any signs of bipolarity in the clinical presentation prior to starting an antidepressant. For TAY who may present with subthreshold symptoms of a bipolar spectrum illness, treatment guidelines for BP NOS do not currently exist [4].

Overall, when working with TAY, general themes of medication management include the following:

- Second-generation antipsychotics are very effective.
- Youth are more sensitive to metabolic side effects.
- Anticonvulsant mood stabilizers are less efficacious in youth compared to adults.
- Lithium has efficacy in mania/mixed episodes and maintenance treatment in youth.
- Treatment of comorbid ADHD with stimulants is safe and efficacious but should be done in the context of a mood stabilizer [37].
- There are limited data providing guidelines on the pharmacological management of BP NOS.

Psychotherapy

There are several empirically supported psychosocial interventions for bipolar spectrum disorders. These include child-and-family-focused cognitive behavioral therapy, multi/individual family psychoeducation, family-focused treatment for adolescents, dialectical behavioral therapy for adolescents, interpersonal and social rhythm therapy for adolescents, and cognitive behavioral therapy for bipolar disorders [19, 91]. Psychosocial interventions that include family psychoeducation plus skill building have been shown to be a well-established treatment in youth with a bipolar spectrum disorder [37]. Family dynamics can contribute to a risk of relapse, especially if the environment is characterized by high levels of expressed emotion. The family can also be a supportive element. Keeping this in mind, it makes sense that an intervention, such as family-focused therapy (FFT), has shown to be an evidence-based approach to treating bipolar youth. Family-focused therapy has components that include psychoeducation, communication training, and problem-solving [59]. In one study, youth who received family-focused therapy had more rapid recovery from their initial mood symptoms, more weeks in remission, and lower YMRS scores over 1 year when compared to youth in the control group [37, 60, 61].

Several forms of psychotherapy for depressed youth can be utilized such as supportive psychotherapy, psychodynamic psychotherapy, and family therapy; however, only cognitive behavioral therapy (CBT) and interpersonal psychotherapy (IPT) have been recognized as evidence-based modalities for depressed adolescents [7]. In the Treatment for Adolescents with Depression Study (TADS), 327 participants of ages 12–17 years were assigned to fluoxetine alone, CBT alone, and combination treatment and assessed at weeks 12, 18, and 36. Fluoxetine alone or in combination with CBT accelerated improvement in depression with combination treatment being superior to monotherapy [53]. The Treatment of SSRI- Resistant Depression in Adolescents (TORDIA) RCT sampled 334 patients aged 12 to 18 years with refractory MDD and randomized participants to (1) switch to a second SSRI, (2) switch to a different SSRI plus CBT, (3) switch to venlafaxine, or (4) switch to venlafaxine plus CBT. The addition of CBT with a switch of medication led to higher response rates compared to a medication switch alone [14]. These studies highlight the benefit of the incorporation of CBT into the treatment of TAY with MDD. IPT for adolescents (IPT-A) focuses on dysfunctional interpersonal communication processes [66] and has shown efficacy in several randomized controlled clinical trials. In a 12-week RCT of depressed adolescents aged 12–18 years, patients who received IPT-A had a decrease in depressive symptoms and overall improvement in social functioning [65].

System-Based Interventions

Treatment of mood disorders in TAY should transcend medication management and psychotherapy and should incorporate a system-based approach. We will review primary systems that intersect the lives of TAY and suggested interventions to assist youth with mood disorders.

Family

Whether it is in the absence of or presence of a family, a youth develops in the context of these relationships. As a TAY enters adulthood, it is important to evaluate the family system and how it affects a youth's clinical course and possible trajectory. Before the family system can be used as an intervention, the structure should be better understood. A clinician should assess who the youth identifies as family, cultural beliefs, generational differences, caregiver styles, and family trauma history [52]. From a cultural standpoint, a provider needs to know if there are cultural barriers to treatment, acculturation issues, and any cultural biases that may influence the transitional period [52]. From a generational standpoint, there are differences related to social norms that may cause a rift between families and TAY. The caregiver style influences how a TAY may or may not be prepared to individuate and how the family can be used as an intervention. A TAY who had overly intrusive parents and limited opportunities to self-advocate will have a different transition into adulthood compared to a TAY who has more permissive parents with too much autonomy without guidance. In both cases, these TAY will struggle with the transition, but the interventions that can be done using the family will differ greatly. In the first case, a clinician may need to work with limiting enmeshment with the TAY and help them gain increased independence. In the latter case, the clinician may have difficulty convincing the patient to allow their family to be available in times of crisis. Family history of trauma can also influence parental behavior. For example, there are noted associations of parents who are victims of childhood sexual abuse with having a higher rate of boundary distortions, permissive parenting, and use of physical punishment [28, 52]. This can affect the family construct, the TAY's health, and how the TAY may wish to engage their family in their treatment during the transitional years.

Once the clinician has a good grasp of the dynamics of the family system, they can consider appropriate interventions. Suggested family-based interventions include the following:

- Determining the level of financial support that can be provided or decreased
- Providing housing options with developmentally appropriate expectations (i.e., living at home while starting a job and also paying a portion of rent, or commuting to college while also contributing to chores and daily upkeep of the home)
- Being an emergency contact
- Establishing role and limitations of confidentiality
- Involving family in psychiatric advance directives or alternative forms of safety planning and crisis management
- Engaging in family therapy if there are concerns that family dynamics are contributing to the clinical presentation
- Engaging in psychoeducation and reviewing expectations regarding recovery and relapse [92]
- Engaging in therapeutic programs or treatment focused on parenting and support for the caregiver [92]

Colleges

Specific factors should be considered when planning for TAY with mood disorders who are college bound. College is a time of increased independence, decreased forced structure by caregivers, and increased exploration of interests. While college can be an exciting time, it can also be quite stressful and challenging for a significant group of students. A national college health survey looked at the impact of depression on undergraduate students. Approximately 40% of students reported feeling so depressed that it was difficult to function, approximately 17% reported depression impacting academic performance, 12% seriously considered suicide, and 2% made a suicide attempt [20]. Mood disorders can negatively affect success in college as discussed earlier in this chapter. Below are interventions to consider for TAY with mood disorders who are college bound:

- If a TAY had a previous 504 or Individualized Education Plan (IEP) related to their mood disorder, consider enrollment in the on-campus disability office [20].
- Educate TAY on the need for student-initiated request for accommodations [20].
- Identify campus-based resources:

  - Investigate the limitations of resources such as number of psychotherapy sessions offered, extent of specialized services, etc.
- Establish outpatient providers near or on campus.
- Identify social supports nearby (family friends, extended family).
- Consider disclosure to specific administration or residential/graduate assistants to allow for increased support on campus [74].
- Review lifestyle choices to maintain mood stability:
  - Per the National Sleep Foundation, minimum sufficient sleep for TAY is 6–11 hours [20, 40].
  - Encourage 150–300 minutes per week of physical activity.
  - Recommend the use of sleep-monitoring apps and logs.
  - Advise avoidance of substance use.

Providers

TAY are at risk of falling out of care, especially in the setting of the transition from a CAP to an adult psychiatrist. This transition should be handled with care, and emphasis should be placed on a warm handoff to the new provider. The previously established clinician of the TAY will likely have a sense of the developmental progression of the patient as well as the course of their illness. Facilitating a conversation with the new provider allows for the transmission of valuable information to assist the adult psychiatrist in ongoing management. This is also discussed in more detail in a separate chapter. Specific to TAY with mood disorders, information on the following would be important to highlight in the transition to the next provider:

- Characteristics of manic episodes (types of risky behaviors usually exhibiting, early warning signs, number of hours of sleep that put patient at risk)
- Typical duration of symptoms when symptomatic
- Nonpharmacological effective interventions (i.e., mindfulness, yoga, CBT, IPT, etc.)
- Comorbid illness and manifestation of these symptoms in symptomatic state vs. euthymic state
- History of suicidal ideation, attempts, or non-suicidal self-injurious behaviors
- History of mood-congruent psychosis
- Dominant mood state
- Effective vs. ineffective maximum dosing and serum levels in failed trials
- History of side effects (metabolic, thyroid, renal, sexual) based on typical classes of medications used, such as mood stabilizers, antidepressants, and antipsychotics

Employment

For TAY with mood disorders who chose to seek employment, it is important to help facilitate the selection of an appropriate job that will allow for stability of their mood. *For example, if Savannah chooses to stay home and work, her clinician should advise her on avoiding a job that reduces her sleep significantly or a job where she has increased access to alcohol. These two factors could increase her risk of a manic episode and relapse related to her alcohol use disorder.* TAY with mood disorders should pay particular attention to work hours, flexibility for modified schedules to accommodate treatment, stress level of position, level of emphasis on work-life balance, number of sick and personal days, benefits related to mental health care, and access to accommodations. Workplace accommodations focus on creating environments that allow for maintaining concentration, increased organizational support, assistance with managing stress, and flexibility in scheduling. In order to obtain accommodations, TAY would need to have a discussion with their employer's human resource or an equal employment officer. Clinicians should work with TAY and coach them on how to request workplace accommodations through the American with Disabilities Act [20], which is discussed in a separate section of this book. In addition, Individualized Education Plans (IEPs) should include transitional plans, and often services such as vocational resources are available. If these services are not in the IEP, the clinician should advise the caregiver to request a meeting to have the IEP revised. Providers should also encourage the use of vocational support programs that focus on résumé building, interview skills, job searching, job coaches, organizational skills, and time management [41].

Special Populations

Foster Care

TAY in foster care tend to have higher rates of polypharmacy, risk of inappropriate prescribing practices, use of antipsychotics, and limited access to evidence-based psychotherapies [49]. This population of TAY also tends to accumulate diagnoses such as posttraumatic stress disorder (PTSD), ODD, conduct, disruptive mood dysregulation disorder (DMDD), and primary psychotic disorders that can confound or inadvertently guide a provider away from a diagnosis of a mood disorder. Youth in foster care are a highly vulnerable population when it comes to diagnosis and treatment. Clinicians should be mindful of prescribing practices given this noted discrepancy.

TAY in foster care tend to have increased adverse childhood experiences (ACEs), which increase the risk for depression in early adulthood. A recent review highlighted the effects of child abuse and neglect on mood disorders and identified associations with increased risk for first mood episode, episode recurrence, greater comorbidities, and increased risks for suicide attempts and ideation [51]. In a 7-year longitudinal study of 243 adolescents of ages 12–18 years, findings showed that childhood maltreatment was associated with an increased risk for more severe trajectories of depressive symptoms [29, 51]. A meta-analysis assessed the effect of childhood maltreatment before the age of 18 years in individuals with bipolar disorder. Those who had experienced a form of maltreatment had greater severity of mania, depression, and psychosis; higher risk of comorbidity with PTSD, anxiety, and substance use disorders; higher risk of suicide attempts; higher risk of rapid cycling; and a greater number of manic and depressive episodes [1]. ACEs also affect attachment and may lead to obstacles with a TAY engaging in a relationship with a mental health provider. TAY in foster care who have had multiple placements are likely to have had multiple mental health providers. This disruption in care can lead to limited continuity and lack of understanding of their developmental and clinical course. These youth also rely on case management and social work services to support their mental health needs. When they age out of foster care, these TAY are at risk of struggling with managing their mental health without the previous supports in place. Establishment of mentoring relationships has shown improved outcomes in health, educational attainment, suicidality, arrests, sexually transmitted disease, and feelings of stress in these youth [22, 48]. Additional supports for foster care TAY include federal programs such as the Education and Training Vouchers Program. This program provides financial assistance to foster care youth and alumni enrolled in educational, vocational, or technical programs [48]. With this in mind, a clinician working with a youth in foster care should know the youth's ACEs profile, collaborate with the case manager/social worker, encourage the establishment of mentors, be aware of available resources, and be mindful of diagnostic and treatment pitfalls.

Ethnic and Racial Minorities

Minority adolescents may experience racism and prejudice, and this can increase risk for MDD [20]. Keeping in mind the developmental stage of TAY, one can imagine the effect that discrimination, marginalization, and subtle biases can have on identity formation. Unfortunately, racial biases do enter the medical field when caring for minority youth. For example, when TAY present with psychotic symptoms, which can be seen with both MDD and bipolar disorder, minority youth are more likely to be misdiagnosed as having schizophrenia [2]. This then limits access to appropriate treatment. On review of data from the National Comorbidity Survey – Adolescent

Supplement, the majority of adolescents with MDD did not receive disorder-specific treatment, with the greatest discrepancy being seen in minority youth [3]. Providers need to be aware of implicit biases and the effect they can have on patient interactions and treatment management.

LGBTQ

Similar to ethnic and racial minority youth, LGBTQ transitional age youth are in the stage of identity formation and have to navigate discrimination and biases. These youth experience higher rates of bullying and victimization, which directly relates to increased rates of depression and suicide [20, 75]. A meta-analysis examined disparities between sexual minority youth and rates of depression and suicidality. Sexual minority youth had higher rates of suicidality and depression symptoms [54]. When working with an LGBTQ youth, it is important to assess experiences with bullying, extent of social supports, and access to LGBTQ alliance organizations.

Case Closing

After a careful assessment and reflection, Savannah and her clinician decided that it was best to attend her local community college while commuting from home. She continued working on weekends at the hair salon. She remained engaged in regular medication management appointments and weekly psychotherapy. Savannah ultimately allowed her mother to be her emergency contact and be involved in crisis management planning. Fortunately, this plan did not have to go into effect, as Savannah was able to maintain her stability. After she assessed factors that contributed to her stability, Savannah decided to attend a 4-year college a few hours way but made sure to be close to extended family. While she lived on campus, she frequently visited her cousins and created a support network while away at college. She did disclose her mental health diagnosis to campus officials and was able to have psychiatric services on site as well as academic accommodations. When Savannah came home for long breaks, she checked in with her previous providers who had been in close communication with her on campus team. She had some moments of increased anxiety around finals, which led to a few nights of minimal sleep. She had been keeping a sleep log and noticed her patterns early. This allowed her to adjust her sleep routine and work with her psychiatrist to adjust her medications. Savannah also routinely went to Alcohol Anonymous meetings and built a community of support to maintain her sobriety. Savannah is managing her treatment, is aware of her risks due to her mental health, and has put supportive interventions in place as she traverses her bridge into adulthood.

References

1. Agnew-Blais J, Danese A. Childhood maltreatment and unfavourable clinical outcomes in bipolar disorder: a systematic review and meta-analysis. Lancet Psychiatry. 2016;3(4):342–9.
2. Akinhanmi MO, Biernacka JM, Strakowski SM, et al. Racial disparities in bipolar disorder treatment and research: a call to action. Bipolar Disord. 2018;20(6):506–14.
3. Avenevoli S, Swendsen J, He JP, et al. Major depression in the National Comorbidity Survey–Adolescent Supplement: prevalence, correlates, and treatment. J Am Acad Child Adolesc Psychiatry. 2015;54(1):37–44.e2.
4. Axelson DA, Birmaher B, Strober MA, et al. Course of subthreshold bipolar disorder in youth: diagnostic progression from bipolar disorder not otherwise specified. J Am Acad Child Adolesc Psychiatry. 2011;50(10):1001–16.e3.
5. Birmaher B. Major depressive disorder. In: McVoy M, Findling RL, editors. Clinical manuel of child and adolescent psychopharmacology. 3rd ed. District of Columbia: American Psychiatric Association Publishing; 2017. p. 224.
6. Birmaher B, Axelson D. Course and outcome of bipolar spectrum disorder in children and adolescents: a review of the existing literature. Dev Psychopathol. 2006;18:1023–35.
7. Birmaher B, Brent D. Depressive and disruptive mood dysregulation disorders. In: Dulcan M, editor. Dulcan's textbook of child and adolescent psychiatry. 2nd ed. Virginia: American Psychiatric Association Publishing; 2016. p. 246–8, 253, 257-258.
8. Birmaher B, Ryan ND, Williamson DE, et al. Childhood and adolescent depression: a review of the past 10 years. Part I. J Am Acad Child Adolesc Psychiatry. 1996;35(11):1427–39.

9. Birmaher B, Arbelaez C, Brent D. Course and outcome of child and adolescent major depressive disorder. Child Adolesc Psychiatr Clin N Am. 2002;11(3):619–37.
10. Birmaher B, Brent D, the AACAP Work Group on Quality Issues. Practice parameter for the assessment and treatment of children and adolescents with depressive disorders. J Am Acad Child Adolesc Psychiatry. 2007;46(11):1503–26.
11. Birmaher B, Axelson D, Goldstein B, et al. Four-year longitudinal course of children and adolescents with bipolar spectrum disorder: The course and outcome of bipolar youth (COBY) study. Am J Psychiatry. 2009b;166(7):795–804.
12. Birmaher B, Axelson D, Goldstein B, et al. Four-Year Longitudinal Course of Children and adolescents with the course and outcome of bipolar youth (COBY) study. Am J Psychiatry. 2009b;166(7):795–804.
13. Blanco C, Okuda M, Wright C, et al. Mental health of college students and their non-college-attending peers: results from the national epidemiologic study on alcohol and related conditions. Arch Gen Psychiatry. 2008;65(12):1429–37.
14. Brent D, Emslie G, Clarke G, et al. Switching to another SSRI or to venlafaxine with or without cognitive behavioral therapy for adolescents with SSRI-resistant depression: the TORDIA randomized controlled trial. JAMA. 2008;299(8):901–13.
15. Bridge JA, Salary CB, Birmaher B, et al. The risks and benefits of antidepressant treatment for youth depression. Ann Med. 2005;37(6):404–12.
16. Bridge JA, Iyengar S, Salary CB, et al. Clinical response and risk for reported suicidal ideation and suicide attempts in pediatric antidepressant treatment: a meta-analysis of randomized controlled trials. JAMA. 2007;297(15):1683–96.
17. Bridge JA, Birmaher B, Iyengar S, et al. Placebo response in randomized controlled trials of antidepressants for pediatric major depressive disorder. Am J Psychiatr. 2009;166(1):42–9.
18. Carlson GA, Klein DN. How to understand divergent views on bipolar disorder in youth. Annu Rev Clin Psychol. 2014;10:529–51.
19. Carlson GA, Pataki C, Meyer SE. Bipolar disorder. In: Dulcan M, editor. Dulcan's textbook of child and adolescent psychiatry, vol. 286. 2nd ed. Virgina: American Psychiatric Association Publishing; 2016. p. 293–4.
20. Chan V, Moore J, Derenne J, et al. Transitional age youth and college mental health. Child Adolesc Psychiatr Clin N Am. 2019;28(3):363–75.
21. Chung WW, Hudziak JJ. The transitional age brain "the best of times and the worst of times". Child Adolesc Psychiatr Clin N Am. 2017;26(2):157–75.
22. Collins ME, Spencer R, Ward R. Supporting youth in the transition from foster care: formal and informal connections. Child Welfare. 2010;89:125–43.
23. Copeland WE, Wolke D, Shanahan L, et al. Adult functional outcomes of common childhood psychiatric problems a prospective, longitudinal study. JAMA Psychiat. 2015;72(9):892–9.
24. Correll CU, Sheridan EM, DelBello MP. Antipsychotic and mood stabilizer efficacy and tolerability in pediatric and adult patients with bipolar I mania: a comparative analysis of acute, randomized, placebo-controlled trials. Bipolar Disord. 2010;12:116–41.
25. Costello EJ, Pine DS, Hammen C, et al. Development and natural history of mood disorders. Biol Psychiatry. 2002;52(6):529–42.
26. Daviss WB, Bentivoglio P, Racusin R, et al. Bupropion sustained release in adolescents with comorbid attention-deficit/hyperactivity disorder and depression. J Am Acad Child Adolesc Psychiatry. 2001;40(3):307–14.
27. Diagnostic and Statistical Manual of Mental Disorders (DSM 5) (2013), Fifth edition. American Psychiatric Association Publishing, Virgina.
28. DiLillo D, Damashek A. Parenting characteristics of women reporting a history of childhood sexual abuse. Child Maltreat. 2003;8(4):319–33.
29. Ellis RER, Seal ML, Simmons JG, et al. Longitudinal trajectories of depression symptoms in adolescence: psychosocial risk factors and outcomes. Child Psychiatry Hum Dev. 2017;48:554–71.
30. Erikson EH. Identity, youth and crisis. New York: W. W. Norton & Company; 1968.
31. Fergusson DM, Boden JM, Horwood LJ. Recurrence of major depression in adolescence and early adulthood, and later mental health, educational and economic outcomes. Br J Psychiatry. 2007;191(4):335–42.
32. Ferro MA, Gorter JW, Boyle MH. Trajectories of depressive symptoms during the transition to young adulthood: the role of chronic illness. J Affect Disord. 2015;174:594–601.
33. Findling RL, McNamara NK, Youngstrom EA, et al. Blind 18-month trial of lithium versus divalproex maintenance treatment in pediatric bipolar disorder. J Am Acad Child Adolesc Psychiatry. 2005;44(5):409–17.
34. Findling RL, Robb A, McNamara NK, et al. Lithium in the acute treatment of bipolar I disorder: a double-blind, placebo-controlled study. Pediatrics. 2015a;136(5):885–94.
35. Findling RL, Chang K, Robb A, et al. Adjunctive maintenance lamotrigine for pediatric bipolar I disorder: a placebo-controlled, randomized withdrawal. J Am Acad Child Adolesc Psychiatry. 2015b;54(12):1020–1031.e3.
36. Findling RL, McNamara NK, Pavuluri M, et al. Lithium for the maintenance treatment of bipolar I disorder: a double-blind, placebo-controlled discontinuation study. J Am Acad Child Adolesc Psychiatry. 2019;58(2):287–296.e4.
37. Goldstein BI, Birmaher B, Carlson GA, et al. The International Society for Bipolar Disorders Task Force report on pediatric bipolar disorder: knowledge to date and directions for future research. Bipolar Disord. 2017;19(7):524–43.
38. Hafeman DM, Rooks B, Merranko J, et al. Lithium versus other mood-stabilizing medications in a lon-

gitudinal study of bipolar youth. J Am Acad Child Adolesc Psychiatry. 2019; in press.
39. Hazell P, O'Connell D, Heathcote D, et al. Tricyclic drugs for depression in children and adolescents. Cochrane Database Syst Rev. 2002;(2):CD002317.
40. Hirshkowitz M, Whiton K, Albert SM, et al. National sleep foundation's sleep time duration recommendations: methodology and results summary. Sleep Health. 2015;1(1):40–3.
41. Hower H, Lee EJ, Jones RN, et al. Predictors of longitudinal psychosocial functioning in bipolar youth transitioning to adults. J Affect Disord. 2019;246:578–85.
42. Hunt J, Eisenberg D, Kilbourne AM. Consequences of receipt of a psychiatric diagnosis for completion of college. Psychiatr Serv. 2010;61(4):399–404.
43. Kessler RC, Berglund P, Demler O, et al. Lifetime prevalence and age-of-onset distributions of DSM-IV disorders in the National Comorbidity Survey Replication. Arch Gen Psychiatry. 2005;62(6):593–602.
44. Kovacs M, Goldston D. Cognitive and social cognitive development of depressed children and adolescents. J Am Acad Child Adolesc Psychiatry. 1991;30(3):388–92.
45. Kowatch RA, Findling RL, Scheffer RE, et al. Pediatric bipolar collaborative mood stabilizer trial. Poster presented at the annual meeting of the American Academy of Child and Adolescent Psychiatry, Boston, 23–28 October 2007.
46. Kowatch RA, Findling RL, Scheffer RE, et al. Pediatric bipolar collaborative mod stabilizer trial. Poster presented at the annual meeting of the American Academy of Child and Adolescent Psychiatry, Boston, 23–28 October 2007.
47. Kozloff N, Cheung AH, Schaffer A, et al. Bipolar disorder among adolescents and young adults: results from an epidemiological sample. J Affect Disord. 2010;125(1–3):350–4.
48. Lee T, Morgan W. Transitioning to adulthood from foster care. Child Adolesc Psychiatr Clin N Am. 2017;26(2):283–96.
49. Lee T, Fouras G, Brown R. Practice parameter for the assessment and management of youth involved with the child welfare system. J Am Acad Child Adolesc Psychiatry. 2015;54(6):502–17.
50. Leibenluft E. Severe mood dysregulation, irritability, and the diagnostic boundaries of bipolar disorder in youths. Am J Psychiatry. 2011;168:129–42.
51. Lippard ETC, Nemeroff CB. The devastating clinical consequences of child abuse and neglect: increased disease vulnerability and poor treatment response in mood disorders. Am J Psychiatry. 2020;177(1):20–36.
52. Livesey CMW, Rostain AL. Involving parents/family in treatment during the transition from late adolescence to young adulthood: rationale, strategies, ethics, and legal issues. Child Adolesc Psychiatr Clin N Am. 2017;26(2):199–216.
53. March JS, Silva S, Petrycki S, et al. The treatment for adolescents with depression study (TADS): long-term effectiveness and safety outcomes. Arch Gen Psychiatry. 2007;64(10):1132–43.
54. Marshal MP, Dietz LJ, Friedman MS, et al. Suicidality and depression disparities between sexual minority and heterosexual youth: a meta-analytic review. J Adolesc Health. 2011;49(2):115–23.
55. Martel A, Fuchs DC. Transitional age youth and mental illness – influences on young adult outcomes. Child Adolesc Psychiatr Clin N Am. 2017;26(2):xiii–vii.
56. Martin A, Young C, Leckman JF, et al. Age effects on antidepressant-induced manic conversion. Arch Pediatr Adolesc Med. 2004;158(8):773–80.
57. McGorry PD, Mei C. Early intervention in youth mental health: progress and future directions. Evid Based Ment Health. 2018;21(4):182–4.
58. Merikangas KR, Cui L, Kattan G, et al. Mania with and without depression in a community sample of US adolescents. Arch Gen Psychiatry. 2012;69(9):943–51.
59. Miklowitz D. Evidence-based psychotherapies for pediatric bipolar disorders. In: Singh MK, editor. Clinical handbook for the diagnosis and treatment of pediatric mood disorders. District of Columbia: American Psychiatric Association Publishing; 2019. p. 227–9.
60. Miklowitz DJ, Chung B. Family-focused therapy for bipolar disorder: reflections on 30 years of research. Fam Process. 2016;55(3):483–99.
61. Miklowitz DJ, Schneck CD, Singh MK, et al. Early intervention for symptomatic youth at risk for bipolar disorder: a randomized trial of family-focused therapy. J Am Acad Child Adolesc Psychiatry. 2013;52(2):121–31.
62. Mojtabai R, Stuart EA, Hwang I, et al. Long-term effects of mental disorders on educational attainment in the National Comorbidity Survey ten-year follow-up. Soc Psychiatry Psychiatr Epidemiol. 2015;50(10):1577–91.
63. Mojtabai R, Olfson M, Han B. National trends in the prevalence and treatment of depression in adolescents and young adults. Pediatrics. 2016;138(6):e20161878.
64. Mueser KT, Penn DL, Addington J, et al. The NAVIGATE program for first-episode psychosis: rationale, overview, and description of psychosocial components. Psychiatr Serv. 2015;66(7):680–90.
65. Mufson L, Weissman MM, Moreau D, et al. Efficacy of interpersonal psychotherapy for depressed adolescents. Arch Gen Psychiatry. 1999;56(6):573–9.
66. Mufson L, Dorta KP, Moreau D, et al. Interpersonal psychotherapy for depressed adolescents. 2nd ed. New York: The Guilford Press; 2004. p. 14.
67. Naicker K, Galambos NL, Zeng Y, et al. Social, demographic, and health outcomes in the 10 years following adolescent depression. J Adolesc Health. 2013;52(5):533–8.
68. Nemeroff CB, Kalali A, Keller MB, et al. Impact of publicity concerning pediatric suicidality data on physician practice patterns in the United States. Arch Gen Psychiatry. 2007;64(4):466–72.
69. O'Donnell LA, Ellis AJ, Van de Loo MM, et al. Mood instability as a predictor of clinical and functional

outcomes in adolescents with bipolar I and bipolar II disorder. J Affect Disord. 2018;236:199–206.
70. Perlis RH, Miyahara S, Marangell LB, et al. Long-term implications of early onset in bipolar disorder: data from the first 1000 participants in the Systematic Treatment Enhancement Program for Bipolar Disorder (STEP-BD). Biol Psychiatry. 2004;55(9):875–81.
71. Propper L, Ortiz A, Slaney C, Garnham J, et al. Early-onset and very-early-onset bipolar disorder: distinct or similar clinical conditions? Bipolar Disord. 2015;17:814–20.
72. Rao U, Hammen CL, Poland RE. Longitudinal course of adolescent depression: neuroendocrine and psychosocial predictors. J Am Acad Child Adolesc Psychiatry. 2010;49(2):141–51.
73. Renaud J, Brent DA, Baugher M, et al. Rapid response to psychological treatment for adolescent depression: a two year follow up. J Am Acad Child Adolesc Psychiatry. 1998;37(11):1184–90.
74. Robb A. Coping with highs and lows: a student with bipolar disorder goes to college. In: Martel A, Derenne J, Leebens PK, editors. Promoting safe and effective transitions to college for youth with mental health conditions. New York: Springer; 2018.
75. Rodgers SM. Transitional age lesbian, gay, bisexual, transgender, and questioning youth: issues of diversity, integrated identities, and mental health. Child Adolesc Psychiatr Clin N Am. 2017;26(2):297–309.
76. Scheyett AM, Rooks A. University students' views on the utility of psychiatric advance directives. J Am Coll Heal. 2012;60(1):90–3.
77. Simon GE, Savarino J, Operskalski B, et al. Suicide risk during antidepressant treatment. Am J Psychiatr. 2006;163(1):41–7.
78. Solomon DA, Keller MB, Leon AC, et al. Recovery from major depression: a 10-year prospective follow-up across multiple episodes. Arch Gen Psychiatry. 1997;54(11):1001–6.
79. Solomon DA, Keller MB, Leon AC, et al. Multiple recurrences of major depressive disorder. Am J Psychiatr. 2000;157(2):229–33.
80. Srebnik DS, La Fond JQ. Advance directives for mental health treatment. Psychiatr Serv. 1999;50(7):919–25.
81. Stringaris A, Cohen P, Pine DS. Adult outcomes of youth irritability: a 20-year prospective community-based study. Am J Psychiatry. 2009;166(9):1048–54.
82. Stringaris A, Santosh P, Leibenluft E, et al. Youth meeting symptom and impairment criteria for manic-like episodes lasting less than four days: an epidemiological enquiry. J Child Psychol Psychiatry. 2010;51(1):31–8.
83. Thapar A, Collishaw S, Pine DS. Depression in adolescence. Lancet. 2012;379(9820):1056–67.
84. Thomas-Lakia T, Levy J, Findling RL. Bipolar disorders. In: McVoy M, Findling RL, editors. Clinical manuel of child and adolescent psychopharmacology. 3rd ed. District of Columbia: American Psychiatric Association Publishing; 2017. p. 264–5, 274, 295–296.
85. Trivedi MH, Fava M, Wisniewski SR, et al. Medication augmentation after the failure of SSRIs for depression. N Engl J Med. 2006;354(12):1243–52.
86. Vaudreuil CAH, Faraone SV, Di Salvo M, et al. The morbidity of subthreshold pediatric bipolar disorder: a systematic literature review and meta-analysis. Bipolar Disord. 2019;21(1):16–27.
87. Vitiello B, Riddle MA, Yenokyan G, et al. Treatment moderators and predictors of outcome in the Treatment of Early Age Mania (TEAM) study. J Am Acad Child Adolesc Psychiatry. 2012;51(9):867–78.
88. Wagner KD, Ambrosini P, Rynn M, et al. Efficacy of sertraline in the treatment of children and adolescents with major depressive disorder: two randomized controlled trials. JAMA. 2003;290(8):1033–41.
89. Wagner KD, Kowatch RA, Emslie GJ, et al. A double-blind, randomized, placebo-controlled trial of oxcarbazepine in the treatment of bipolar disorder in children and adolescents. Am J Psychiatry. 2006;163(7):1179–86.
90. Wagner KD, Redden L, Kowatch RA, et al. A double-blind, randomized, placebo-controlled trial of divalproex extended-release in the treatment of bipolar disorder in children and adolescents. J Am Acad Child Adolesc Psychiatry. 2009;48(5):519–32.
91. Weinstein SM, West AE, Pavuluri M. Psychosocial intervention for pediatric bipolar disorder: current and future directions. Expert Rev Neurother. 2013;13(7):843–50.
92. Wilens TE, Rosenbaum JF. Transitional aged youth: a new frontier in child and adolescent psychiatry. J Am Acad Child Adolesc Psychiatry. 2013;52(9):887–90.
93. Wilens TE, Biederman J, Millstein RB, et al. Risk for substance use disorders in youths with child- and adolescent- onset bipolar disorder. J Am Acad Child Adolesc Psychiatry. 1999;38(6):680–5.
94. Wilson S, Hicks BM, Foster KT. Age of onset and course of major depressive disorder: associations with psychosocial functioning outcomes in adulthood. Psychol Med. 2015;45(3):505–14.
95. Zimmermann P, Brückl T, Nocon A, et al. Heterogeneity of DSM-IV major depressive disorder as a consequence of subthreshold bipolarity. Arch Gen Psychiatry. 2009;66(12):1341–52.
96. Zisook S, Lesser I, Stewart JW, et al. Effect of age at onset on the course of major depressive disorder. Am J Psychiatry. 2007;164(10):1539–46.

6 Substance Use Disorders

Colin W. Burke, Elizabeth S. Firmin, Timothy E. Wilens, and Amy M. Yule

Key Points

- Compared with other age groups, transitional age youth (TAY) have the highest rates of substance misuse and substance use disorders (SUDs) across all substances, the highest rates of access to substances, the lowest perceived risk of substance use, and the lowest rates of engagement in specialty SUD treatment.
- Substance use among TAY leads to significant morbidity and mortality, as well as impacts on cognitive functioning, family and social relationships, educational attainment, and life satisfaction. Many of these impacts can persist well into adulthood.
- TAY are particularly vulnerable to problematic substance use due to the unique confluence of psychological and neurocognitive developmental factors, burgeoning independence and legal autonomy, and changing social contexts during this time of life.
- Given the extent of substance use among TAY, screening for problematic use should be a routine part of practice in a broad range of clinical settings, and providers should be familiar with screening tools and local resources for referral to further specialty treatment as indicated.
- Providers should seek to place substance use in a broader social, medical, psychiatric, systems-based, and cultural context in order to leverage multimodal and targeted treatment interventions.
- There are a number of evidence-based psychosocial and psychopharmacological treatments for TAY SUD.

C. W. Burke (✉)
Massachusetts General Hospital, Boston, MA, USA

Harvard Medical School, Boston, MA, USA
e-mail: colin.burke@mgh.harvard.edu

E. S. Firmin
Clinical and Research Programs in Pediatric Psychopharmacology & Adult ADHD, Massachusetts General Hospital, Boston, MA, USA

T. E. Wilens
Harvard Medical School, Boston, MA, USA

Clinical and Research Programs in Pediatric Psychopharmacology & Adult ADHD, Massachusetts General Hospital, Boston, MA, USA

A. M. Yule
Harvard Medical School, Boston, MA, USA

Clinical and Research Programs in Pediatric Psychopharmacology & Adult ADHD, Massachusetts General Hospital, Boston, MA, USA

Boston Medical Center, Boston, MA, USA

Boston University School of Medicine, Boston, MA, USA

V. Chan, J. Derenne (eds.), *Transition-Age Youth Mental Health Care*,
https://doi.org/10.1007/978-3-030-62113-1_6

- Whenever possible, families and other supports should be involved in the treatment with the consent of the TAY patient. Even in cases where no consent is given, or the TAY patient will not engage, families and supports can be engaged in evidence-based parent guidance independent of the TAY's individual treatment.
- Treatment of SUD among TAY should be team-based and multidisciplinary, both to provide appropriate wraparound services and to diffuse stress and risk of burnout among members of the treatment team.
- It is developmentally normative for TAY to have diminished or variable motivation to change; treatment conducted in a patient-centered and harm reduction-oriented framework is more likely to be effective than rigid insistence on abstinence or a punitive, paternalistic approach.

Background

Perhaps more than any other time of life, early adulthood is a time of great personal growth, exploration of new experiences, and identity formation. As we will see throughout this chapter, the groundwork for these changes is laid by an interconnected set of social, biological, and psychological changes that confer increased autonomy and pliability at this crucial time of life. This chapter will also explore the ways in which these same forces can create a "perfect storm" for vulnerability to problematic substance use among TAY, which can have significant and lasting impacts on long-term health, well-being, and functioning. Further, this time of life spans a transitional period in the development of personal and family relationships, as well as formal legal status, which can complicate the efforts of families and treatment providers seeking to assist TAY struggling with problematic substance use.

Recent years have seen a significant increase in public awareness of the effects of substance use on individuals and communities. It is now commonplace to hear of the epidemic proportions of the problem, particularly in reference to opioid-related overdose and deaths. In response to this increased awareness, government agencies, healthcare systems, and philanthropists have begun to channel increased resources toward identifying and treating individuals with problematic substance use and reducing public stigma for those seeking treatment. Less commonly reported, however, is the disproportionate impact of substance use among TAY and the relatively worse engagement, retention, and treatment outcomes of TAY in traditional adolescent- or adult-oriented treatment programs. In other words, despite a global increase in focus on the effects of substance use in society, TAY struggling with substance use remain an under-recognized and highly vulnerable group. Given that the majority of individuals with problematic substance use begin use during the TAY years [73], this is a critically important time of life in which to identify and intervene upon substance use.

Substance use can be conceptualized as existing along a continuum, from isolated episodes of trying substances at one end to diagnosable substance use disorder (SUD, as defined by the *Diagnostic and Statistical Manual of Mental Disorders, 5th Ed* [DSM-5]) at the other. For the purposes of this chapter, we will use the term "substance misuse" to signify patterns of substance use behavior which raise concern or create some level of functional or relational impairment (such as underage or binge drinking, non-prescribed or inappropriate use of prescription medications, or use of illicit substances), but do not meet formal criteria for SUD based on time course or severity. We will use the term "problematic substance use" to signify a broader category encompassing both substance misuse and SUD.

Epidemiology

There is no comprehensive national survey that captures data on substance use among TAY between the ages of 16 and 26 years. Monitoring the Future, an annual national survey funded by the National Institute on Drug Abuse (NIDA), collects data on 8th, 10th, and 12th graders and, separately, college-age youth. The National Survey on Drug Use and Health (NSDUH) separates youth ages 18–25 years ("young adults") for comparison against adolescent (ages 12–17 years) and adult populations (ages 26+ years), providing a useful approximate comparison of TAY against other age groups. Given the utility of comparing age groups across a single survey, we have summarized the results of the 2018 NSDUH survey in the tables below.

As seen in Fig. 6.1, as compared with both adolescent and adult populations, young adults have the highest overall past-year rates of SUD, and the highest past-year rates of disordered use of every substance queried. Perhaps most notable are the rates of any SUD, which are four times higher among young adults than among adolescents and over two times higher among young adults than among adults. Similarly striking are the numbers for alcohol use disorder, which are over six times higher among young adults than among adolescents and nearly twice as high among young adults than among adults. Taken together, these data make clear the disproportionate burden of SUD borne by TAY.

Substance misuse – again, defined as problematic use which may not rise to the level of full SUD – has a similarly disproportionate effect on young adults. As seen in Fig. 6.2, past-year rates of binge alcohol use (defined as five or more standard drinks in a single occasion for men and four or more for women), non-medical use of prescription stimulants, and opioid misuse are highest among young adults, as compared to adolescents and adults.

Perhaps not surprisingly based upon these prevalence data, young adults have the highest rates of identified need for SUD treatment –

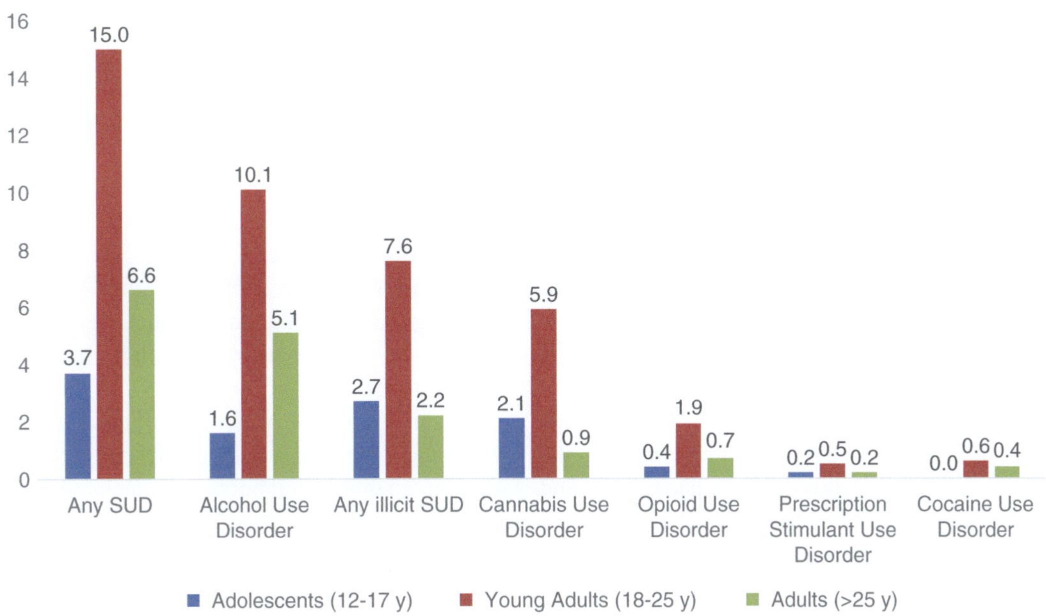

Fig. 6.1 Rates (as percentages) of any SUD and individual SUDs in the past year by age group [91]

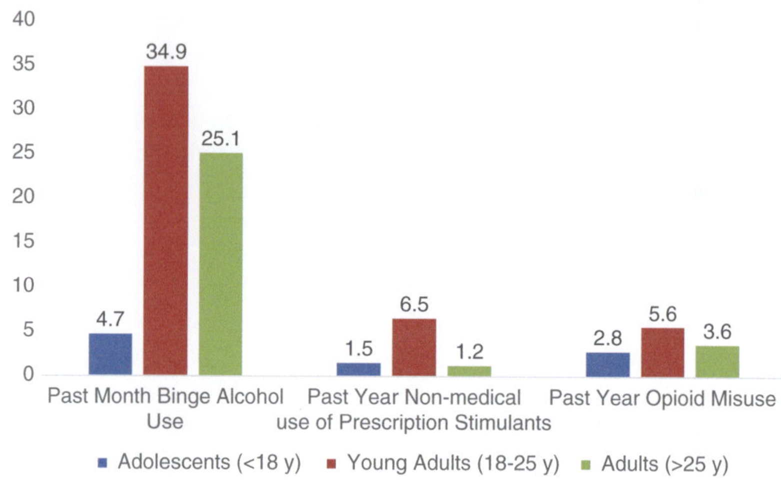

Fig. 6.2 Rates (as percentages) of substance misuse by age group [91]

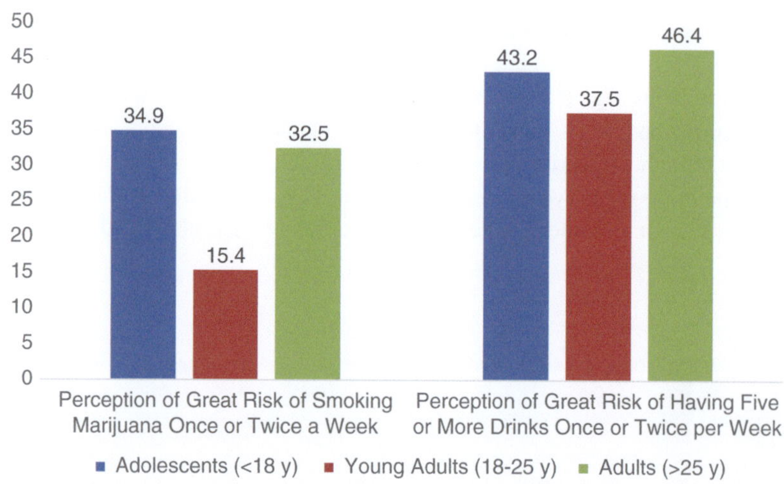

Fig. 6.3 Perception of risk of substances (as percentages), by age group [90]

according to NSDUH, over double those of adults and nearly five times those of adolescents (15.3% compared with 7.0% and 3.8%, respectively). What may come as a surprise, however, is that despite this high level of need, young adults have the lowest rates of having treatment needs met with specialty substance use treatment in the past year – 6.3% versus 8.8% for adolescents and 12.9% for adults. In addition, as seen in Figs. 6.3 and 6.4, young adults have the lowest perception of risk associated with smoking marijuana or drinking alcohol and the highest rates of passive access to marijuana and other substances.

In addition to these findings, the annual Monitoring the Future survey (National Institute on Drug Abuse) has documented a striking increase in lifetime nicotine vaping in recent years among 12th graders, from 33.8% of 12th graders in 2016 to 45.6% in 2019. This is occurring at the same time as rates of lifetime cigarette smoking among 12th graders have declined from 28.3% in 2016 to 22.3% in 2019. Although there is less longitudinal data available for THC vaping, the survey also found that 3.5% of 12th graders reported daily THC vaping and 14% reported past month use [66].

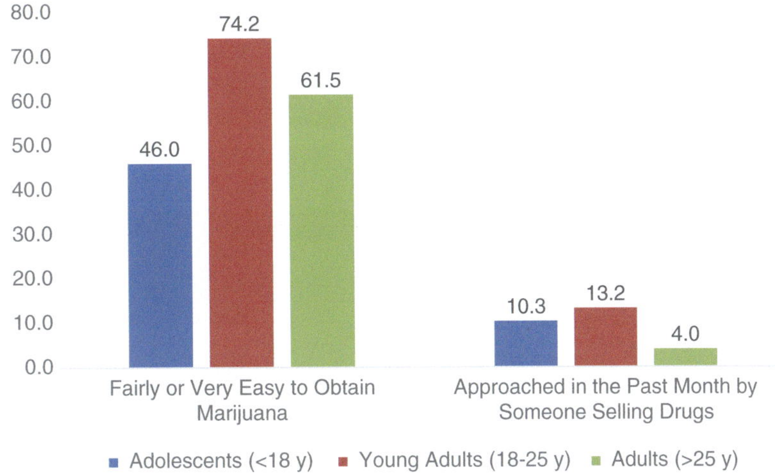

Fig. 6.4 Passive access to substances (as percentages), by age group [90]

Impacts of Substance Use Among TAY

Were substance use harmless, these data regarding the high prevalence of substance use among TAY might not be so alarming. However, a growing body of evidence has begun to create a clear picture of the short- and long-term impacts of substance use during these transitional years. Substance use impacts various domains of life in complex, intersecting, and often mutually compounding ways. To date, much of the research in TAY has focused on alcohol and marijuana use, which is reflected in the information presented here.

Cognitive Impacts

The evidence base for cognitive impacts of substance use among TAY is strongest for alcohol and marijuana. The emerging literature in this area paints a picture of both short-term and long-term cognitive impacts of alcohol and marijuana use, reflecting vulnerability due to ongoing neurocognitive development during these transitional years (as will be discussed subsequently in this chapter) in the setting of high access to substances, which can persist into adulthood. This is particularly troubling given that these transitional years are a time in which future trajectories are to a large degree set, as TAY are called upon to "launch" into novel academic, occupational, and social settings, calling upon higher-level cognitive functioning to lay the foundation for future success and fulfillment.

Alcohol use in late adolescence has been linked to lower visuospatial functioning and poorer verbal learning and memory [43, 67]. Cannabis use has been shown to have immediate negative impacts on delayed-memory recall and perceptual reasoning and to have delayed-onset, neurotoxic effects on inhibitory control and working memory among younger teens [62]. In addition, early-onset cannabis use has been linked to decreased verbal IQ and decreased executive functioning [12]. Further, a neuroimaging study has shown differences in gray matter volume in the temporal lobes, posterior cingulate, lingual gyri, and cerebellum which were linked with concurrent decreases in perceptual reasoning and future generalized anxiety symptoms among adolescents with even extremely low-level cannabis use (one or two lifetime instances of cannabis use) [72]. Findings from Gruber and Sagar [42] and Lisdahl et al. [52] suggest that the potential for neurobiological changes and severe cognitive deficits are particularly noxious with onset of use before age 16 years. Put together, these data form a picture of significant negative impacts of alcohol and marijuana use on memory, reasoning, and executive functioning among TAY, which impact their functioning not only at the time of use, but in some cases for years thereafter.

Social and Developmental Impacts

In addition to these neurocognitive impacts, substance use among TAY impacts individual development, family relationships, and societal productivity in significant ways, causing elevated levels of disability, family discord, worse outcomes in school and at work, and diminished life satisfaction for TAY. Evidence has shown that substance use is a leading cause of global disability in this age group [37]. As of 2006 underage drinking was estimated to result in $27 billion in annual costs in the United States, mostly associated with loss of productivity due to early mortality [9]. With regard to families, alcohol and marijuana use in adolescence have been linked to poorer relationships between young adults and their parents [89], a research finding which is certainly borne out in clinical practice. On an individual level, early-onset and more frequent cannabis use in adolescence has been associated with decreased high school graduation (controlled for early adolescent academic achievement) [12]. In addition, data from New Zealand illustrate links between cannabis use between ages 14 and 25 years and lower levels of degree attainment at age 25 years, lower income at age 25 years, higher levels of welfare dependence, higher unemployment, lower levels of relationship satisfaction, and lower levels of life satisfaction, even when controlling for a wide range of possible confounding factors [32].

Physical Impacts

Perhaps the most widely publicized physical impacts of substance use among TAY are morbidity and mortality related to substance-induced intoxication. In the general population, motor vehicle crashes are the leading cause of death from birth until age 30 years [13]. This high risk of mortality is coupled with high rates of comorbidity between motor vehicle accidents and substance use and dependence [29]. According to the CDC, in 2016 26% of alcohol-intoxicated drivers (with blood alcohol content above the legal driving limit) involved in fatal automobile accidents were between the ages of 21 and 24 years [17]. However, alcohol is far from the only culprit in intoxication-related deaths; between 2015 and 2016, the largest increase in opioid overdose deaths was among males age 15–24 years [81]. Risk factors for overdose among TAY include injection substance use, opioid use, tranquilizer use, use of multiple substances, history of psychopathology, prior incarceration, unstable housing, and having witnessed an overdose [53].

Infectious diseases present another physical health risk associated with substance use, both through injection use and through other risky behaviors such as unprotected sex which might occur while intoxicated. After a decline in the number of cases of acute hepatitis C in the United States in the early 2000s, the incidence has been steadily increasing since 2011 [14]. The largest increase in rate of hepatitis C occurred among individuals 20–29 years of age who also have the highest rate of acute hepatitis C relative to other age groups. A recent study using national surveillance data found increases in opioid injection mirrored increases in reported cases of acute hepatitis C infection among demographic subgroups suggesting the increases in acute hepatitis C infection were related to opioid injection drug use [99]. It is important to note that hepatitis C is spread not only through shared syringes but also through the sharing of other injection paraphernalia such as "cookers" and cotton filters [92].

In 2018, the CDC noted that "In 2014, persons aged 13–29 years represented 23% of the U.S. population, yet accounted for 40% of diagnoses of human immunodeficiency virus (HIV) infection during the same year" [71]. Among this group, rates of HIV diagnosis were highest in those 22–23 years old [71]. According to the CDC, while the majority of new HIV infections in youth were related to sexual contact, intravenous substance use remains a significant risk factor, with 4% of new cases in young men and 11% of new cases in young women attributable at least in part to intravenous substance use [16].

The discussion of physical harms associated with substance use has broadened even further in recent years, given the appearance of novel drug delivery devices, most notably portable electronic vaporizing devices for nicotine and tetrahydrocannabinol (THC), the psychoactive ingredient in marijuana. A recent outbreak of acute respiratory illness in young people using electronic vaping devices has shed light on risks associated with novel and unregulated devices and substance formulations which hold particular appeal to adolescents and young adults [50].

Unique Features Related to Substance Use Among TAY

The years of late adolescence and early adulthood present a "perfect storm" of biological, psychological, and sociocultural factors which increase vulnerability to problematic substance use and complicate treatment. While this period of rapid change and pliability confers risk, conversely it also holds great promise for intervention and prevention. In fact, research suggests that for every year of delayed onset of alcohol and other drug use, there are significant decreases in risk of later development of SUD [38, 39]. The hope is that an understanding of the complexities outlined below can inform comprehensive and practical treatment strategies, recognizing both the risk and the promise of these transitional years.

Psychological Developmental Vulnerabilities

The years of late adolescence and early adulthood are commonly a time for trying on new roles; forming identity in relation to one's self, family, and friends; and re-contextualizing the formative bonds of one's childhood and adolescent years. In this context of low responsibility and high independence, it is culturally normative for TAY to use their increased autonomy and decreased oversight to try a variety of new experiences. For some, this will include trying substances, which will be felt by some to "enhance the good times and mitigate the bad" [6] during this potentially stressful period. From a psychological perspective, substance use during this period of life contains a twofold danger. First, for a subset of TAY, substances themselves may become integrated as foundational aspects of identity, especially in peer groups or relationships in which the procuring and using of substances takes on a central role. Second, and more insidiously, substance use may become integrated into young peoples' understanding of social interactions, recreational activities, and romantic relationships, making it hard to disentangle the pleasure and joy of relationships themselves from the reinforcing and ultimately maladaptive effects of substances. TAY suffering from anxiety, depression, or other psychiatric comorbidities may be particularly susceptible to these effects.

Neurocognitive Developmental Vulnerabilities

TAY also face a set of cognitive developmental discrepancies which appear to increase the risk associated with substance use. As described in a review by [11], human and animal studies have shown evidence of differential brain development in adolescence and young adulthood, with "bottom-up" limbic circuits (including the mesolimbic circuit, which is instrumental in addiction and response to reward) developing earlier than higher cortical/frontal circuits which govern planning and impulse control. In other words, the "gas pedal" areas of the brain – those involved in processing rewards and motivating further reward-seeking – reach maturity before the "brakes," those areas that help to inhibit impulsive action and weigh the risks involved in substance use and other risky behaviors, are fully developed. This may provide a neurobiological basis for increased vulnerability to problematic substance use and risky behaviors among adolescents and young adults.

Legal Status, Consent, and Family Support

Changes in legal status during the transitional years have significant implications for treatment. In most instances, family involvement remains a key component to treatment for SUDs among TAY. However, practitioners must be vigilant of the way in which this family involvement is introduced and managed and must be familiar with the consent laws that govern the provision of substance use treatment for TAY.

For TAY in the age of majority, consent is required for engaging family for non-emergent treatment, as for any other psychiatric or medical condition. Complications arise in the treatment of minors; consent law for the treatment of minors with problematic substance use varies by state, and practitioners should familiarize themselves with existing local statues. As a general overview, Kerwin et al. [47] surveyed the patchwork national landscape of consent laws and found that, at that time, 45 states accepted minor consent (or accepted consent from *either* the minor patient *or* a parent) for outpatient SUD treatment. Further complicating things, the age definitions of "minor" varied by state, with the lower limit of majority age ranging from ages 12 to 16 years. Given variable laws regarding consent, this is a complex and highly geographically specific issue with important implications for treatment.

Notwithstanding the details of consent laws, the involvement of family supports is a potentially delicate affair in this population. Though we strongly recommend family involvement, unless there is a clinical emergency which requires immediately contacting family, we generally recommend a collaborative approach, wherein TAY are invited in one-on-one discussion to share any concerns they have about family involvement and are given an opportunity to explore the pros and cons of such involvement in a supported environment. In addition, TAY may agree to consent for contact with families about certain specific topics such as scheduling appointments and confirming attendance, which can give an opening to family involvement in treatment. In conversations with TAY about consent for family contact, it is often helpful to draw guidance from the spirit and techniques of motivational interviewing [57], utilizing respectful and reflective listening to draw out ambivalence and supporting the aspects of family involvement which might be of immediate or direct benefit. For instance, reducing tension and arguments with parents, unburdening oneself of anxiety-producing secrets, and eliciting more effective support from worried family members can be valuable goals to our patients. For many TAY, reframing family involvement as a way to channel existing parental anxieties into more directed and purposeful support, with the patient in the "driver's seat" as a central stakeholder in the treatment rather than a passive recipient of diffuse worry, is an appealing idea. These conversations are often best introduced in a treatment setting with a caring provider as facilitator.

Even for TAY with significant ambivalence about family involvement, or for families of TAY who are not yet willing to engage in treatment, we have found great benefit from offering separate parental education and supports as part of a comprehensive outpatient treatment program. Facilitated family education and support groups allow for parents to learn about the general principles of SUDs, communication strategies, and treatment and to gain support from families facing the challenge of supporting loved ones in the TAY age range struggling with substance use. The fact that these groups do not include the transmission of any confidential information about patients by the treatment team allows for them to operate in parallel with the individual treatment planning for TAY – they serve as an augmentation rather than replacement for direct family involvement in the treatment.

Educational Status

The transitional years represent the first time of life at which diversity of educational and vocational endeavors is the rule rather than the exception. Differences in substance misuse have been found between TAY who go on to graduate high school and attend college and those who do not. Non-college attending TAY are more likely to have non-alcohol SUDs and have worse SUD treatment outcomes than their college-attending peers [8]. Schepis et al. [79] revealed that prescription opioid misuse was higher among non-school attending young adults and particularly those who did not complete high school, while conversely prescription stimulant misuse was highest among full-time college students and college graduates. These findings also highlight the importance of peer environment given that TAY are more likely to obtain substances from peers and family members rather than from a physician or other source [78]. This college/non-college dichotomy is likely a superficial marker for a much more complex set of risk factors related to family structures, socioeconomic status, peer environments, and many other factors; however, clinicians should be aware of the implications of the college/non-college dichotomy as they go about formulating individual patient cases.

Initial Clinical Approach to Problematic Substance Use Among TAY

General Approach

In approaching the clinical treatment of SUDs among TAY, it is important to highlight that *context matters*. The approach taken by a primary care provider during an annual well-check will differ from the approach of a specialist seeing a patient referred specifically for SUD treatment, with infinite variations in between. Some settings may call for screening, brief intervention, and referral to specialty care, while others will call for more comprehensive substance use history-taking, formulation, and longitudinal treatment. The availability of specialty SUD treatment services varies widely by region, meaning that a case which might be overseen by a SUD specialist in one part of the country may be managed by a primary care doctor or general psychiatrist in another.

Screening

Given the high prevalence and significant sequelae of problematic substance use among TAY, screening for substance use should be routine practice for providers seeing TAY in a wide range of contexts including outpatient, inpatient, and emergency department visits. Screening allows providers to quickly and reliably identify youth who are at risk for developing SUDs, monitor for concerning changes in substance use over time, and triage those who have already developed problematic use for further treatment. In fact, the Substance Abuse and Mental Health Services Administration has recommended broad screening for substance use as a cornerstone of the Screening, Brief Intervention, and Referral to Treatment (SBIRT) approach (more information available at samhsa.gov/sbirt). There are a number of screening tools approved for this population, each with distinct features which aid in selection depending upon context. Though a number of screening tools including the Screening to Brief Intervention (S2BI), the NIAAA's Adolescent Substance Abuse Subtle Screening Inventory-A2 (SASSI A2), and the Brief Screener for Tobacco, Alcohol and Other Drugs (BSTAD) are validated for adolescent substance use screening, here we will focus on screening tools validated or studied for TAY substance use specifically or for both adolescent and adult substance use. Please see Table 6.1 for an overview of screening tools.

Several tools screen for use of alcohol, the most common substance of use among TAY. The CAGE screening tool, which asks about problematic patterns of alcohol use, has high sensitivity and specificity with adolescent reporting and parent reporting of the CAGE questions [25]. The Alcohol Use Disorders Identification Test (AUDIT) and its abbreviated counterpart – the AUDIT-C – have shown efficacy in youth after modifications such as changing the wording to adapt the screener to a youth population [18, 74]. Other researchers have found that adjusting the cut-point of the AUDIT produces more reliable results in younger age groups. For adolescents, a cut-point of 2 can be used to identify an alcohol

Table 6.1 Substance use screening tools for TAY

Tool	Substances screened	Population	Administration method
S2BI	Alcohol and drugs	Adolescents and adults	Self-report or clinician
SASSI A2	Alcohol	Adolescents and adults	Self-report
BSTAD	Alcohol and drugs	Adults	Self-report or clinician
CAGE	Alcohol	Adults	Clinician
AUDIT	Alcohol	Adults	Clinician
CRAFFT	Alcohol and drugs	Adolescents	Self-report or clinician
NIDA-Modified Assist	Alcohol and drugs	Adolescents[a] and adults	Clinician

[a]Adolescent modifier available

problem, while a cut-point of 3 suggests disordered use [49]. For TAY ages 18–20, a cut-point of 10 may be more appropriate [46].

Comprehensive substance use screening tools include the CRAFFT which more broadly queries about substance use within the last 12 months and assesses impairment related to substance use. Another comprehensive tool useful with TAY is the NIDA-Modified Assist, which additionally allows for an Adolescent Modifier [65].

Diagnosis

Diagnosis of a SUD is based upon DSM-5 criteria [2]. As described in the DSM, the criteria can be broken down into five categories, impaired control, social impairment, risky use, tolerance, and withdrawal, with 11 total criteria spread among these categories. A diagnosis of SUD can be made with only two symptoms from this list within a 12-month period. According to the DSM, mild SUD is characterized by the presence of 2–3 symptoms, moderate by 4–5 symptoms, and severe by 6 or more symptoms. There are no differences between the diagnostic criteria for adolescents and adults. Winters et al. [97] have also noted that criteria related to tolerance, withdrawal, and hazardous use may have limited or developmentally mediated applicability to adolescent substance use which might lead to underdiagnosis, while the two-criteria threshold for SUD may lead to overdiagnosis in the adolescent population. Despite these and other valid caveats, the DSM remains the gold standard for diagnosis of SUD in TAY populations.

Assessment and Formulation

Assessment of Functional Impairment

For those youth screening positive for problematic substance use or meeting criteria for SUD, it is helpful to gather further objective data to assess for severity of illness and impairment. In addition to the DSM thresholds for SUD severity, the Global Assessment of Individual Needs (GAIN) provides a range of instruments, from brief screening to comprehensive biopsychosocial assessment, which can assist in viewing substance use in the larger context of overall functioning and psychiatric and physical health. The American Society of Addiction Medicine (ASAM) offers a text entitled *The ASAM Criteria: Treatment Criteria for Addictive, Substance-Related, and Co-Occurring Conditions*, which also contains resources for assessing functional impairment related to substance use.

History and Formulation

Though each TAY will bring different specifics in terms of life experiences, type and severity of substance use, and complicating factors, we find that the areas listed in Fig. 6.5 are a good starting place for gaining a comprehensive view of the challenges and strengths TAY bring to treatment. Given the sensitive nature of much of this information and the common challenges of mistrust or ambivalence on the part of TAY early in treatment, it is expected that some of this information may not be available or may only be discussed in a limited fashion, until a trusting treatment relationship is established.

Toxicology Screening

Toxicology screening can provide further useful data in the initial assessment and in follow-up. Objective toxicological testing can assist in identifying additional substances of use which have not yet been disclosed, help to clarify patterns of use and abstinence, and provide further information on adherence patterns to prescribed controlled substances. As with any test, of course, the interpretation of results is critical. Clinicians should be familiar with issues related to (1) confirmation of results, (2) timing of positive results,

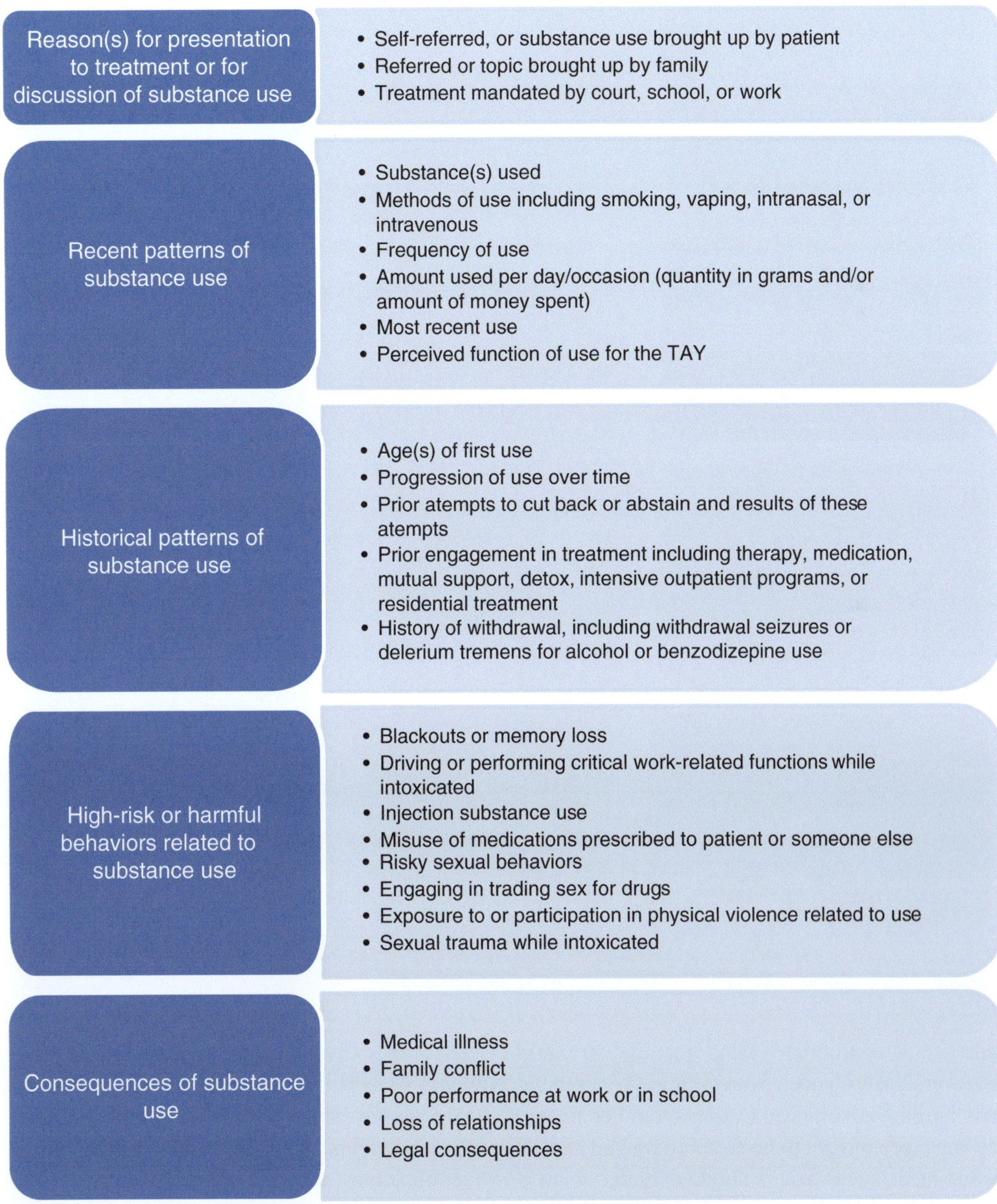

Fig. 6.5 Salient categories for history and formulation of SUD in TAY, with examples

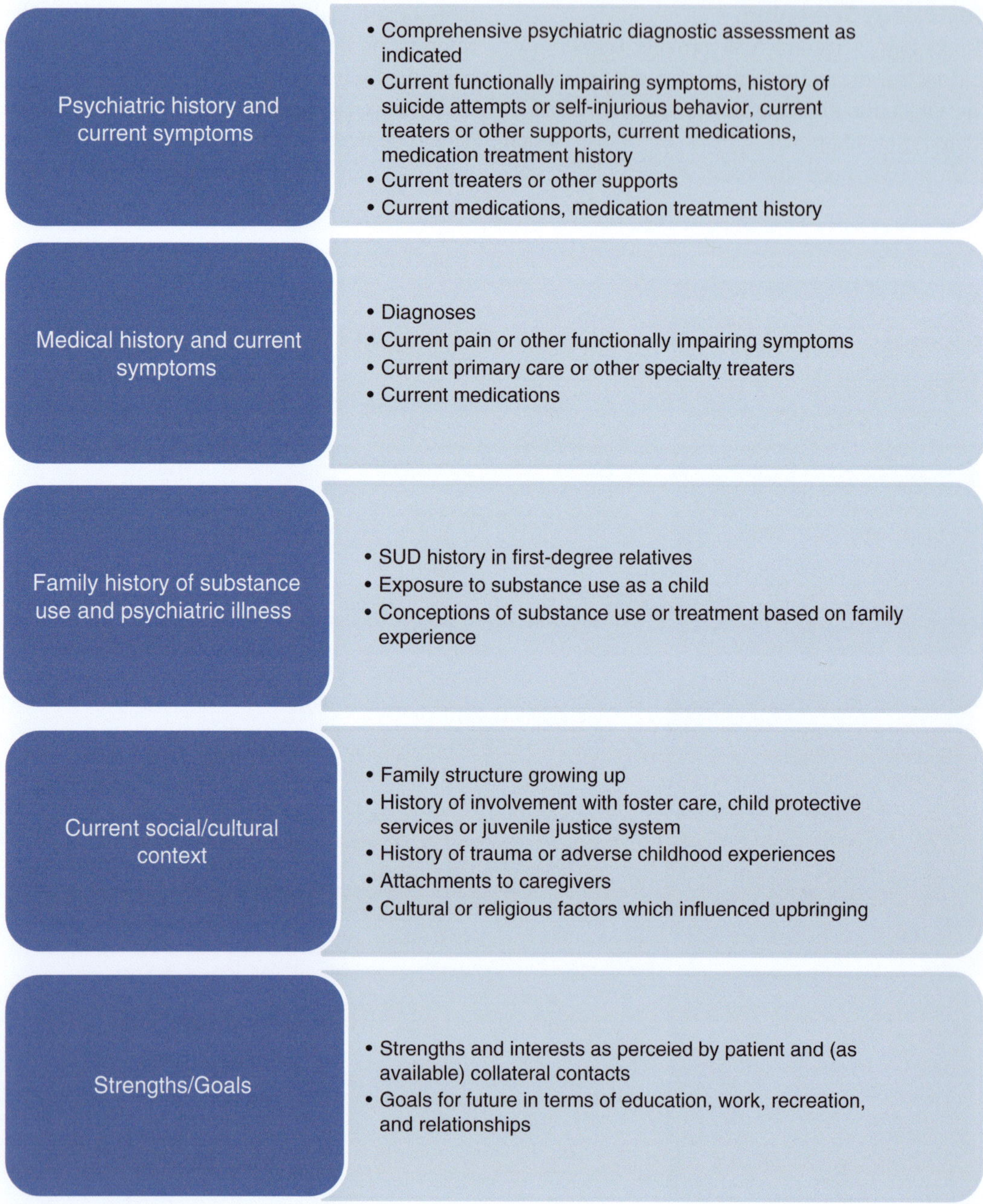

Fig. 6.5 (continued)

and (3), as appropriate, using quantitative markers to track substance use over time. As a general note, urine toxicological testing should be treated as one piece of data to be factored into an overall assessment, rather than a single defining or overriding source of objective data. If questions arise, laboratory personnel can often be very helpful with specific questions about results or procedures related to toxicological testing, including issues related to best practices for obtaining, storing, and ensuring integrity of urine samples, as well as interpretations of study results. As an alternative, clinicians may use structured interviews as a means of establishing diagnoses as they have been found to have high sensitivity, specificity, and agreement with urine toxicology screens [35].

Confirmatory Testing

Due to cost, efficiency of testing, and relative ease of use, most initial toxicological screenings are performed by urine immunoassay. For patients who are well-known and for whom results match with reported use, this can be an efficient and effective method of screening. However, providers should be aware of the potential for false-positive results based on cross-reactivity between prescribed or over-the-counter medications and substances of misuse. Cross-reactivity is a complex issue given differences between available immunoassay kits and variable levels of guidance on this issue in the literature and immunoassay package inserts [76]. Consultation with local laboratory personnel is likely to be quite helpful in determining common patterns of cross-reactivity for a particular immunoassay kit. Given this possibility of false-positive results, for new patients or those for whom there is a discrepancy between subjective reporting and urine immunoassay results, it is useful to obtain confirmatory testing via urine gas chromatography-mass spectrometry (GC-MS) testing as available. GC-MS testing is considered the gold standard for confirmatory testing and can provide clarity in difficult situations when there is concern for false-positive results on immunoassay. Downsides include a time delay in obtaining results and increased cost of GC-MS testing. Toxicology testing can additionally be done with alternative biological samples including serum, saliva, hair, and meconium. The window of detection of substance use, types of substances detected, and cost of testing varies by sample type, and practitioners should consult with local laboratory representatives to clarify these parameters as needed.

Timing

Since urine toxicological screening is a cross-sectional, point-in-time measure, clinicians should be familiar with rough guidelines for the timing of positive and negative results, to better understand the meaning of what they are and, as importantly, are not seeing in urine toxicology results.

With the caveat that individual metabolism, pharmacokinetics, duration and frequency of use, and other factors can influence timing of results, Moeller et al. [61] provide a summary of rough guidelines for detection times for various substances, listed in Table 6.1. Within these timeframes, we would expect that urine immunoassay would return positive for the substances listed. These should be taken more as rough guides than as set-in-stone and should not take the place of confirmatory testing. Particularly of note is the apparent wide variation in half-life of increasingly prevalent synthetic substances of misuse such as fentanyl, a synthetic opioid which in clinical experience appears to have a significantly longer half-life than other short-acting opioids such as heroin. Examples such as these remind us that clinicians must remain aware of regional trends in substances of misuse and novel substances and forms of ingestion which might affect the interpretation of test results (Table 6.2).

Table 6.2 Urine immunoassay detection times of common substances

Substance	Duration of detectability in urine
Alcohol	7–12 hours
Amphetamine/ methamphetamine	48 hours
Benzodiazepine (short-acting, e.g., lorazepam)	3 days
Benzodiazepine (long-acting, e.g., diazepam)	30 days
Cocaine metabolites	2–4 days
Marijuana:	
Single use	3 days
4× per week	5–7 days
Daily use	10–15 days
Long-term, heavy use	>30 days
Opioids[a]*:*	
Codeine	48 hours
Heroin	48 hours
Methadone	3 days
Oxycodone	2–4 days

Adapted from [60]

[a]Of note, some immunoassays list results for *opiates*, meaning naturally derived substances such as morphine and heroin (which is semisynthetic but metabolized to morphine), and report separately or exclude synthetic or semisynthetic *opioids* such as oxycodone, hydromorphone, fentanyl, methadone, or buprenorphine, which may be tested for separately

Quantitative Measures

For some substances, a quantitative measure of drug level can provide meaningful information for longitudinal tracking. We have found this particularly true for marijuana, for which, as Table 6.2 shows, urine toxicological screening can be quite nonspecific when it comes to heavy use. For tracking progression in treatment for marijuana use, quantitative test results can be more useful as a relative measure rather than an absolute one – that is, given variability in potency, delivery method, and use patterns, it is most useful to obtain a baseline quantitative delta-9-tetrahydrocannabinol level and compare subsequent measures against this baseline to track an individual's changes in use, rather than comparing cross-sectional levels across patients. As with GC-MS confirmatory testing, the potential downsides here are the delay to receiving results and the cost of quantitative testing.

Medical Screening and Prevention

Given the higher likelihood of risk factors for infectious diseases and other medical illness among youth with problematic substance use, clinicians should screen for high-risk activities such as intravenous substance use and unprotected sex and should routinely screen for HIV, hepatitis B and C, sexually transmitted infections, and pregnancy in youth with elevated risk. In addition, a discussion of sexual practices and contraception can play a prominent role in these discussions, and a frank discussion of the risk of unintended pregnancy can at times be an additional motivator for behavior change.

The CDC recommends prophylactic treatment for HIV, known as pre-exposure prophylaxis, or PrEP, for youth with significantly elevated risk of HIV infection, such as those having unprotected sex (especially with partners known to have HIV or at high risk for HIV) or patients recently diagnosed with sexually transmitted infections [15]. These medications can be prescribed by a psychiatrist, or patients can be referred to their primary care clinician for treatment.

Treatment of Substance Use Disorders and Comorbid Conditions Among TAY

Levels of Care

After triaging for and addressing any emergent concerns, one of the first major questions that arises in addressing problematic substance use is the appropriate level of care. This decision relies on multiple factors, including the severity of use, the level of engagement/motivation of the patient, the availability of external supports, the presence or absence of comorbid medical or psychiatric illness, and the availability of local resources. Common levels of care for TAY SUD are described below. For more detailed information on levels of care, the American Society of Addiction Medicine (ASAM) offers a text entitled *The ASAM Criteria: Treatment Criteria for Addictive, Substance-Related, and Co-Occurring Conditions* which offers further detail and assistance in triaging for levels of care. For a searchable database of local resources, SAMHSA's Behavioral Health Treatment Services Locator can be accessed online through SAMHSA's website, samhsa.gov.

Outpatient SUD Treatment

Outpatient care is the "backbone" of a comprehensive treatment plan. Care is delivered in a general practice or specialty SUD setting, with varying availability of wraparound services, potentially including individual therapy, psychopharmacological and general medical services, individual and family treatment groups, parent guidance, case management, social work services, and peer recovery supports. Treatment approaches vary depending upon the program and may incorporate elements of motivational enhancement, contingency management, community reinforcement, twelve-step facilitation, or others. The frequency of treatment varies widely depending upon severity of illness and availability of resources, and the duration of treatment is generally indefinite. Patients can be "stepped up" to higher levels of care as needed and then return to their outpatient treatment team for ongoing longitudinal care.

Partial Hospitalization/Intensive Outpatient Programs

Partial Hospitalization Programs and Intensive Outpatient Programs (PHPs and IOPs, respectively) are outpatient programs which provide more intensive and time-limited treatment. Patients generally attend treatment for 3–5 days or portions of days per week (requiring transportation to and from treatment and a place to stay in the evenings), with treatment lasting on the order of weeks. Of particular note is the fact that IOPs generally focus specifically on SUD treatment, while PHPs are generally able to provide broader "dual-diagnosis" treatment for SUD and co-occurring psychiatric disorders, given the high rates of co-occurring psychiatric illness in TAY with SUD. This level of care acts as an intermediate step between outpatient clinic and inpatient hospitalization and potentially allows for patients to participate in school, work, or family activities during treatment (depending on the hours of programming).

Medically Monitored Detoxification

Medically monitored detoxification ("detox") is an acute inpatient setting which allows for monitored and medication-assisted treatment of withdrawal from substances including alcohol, opioids, and benzodiazepines. These programs are time-limited and focus on physiological detoxification, with widely variable access to wraparound services and ability to link to ongoing care.

Inpatient Dual Diagnosis

Inpatient dual diagnosis facilities are acute inpatient settings which ideally allow for medically monitored detoxification and simultaneous treatment of co-occurring psychiatric disorders. Of note is the fact that, due to high demand and relatively limited length of stay, the ability to assess and treat longitudinal psychiatric conditions and assess responses to treatment may be limited in these settings. Compared with pure medically monitored detoxification settings, dual diagnosis units tend to have greater access to social work and case management for referral to ongoing residential or outpatient care upon discharge, as well as clinical treatment staff with experience diagnosing and treating psychiatric illness.

Residential Treatment

Residential SUD treatment programs are generally longer-term settings which allow for patients to gain skills and pursue recovery in a stable and controlled environment. In general, these settings tend to be particularly useful for patients with high-risk or chaotic social environments. Residential treatment programs are extremely variable in terms of length of stay; treatment orientation; approach to and acceptance of medically assisted SUD treatment; availability of psychiatric or medical treatment, additional wrap-around services, or family supports; and acceptance of insurance for payment. In general, patients and outpatient providers should be sure to investigate potential residential treatment programs thoroughly along these axes, to ensure that the treatment philosophy and logistical components of the program match patient, family, and provider goals for residential treatment.

Outpatient Treatment Interventions

Regardless of the exact theoretical background of a treatment program, treatment for problematic substance use for TAY is ideally a comprehensive, multidisciplinary endeavor involving some combination of individual therapy, pharmacological consultation/management, family work, group work, peer recovery supports, and case management. Though not all TAY will require all of these interventions, having access to services in each of these areas allows for a tailored and flexible approach to treatment for the majority of patients. Given high rates of co-occurring psychiatric illness in TAY with SUD, all new TAY patients should be screened for co-occurring conditions, with recommendations for ongoing psychiatric care as appropriate. In addition, given the complex and at times frustrating nature of this work, having a multidisciplinary team to share delegation of work and collaborate on solving difficult issues helps to prevent burnout among providers and encourages a well-rounded approach to treatment. In general, given the trend of variable motivation to change and the developmental and neurocognitive factors previously described, treatment tends to focus on a "harm reduction" model, in which emphasis is placed on reducing risky and problematic substance use rather than on strict abstinence from substances.

Psychosocial and Therapy-Based Interventions

The guiding spirit and approach of motivational interviewing [57] is a useful framework for encounters focused on SUD among TAY, regardless of the context or specific goals. There is a great deal of high-quality writing and training about motivational interviewing available – as a start, basic references and links to training can be found at the website of the Motivational Interviewing Network of Trainers, motivationalinterviewing.org. Briefly, the approach outlined by Miller and Rollnick emphasizes the importance of taking a respectful, collaborative, nonjudgmental, and compassionate approach to these conversations, seeking to draw out the patient's motivations for change and supporting these motivations with targeted assistance. These conversations are built on a bedrock of engagement and active listening, with the provider seeking permission to provide pertinent information, referrals, or treatment planning as appropriate. Especially given the developmental factors outlined previously in this chapter – most notably the high value many TAY place on autonomy – paternalistic or punitive approaches are unlikely to be productive and run the risk of increasing resistance and/or avoidance of treatment altogether.

Compared with the research on treatment programs for adolescents and adults, the evidence base for treatment of problematic substance use among TAY is relatively sparse. However, studies point toward particular outpatient interventions which have promise and possible alterations to existing treatments that take into account the unique developmental needs of TAY.

The Adolescent Community Reinforcement Approach (A-CRA) [36] is a skills-based approach focused on working with adolescents in the context of their social support networks by supporting prosocial activities and improving family communication. It involves work both with adolescents and their families, separately and together, and has been shown to be an effective intervention for adolescents [27]. However, results with TAY have been more mixed. Smith et al. [84] found that this intervention was less effective for emerging adults than for adolescents in an adolescent-focused treatment program. In a later study, Smith et al. [83] found that A-CRA with an enhanced peer-support element resulted in better outcomes than standard A-CRA for a population of emerging adults.

Contingency management (CM) is a model based on operant conditioning, which generally involves providing rewards (or the possibility of reward) for positive treatment outcomes such as attendance, negative urine toxicology screens, or other desired goals. Stanger et al. [86] reviewed the literature on the use of CM with adolescent patients and found generally positive results, at least during the course of active treatment. Though little research focuses on the application of CM to TAY populations, elements of this approach are often adapted into individual and family work with TAY, leveraging desired outcomes, privileges, and rewards to motivate engagement in treatment and progress toward treatment goals.

For college students, the brief alcohol screening intervention for college students (BASICS), a brief face-to-face intervention, has been shown in a review [31] to lower alcohol consumption and negative consequences related to alcohol use.

Bergman et al. [6] outline general modifications to outpatient approaches to better meet the needs of TAY with problematic substance use, which can be applied widely across theoretical approaches. These modifications include moving toward a harm-reduction approach as opposed to an abstinence-only approach, offering alternative means of communication such as text messaging (as appropriate and after review of relevant privacy-related issues), engaging support systems separately through parent coaching/guidance, and finding ways to positively intervene on patients' social networks. These modifications seek to recognize and respect the issues of autonomy, developing social and legal status, and changing family relationships as highlighted previously in this chapter.

Pharmacological Interventions

In general, even for medications which have FDA approval for adult populations, use in young adult populations (ages 18–25 years) is relatively less well-studied. Providers should be familiar with the range of FDA-approved and off-label medications used to treat problematic substance use among TAY. Squeglia et al. [85] compiled a review of pharmacological treatments for youth SUD; in addition, for clinicians seeking more information including guidelines, trainings, and resources on medication management of SUDs targeted to general practitioners, the SAMHSA-funded Providers Clinical Support System is a resource. Here, we will offer a brief overview of evidence-based psychopharmacological treatments specific to TAY SUD.

Alcohol Use Disorder

Naltrexone, an opioid receptor antagonist, is FDA-approved for the treatment of alcohol use disorder (and, as will be discussed subsequently, opioid use disorder) in patients ages 18 years and above. The putative mechanism for the effect of naltrexone on drinking has to do with modulation of the endogenous opioid and downstream dopamine reward system, which is activated by alcohol use. A small study of naltrexone in adolescents ages 15–19 years completed by Miranda et al. [58] showed that a short course of naltrexone led to reduced levels of drinking, heavy drinking, and craving for alcohol among treated adolescents. A study of naltrexone among young adults ages 18–25 with binge-pattern alcohol use completed by O'Malley et al. [70] showed no reduction in total drinking days or frequency of drinking, but did show reduction of drinks per occasion in the young adults taking naltrexone. This result suggests potential for use of naltrexone in populations with problematic binge alcohol use, including college-attending young adults.

Opioid Use Disorder

Buprenorphine, commonly prescribed as Suboxone (buprenorphine/naloxone), is a partial opioid agonist which is FDA-approved for the treatment of opioid use disorder (OUD) for youth ages 16 years and above. In addition to the evidence base for buprenorphine in the treatment of adult OUD, [54] showed that a 28-day buprenorphine detoxification resulted in significantly better retention in treatment and reduced use of opioids compared with clonidine detoxification in a group of adolescents ages 16–18 years. Among TAY, two studies have shown that a longer duration of buprenorphine treatment – 12 weeks vs 14 days in a study Woody et al. [98] and 56 days vs 28 days in a study by Marsch et al. [55] – resulted in better retention in treatment and decreased opioid use. Putting these results together, evidence suggests that buprenorphine is effective in treating OUD among younger populations and that a relatively longer period of treatment has better results than a rapid detoxification and taper among TAY. However, despite these promising results, it is important to note that TAY have been shown to have significantly lower retention in buprenorphine treatment and generally worse outcomes as compared to older adult populations [80], suggesting that TAY may need a different approach. Buprenorphine has recently been approved in a once-monthly, long-acting injectable form which may reduce barriers to adherence, though studies on outcomes of treatment with this new formulation among TAY are needed.

Naltrexone is an opioid receptor agonist which is available in both oral and long-acting injectable form and is FDA-approved for the treatment of OUD for those ages 18 years and above. A small case series by Fishman et al. [33] suggested that long-acting injectable naltrexone could have promise for decreased opioid use among TAY. Innovative models of care delivery for naltrexone extended release are currently being studied, including home-based administration of the medication, to improve TAY retention in OUD treatment [94].

Cannabis Use Disorder

N-Acetylcysteine (NAC) is a natural compound available over-the-counter in the United States that is thought to modulate the glutamate system, which is active in reward processing and craving. In a study completed by Gray et al. [40], youth ages 15–21 years treated with NAC had significant reductions in positive urine cannabis screening compared with controls during the treatment period. A subsequent study of NAC for cannabis use disorder in adults ages 18–50 years [41] showed no significant effect of NAC on cannabis use across this broad adult population; however, a small subgroup analysis of results among participants ages 18–21 years showed positive results consistent with the prior study in adolescents (though the study was not powered to show statistical significance for this subgroup). These results suggest that NAC may be a uniquely effective intervention for youth with cannabis use disorder; research into this question is ongoing.

Recovery Supports

Peer relationships are important for TAY, and social interactions and events often become intimately linked to substance use for many TAY struggling with SUDs. As TAY with SUD begin to make changes in their substance use, they may feel socially isolated and often need formal support to identify options for social activities that do not involve substance use. In recognition of this, the ACRA protocol includes procedures focused on understanding barriers to prosocial activities and formally helps TAY identify activities of interest to them [36].

Organized groups such as peer-led mutual help organizations and recovery high school and college programs can facilitate TAY engagement with activities that support recovery and peers who are not using substances. The mutual help 12-step program Alcoholics Anonymous has groups specifically for young people and is the largest mutual help organization in the United States with over 65,000 groups in the United States and Canada. Active involvement in a mutual help group has been shown to be as beneficial for TAY as it is for older adults [45]. Active involvement includes identifying oneself as a member of a mutual help group, sharing at the meeting, and having a sponsor. In contrast to mutual help organizations, formal recovery support within the academic setting is less commonly available but quickly growing with increased recognition of the importance of this type of recovery support for TAY. Recovery high schools promote recovery and provide academic as well as therapeutic support in a structured setting. These schools are generally small and are often embedded structurally and organizationally within another school or another set of alternative school programs [59]. Collegiate recovery programs have been developing independently on college campuses and can therefore vary in the structure and support provided [51]. Services can include drug and alcohol-free housing, on-site peer-led meetings, and counseling.

Psychiatric Comorbidities

SUD and psychiatric disorders commonly co-occur, particularly in the TAY population. In 2017 2.4 million TAY in the United States had a co-occurring SUD and psychiatric disorder [90]. Rates of substance use are significantly higher in adults with a psychiatric disorder when compared to those without. For example, the prevalence of past-year illicit drug use was 16% for adults without a mental illness, 37% for those with any mental illness, and 49% for those with a serious mental illness [90]. Among individuals in treatment, the prevalence of co-occurring SUD and psychiatric disorders is higher in individuals in SUD treatment relative to individuals in mental health treatment. Nonetheless, since the prevalence of SUD in TAY in mental health treatment is significantly higher than the prevalence of SUD in TAY with no psychiatric disorder, it is important to identify and treat co-occurring disorders in both settings.

Substance use can cause psychiatric symptoms both when an individual is intoxicated and while they are experiencing withdrawal symptoms. For example, acute intoxication with cannabis, particularly cannabis products with high levels of tetrahydrocannabinol, can cause anxiety and paranoia [95]. Symptoms of cannabis withdrawal also include anxiety, irritability, depressed mood, and insomnia. It is therefore important to determine if an individual had psychiatric symptoms and/or a disorder before ever using substances and whether the psychiatric symptoms persist during periods with no substance use. There is a higher likelihood that an individual has a co-occurring psychiatric disorder as opposed to a substance-induced psychiatric disorder if psychiatric symptoms predate substance use and have been present in the absence of substance use and/or the individual has a family history of the same psychiatric disorder [28]. Regardless of whether the psychiatric disorder is co-occurring with the SUD or is substance induced, clinicians need to consider co-occurring psychiatric symptoms when engaging TAY in SUD treatment. For example, symptoms of anxiety may impact a TAY's willingness to engage in group therapy, or symptoms of depression may impact their motivation to follow up with treatment recommendations. TAY with SUD and psychiatric symptoms also benefit from close monitoring, since research indicates some substance-induced psychiatric disorders can transition to a co-occurring psychiatric disorder over time. For example, one registry study found 24–32% of individuals with substance-induced psychosis subsequently developed a schizophrenia spectrum disorder or bipolar disorder [87].

Treatment for co-occurring SUD and psychiatric disorders in TAY should address both disorders simultaneously through integrated treatment, ideally by the same clinician or clinical team. Although there have been treatments developed for adults that address both disorders simultaneously, such as group therapy for adults with bipolar disorder and a co-occurring SUD [96], to our knowledge, similar protocols have not been developed for TAY. Integrated treatment in TAY therefore involves evaluating the role for medication and therapy for both the SUD and psychiatric disorder and considering the influence of one disorder on treatment targeted to the other disorder. For example, when prescribing medication, clinicians should consider the risk for adverse effects if TAY misuse substances while taking the prescribed medication. Or, as noted above, clinicians might consider how psychiatric symptoms may impact engagement in SUD treatment. Treatment for one disorder can also influence both disorders, and evidence-based therapies for SUD, such as cognitive behavioral therapy, have been shown to improve symptoms of the SUD and psychiatric disorder in adolescents with co-occurring disorders such as major depressive disorder [20–22, 26] and attention-deficit/hyperactivity disorder [77]. More research is needed to evaluate the role of pharmacotherapy for TAY with co-occurring disorders. However, medication for psychiatric disorders should not be arbitrarily withheld because of the presence of substance misuse or a co-occurring SUD. Furthermore, particularly for co-occurring psychiatric disorders with moderate to severe impairment, the risks and benefits of medication as part of a multimodal treatment plan for the co-occurring disorders should be reviewed. Finally, consideration should be given to safeguarding, storage, and management of medications, utilizing the TAY patient's available supports and/or guardians as appropriate.

Special Populations

Homeless and Unstably Housed TAY

Homelessness among TAY is a widespread problem, with a national prevalence of homelessness of over 4% for families with youth aged 13–17 years and nearly 10% for young adults aged 18–25 years [63]. Substance use is disproportionately common in this population [4, 30, 48] and is linked to a range of negative outcomes including higher rates of trauma and post-traumatic stress disorder (PTSD) [5]; sexual risk behavior and sexual victimization [44]; comorbid psychiatric illness including mood disorders, ADHD, anxiety disorders, and conduct disorder [64, 82]; incarceration [68]; and poor perceived physical health [69]. While the search for effective interventions to target substance use among homeless TAY is an active area of research, a recent Cochrane review found no consistent benefit from previously evaluated focused therapeutic interventions on substance misuse in this population as compared with standard drop-in and case management services [19]. These results highlight the need for further development and evaluation of services for SUD treatment in this highly vulnerable population.

Immigrant and Culturally Underrepresented TAY

The effects of immigration on youth substance use are complex. In what has been termed the "immigrant paradox," studies have found that first-generation immigrant youth are less likely to use substances than their non-immigrant counterparts, but that their substance use tends to increase to match non-immigrant peer use with increased exposure to US American society [7, 34]. This effect appears to be mediated by a wide range of factors including family and school environments and in one study was shown to affect White, Hispanic, and Asian immigrants more than Black immigrants [10]. Also important to note is the fact that undocumented immigrants, including young people with Deferred Action for Childhood Arrivals (DACA) status, are not eligible for insurance through Medicare, Medicaid, or the Children's Health Insurance Program (CHIP), which can create significant barriers to accessing SUD care, though a small number of states do use state funds to provide care to children with undocumented status [3]. Though it should not affect treatment decision-making, providers should also be aware that, under federal immigration law, being a "drug abuser or addict" is potentially grounds for deportation of any immigrant to the United States [93] which may cause difficulty in outreaching and engaging undocumented youth and families in SUD treatment.

More broadly, research does show that youth in ethnic and cultural minority groups face barriers to treatment for SUDs. For instance, Black adolescents with SUDs are less likely to receive specialty SUD treatment services than their White counterparts, and Latinx adolescents are less likely to receive informal SUD services [1]. On a more hopeful note, a meta-analysis by Steinka-Fry et al. [88] showed that culturally sensitive SUD treatments can result in better outcomes for racial/ethnic minority youth, suggesting that targeted treatment interventions can help to overcome these disparities. In general, the literature in this area underscores the importance of incorporating an understanding of cultural factors and potential barriers into assessments and individualized SUD treatment plans for TAY in ethnic or cultural minority groups.

LGBTQ Youth

Sexual minority youth (SMY; a designation which includes those identifying lesbian, gay, and bisexual) have significantly higher rates of lifetime substance use compared with their heterosexual peers, with average rates of substance use being 190% higher in general among SMY and rates ranging to 340% higher for bisexual youth and 400% higher for female SMY [56]. Gender minority youth (GMY, including transgender and gender non-conforming youth) have 42–80% higher odds of past-year substance use compared with cisgender youth [75]. Further, gender- or sexuality-based harassment appears to independently contribute to higher rates of substance use among LGBT youth [23]. A recent review found only two prior studies of specialized SUD treatment for sexual and gender minorities [24], highlighting the need for further research into specialized treatments for SUD among LGBTQ youth.

Summary

TAY are at particularly high risk for problematic substance use given the complex intersection of developmental, neurocognitive, social, and legal factors which are active at this time of life. Substance use during these years can have significant and long-term consequences on health and well-being, but early intervention and engagement can improve outcomes for SUD treatment. Given the high prevalence of problematic substance use, all TAY should be screened for substance use and triaged to further care as appropriate. A range of evidence-based psychosocial and psychopharmacological interventions have been shown to be effective for problematic substance use among TAY, though engaging and retaining TAY in treatment may require a reorientation of practitioners and systems toward a harm reduction framework which can flex with TAY patients' developmentally normative ambivalence and variable motivation to change. Further, given significant levels of co-occurring psychiatric illness, all TAY with problematic substance use should be assessed for psychiatric illness and triaged to treatment as appropriate. As with many aspects of the treatment of TAY, treating problematic substance use in this population can be complex and challenging, but with the appropriate multidisciplinary approaches and patient-centered approach, it can also be incredibly rewarding for treaters and life-altering for patients and their families.

Acknowledgments This work was supported by the American Academy of Child and Adolescent Psychiatry Physician Scientist Program in Substance Abuse 5K12DA000357-17.

Dr. Colin Burke is currently receiving grant support from the Massachusetts General Hospital Louis V. Gerstner III Research Scholar Award and the Harvard Medical School Norman E. Zinberg Fellowship in Addiction Psychiatry Research.

Dr. Amy Yule received grant support from the Massachusetts General Hospital Louis V. Gerstner III Research Scholar Award from 2014 to 2016. Dr. Yule is currently receiving funding through the American Academy of Child and Adolescent Psychiatry Physician Scientist Program in Substance Abuse 5K12DA000357-17 and the NIH (NIDA). She was a consultant to Phoenix House from 2015 to 2017 and is currently a consultant to the Gavin House and Bay Cove Human Services (clinical service).

Dr. Timothy Wilens is Chief, Division of Child and Adolescent Psychiatry, and (Co-)Director of the Center for Addiction Medicine at Massachusetts General Hospital. He receives grant support from the following sources: NIH (NIDA) and Ironshore. Dr. Wilens has published a book, *Straight Talk About Psychiatric Medications for Kids* (Guilford Press), and co/edited books: *ADHD in Adults and Children* (Cambridge University Press), *Massachusetts General Hospital Comprehensive Clinical Psychiatry* (Elsevier), and *Massachusetts General Hospital Psychopharmacology and Neurotherapeutics* (Elsevier). Dr. Wilens is co-/owner of a copyrighted diagnostic questionnaire (Before School Functioning Questionnaire) and has a licensing agreement with Ironshore (BSFQ Questionnaire). He is or has been a consultant for Kempharm, Otsuka, Ironshore, and Vallon and serves as a clinical consultant to the US National Football League (ERM Associates), US Minor/Major League Baseball, Phoenix House, and Bay Cove Human Services.

Elizabeth Firmin has no conflicts of interest to report.

References

1. Alegria M, Carson NJ, Goncalves M, Keefe K. Disparities in treatment for substance use disorders and co-occurring disorders for ethnic/racial minority youth. J Am Acad Child Adolesc Psychiatry. 2011;50(1):22–31. https://doi.org/10.1016/j.jaac.2010.10.005.
2. American Psychiatric Association. Diagnostic and statistical manual of mental disorders: DSM-5. 5th ed. Arlington: American Psychiatric Publishing; 2013.
3. Artiga S, Diaz M. Health coverage and care of undocumented immigrants. 2019. Retrieved from https://www.kff.org/disparities-policy/issue-brief/health-coverage-and-care-of-undocumented-immigrants/.
4. Baer JS, Ginzler JA, Peterson PL. DSM-IV alcohol and substance abuse and dependence in homeless youth. J Stud Alcohol. 2003;64(1):5–14. https://doi.org/10.15288/jsa.2003.64.5.
5. Bender K, Ferguson K, Thompson S, Komlo C, Pollio D. Factors associated with trauma and posttraumatic stress disorder among homeless youth in three U.S. cities: the importance of transience. J Trauma Stress. 2010;23(1):161–8. https://doi.org/10.1002/jts.20501.
6. Bergman BG, Kelly J, Nargiso JE, McKowen JW. "The age of feeling in-between": addressing challenges in the treatment of emerging adults with substance use disorders. Cogn Behav Pract. 2015;23:270–88.

7. Blake SM, Ledsky R, Goodenow C, O'Donnell L. Recency of immigration, substance use, and sexual behavior among Massachusetts adolescents. Am J Public Health. 2001;91(5):794–8. https://doi.org/10.2105/ajph.91.5.794.
8. Blanco C, Okuda M, Wright C, Hasin DS, Grant BF, Liu SM, Olfson M. Mental health of college students and their non-college-attending peers: Results from the National Epidemiologic Study on Alcohol and Related Conditions. Arch Gen Psychiatry 2008;65(12):1429–37.
9. Bouchery EE, Harwood HJ, Sacks JJ, Simon CJ, Brewer RD. Economic costs of excessive alcohol consumption in the U.S., 2006. Am J Prev Med. 2011;41(5):516–24. https://doi.org/10.1016/j.amepre.2011.06.045.
10. Bui HN. Racial and ethnic differences in the immigrant paradox in substance use. J Immigr Minor Health. 2013;15(5):866–81. https://doi.org/10.1007/s10903-012-9670-y.
11. Casey BJ, Jones RM. Neurobiology of the adolescent brain and behavior: implications for substance use disorders. J Am Acad Child Adolesc Psychiatry. 2010;49(12):1189–201; quiz 1285. https://doi.org/10.1016/j.jaac.2010.08.017.
12. Castellanos-Ryan N, Pingault JB, Parent S, Vitaro F, Tremblay RE, Seguin JR. Adolescent cannabis use, change in neurocognitive function, and high-school graduation: a longitudinal study from early adolescence to young adulthood. Dev Psychopathol. 2017;29(4):1253–66. https://doi.org/10.1017/S0954579416001280.
13. Centers for Disease Control and Prevention. Motor vehicle injuries. 2017. Retrieved from https://www.cdc.gov/winnablebattles/report/motor.html.
14. Centers for Disease Control and Prevention. Surveillance for viral hepatitis – United States, 2015. 2017, 2017/06/19. Retrieved from https://www.cdc.gov/hepatitis/statistics/2015surveillance/index.htm.
15. Centers for Disease Control and Prevention. Preexposure prophylaxis for the prevention of HIV infection in the United States – 2017 update: a clinical practice guideline. 2018. Retrieved from https://www.cdc.gov/hiv/pdf/risk/prep/cdc-hiv-prep-provider-supplement-2017.pdf.
16. Centers for Disease Control and Prevention. HIV and youth. 2019, 2019/11/12. Retrieved from https://www.cdc.gov/hiv/group/age/youth/index.html.
17. Centers for Disease Control and Prevention. Motor vehicle safety: get the facts. 2019, 2019/03/22. Retrieved from www.cdc.gov/motorvehiclesafety/impaired_driving/impaired-drv_factsheet.html.
18. Chung T, Colby SM, Barnett NP, Rohsenow DJ, Spirito A, Monti PM. Screening adolescents for problem drinking: performance of brief screens against DSM-IV alcohol diagnoses. J Stud Alcohol. 2000;61(4):579–87. https://doi.org/10.15288/jsa.2000.61.579.
19. Coren E, Hossain R, Pardo Pardo J, Bakker B. Interventions for promoting reintegration and reducing harmful behaviour and lifestyles in street-connected children and young people. Cochrane Database Syst Rev. 2016;(1):CD009823. https://doi.org/10.1002/14651858.CD009823.pub3.
20. Cornelius JR, Bukstein OG, Douaihy AB, Clark DB, Chung TA, Daley DC, et al. Double-blind fluoxetine trial in comorbid MDD-CUD youth and young adults. Drug Alcohol Depend. 2010;112(1–2):39–45. S0376-8716(10)00184-5 [pii]. https://doi.org/10.1016/j.drugalcdep.2010.05.010.
21. Cornelius JR, Bukstein OG, Wood DS, Kirisci L, Douaihy A, Clark DB. Double-blind placebo-controlled trial of fluoxetine in adolescents with comorbid major depression and an alcohol use disorder. Addict Behav. 2009;34(10):905–9. https://doi.org/10.1016/j.addbeh.2009.03.008.
22. Cornelius JR, Douaihy AB, Kirisci L, Daley DC. Longer-term effectiveness of Cbt in treatment of comorbid Aud/Mdd adolescents. Int J Med Biol Front. 2013;19(2).
23. Coulter RWS, Bersamin M, Russell ST, Mair C. The effects of gender- and sexuality-based harassment on lesbian, gay, bisexual, and transgender substance use disparities. J Adolesc Health. 2018;62(6):688–700. https://doi.org/10.1016/j.jadohealth.2017.10.004.
24. Coulter RWS, Egan JE, Kinsky S, Friedman MR, Eckstrand KL., Frankeberger J, et al. Mental health, drug, and violence interventions for sexual/gender minorities: a systematic review. Pediatrics. 2019;144(3). https://doi.org/10.1542/peds.2018-3367.
25. Couwenbergh C, Van Der Gaag RJ, Koeter M, De Ruiter C, Van den Brink W. Screening for substance abuse among adolescents validity of the CAGE-AID in youth mental health care. Subst Use Misuse. 2009;44(6):823–34. https://doi.org/10.1080/10826080802484264.
26. Deas D, Randall CL, Roberts JS, Anton RF. A double-blind, placebo-controlled trial of sertraline in depressed adolescent alcoholics: a pilot study. Hum Psychopharmacol. 2000;15(6):461–9. https://doi.org/10.1002/1099-1077(200008)15:6<461::AID-HUP209>3.0.CO;2-J.
27. Dennis M, Godley SH, Diamond G, Tims FM, Babor T, Donaldson J, et al. The Cannabis Youth Treatment (CYT) study: main findings from two randomized trials. J Subst Abuse Treat. 2004;27(3):197–213.
28. Dennison SJ. Substance use disorders in individuals with co-occurring psychiatric disorders. In: Ruiz P, Strain EC, editors. Lowinson and Ruiz's substance abuse: a comprehensive textbook. 5th ed. Philadelphia: Lippincott Williams & Wilkins; 2011. p. 721–9.
29. Derakhshanfar H, Kalantari Meibodi M, Kariman H, Arhamidolatabadi A, Safari S. Substance abuse among drivers of motor vehicle collisions. Trauma Mon. 2012;17(1):236–8. https://doi.org/10.5812/traumamon.4182.
30. Edidin JP, Ganim Z, Hunter SJ, Karnik NS. The mental and physical health of homeless youth: a literature review. Child Psychiatry Hum Dev. 2012;43(3):354–75. https://doi.org/10.1007/s10578-011-0270-1.

31. Fachini A, Aliane PP, Martinez EZ, Furtado EF. Efficacy of brief alcohol screening intervention for college students (BASICS): a meta-analysis of randomized controlled trials. Subst Abuse Treat Prev Policy. 2012;7:40. https://doi.org/10.1186/1747-597X-7-40.
32. Fergusson DM, Boden JM. Cannabis use and later life outcomes. Addiction. 2008;103(6):969–76; discussion 977-968. https://doi.org/10.1111/j.1360-0443.2008.02221.x.
33. Fishman MJ, Winstanley EL, Curran E, Garrett S, Subramaniam G. Treatment of opioid dependence in adolescents and young adults with extended release naltrexone: preliminary case-series and feasibility. Addiction. 2010;105(9):1669–76. https://doi.org/10.1111/j.1360-0443.2010.03015.x.
34. Gfroerer JC, Tan LL. Substance use among foreign-born youths in the United States: does the length of residence matter? Am J Public Health. 2003;93(11):1892–5. https://doi.org/10.2105/ajph.93.11.1892.
35. Gignac M, Wilens TE, Biederman J, Kwon A, Mick E, Swezey A. Assessing cannabis use in adolescents and young adults: what do urine screen and parental report tell you? J Child Adolesc Psychopharmacol. 2005;15(5):742–50. https://doi.org/10.1089/cap.2005.15.742.
36. Godley SH, Meyers RJ, Smith JE, Karvinen T, Titus JC, Godley MD, et al. The adolescent community reinforcement approach for adolescent Cannabis users, Cannabis Youth Treatment (CYT). Retrieved from Substance Abuse and Mental Health Services Administration (DHHS/PHS). Rockville, MD: Center for Substance Abuse Treatment; 2001.
37. Gore FM, Bloem PJ, Patton GC, Ferguson J, Joseph V, Coffey C, Sawyer SM, Mathers CD. Global burden of disease in young people aged 10-24 years: A systematic analysis. Lancet 2011;377(9783):2093–102.
38. Grant BF, Dawson DA. Age at onset of alcohol use and its association with DSM-IV alcohol abuse and dependence: results from the National Longitudinal Alcohol Epidemiologic Survey. J Subst Abuse. 1997;9:103–10. https://doi.org/10.1016/s0899-3289(97)90009-2.
39. Grant BF, Dawson DA. Age of onset of drug use and its association with DSM-IV drug abuse and dependence: results from the National Longitudinal Alcohol Epidemiologic Survey. J Subst Abuse. 1998;10(2):163–73. https://doi.org/10.1016/s0899-3289(99)80131-x.
40. Gray KM, Carpenter MJ, Baker NL, DeSantis SM, Kryway E, Hartwell KJ, et al. A double-blind randomized controlled trial of N-acetylcysteine in cannabis-dependent adolescents. Am J Psychiatry. 2012;169(8):805–12. https://doi.org/10.1176/appi.ajp.2012.12010055.
41. Gray KM, Sonne SC, McClure EA, Ghitza UE, Matthews AG, McRae-Clark AL, et al. A randomized placebo-controlled trial of N-acetylcysteine for cannabis use disorder in adults. Drug Alcohol Depend. 2017;177:249–57. https://doi.org/10.1016/j.drugalcdep.2017.04.020.
42. Gruber SA, Sagar KA. Marijuana on the mind? The impact of Marijuana on cognition, brain structure, and brain function, and related public policy implications. Policy Insights Behav Brain Sci. 2017;4(1):104–11.
43. Hanson KL, Cummins K, Tapert SF, Brown SA. Changes in neuropsychological functioning over 10 years following adolescent substance abuse treatment. Psychol Addict Behav. 2011;25(1):127–42. https://doi.org/10.1037/a0022350.
44. Heerde JA, Hemphill SA. Sexual risk behaviors, sexual offenses, and sexual victimization among homeless youth: a systematic review of associations with substance use. Trauma Violence Abuse. 2016;17(5):468–89. https://doi.org/10.1177/1524838015584371.
45. Hoeppner BB, Hoeppner SS, Kelly JF. Do young people benefit from AA as much, and in the same ways, as adult aged 30+? A moderated multiple mediation analysis. Drug Alcohol Depend. 2014;143:181–8. https://doi.org/10.1016/j.drugalcdep.2014.07.023.
46. Kelly SM, Gryczynski J, Mitchell SG, Kirk A, O'Grady KE, Schwartz RP. Validity of brief screening instrument for adolescent tobacco, alcohol, and drug use. Pediatrics. 2014;133(5):819–26. https://doi.org/10.1542/peds.2013-2346.
47. Kerwin ME, Kirby KC, Speziali D, Duggan M, Mellitz C, Versek B, McNamara A. What can parents do? A review of state laws regarding decision making for adolescent drug abuse and mental health treatment. J Child Adolesc Subst Abuse. 2015;24(3):166–76. https://doi.org/10.1080/1067828X.2013.777380.
48. Kipke MD, Montgomery SB, Simon TR, Iverson EF. "Substance abuse" disorders among runaway and homeless youth. Subst Use Misuse. 1997;32(7–8):969–86. https://doi.org/10.3109/10826089709055866.
49. Knight JR, Sherritt L, Shrier LA, Harris SK, Chang G. Validity of the CRAFFT substance abuse screening test among adolescent clinic patients. Arch Pediatr Adolesc Med. 2002;156(6):607–14. https://doi.org/10.1001/archpedi.156.6.607.
50. Krishnasamy VP, Hallowell BD, Ko JY, Board A, Hartnett KP, Salvatore PP, et al. Update: characteristics of a nationwide outbreak of E-cigarette, or vaping, product use-associated lung injury - United States, august 2019–January 2020. MMWR Morb Mortal Wkly Rep. 2020;69(3):90–4. https://doi.org/10.15585/mmwr.mm6903e2.
51. Laudet A, Harris K, Kimball T, Winters KC, Moberg DP. Collegiate recovery communities programs: what do we know and what do we need to know? J Soc Work Pract Addict. 2014;14(1):84–100. https://doi.org/10.1080/1533256X.2014.872015.
52. Lisdahl KM, Gilbart ER, Wright NE, Shollenbarger S. Dare to delay? The impacts of adolescent alcohol and marijuana use onset on cognition, brain structure, and function. Front Psych. 2013;4:53. https://doi.org/10.3389/fpsyt.2013.00053.
53. Lyons RM, Yule AM, Schiff D, Bagley SM, Wilens TE. Risk factors for drug overdose in young people: a systematic review of the literature. J Child Adolesc

Psychopharmacol. 2019;29(7):487–97. https://doi.org/10.1089/cap.2019.0013.
54. Marsch LA, Bickel WK, Badger GJ, Stothart ME, Quesnel KJ, Stanger C, Brooklyn J. Comparison of pharmacological treatments for opioid-dependent adolescents: a randomized controlled trial. Arch Gen Psychiatry. 2005;62(10):1157–64. 62/10/1157 [pii]. https://doi.org/10.1001/archpsyc.62.10.1157.
55. Marsch LA, Moore SK, Borodovsky JT, Solhkhah R, Badger GJ, Semino S, et al. A randomized controlled trial of buprenorphine taper duration among opioid-dependent adolescents and young adults. Addiction. 2016;111(8):1406–15. https://doi.org/10.1111/add.13363.
56. Marshal MP, Friedman MS, Stall R, King KM, Miles J, Gold MA, et al. Sexual orientation and adolescent substance use: a meta-analysis and methodological review. Addiction. 2008;103(4):546–56. https://doi.org/10.1111/j.1360-0443.2008.02149.x.
57. Miller W, Rollnick S. Motivational interviewing: helping people change. 3rd ed. New York: The Guilford Press; 2013.
58. Miranda R, Ray L, Blanchard A, Reynolds EK, Monti PM, Chun T, et al. Effects of naltrexone on adolescent alcohol cue reactivity and sensitivity: an initial randomized trial. Addict Biol. 2014;19(5):941–54. https://doi.org/10.1111/adb.12050.
59. Moberg DP, Finch AJ. Recovery high schools: a descriptive study of school programs and students. J Groups Addict Recover. 2008;2:128–61. https://doi.org/10.1080/15560350802081314.
60. Moeller KE, Kissack JC, Atayee RS, Lee KC. Clinical interpretation of urine drug tests: what clinicians need to know about urine drug screens. Mayo Clin Proc. 2017;92(5):774–96. https://doi.org/10.1016/j.mayocp.2016.12.007.
61. Moeller KE, Lee KC, Kissack JC. Urine drug screening: practical guide for clinicians. Mayo Clin Proc. 2008;83(1):66–76. https://doi.org/10.4065/83.1.66.
62. Morin JG, Afzali MH, Bourque J, Stewart SH, Seguin JR, O'Leary-Barrett M, Conrod PJ. A population-based analysis of the relationship between substance use and adolescent cognitive development. Am J Psychiatry. 2019;176(2):98–106. https://doi.org/10.1176/appi.ajp.2018.18020202.
63. Morton MH, Dworsky A, Matjasko JL, Curry SR, Schlueter D, Chavez R, Farrell AF. Prevalence and correlates of youth homelessness in the United States. J Adolesc Health. 2018;62(1):14–21. https://doi.org/10.1016/j.jadohealth.2017.10.006.
64. Narendorf SC, Cross MB, Santa Maria D, Swank PR, Bordnick PS. Relations between mental health diagnoses, mental health treatment, and substance use in homeless youth. Drug Alcohol Depend. 2017;175:1–8. https://doi.org/10.1016/j.drugalcdep.2017.01.028.
65. National Institute on Drug Abuse. NIDA drug screening tool: NIDA-modified ASSIST (NM ASSIST). Retrieved from https://www.drugabuse.gov/nmassist/.
66. National Institute on Drug Abuse. Monitoring the future 2019 survey results: vaping. 2019. Retrieved from https://www.drugabuse.gov/related-topics/trends-statistics/infographics/monitoring-future-2019-survey-results-vaping.
67. Nguyen-Louie TT, Castro N, Matt GE, Squeglia LM, Brumback T, Tapert SF. Effects of emerging alcohol and marijuana use behaviors on adolescents' neuropsychological functioning over four years. J Stud Alcohol Drugs. 2015;76(5):738–48. https://doi.org/10.15288/jsad.2015.76.738.
68. Nyamathi A, Hudson A, Greengold B, Leake B. Characteristics of homeless youth who use cocaine and methamphetamine. Am J Addict. 2012;21(3):243–9. https://doi.org/10.1111/j.1521-0391.2012.00233.x.
69. Nyamathi A, Hudson A, Greengold B, Slagle A, Marfisee M, Khalilifard F, Leake B. Correlates of substance use severity among homeless youth. J Child Adolesc Psychiatr Nurs. 2010;23(4):214–22. https://doi.org/10.1111/j.1744-6171.2010.00247.x.
70. O'Malley SS, Corbin WR, Leeman RF, DeMartini KS, Fucito LM, Ikomi J, et al. Reduction of alcohol drinking in young adults by naltrexone: a double-blind, placebo-controlled, randomized clinical trial of efficacy and safety. J Clin Psychiatry. 2015;76(2):e207–13. https://doi.org/10.4088/JCP.13m08934.
71. Ocfemia MCB, Dunville R, Zhang T, Barrios LC, Oster AM. HIV diagnoses among persons aged 13-29 years - United States, 2010–2014. MMWR Morb Mortal Wkly Rep. 2018;67(7):212–5. https://doi.org/10.15585/mmwr.mm6707a2.
72. Orr C, Spechler P, Cao Z, Albaugh M, Chaarani B, Mackey S, et al. Grey matter volume differences associated with extremely low levels of Cannabis use in adolescence. J Neurosci. 2019;39(10):1817–27. https://doi.org/10.1523/JNEUROSCI.3375-17.2018.
73. Poudel A, Gautam S. Age of onset of substance use and psychosocial problems among individuals with substance use disorders. BMC Psychiatry. 2017;17(1):10. https://doi.org/10.1186/s12888-016-1191-0.
74. Reinert DF, Allen JP. The alcohol use disorders identification test: an update of research findings. Alcohol Clin Exp Res. 2007;31(2):185–99. https://doi.org/10.1111/j.1530-0277.2006.00295.x.
75. Reisner SL, Greytak EA, Parsons JT, Ybarra ML. Gender minority social stress in adolescence: disparities in adolescent bullying and substance use by gender identity. J Sex Res. 2015;52(3):243–56. https://doi.org/10.1080/00224499.2014.886321.
76. Reschly-Krasowski JM, Krasowski MD. A difficult challenge for the clinical laboratory: accessing and interpreting manufacturer cross-reactivity data for immunoassays used in urine drug testing. Acad Pathol. 2018;5:2374289518811797. https://doi.org/10.1177/2374289518811797.
77. Riggs PD, Winhusen T, Davies RD, Leimberger JD, Mikulich-Gilbertson S, Klein C, et al. Randomized controlled trial of osmotic-release methylphenidate with cognitive-behavioral therapy in adolescents with attention-deficit/hyperactivity disorder and substance use disorders. J Am Acad Child Adolesc Psychiatry. 2011;50(9):903–14. S0890-8567(11)00527-2 [pii]. https://doi.org/10.1016/j.jaac.2011.06.010.

78. Schepis TS, Krishnan-Sarin S. Sources of prescriptions for misuse by adolescents: differences in sex, ethnicity, and severity of misuse in a population-based study. J Am Acad Child Adolesc Psychiatry. 2009;48(8):828–36. https://doi.org/10.1097/CHI.0b013e3181a8130d.
79. Schepis TS, Teter CJ, McCabe SE. Prescription drug use, misuse and related substance use disorder symptoms vary by educational status and attainment in U.S. adolescents and young adults. Drug Alcohol Depend. 2018;189:172–7. https://doi.org/10.1016/j.drugalcdep.2018.05.017.
80. Schuman-Olivier Z, Weiss RD, Hoeppner BB, Borodovsky J, Albanese MJ. Emerging adult age status predicts poor buprenorphine treatment retention. J Subst Abuse Treat. 2014;47(3):202–12. https://doi.org/10.1016/j.jsat.2014.04.006.
81. Seth P, Scholl L, Rudd RA, Bacon S. Overdose deaths involving opioids, cocaine, and psychostimulants - United States, 2015–2016. MMWR Morb Mortal Wkly Rep. 2018;67(12):349–58. https://doi.org/10.15585/mmwr.mm6712a1.
82. Slesnick N, Prestopnik J. Dual and multiple diagnosis among substance using runaway youth. Am J Drug Alcohol Abuse. 2005;31(1):179–201. https://doi.org/10.1081/ada-200047916.
83. Smith DC, Davis JP, Ureche DJ, Dumas TM. Six month outcomes of a peer-enhanced community reinforcement approach for emerging adults with substance misuse: a preliminary study. J Subst Abuse Treat. 2016;61:66–73. https://doi.org/10.1016/j.jsat.2015.09.002.
84. Smith DC, Godley SH, Godley MD, Dennis ML. Adolescent community reinforcement approach outcomes differ among emerging adults and adolescents. J Subst Abuse Treat. 2011;41(4):422–30. https://doi.org/10.1016/j.jsat.2011.06.003.
85. Squeglia LM, Fadus MC, McClure EA, Tomko RL, Gray KM. Pharmacological treatment of youth substance use disorders. J Child Adolesc Psychopharmacol. 2019;29(7):559–72. https://doi.org/10.1089/cap.2019.0009.
86. Stanger C, Lansing AH, Budney AJ. Advances in research on contingency management for adolescent substance use. Child Adolesc Psychiatr Clin N Am. 2016;25(4):645–59. https://doi.org/10.1016/j.chc.2016.05.002.
87. Starzer MSK, Nordentoft M, Hjorthoj C. Rates and predictors of conversion to schizophrenia or bipolar disorder following substance-induced psychosis. Am J Psychiatry. 2018;175(4):343–50. https://doi.org/10.1176/appi.ajp.2017.17020223.
88. Steinka-Fry KT, Tanner-Smith EE, Dakof GA, Henderson C. Culturally sensitive substance use treatment for racial/ethnic minority youth: a meta-analytic review. J Subst Abuse Treat. 2017;75:22–37. https://doi.org/10.1016/j.jsat.2017.01.006.
89. Stormshak EA, DeGarmo DS, Chronister KM, Caruthers AS, Stapleton J, Falkenstein CA. The impact of substance use during middle school and young adulthood on parent-young adult relationships. J Fam Psychol. 2019;33(7):797–808. https://doi.org/10.1037/fam0000549.
90. Substance Abuse and Mental Health Services Administration. Key substance use and mental health indicators in the United States: results from the 2017 National Survey on Drug Use and Health. (HHS Publication No. SMA 18-5068, NSDUH Series H-53). Rockville, MD: Center for Behavioral Health Statistics and Quality, Substance Abuse and Mental Health Services Administration. 2018. Retrieved from https://www.samhsa.gov/data/report/2017-nsduh-annual-national-report.
91. Substance Abuse and Mental Health Services Administration. Key substance use and mental health indicators in the United States: results from the 2018 National Survey on Drug Use and Health. (HHS Publication No. PEP195068, NSDUH Series H54). Rockville, MD: Center for Behavioral Health Statistics and Quality, Substance Abuse and Mental Health Services Administration. 2019. Retrieved from https://www.samhsa.gov/data/sites/default/files/cbhsq-reports/NSDUHNationalFindingsReport2018/NSDUHNationalFindingsReport2018.htm.
92. Thorpe LE, Ouellet LJ, Hershow R, Bailey SL, Williams IT, Williamson J, et al. Risk of hepatitis C virus infection among young adult injection drug users who share injection equipment. Am J Epidemiol. 2002;155(7):645–53.
93. United States Code. Deportable aliens (§1227). (1227). United States Code. 2019. Retrieved from https://uscode.house.gov/view.xhtml?req=granuleid:USC-prelim-title8-section1227&num=0&edition=prelim.
94. Vo HT, Burgower R, Rozenberg I, Fishman M. Home-based delivery of XR-NTX in youth with opioid addiction. J Subst Abuse Treat. 2018;85:84–9. https://doi.org/10.1016/j.jsat.2017.08.007.
95. Volkow ND, Wang GJ, Telang F, Fowler JS, Alexoff D, Logan J, et al. Decreased dopamine brain reactivity in marijuana abusers is associated with negative emotionality and addiction severity. Proc Natl Acad Sci U S A. 2014;111(30):E3149–56. https://doi.org/10.1073/pnas.1411228111.
96. Weiss RD, Griffin ML, Kolodziej ME, Greenfield SF, Najavits LM, Daley DC, et al. A randomized trial of integrated group therapy versus group drug counseling for patients with bipolar disorder and substance dependence. Am J Psychiatry. 2007;164(1):100–7. https://doi.org/10.1176/appi.ajp.164.1.100.
97. Winters KC, Martin CS, Chung T. Substance use disorders in DSM-V when applied to adolescents. Addiction. 2011;106(5):882–4; discussion 895-887. https://doi.org/10.1111/j.1360-0443.2010.03334.x.
98. Woody GE, Poole SA, Subramaniam G, Dugosh K, Bogenschutz M, Abbott P, et al. Extended vs short-term buprenorphine-naloxone for treatment of opioid-addicted youth: a randomized trial. JAMA. 2008;300(17):2003–11. 300/17/2003 [pii]. https://doi.org/10.1001/jama.2008.574.
99. Zibbell JE, Asher AK, Patel RC, Kupronis B, Iqbal K, Ward JW, Holtzman D. Increases in acute hepatitis C virus infection related to a growing opioid epidemic and associated injection drug use, United States, 2004 to 2014. Am J Public Health. 2018;108(2):175–81. https://doi.org/10.2105/AJPH.2017.304132.

7 Anxiety Disorders

Kevin L. Sun, Vinita Shivakumar, and Anita R. Kishore

Key Points

- 1 out of every 3 to 5 youth will have had an anxiety disorder by the age of 26 years.
- Anxiety disorders affect TAY in various domains of life, including interpersonal relationships, educational and employment outcomes, central nervous system development, and psychiatric sequelae.
- Since TAY with anxiety disorders may have heightened concerns about finances and privacy, mental healthcare practitioners should explicitly address issues of service fees, confidentiality, and billing.
- Thorough social history-taking (using the HEEADSSS psychosocial interview), family history-taking (assessing for parental anxiety and parenting style), and collateral information-gathering are critical for identifying risk factors for and contributors to anxiety symptoms.
- Treatment should begin with psychotherapy—preferably cognitive behavioral therapy, which has the most evidence of effectiveness, and family therapy if appropriate. Other therapy modalities include short-term psychodynamic psychotherapy, interpersonal therapy, mindfulness-based interventions, acceptance and commitment therapy, and dialectical behavior therapy.
- If medication is indicated, we recommend selective serotonin reuptake inhibitors due to their demonstrated effectiveness and tolerability in children, adolescents, and adults.
- Parent-focused and early childhood interventions by pediatricians, child psychiatrists, and other healthcare professionals can reduce the risk of anxiety disorders later in life.
- The relatively low-anxiety middle childhood period may be an optimal time for prophylaxis against generalized anxiety disorder, panic disorder, and agoraphobia in TAY.
- School-based, peer-delivered, community-based, and online intervention models are being developed around the world, with preliminary evidence showing effectiveness towards reducing anxiety symptoms, increasing mental health literacy, and reducing stigma around help-seeking behaviors.

K. L. Sun · V. Shivakumar · A. R. Kishore (✉)
Department of Psychiatry and Behavioral Sciences, Stanford University School of Medicine, Stanford, CA, USA
e-mail: akishore@stanford.edu

V. Chan, J. Derenne (eds.), *Transition-Age Youth Mental Health Care*, https://doi.org/10.1007/978-3-030-62113-1_7

Introduction

Anxiety is a normal emotion of everyday life. In reaction to important, stressful, unfamiliar, or dangerous situations, anxiety can be experienced as feelings of worry, fear, irritability, alarm, or unease. It may manifest as physical symptoms, including muscle tension, cramps, stomachaches, and headaches. Other common physiological responses are flushing, sweating, and hyperventilating. Short-term behavioral changes, especially to sleep, appetite, and social interaction, may occur as well.

However, when these feelings, physical symptoms, physiological responses, and behavioral changes become persistent, irrational, and uncontrollable, they can prevent individuals from living their everyday lives. As a result, self-care, work performance, and relationships with others may suffer. Anxiety that interferes with daily functioning is no longer within normal limits. Such levels of anxiety warrant medical evaluation, since anxiety disorders are real, serious, and common medical conditions.

For a variety of reasons that we will explore in this chapter, transition-age youth (TAY) are especially at risk for the progression of everyday anxiety to diagnosed anxiety disorders. Indeed, the most prominent increase in prevalence of anxiety disorders is during the transition to early adulthood. Given little evidence of attenuation over time [1], this presents a public health concern.

Background and Significance

In this section, we first describe the anxiety that is frequently experienced during the transition to adulthood. We do so by explaining how the fundamental tasks of TAY development can so often provoke anxiety. These developmental factors of anxiety will serve as baseline knowledge for the chapter's later treatments of epidemiology, assessment, treatment, barriers to treatment, and outreach and prevention. Then, we briefly define anxiety disorders and explain their significance to TAY. By acknowledging the impact of anxiety disorders on quality of life and psychiatric sequelae, we justify our call to action: mental healthcare practitioners must provide holistic and evidence-based care in order to prevent, treat, and screen for anxiety disorders in TAY.

Everyday Anxiety in Transition-Age Youth

Since the transition from youth to adulthood involves new responsibilities, stressors, and experiences, anxiety during this period of life is to be expected. The fundamental tasks of *identity formation*, *separation and individuation*, and *achieving intimacy* are intrinsic to the TAY developmental period. Since these tasks are nontrivial, it is worth looking at each of them through the lens of anxiety.

Identity formation involves integrating identities, articulating goals, and consolidating personal values. While this is occurring, it is often the case that parents, peers, and mentors project their own expectations and value systems. When these expectations and values of others are not aligned with the individual's, the individual may feel different or inadequate, leading to unease, shyness, and fears of social situations. Other common stressors associated with identity formation involve the new kinds of work with which TAY engage: more intensive academics, presentations and public speaking, and applications to schools and jobs. Some amount of nervousness is completely normal for these important career steps. Furthermore, the unavoidable challenges faced during their learning experiences can lead to self-doubt and worry, affecting TAY's self-esteem and goal-setting.

Separation from parents and guardians involves the tapering of parental scaffolding and decision-making, and *individuation* requires TAY to take on new responsibilities. Youth are expected to deal with this novelty despite not having achieved full cognitive maturity [2, 3]. Tasks that seem mundane to adults—paying credit card bills, scheduling medical appointments, and taking transportation to work—are not yet routine to TAY; in fact, setting up one's own routines is a necessary skill to learn during their transition years. At first, the number of tasks juggled by adults can be overwhelming for TAY. More importantly, the self-initiation, self-advocacy, and social skills needed—to open a new credit card, set up a first-time medical appointment, or buy a car—are often new and difficult. Many TAY find these experiences uncomfortable or even fear-inducing and may avoid them.

Achieving intimacy involves developing and committing to mature relationships, which require trust, self-disclosure, and concern for each other. Sexual and romantic intimacy becomes an omnipresent issue during the transition ages. The development of these forms of intimacy requires self-initiation and social skills, posing difficulties for anxious youth. Traumatic outcomes of these intimacies—that is, sexual assault, intimate partner violence, abuse, and sudden or complicated breakups—can lead to an increase in anxiety symptoms and avoidance of the people, places, and relationship dynamics involved. Just as important as romantic relationships are substantive friendships, which are developed, strengthened, and ended during this time. The forging of new friendships in new settings and the endings of unhealthy friendships can create discomfort and stress in youth, who subsequently may practice avoidant behaviors around making friends.

In summary, youth during their transition years are defining their identities and work goals, growing their responsibilities, and building mature relationships. As these tasks present important, stressful, unfamiliar, and dangerous situations to youth, anxiety can be a natural reaction. However, when the sheer number of these situations becomes overwhelming, when the trauma from these situations is serious, or when youth have risk factors predisposing them to anxiety disorders, anxiety as a natural reaction may eventually reach a "chronic, high-pitched state" that requires medical intervention [4].

Significance of Anxiety Disorders

The anxiety that is typical during the transition to adulthood becomes significant when it affects youths' emotional well-being and daily functioning, negatively impacting their chances to successfully transition to adulthood.

Table 7.1 Symptoms of common anxiety disorders

Symptoms of potential anxiety disorder	Potential anxiety disorder diagnosis
Persistent, unsubstantiated worry that is difficult to control, causes significant distress, and interferes with daily functioning	Generalized anxiety disorder
Avoidance of social situations for fear of being judged, humiliated, or rejected	Social anxiety disorder
Seemingly out-of-the-blue panic attacks and preoccupation with fear of the next panic attack	Panic disorder
Fear of being in situations from which escape might be difficult or embarrassing, or in which help may not be available in the event of a panic attack	Agoraphobia
Fear and avoidance of an object, place, or situation, despite little or no threat of danger	Specific phobia

The five most common anxiety disorders in transition-age youth are generalized anxiety disorder, social anxiety disorder, panic disorder, agoraphobia, and specific phobia [1]. Table 7.1 briefly describes symptoms of these anxiety disorders [5]. The clinical presentations of these anxiety disorders will be further discussed in the "Assessment" section of this chapter.

To our knowledge, there is no clear research that examines whether clinical presentations of anxiety disorders are unique in TAY. The best data we have concern the prevalence of anxiety disorders during this period (see "Epidemiology" section), followed by the impact of anxiety disorders on the quality of life and longitudinal outcomes of TAY.

The impact of anxiety disorders extends across many important domains of life. As might be expected, TAY with anxiety disorders have been shown to have issues with interpersonal relationships, including higher levels of parent-child attachment disorganization and peer relationship dysfunction [6]. In terms of education, they are more likely to drop out of high school [7] and less likely to enter university [8, 9]. TAY with higher levels of anxiety have been shown to have more severe Internet addiction behaviors [10], but not substance dependence [11, 12]. From a physical health standpoint, a diagnosis of generalized anxiety disorder is associated with the presence of migraine in TAY [13]. Chronic anxiety disorder during early adolescence is associated with DNA hypermethylation in central nervous system development pathways over time [14]. And, at the brain circuitry level, TAY with anxiety symptoms exhibit amygdala hyperactivity during emotion processing, which is related to self-reported poorer quality of life [15]. In a similar vein, college students with social anxiety were found to have decreased levels of attentional control and increased rumination, the latter of which predicted increased depression [16].

A link between anxiety disorders in TAY and psychiatric sequelae over time is well demonstrated. TAY with baseline specific phobia were followed up for 10 years and were found to have a fourfold risk of developing panic disorder, generalized anxiety disorder, and obsessive-compulsive disorder [17]. Social anxiety disorder has been implicated as a risk factor of subsequent depressive disorders and of a more malignant course in adolescents who are already depressed [18]. In general, youth aged 20–29 years with anxiety disorders are more likely to have anxiety disorders and depression 10 years later [19]. Importantly, anxiety disorders have been linked to suicide. Studies have found that the odds of suicidal ideation and the rate of suicide attempts in TAY are four to eight times higher with generalized anxiety disorder and panic disorder, and the risk increases with multiple anxiety disorders [20, 21]. Other studies show that the relationship to suicidality depends on the anxiety disorder being comorbid with other disorders [22].

All in all, the literature shows that anxiety disorders significantly affect the lives of TAY, both during their transition years and long after. Returning to the ideas of development, we recognize that anxiety disorders must be treated thoroughly and holistically, addressing upstream issues in addition to downstream symptoms and behaviors. If we can understand that this period of development at once provokes anxiety and creates a lasting impact on future mental health outcomes, then we can affirm the need for more empathy and effort in how we practice mental healthcare for anxious TAY.

Epidemiology

In the previous section, we established that the transition-age period is fundamentally a risky time for the development of anxiety disorders, and we described the significant impact that anxiety disorders make on the lives of TAY.

These issues present a serious public health concern and warrant an epidemiological approach. A thorough examination of prevalence, risk factors, and higher-risk groups of anxiety disorders within the transition-age period can help prevent the onset of anxiety in late adolescence and attenuate the effect of anxiety on adulthood.

Discussing the epidemiology of anxiety disorders in TAY is difficult for several reasons. First, there are few studies that cross the age boundary of 18 years; research either focuses on adolescents up to the age of 18 years or discusses “adults” defined as people aged 18 years and above. Any conclusions we present must combine the findings of multiple studies with different methodologies, a fact that presents self-evident limitations.

Second, the literature is often specific to young adults in higher education, since college and university students are more easily recruited into research studies of TAY. As a result, research on the 42.9% of 16- to 24-year-olds who are not enrolled in any school is far harder to come by [23]. This lack of visibility is concerning, as we may surmise that healthcare access and mental health service utilization are lower in these youth. Future investigations of anxiety in non-college-attending youths are crucial to our general understanding of TAY and to our efforts at mental health outreach, healthcare navigation, and prevention for these individuals. Mental health research in TAY must take into account the enormous variety in socioeconomic factors and seek ways to address the disparities in research.

Finally, large-scale epidemiological studies of anxiety disorders in TAY may be out of date. It must be mentioned that the past decade has brought enormous changes to how and with what frequency TAY interact with each other. The advent of social media, massively multiplayer online gaming, and on-demand media consumption has coincided with the childhoods of the transition-age youth discussed in this book. This fact, combined with the fact that anxiety very often manifests first during childhood or late adolescence, suggests that the transition-age youth discussed here may have very different prevalence rates and risk factors of anxiety, compared to transition-age youth from just a decade ago. Literature presented here must be considered with this caveat in mind. Future research presenting new data about prevalence, incidence, and risk is needed to examine the impact of these new twenty-first-century behaviors on the development of anxiety disorders.

Acknowledging these difficulties, we summarize the extant literature around the prevalence of anxiety disorders. Then, we discuss the risk factors that have the strongest evidence of contributing to the development of anxiety.

Prevalence

In general, anxiety and anxiety disorders are very common in TAY. Between 2001 and 2003, the past-year prevalence of any anxiety disorder among American adults (aged 18 years and above) was 19.1% [24]. In 2008, among American college students, 61.9% reported feeling overwhelming anxiety at some point in the past year, and 19.7% were diagnosed or treated for an anxiety disorder [25].

Historical data have demonstrated two peaks in the age distribution of prevalence: during childhood—predominantly in the form of separation anxiety—and during the transition from adolescence to early adulthood [26, 27]. More recently, two large longitudinal studies provide the best data to estimate prevalence of anxiety disorders in US TAY. The first is the National Comorbidity Survey Replication Adolescent Supplement (NCS-A). The NCS-A was a face-to-face survey of 10,123 adolescents aged 13–18 years, conducted between 2001 and 2004 [28]. From the NCS, the following points emerge:

- Prevalence of any anxiety disorder (including posttraumatic stress disorder) was 31.9%.
- Prevalence of any anxiety disorder was higher in females (38.0%) than males (26.1%).
- Prevalence was similar between 13- and 14-year-olds (31.4%) and 17- and 18-year-olds (32.3%).
- Generalized anxiety disorder, social phobia (social anxiety disorder), and panic disorder modestly increased in prevalence across adolescence. Specific phobia and separation anxiety disorder decreased in prevalence, and agoraphobia remained about the same.
- The anxiety disorders most likely to involve severe impairment (excluding posttraumatic stress disorder) were social phobia (1.3%), generalized anxiety disorder (0.9%), specific phobia (0.6%), and separation anxiety disorder (0.6%).

The second is the Great Smoky Mountains Survey, which began in the early 1990s to follow 1,420 participants living in the southeastern United States across 20 years starting from ages 9 to 13 [1]. Highlighted findings from this survey include the following:

- Replicating previous findings, the overall pattern was U-shaped, with a trough in prevalence during middle childhood, followed by increasing prevalence beginning around age 15 years and continuing into the transition-age period.
- By age 26 years, the cumulative 3-month prevalence rate of any anxiety disorder was 22.7%.
- Prevalence of generalized anxiety disorder steadily increased across the transition-age period: from about 1.5% to 4% in females and from about 0.5% to 3% in males.
- Prevalence of panic disorder and agoraphobia made a sudden jump between ages 16 and 19 years, from near 0% to about 1–3%, then remained constant through the age of 26 years.

- Social anxiety disorder and specific phobia were relatively uncommon across development ($\leq 1\%$).
- 13.8% of those with an anxiety disorder met criteria for 2 or more anxiety disorders at any point in time.

Though the findings of these two studies are not entirely aligned, they present some clear takeaways. First, one out of every three to five TAY will have had an anxiety disorder by the age of 26 years. Second, the trends in the onset of generalized anxiety disorder and panic disorder suggest the need for prevention during the relatively low-anxiety middle childhood period. Third, females are at a higher risk of developing anxiety disorders than males. These points lead us to a discussion of risk factors for anxiety disorders.

Risk Factors

The risk factors for anxiety disorders can be divided into three categories: genetic, environmental, and temperamental. The relative importance of these types is likely unique to each individual, and clinicians should take into account all three types during their assessments (see "Assessment" section).

Genetic risk factors have been investigated through family studies, which have shown certain anxiety disorders to be heritable. Transmission of the same disorder from parent to offspring was observed in studies of panic disorder [29, 30], social anxiety disorder [31], and specific phobia [32]. In general, rates of any anxiety disorder are higher in offspring of affected parents (21–68%) compared with offspring of neurotypical parents (0–26%) [33]. Furthermore, parents with major depressive disorder are more likely to have offspring with anxiety disorders [34].

Environmental risk factors include parenting behaviors, life events, and interpersonal relationships. Parental factors that increase risk for anxiety in 12- to 18-year-olds include less warmth, more interparental conflict, overinvolvement, and greater hostility [35]. Difficult life events such as parental separation and poverty before age 5 years predict the development of anxiety disorders at age 15 years [36]. Peer-peer interactions are also likely contributors, and peer rejection and exclusion at the start of high school has been linked to later social anxiety disorder [37]. Important to consider are the results of twin studies, which have shown that unique, unshared environmental factors play a greater role in the development of anxiety than shared environmental factors do [38, 39]. This suggests that unshared life events and distinct interpersonal relationships more significantly impact anxiety than shared parenting behavior does. Nevertheless, all factors undoubtedly contribute.

Temperamental risk factors with the most research evidence to support their impact are behavioral inhibition and anxiety sensitivity. Behavioral inhibition is the persistent tendency to withdraw or act reticent in novel situations or with unfamiliar people [40]. Toddlers and children who exhibit behavioral inhibition are more likely to later develop social anxiety disorder [41, 42]. Anxiety sensitivity is the tendency to interpret physiological arousal as having negative consequences, leading to a "fear of fear" cycle [43]. In TAY, anxiety sensitivity has been shown to predict later onset of panic attacks and development of anxiety disorders [44, 45].

While it is convenient to separate these various risk factors for our conceptual understanding, in reality they interact in complicated, variable ways. Genetics and temperament may potentiate the effect of environmental factors on anxiety. Reciprocally, environmental factors may affect epigenetics and the microbiome, both of which have been linked to anxiety [46, 47] and are possibly heritable [48]. For this reason, the assessment of TAY should be holistic. Rather than consider these risk factors as criteria to be checked, clinicians should take advantage of them as guideposts for thorough social and family history-taking during the evaluation for anxiety disorders.

Acknowledging these risk factors is especially important for the mental healthcare of TAY populations at higher risk of anxiety disorders. At one university, transfer students were found to be significantly more anxious than non-transfers, but the reasons for this were not explored [49]. Various studies have found that TAY of sexual minorities display higher symptoms of anxiety [50–52]. TAY with autism spectrum disorder are also prone to anxiety [53, 54].

In concluding this section on epidemiology, we underscore the need for further research and prevention measures. In this new era of online hyperconnectivity, new prospective longitudinal studies are warranted for comparison of prevalence numbers with those of the NCS-A and the Great Smoky Mountains Study, and for investigation of new kinds of risk factors. While these studies are being conducted for the future, we must intervene in the present. We now know that the middle childhood period may be an optimal time for prophylaxis against generalized anxiety disorder, panic disorder, and agoraphobia. We know that women must be better supported and heard, so that the gender gap in prevalence of anxiety disorders may close. And we know that outreach to TAY should make sure transfer students, LGBTQ+ people, and neurodivergent youth feel welcome and included. By understanding epidemiology, we can design more impactful approaches to help TAY with their anxiety (see "Outreach and Prevention" section).

Assessment

Effective treatment of anxiety disorders requires a thorough assessment of not only the patient's symptoms but also the patient's personal characteristics and functioning. Here, we discuss the guiding principles for the assessment of anxiety disorders in TAY, including clarification of treatment logistics, routine screening, differential diagnosis and evaluation, social and family history, and use of collateral information.

Treatment Logistics

The act of seeking mental healthcare alone can be anxiety-provoking, especially for TAY. Some concerns may stem from the novelty of the situation; TAY are likely to be navigating mental healthcare on their own for the first time, possibly without their parents' knowing. Seeking care without parental help, anxious youth may have questions about finances and privacy, including issues of service fees, confidentiality, and billing. The complexity of these issues adds an understandable burden to the process of self-initiating health-seeking behavior. Mental healthcare practitioners, on first meeting a transition-age person, must acknowledge these issues and explicitly address these concerns. By clearing the air of these worries about the process, healthcare practitioners and TAY can build trust and work out the logistics necessary for a sustained therapeutic relationship.

Screening and Diagnosis

It is recommended that all TAY be routinely screened for anxiety symptoms due to the high prevalence of anxiety disorders in this age group. Screening can consist of interview questions and/or tools for rating symptoms and functioning. The general clinical interview is one of the most important means of gathering information as it allows providers to gain a comprehensive understanding of the patient. Starting with a broad approach and informal conversation is also a good means of establishing rapport. This is especially important with TAY, as they are more likely to camouflage their symptoms and rationalize their avoidance of stressful situations. Apart from beginning with general topics, potential means of establishing rapport include avoiding any signs of disapproval and providing normalizing psychoeducation.

For patients who self-report anxiety symptoms, or if indicated by screening, there are a variety of established interview schedules and clinician-administered scales based on DSM criteria that can be used to supplement the clinical interview to establish a diagnosis and/or to assess symptom severity and functional impairment (Table 7.2). As tools, they are generally categorized for children or adults; therefore, assessing TAY often involves utilizing multiple resources.

Table 7.2 Assessment tools for anxiety in children and adults

Semi-structured interviews	Anxiety scales	Ratings of global function
Primarily categorical diagnostic interview questions	Primarily self-report questionnaires for symptom presence and severity [55]	Primarily measures of overall functioning or treatment progress [56]
Anxiety Disorders Interview Schedule (ADIS) [57] K-SADS-PL DSM-5 [58]	Multidimensional Anxiety Scale for Children (MASC) Screen for Child Anxiety Related Disorders (SCARED) Spence Children's Anxiety Scale (SCAS) Youth Anxiety Measure for DSM-5 (YAM-5) Generalized Anxiety Disorder Screener (GAD-7) Clinically Useful Anxiety Outcome Scale (CUXOS) Hamilton Rating Scale for Anxiety (HAM-A)	Clinical Global Impression Scale (CGI) Children's Global Assessment Scale (CGAS)

It should be noted that the structured interview style may feel artificial or uncomfortable to TAY patients, so the prior establishment of rapport is critical.

Gathering together all information from the clinical interview and the assessment tools, clinicians may arrive at a diagnosis of an anxiety disorder or multiple disorders. Characteristic clinical presentations of anxiety disorders include:

- *Generalized anxiety disorder*: excessive uncontrollable worry about a variety of topics accompanied by cognitive/physical symptoms such as restlessness, fatigue, impaired concentration
- *Social anxiety disorder*: disproportionate fear specific to social situations due to feelings of being noticed or scrutinized, leading to avoidance of social situations
- *Panic disorder*: recurrent unexpected panic attacks and fear of having more attacks, leading to avoidance of situations that may provoke an attack
- *Agoraphobia*: marked fear about situations in which escape or receiving help may be difficult such as using public transportation, being in open or enclosed spaces, being in a crowd
- *Specific phobias*: unreasonable excessive fear instantaneously triggered by specific object or situation that significantly impacts functioning
- *Substance-induced anxiety disorder*: anxiety or panic within a month of ingestion of a substance known to cause anxiety

Differential Diagnosis

As always, it is important to create a differential diagnosis of somatic, psychiatric, and substance-induced conditions that may mimic or contribute to anxiety. General medical conditions such as hyperthyroidism, migraine, asthma, seizure disorders, pheochromocytoma, and substance use including caffeine, levothyroxine, and steroids should be assessed. Psychiatric disorders such as attention deficit hyperactivity disorder, psychotic disorders, developmental disorders such as autism spectrum disorder, learning conditions, bipolar disorder, and depression can all present with some symptoms similar to those seen in anxiety disorders. These include restlessness, social withdrawal, and persistent worries about performance.

Social History

Taking a thorough social history is a prerequisite for an effective clinical interview. While any anxiety disorder treatment requires a holistic view of the patient, this is especially crucial for TAY as their rapidly changing circumstances may be large contributors to their symptoms. Furthermore, as TAYs adjust to separation and individuation, the skills and coping mechanisms they learn through treatment can have compounding downstream and potentially multigenerational effects. We recommend the HEEADSSS psychosocial interview for adolescents, a commonly used tool [59]. Example opening questions for each section include:

- *Home and environment:* Where do you live, and who lives there with you?
- *Education and employment:* Are you in school? Do you work now? What are you good at/what's hard for you?
- *Eating:* What do you like and not like about your body?
- *Activities:* What do you do for fun? What things do you do with your friends, and what do you do in your free time?
- *Drugs:* Many young people experiment with drugs, alcohol, or cigarettes. Have you or your friends ever tried them? What have you tried?
- *Sexuality:* Are you involved in a relationship? How was that experience for you? How do you see yourself in terms of sexual preference?
- *Suicide/depression:* Have you ever thought about hurting yourself? Have you ever tried?
- *Safety:* Have you ever been seriously injured? Do you use safety equipment (seatbelt, helmet)? Is there violence at your school/neighborhood?

Family History

Family history is also important to gather, in order to evaluate for risk factors associated with genetics and parenting style [60]. For children, psychiatric evaluation generally requires a family assessment, which at minimum includes obtaining family history from a caregiver and observing the child interact with a caregiver. This is because family, though often the child's primary resource for healing, can also be the primary source of distress. While this level of assessment is often not possible for TAY who live away from parents, the importance of family in the patient's life is often still true for this population. Therefore, it is important for providers to ask patients about their interactions with their family and to observe whether there is a relationship between interfamilial interactions and their anxiety disorder. Family history should include specific questions on parenting style (authoritarian or permissive), changes such as separation or divorce, and parental unavailability. The family evaluation should provide enough data to characterize the family's structure, level of communication, belief system, and regulatory functioning.

Collateral Information

If appropriate and feasible (and approved in the case of non-minors), obtain collateral information from parents, school personnel, roommates, and/or romantic partners. Information about anxiety symptoms from multiple sources is important to counteract incomplete agreement among informants. Others' perceptions of the impact on functioning can supplement the youth's self-experience [58]. Furthermore, the perspectives of others can provide insight into the youth's developmental progress, the knowledge of which enables developmentally appropriate therapy. Finally, establishing relationships with collateral contacts can allow the mental health practitioner to suggest collaborative treatment strategies. By leveraging the youth's connections with others, clinicians can provide care that is more accessible, acceptable, and sustainable.

Treatment

Treatment of TAY with anxiety disorders is multimodal. Providers should consider "education of the patient about the anxiety disorder, consultation with primary care physicians and other providers, cognitive-behavioral interventions, psychodynamic psychotherapy, family therapy, and pharmacotherapy" [61]. Underlying all treatment modalities is the therapeutic alliance, in which provider and patient take a collaborative strength-based approach to effecting positive change in the patient's life. In this section, we discuss general considerations for treatment and then introduce each potential therapeutic modality for clinicians' independent research.

General Considerations

For planning the treatment of anxiety disorders, clinicians should reference the *Practice Parameter for the Assessment and Treatment of Children and Adolescents with Anxiety Disorders*, released by the American Academy of Child and Adolescent Psychiatry [61]. From this practice parameter and our own clinical judgment, we provide the following general considerations:

- *The earlier the better:* Treatment should begin as early as possible. It has been shown that earlier treatment leads to better longitudinal outcomes [62]. This consideration relies on frequent screening, building rapport, and communicating effectively with the patient.
- *Goals of care:* Treatment should begin with a discussion of goals of care. Given that transition to adulthood is naturally anxiety-provoking, clinicians should set expectations early on, so that patient and provider have a common scale with which to measure progress. It is helpful to have both short- and long-term goals: for example, learning and implementing a particular coping strategy in the short term, and reducing symptom frequency, intensity, or duration in the long term. The discussion should also be frequently revisited so as to help patients reflect upon their achievements and learn self-monitoring strategies.
- *High rate of service disengagement:* It is well known that TAY have lower levels of engagement with mental healthcare services [63]. While there are a multitude of structural factors that contribute to this higher rate of service disengagement, there are also individual factors and attitudes specific to TAY that contribute to this phenomenon (see "Barriers to Treatment" section). It is important to address these thought patterns and to help patients appreciate their strengths and progress.
- *Factors to consider for treatment selection:* Treatment selection should be based on psychosocial stressors, risk factors, severity of symptoms, impairment of disorder and comorbid disorders, developmental functioning, and family functioning. In addition, the provider's own training, patient's access to care, and affordability of treatment should be considered.
- *Monitoring:* It is recommended that both functional impairments and symptom reduction be monitored during treatment as residual anxiety disorder symptoms can increase the risk for relapse of the same or a comorbid anxiety disorder.

Based on studies and practice parameters, we recommend that the treatment of anxiety disorders of mild severity should begin with psychotherapy, most commonly cognitive behavioral therapy. This method allows providers to intentionally communicate and share understanding of the patient's difficulties, as well as acknowledge strengths. This method also facilitates the necessary development of resilience and self-management skills. We also recommend family therapy for TAY with relevant risk factors. For patients with greater symptom severity, other adjunctive treatments targeted at specific symptoms should be considered (see section "Potential Treatment Modalities").

If initial psychotherapy does not yield significant amelioration, medication should be started. We also consider medications at the outset—either before starting therapy or concurrently—in cases of greater functional impairment or symptom severity, or if psychotherapy is not possible [64]. Medication treatment should last at least 12 months after the patient begins to feel better. If the patient's symptoms are stable for 1 year, prescribing providers should converse with TAY and families to determine if medication should be continued or tapered under supervision [65]. Patient and family preferences must play a big role in all decisions.

Potential Treatment Modalities

Modality #1: Resilience and Self-Management Skills Development

Since this period of life features significant changes, TAY must be equipped with strategies that help them deal with stress during novel situations [66]. In addition, as TAY begin to self-manage their daily behaviors without their parents' scaffolding, they must receive help in developing healthy sleep habits, nutrition, exercise, financial responsibility, and relationships. Developing these skills of resilience and self-management, TAY can address potential contributing factors of anxiety: avoidance and risk-taking behaviors, poor sleep and diet, sedentary indoors lifestyle, social isolation, and "failure to launch" in general [67].

Modality #2: Family Therapy

Since one-third of all 18- to 34-year-olds live in their parents' home [68], and since parental anxiety and parenting styles are risk factors for anxiety in their children [69], it is essential that family therapy be considered as treatment for TAY. Approaching issues as they arise in the family structure and process, rather than only in the individual, the clinician gains a more dynamic view into stressors and behaviors that contribute to anxiety. Furthermore, the clinician can leverage the strengths of the existing parent-child and/or parent-parent relationships in their suggestions of family-based interventions.

Modality #3: Cognitive Behavioral Therapy (CBT)

Adaptive coping skills are at the core of CBT. These skills are gained through psychoeducation about the anxiety disorder and cognitive restructuring, as well as through exposure to feared stimuli and somatic management skills training (e.g., relaxation and deep breathing). Importantly, CBT also involves coordinating relapse prevention plans. For treating specific anxiety disorders, CBT modifications, such as social skills training for social anxiety [70] and interoceptive exposure for panic disorder [71], have been shown to be of benefit.

Cognitive behavioral therapy is supported by numerous randomized controlled trials and is considered the first-line psychotherapy for anxiety disorders in youth [61]. The principal evidence base is the Child-Adolescent Anxiety Multimodal Study (CAMS), the largest clinical trial for treatment of anxiety, which showed that CBT, medication (sertraline), and combination treatment are all more effective than placebo, and the combination is more effective than monotherapies [72]. Importantly, short-term outcomes for CBT in youth are among the most favorable [73].

However, subsequent studies have shown that relapse occurred in almost half of youth responders, suggesting that further research is necessary to determine treatment optimization for nonresponders as they go on to develop increasing impairment in adulthood. Further, there are no specific guidelines for CBT in TAY, even though research shows that individually tailored, developmentally sensitive approaches to CBT are the most effective. It has been suggested that CBT for TAY should focus on contextual factors such as family environment, peer interaction, and age-appropriate settings including dorms and parties [74].

Modality #4: Short-Term Psychodynamic Psychotherapy

Psychodynamic psychotherapy views anxiety as a sign of internal, unconscious distress and conflict that needs to be consciously understood and addressed. Supportive and expressive techniques are used to decrease internal conflict and allow regulation of impulses and affect.

Benefits of this modality in TAY are that it may increase insight into typical behavior patterns, defenses, and responses to thoughts or conflict. It may also help youth work through underlying fears and difficult memories that impact their trust in others and separation from guardians. By acknowledging the challenges of childhood, clinicians can build a therapeutic alliance with TAY in which they feel understood and more expressive [75].

Modality #5: Interpersonal Therapy (IPT)

Interpersonal therapy is a short-term treatment focused on how interpersonal events affect the patient's emotional state. By framing difficulties in interpersonal terms, problematic relationships can be addressed. This intentional focus on social interactions may be particularly beneficial for TAY as they navigate their identity, role confusion, and formation of intimacy. Although this psychotherapy was originally specifically for treating depression, it has since been shown to be effective for anxiety disorders and used for other conditions [76].

Modality #6: Mindfulness-Based Interventions (MBIs)

Structured mindfulness-based approaches are gaining traction as interventions for children and adolescents and have been dubbed "third wave therapies." The third wave of cognitive behavioral therapy refers to a set of new approaches that deals with the individual's relationship to thought and emotion. These approaches combine classic CBT's focus on maladaptive thinking patterns with new areas of interest: acceptance, values, goals, metacognition, and mindfulness [77]. Mindfulness, adapted from Eastern Buddhist traditions, refers to the practice of paying attention purposefully and non-judgmentally [78].

Mindfulness-Based Stress Reduction (MBSR)—the first MBI to gain empirical support—consists of various mind-body meditative practices, such as sitting meditation, body scans, and yoga, in an 8-week group format [79]. Mindfulness-Based Cognitive Therapy (MBCT) is an adapted form of MBSR that adds a component of cognitive therapy. The potential benefits of this treatment include improvement of self-regulation and emotional awareness [80]. There is evidence to suggest that it can be a useful adjunct to behavioral and medical interventions for children, adolescents, and their parents, and that it supports the reduction of anxiety and depression symptoms [81]. However, overall research is limited with mixed results from meta-analyses [82].

Modality #7: Acceptance and Commitment Therapy (ACT)

Acceptance and commitment therapy is another third-wave therapy that incorporates mindfulness, acceptance of experiences without judgment, and a commitment to change as means of coping with unwanted thoughts or feelings. There is growing interest in ACT as a school-based intervention for anxious youth in particular [83]. Preliminary evidence is promising [84, 85], but more research of ACT's effectiveness for TAY needs to be conducted.

Modality #8: Dialectical Behavior Therapy (DBT)

Dialectical behavior therapy is another third-wave therapy and was originally developed for the treatment of patients hospitalized after self-harm. It is based on the concept that a unified view of life requires acceptance of opposing forces, such as the contrast between acceptance and change (i.e., "radical acceptance"). Often a mixture of individual and group therapy, DBT helps patients identify their reactions to conflict and commit to change. It does so by combining skills of mindfulness, interpersonal effectiveness, and emotional regulation. DBT has mainly been shown to be effective for borderline personality disorder [86]. There is a dearth of literature for use in anxiety disorders, but its efficacy in emotional regulation skills has led to the suggestion of its use as an adjunct or in cases of treatment-resistant anxiety [87, 88].

Modality #9: Medications

When anxiety disorder symptoms are moderate or severe, when impairment makes participation in psychotherapy difficult, or when psychotherapy results in a partial response, then treatment with medication is recommended. Selective serotonin reuptake inhibitors (SSRIs) have emerged as the first-line medication for treating anxiety in children and adolescents. Multiple randomized controlled trials support their efficacy, both alone and in combination, for the treatment of anxiety disorders in youth.

Considerations when prescribing SSRIs include the following:

- There is no empirical evidence for a particular SSRI being more effective. Clinically, the choice depends on side effect profile, duration of action, and response in first-degree relatives with anxiety. If SSRIs need to be switched, they should be cross-tapered.
- SSRIs are generally well tolerated. Mild and transient effects include gastrointestinal symptoms, increased motor activity, and insomnia.
- Importantly, SSRIs have a regulatory boxed ("black-box") warning for increased risk of suicidality [89]. This was based on a pooled analysis of 24 short-term placebo-controlled trials of 9 antidepressants (including SSRIs) in children and adolescents with systematic psychiatric disorders [90]. This is a low-frequency event, and multiple subsequent studies have not been able to show a correlation between antidepressant use and suicidality [91]. Nevertheless, the use of SSRIs requires prior consent and a close monitoring strategy.
- Visit frequency may be reduced after an effective dose of medication has been reached. It is important to note that both psychotherapy and pharmacotherapy may not result in full remission of symptoms. After symptoms have been stable and reduced for a year on medication maintenance, gradual tapering can be initiated with observation for any recurrence.
- There are no specific dosing schedules for youth, but it is recommended to "start low, go slow." If the patient tolerates the lowest available dose for a week, then the dose can be incrementally increased to initial therapeutic dose. If symptoms do not ameliorate in 6–8 weeks, the dose can be incrementally increased and assessed until the maximum dose is reached or side effects become intolerable. Dosages for children are often similar to those for adults [92].
- Positive synergistic effects have been shown when SSRIs are combined with psychotherapy. In our discussion of the CBT modality above, we pointed out the CAMS study's findings: SSRIs alone are effective, but SSRIs in combination with CBT are even more effective [72].

There is less data on other medications, and their use should be carefully considered.

- *Serotonin norepinephrine reuptake inhibitors* (e.g., venlafaxine) or *buspirone* (partial postsynaptic serotonin agonist, full presynaptic serotonin agonist) can be used as an alternative alone or in combination with SSRIs [65].
- *Benzodiazepines* (GABA agonists) have been identified as helpful anxiolytics in acute-phase treatment [93]. However, due to their addictive potential and the lack of longitudinal research, they are primarily used as short-term adjuncts to SSRIs [64].
- *Tricyclic antidepressants* are not generally recommended, due to their unfavorable side effect profile (cardiac abnormalities, constipation, sedation) and their lack of demonstrated effectiveness [94]. There is only marginal evidence of their effectiveness at treating depression in adolescents [95].
- Current guidelines do not recommend low-potency antipsychotics, beta-blockers, or antihistamines for pharmacological treatment of anxiety disorders in adolescents. However, propranolol can be effective in certain specific circumstances of anxiety, such as performance anxiety [96].

Overall, whenever considering initiation of pharmacotherapy for TAY with anxiety disorders, a risk-benefit ratio must be carefully assessed. CBT is preferred for mild symptoms as it has a more favorable side effect profile. Further, since there is a lack of longitudinal studies of antianxiety pharmacotherapies in youth, current guidelines recommend medication-free trials once a patient has had stable reduction in symptoms for a year on an SSRI. However, multimodal treatment remains very important in anxiety disorders, with evidence of effectiveness using combination CBT and SSRI therapy. Therefore, in patients with more severe symptoms, pharmacotherapy is an important modality to consider.

Barriers to Treatment

In the previous two sections, we discussed how to assess for and treat anxiety disorders in TAY. Although this knowledge is helpful for providing the best care possible to anxious TAY, our efforts are stymied by inaccessibility and underutilization. The 2001–2002 National Epidemiological Survey on Alcohol and Related Conditions found that among TAY aged 18–24 years with anxiety disorders, only 15.9% in college and 12.4% not in college had received any past-year mental health treatment [97]. Higher rates were found in the 2007–2009 Healthy Minds Survey, which included college students older than 26: 50–60% of students with panic disorder or generalized anxiety disorder received medication or therapy in the past year. However, only 15–20% of students with anxiety disorders were *currently* undergoing therapy or counseling [98].

These findings beg the question: how does anxiety affect access to care in TAY? Plenty of literature exists around large-scale, systemic barriers: the shortage of child- and adolescent-focused mental health practitioners, much less those that are TAY-focused [99]; the financial cost with or without insurance [100, 101]; and stigma around mental health [102]. Yet scarce literature exists that examines how anxiety interacts with these factors to uniquely affect access to care.

Here, we attempt to take the perspective of the anxious TAY. We reproduce the self-reported attitudes of TAY from the Healthy Minds Survey, and then we suggest how anxiety may underlie or exacerbate these attitudes and behaviors. We justify this approach by leaning on a key concept of cognitive behavioral therapy: that thoughts, feelings, and behaviors are interconnected. Knowing that TAY practice avoidant *behaviors* of mental health services, we can use the *thoughts* that TAY provide through surveys to interpolate their *feelings* of anxiety. By doing this, we can understand why TAY view services unfavorably [103] and are so likely to terminate treatment early [104, 105].

The following quotes come from the Healthy Minds Study survey, which collected 13,105 online responses from college students at 26 institutions [106]. The relevant analysis focused on students with a mood disorder, anxiety disorder, or suicidal ideation who reported no treatment in the past year, despite feeling low stigma and positive beliefs about treatment. These students provided various reasons for not receiving treatment. These quotes are accompanied by the percentages of students who endorsed them and by our suggestions of how anxiety specifically may interact with each quoted attitude.

> I prefer to deal with these issues on my own (55%).

Self-reliance is an important and desirable trait in TAY who are individuating. With their own power, they must practice problem-solving and coping skills, as these are essential for resilience in the face of adult challenges. However, TAY with clinically significant levels of anxiety need at least some support with addressing their distress and functional impairment. This disagreement between needs and thoughts may have roots in anxious feelings about confidentiality, attitudes towards healthcare professionals' recommendations, and self-medication behaviors for supposed lessening of anxiety.

Confidentiality

As we have discussed previously, TAY, who are navigating mental healthcare on their own for the first time, may have concerns about privacy while on parents' insurance. Indeed, some insurance companies may send an invoice to the parents who are the policyholders, after their child pays a co-pay for mental health services [107]. There are a variety of reasons that anxious TAY may not want their parents to know about treatment:

- Their anxiety may be linked to behaviors (i.e., substance use, Internet addiction), identities (i.e., sexual minorities), or experiences (i.e., sexual assault, emotional abuse) that would provoke negative reactions from their parents.

- Their anxiety may be linked to their parents' parenting style, which was previously mentioned as a risk factor for anxiety disorders.
- They may feel anxious about their parents' well-being, which could supposedly worsen if they were to find out about their child's functional impairment.
- They may be preoccupied with individuating from their parents out of conflict or necessity.

Outreach to TAY should acknowledge these reasons, address concerns about billing, and propose confidential treatment as an approach to handling these parent-related issues. Towards these aims, we take the same positions as those endorsed by the Society for Adolescent Health and Medicine, the American Academy of Pediatrics, and the American College of Obstetricians and Gynecologists [108]. Programs should consider all legal options for delivering confidential services. Mental healthcare professionals can help their TAY patients contact their insurance providers for policy information and for procedures to avoid unwanted disclosure. At a systems level, we encourage legislation to eliminate the sending of explanation of benefit notifications and other similar notices when TAY insured as dependents obtain sensitive services.

Attitudes Towards Treatment Recommendations

TAY's high rates of attrition and underutilization of mental health services can be partially explained by youths' attitudes towards the mental healthcare they receive. Anxious TAY may feel that treatment is too risky or difficult and therefore not worth seeking. We suggest the following reasons:

- TAY with social anxiety disorder, panic disorder, and agoraphobia may have difficulty trusting unfamiliar healthcare professionals or group therapy settings.
- The practiced avoidant behaviors of anxiety disorders in general can affect youths' willingness to try their treatment recommendations.
- The disabling physiological responses of anxiety disorders can affect youths' abilities to carry out treatment recommendations, despite their best efforts.

Treatment of TAY should acknowledge that this is a tricky dance between professional and client. Trust can be gained by following guiding principles for participatory action research with marginalized youth: situated problem- and inquiry-based approach, genuine collaboration, and commitment to active intervention [109]. Empowerment and self-belief can be gained through motivational interviewing, which can improve initial engagement and overall symptom reduction according to preliminary evidence [110]. Finally, realistic progress can be made through gentle pushing and a stepwise approach, as in exposure therapy [111].

Self-Medication Behaviors

Substance use is high among TAY, and self-treatment of anxiety is a significant reason provided [112]. The 2015 College Prescription Drug Study examined the nonmedical use of prescription drugs in 3,918 students. When they asked students why they use, "to relieve anxiety" was endorsed by 35.1% of pain medication users, 48.8% of sedative users, and 9.3% of stimulant users [113]. Cannabis has also been perceived to help with anxiety by 61.8% of "medical" users [114]; alcohol, by socially anxious individuals [115].

Unfortunately, the reality is that these self-treatment behaviors often heighten levels of anxiety and increase risk for development of anxiety disorders [116–119].

However, treatment of TAY should not shame them for their self-medication behaviors. Instead, these behaviors can be leveraged to explore their deeper reasons for drug use and to understand their goals of care. Outreach efforts to TAY also benefit from understanding these behaviors. Campaigns to address substance use disorders can offer TAY other ways of coping with their anxieties.

I don't have time (51%).

During this period of transition, youth often feel overwhelmed by their responsibilities. The way they work in higher education and in their first jobs is new and different from their childhood schoolwork. The perceived significance of their work—earning good grades in difficult higher education schoolwork, hunting for jobs, or performing well at work—may be greater. Along with these work-related stressors, they may have time committed to newly developing relationships.

TAY who are already anxious about these responsibilities may find the extra commitment of mental health services to be too much to handle. They may also feel anxiety around having to figure out the logistics to access care. Without their parents' support and scaffolding, they may think that navigating the process is daunting and time-consuming.

Outreach to TAY must bill itself as being accessible and convenient. Lengths and frequency of appointments should be reasonable and respectful of TAY's time and stress. When youth do begin treatment, the topics of time management and work-life balance are critical to explore.

Stress is normal in college/graduate school (51%).

It takes maturity and strength to accept stress as a normal part of life and to consider a healthy level of stress as a positive motivating factor. Youth who report this belief likely understand the need for coping skills and stress management to function. However, in TAY with anxiety disorders, providing this reason for not seeking treatment leaves us with more questions than answers.

First, we wonder if these anxious TAY are accurately distinguishing between stress and anxiety. Do they believe that stressors are universally experienced, that their levels of anxiety around these stressors are normal, or both? Do they have insight into their impaired levels of functioning, or do they believe their functioning is within normal limits of college students? It seems that outreach to TAY should equip them with a clear lexicon, separating stressful experiences from anxious feelings and impaired functioning.

Second, this statement may suggest a lack of a nuanced understanding of how stress interferes with functioning. In TAY with ongoing cognitive and emotional growth, the idea of normal functioning is still dynamic during their transition to adulthood. Older adults, on the other hand, have decades of experience of their own normal functioning, so a departure from normality is more noticeable to themselves. Since TAY's self-awareness of any abnormal functioning may be less developed, they may believe their functional impairment to be a "normal" response to the high level of stress common to everyone. Treatment of TAY should involve an exploration of what "normal functioning" means to them, thus establishing baselines for future self-assessments.

Third, the use of the word "normal" is notable in and of itself. By leaning on the word "normal" to justify avoiding treatment, TAY may be suggesting significant levels of *personal stigma.* These negative attitudes towards people with mental health problems may make them unwilling to acknowledge their own issues, for fear of harming their own self-esteem [120]. Indeed, a different analysis using the same Healthy Minds survey found that personal stigma was negatively associated with several measures of help-seeking [121]. Fascinatingly, the survey participants who endorsed this reason also said they felt low *public* stigma towards mental health treatment. So why would TAY feel ashamed to begin treatment? We suggest a simple reason for anxious TAY: they do not wish to see themselves as being abnormal. Even if their peers withhold judgment and are supportive, and even if these anxious TAY have positive opinions about the benefit of treatment, they may not want to label themselves as needing help. This fear of deviating from the norm is understandable, considering that the transition years focus so heavily on consolidating identity and forming intimate relationships.

Outreach to TAY, in addition to continuing stigma reduction measures, should work to confront this personal stigma. Language that uses the term "typical" instead of "normal" and that describes young adult development as a growth process can give TAY better perspective on their issues. Examples of celebrities who are valued for their extraordinary lives and are proud to seek mental health treatment may help tackle the anxiety around being "abnormal" for needing mental health treatment.

> I question how serious my needs are (47%).

Similar to the quote before, this quote at first seems to convey maturity and self-awareness, but it may in fact suggest personal stigma or self-stigma (negative attitudes towards oneself). An example attitude from the Self-Stigma of Seeking Help Scale is "I would feel inadequate if I went to a therapist for psychological help" [122]. Unfortunately, the anxiety around self-judgment can lead to self-denial and neglect. This sets up anxious TAY for further exacerbation of anxiety symptoms and more severe functional impairment.

Outreach to TAY should address the sentiments behind this quote explicitly, by highlighting the courage and self-belief required to seek treatment. As high as the risk of anxiety disorders is in TAY, there should be no need for them to be their own gatekeepers.

In summary, this section framed barriers to treatment of anxiety disorders in TAY's own words. By wrestling with these quotes, we better understand their inhibitions and avoidances. With their perspectives, we can more empathetically and collaboratively create treatment and outreach approaches that target upstream factors of anxiety and systemic issues of accessibility. Working at both levels, we can make help-seeking behaviors convenient, confidential, desirable, participatory, and effective for TAY with anxiety.

Outreach and Prevention

Having identified risk factors of anxiety in the "Epidemiology" section, and having highlighted anxious attitudes that prevent help-seeking in the "Barriers to Treatment" section, we must now work to address upstream factors and ease accessibility. How can we do outreach to TAY, especially to at-risk groups, in a way that acknowledges and eases their concerns? And how can we prevent the peak prevalence of anxiety during the transition period when it is by definition a time of significant change?

This section presents notable examples of interventions at various levels: early childhood, school settings, peer support, community centers, and online. Looking at each of these situations where TAY spend significant time and effort, we identify how we can leverage people, programming, and rhetoric to craft situation-specific approaches to reaching out and preventing anxiety. Before this exploration of interventions, we begin by suggesting best practices for all measures taken.

Best Practices

We highly recommend the Best Practice Framework used by Australia's headspace model, which we will introduce more fully in the "Community-Based Interventions" subsection [123]. The headspace summary framework consists of four overarching outcomes: accessible, acceptable, appropriate, and sustainable.

Accessible practices are those that are affordable, convenient, timely, non-stigmatizing, flexible, inclusive, and awareness-raising. All young people up to the age of 26 years should feel welcome and accommodated in terms of time, finances, and means of access.

Acceptable practices ensure that interventions are youth-friendly, confidential, respectful, engaging, responsive, competent, and collaborative. This way, service providers and youth can together participate in effective care.

Appropriate practices allow for services that are early, comprehensive, developmentally appropriate, suitable to the stage of illness and complexity of presentation, evidence-based, and quality-assured. Such services necessitate thorough assessments and reasonable treatment plans.

Sustainable practices are community embedded, integrated within a network, effectively managed, and advocates for young people's wellbeing. Sustainability requires community partnerships, promotional campaigns, financial responsibility, and active problem-solving.

Using these best practice outcomes as objectives to be achieved and measures for self-assessment, outreach and prevention measures can be designed, evaluated, and improved. Such a design process that is grounded in best practices can yield more effective impact on mental healthcare for anxious TAY.

Early Childhood Interventions

In the "Epidemiology" section, we noted that parental anxiety and parenting styles have been identified as risk factors for later anxiety disorders. We also discussed how temperamental indicators, especially behavioral inhibition, can manifest as early as in the toddler years, and how anxiety disorders often arise during the elementary school years. Taking this all together, we see clear opportunities for prevention during early childhood.

For longitudinal outcomes, psychiatric treatment of childhood anxiety is critical. There is clear evidence of benefit from the Child/Adolescent Anxiety Multimodal Extended Long-term Survey [124]. Participants had a mean age of 10.7 years before treatment randomization and were diagnosed with an anxiety disorder [125]. The options for 12-week treatment included cognitive behavioral therapy, sertraline, combined cognitive behavioral therapy and sertraline, and pill placebo. At follow-up assessment, with the participants now averaging 17.6 years of age, there was clear evidence of better functioning, increased life satisfaction, and increasing rates of employment in the cognitive behavioral therapy group compared to the pill placebo group. Trajectories for the sertraline group, on the other hand, did not significantly differ from placebo; the combined therapy and sertraline group only differed from placebo in terms of employment outcomes. These findings underscore the importance of early intervention, targeting the first peak in prevalence of anxiety during the elementary school years, so that anxiety disorders do not persist into the TAY years.

Children who most need the interventions are those with genetic and temperamental risk factors. Unfortunately, literature around such risk reduction programs is sparse. A 2017 systematic review found only 2 studies that researched the effect of prevention programs on the onset of anxiety disorders in at-risk children younger than 13 [126]. These studies focused on children of parents with diagnosed anxiety disorders. Significant benefit was demonstrated: at 12-month follow-up after the program, only 5% of children in the intervention group had developed an anxiety disorder, compared to 31% in the control group [127]. The specific intervention was a family-based cognitive-behavioral intervention called Coping and Promoting Strength [128]. This highlights the importance of family therapy for the risk reduction of anxiety disorders in early adolescence.

Taken together, this literature affirms the critical work of child/adolescent psychiatrists and child-focused mental health professionals. Engaging parents, these practitioners can make a significant impact on family dynamics, children's mental health, and TAY's functioning and wellbeing years later.

School-Based Interventions

For most youth, school is the primary site of forming identity and building relationships. It is also a place rife with environmental risk factors for the development of anxiety. Since youth spend so many significant hours in school, and since so many youth develop anxiety disorders by the age of 26 years, it is necessary from a public health standpoint to ideally intervene at the kindergarten-through-grade-12 school level.

Since there exists a trough period in prevalence of anxiety disorders before the second peak of young adulthood (see "Epidemiology" section), outreach and prevention for TAY should begin in middle school, if not earlier. A 2019 systematic review found 20 studies that examined American middle and high school-based interventions for anxiety [129]. These interventions ranged from universal programs administered by teachers to targeted interventions administered by clinicians placed in schools. Of these 20 interventions, 15 were group sessions, and 17 used traditional programs such as cognitive behavioral therapy. Results of a meta-analysis showed significant reductions in anxiety symptoms after intervention compared to control. However, efficacy of the programs was highly variable, and the reductions in symptoms were no longer present 6 months after intervention.

These findings suggest the potential usefulness of prevention and intervention programs in school, and they bring up questions for research and program development. First, both universal and targeted approaches were found to be effective. Feiss et al. suggest a curriculum-embedded health unit as universal treatment, in addition to elective courses and after-school activities as targeted treatment. This idea provides both prevention during school hours and outreach after-hours, and it allows for students with greater symptoms to receive more help. However, such an idea must ensure that students who use the targeted treatment are not stigmatized by others and that group sessions are completely confidential and inclusive.

Second, both trained schoolteachers and mental health professionals were found to provide effective interventions. This supports the feasibility of teacher-led curricular changes that increase literacy around anxiety and equip students with resilience strategies. However, whether these changes can lower anxious TAY's self-reported barriers to treatment remains to be seen.

Third, it is important to recognize that the effects of intervention did not persist after 6 months. This fact suggests the need for longitudinal programming, giving students the chance to practice anxiety reduction skills in the face of different stressors. Furthermore, we suggest that broader changes are necessary at the level of school culture. As organizations, schools too should strive towards the best practices identified above, in order to lessen students' potential anxiety around their school experience.

All in all, the preliminary evidence for school-based interventions is promising. Further research, especially examining the impact of mental health curriculum on the later incidence of anxiety disorders, remains to be conducted.

Peer Support Services

Peers can provide invaluable support towards outreach efforts. Given that anxious TAY self-report believing that "stress is normal," peers can affirm that statement by citing their own experiences of stress, all the while demonstrating to TAY that stress impacted their own mental health significantly. Furthermore, since TAY report the attitude "I prefer to deal with these issues on my own," peers can pass down knowledge to TAY about the self-management skills that worked for them. In other words, as nonprofessionals, peers can feel more relatable and empowering.

Peer support services is a specific peer model where TAY who have experienced mental health challenges provide support to other TAY, who are currently seeking help for similar challenges. These types of services are in the early stages of development in the United States. A 2017 scoping review found 30 such programs with peers who played various roles, from supporting clinical interventions to delivering services entirely themselves [130]. Data concerning consumer outcomes is still limited, however. Still, it is worth examining how peers can be valuable for helping anxious TAY.

The scoping review found that the most common roles played by peers were as follows:

- *Instruction, skills development, and mentoring* (24 programs): Coaching TAY on symptom management and resilience strategies, peers can equip TAY with the skills "to deal with their issues on their own."
- *Emotional support* (18 programs): Beautifully, peers have provided TAY with understanding, affirmation, and hope. By lending their ears and making TAY feel appreciated, peers can address the attitude held by TAY with anxiety disorders: "I question how serious my needs are."

- *Information and education* (17 programs): Peers have helped increase mental health literacy in their TAY clients, and they have served as navigators for their clients' treatment options and community resources. These services are convenient and forward-looking, helping to break down the self-reported barrier "I don't have time." Furthermore, by demonstrating their acquired knowledge and passion for mental health, peers confront this attitude of not having the time for mental healthcare.
- *Advocacy* (15 programs): Peers fundraised and campaigned for mental health services at organizational and system levels. Taking this role, peers help make visible the needs of anxious TAY, and they inspire the investment of resources into prevention measures.

From these roles, we can see that peers with recent, prior experience with mental healthcare have insight into what TAY need, seek out, and avoid. Peers reduce stigma, ease skepticism towards treatment, and inspire culture change, leading to likelier help-seeking by those who follow them closely in age.

Community-Based Interventions

As TAY separate from parents and individuate, they may wish to seek out resources on their own, outside of their parents' health insurance and purview. Furthermore, as they begin forming mature relationships, they may long for human connection outside of what they can find at schools. Community centers leverage these TAY developmental needs in their accessible, appropriate outreach to TAY, engaging them in TAY-acceptable care.

A 2019 scoping review describes key attributes of integrated community-based youth service hubs for mental health [131]. The eight programs that met inclusion criteria for review were as follows: headspace and Orygen Specialist Program (formerly Orygen Youth Health) in Australia, Jigsaw in Ireland, Forward Thinking Birmingham (formerly Youthspace) in the United Kingdom, Youth One Stop Shops (YOSS) in New Zealand, and YouthCan IMPACT, Foundry, and ACCESS Open Minds in Canada. The Australian headspace model deserves to be highlighted here for the research concerning its organizational characteristics, its relevance to anxiety in TAY, and its success at outreach and prevention. Some notable facts about headspace include the following:

- The program has over 110 centers across the country [132], all of which follow the Best Practice Framework that we have described previously.
- A total of 99,892 youth accessed a headspace center in the 2018–2019 financial year [133]. These included members of marginalized groups, such as indigenous youth and LGBTQ+ youth [134].
- The peak age of presentation at headspace is at the beginning of the transition to adulthood (ages 15–17 years), and the most common presenting problems are mood and anxiety symptoms and disorders [135].
- The most common mental health treatments provided in headspace centers are cognitive behavioral therapy, supportive counseling, and psychoeducation [136].
- Other core services include drug and alcohol services, primary care, and vocational assistance, all three of which we have described as impacting anxiety.
- Preliminary outcomes research has been positive, with TAY experiencing significant improvement in functioning and spending fewer days absent from school and employment [134].
- Models similar to headspace have been adopted in culturally appropriate ways in various countries, including several of the eight mentioned above. New models are currently in development. In the Netherlands, for example, @ease has recently been launched [137].

It should be recognized that all of these programs exist in countries with universal healthcare systems in addition to private sector services. Furthermore, these countries all have smaller populations than the United States. This fact points out the importance of reaching out to TAY in ways outside of the healthcare system.

On the other hand, it should be noted that community-based service hubs cannot exist in isolation from other forms of mental healthcare. After all, 40% of headspace clients do not show significant symptomatic and/or functional improvement from care offered in the center. These clients may instead require outreach care, specific disorder-based expertise, and acute services [133]. Therefore, community-based interventions should vet other mental health services as TAY-friendly and then establish partnerships and a referral system. By doing so, they can help navigate TAY to appropriate treatment.

Furthermore, compared to school-based interventions, community centers must make greater efforts to increase awareness of their existence among TAY. Information about headspace is disseminated to local schools, at community events, to local services and agencies, and to tertiary education institutions. Community activities targeted at youth are also organized outside of the centers [138]. These promotional efforts are critical for gaining the trust of anxious TAY who are concerned about confidentiality, affordability, and appropriateness of care.

Online Interventions

Today's youth—both children and TAY—are hyper-connected through the Internet [139]. There is an abundance of literature associating problematic social media usage with poor mental health outcomes [140–142]. However, online activity is an inevitable way of life for youth, who use the Internet to gather information, consume content, and interact with each other through social media. Furthermore, online activity can be a coping strategy for mental health symptoms [143]. Rather than shame them for their behaviors, we must meet them where they are. Acknowledging the significant time spent by youth online, we can leverage online platforms for stigma reduction, education, and accessible therapeutic interventions.

There is likely benefit of using social networks for outreach and anxiety awareness campaigns, as evidence of their positive effects on stigma reduction grows. A 2015 systematic review examined 30 studies of suicide prevention through social media, and it highlighted social media's scalability, accessibility, and peer support [144]. These benefits are reflected in a study of the 2009–2014 Time to Change mental health anti-stigma program in England. The program's social marketing campaign grew the Time to Change online audience from 50,000 people in July–September 2010 to more than 250,000 in September–December 2014; the vast majority of these people accessed the Facebook webpage or the Twitter account [145]. This rapid growth of interest in an online mental health campaign demonstrates the dual nature of social media as both informative and attractive.

In addition to the vast number of users, the vast number of *data* on social media can also be useful for understanding and reducing stigma. A 2017 computational modeling of Reddit content, comparing anxiety-related posts to control posts, found two- and three-word phrases that were more common to anxiety-related posts than control posts [146]. The common two-word phrases were to be expected, including "self-esteem," "heart rate," "physical symptoms," and "social media." However, three-word phrases in the anxiety community were predominantly phrases seeking commonality and advice: "does anyone else," "wondering if anyone," "has anyone else," "wanted to share," and "in high school." Other phrases describe the struggle with anxiety disorders: "no matter how," "stop thinking about," and "get rid of." These findings demonstrate that social media can serve as a space for anxious TAY to express themselves, feel understood, and seek out hope from others. Although outcomes research concerning Reddit remains to be performed, these preliminary language modeling results suggest the potential of the Internet as a safe and confidential setting for group therapy or peer support for anxiety.

In addition to stigma reduction, studies have looked at literacy outcomes of online psychoeducation. Two randomized controlled trials used a brief video as a direct-to-consumer marketing campaign for social anxiety disorder. They found some meaningful impact on knowledge about social anxiety disorder and cognitive behavioral therapy [147]. A 2018 systematic review examined other studies of information and communication technologies-based interventions on mental health literacy among youth [148]; it found one study that showed increased anxiety literacy in TAY. This was a randomized controlled trial with 67 Australian TAY (18–25 years old), who received 3 weeks of either online psychoeducation or online attention-matched control information. Interestingly, anxiety literacy significantly increased, but not depression literacy [149], suggesting greater prior knowledge of depression among youth. Clearly, greater research is needed to determine the efficacy of online psychoeducation interventions.

Besides education and stigma reduction, the Internet can provide accessible means of telemedicine and therapy. The convenience, the familiarity of one's own computer, and the perceived relative safety in one's own home can address the concerns endorsed by many TAY with anxiety disorders. Technology-delivered interventions for anxiety in children and adolescents are actively being developed. A 2018 systematic review identified 20 technology-delivered interventions targeting anxiety disorders in youth 6–18 years old [150]. Most were computer- or Internet-based cognitive behavioral therapy (8 different programs, most therapist-assisted), and the rest were attention bias modification training (7 trials, all unguided), cognitive bias modification training (2, unguided), and video games for treating anxiety (3, unguided). Of these, technology-delivered cognitive behavioral therapy delivered the most effective treatment, with effect sizes comparable to those for face-to-face cognitive behavioral therapy [151]. This review has these implications: Mental healthcare professionals' expert guidance remains important for effective care, though whether this guidance is delivered in-person or online matters less for outcomes. Still, further development of these interventions is still required, as is subsequent research into utilization rates among TAY.

Summary

In summary, our exploration of outreach and prevention methods has extended across many domains of youths' lives. Since anxiety disorders are so prevalent, and the barriers to treatment are substantial, a multipronged public health approach is not just reasonable, but necessary. Evidence is mounting that early, school-based, peer-delivered, community-based, and technology-delivered interventions are all effective, thanks to the tremendous efforts of mental health champions and practitioners from various walks of life. As we continue to work towards accessible, acceptable, appropriate, and sustainable practices for serving TAY, let us meet anxious youth where they are, all the while creating culture change around anxiety.

Conclusion

This chapter has highlighted numerous twenty-first-century advances in the mental healthcare of TAY with anxiety disorders. Through large epidemiological studies, we are beginning to understand that the transition to adulthood is inherently an anxiety-inducing period. Towards addressing this, progress has been made in the realms of both public health and clinical practice. To prevent the development of everyday anxiety into anxiety disorders in TAY, effective interventions involving parents, teachers, peers, community centers, and technology are being implemented across childhood and young adulthood. When TAY do present with anxiety disorders, thorough assessment tools and evidence-based therapeutic methods can be used to significantly improve their functioning and distress.

Still, there remains much to be learned about anxious TAY. In reviewing the literature, we found few studies that looked specifically at anxiety disorders in TAY. Instead, studies tended to be bounded by the age of 18 years. Because 18 years is not a relevant cutoff in the epidemiology of anxiety disorders, and since the transition ages of 16–26 years present a unique set of challenges, future research must focus on TAY cohorts. Furthermore, studies tended to mix together depression and anxiety outcomes. Though highly comorbid with depression, anxiety disorders deserve to be independently investigated. After all, literacy around anxiety has been found to be lower than that around depression. In addition, anxiety may present unique barriers to treatment.

The need for more research and more prevention is dire. TAY with anxiety disorders are known to experience "failure to launch," remaining at home and depending on their parents [152]. Since anxiety disorders are so prevalent, it is no wonder that in 2014, adults aged 18 to 34 years were more likely to be living in their parents' home than with a domestic partner in their own household [68]. Furthermore, for TAY who do end up forming intimate relationships and starting families of their own, anxiety may make an intergenerational, multigenerational impact. After all, parental anxiety and parenting styles are risk factors for the development of anxiety disorders in children.

Therefore, mental healthcare of TAY with anxiety disorders not only has health-related implications, but also makes societal impact. Reflecting this, our chapter serves as both a summation of knowledge and a call to action. Our dream is the provision of holistic and evidence-based care throughout youths' lives and communities, meeting them where they and their anxiety are. By destigmatizing and addressing TAY's fears, worries, symptoms, and behaviors, we empower our society's new adults to be confident, resilient, and responsible individuals.

References

1. Copeland WE, Angold A, Shanahan L, Costello EJ. Longitudinal patterns of anxiety from childhood to adulthood: the Great Smoky Mountains Study. J Am Acad Child Adolesc Psychiatry. 2014;53(1):21–33. https://doi.org/10.1016/j.jaac.2013.09.017.
2. Giedd JN. The teen brain: insights from neuroimaging. J Adolesc Health. 2008;42(4):335–43. https://doi.org/10.1016/j.jadohealth.2008.01.007.
3. Casey BJ, Getz S, Galvan A. The adolescent brain. Dev Rev. 2008;28(1):62–77. https://doi.org/10.1016/j.dr.2007.08.003.
4. Pruitt DB, American Academy of Child and Adolescent Psychiatry. Your adolescent: emotional, behavioral, and cognitive development from early adolescence through the teen years. 1st ed. New York: HarperCollins; 1999.
5. Anxiety and Depression Association of America: Understand the Facts. 2018. https://adaa.org/understanding-anxiety. Accessed 1 July 2020.
6. Brumariu LE, Obsuth I, Lyons-Ruth K. Quality of attachment relationships and peer relationship dysfunction among late adolescents with and without anxiety disorders. J Anxiety Disord. 2013;27(1):116–24. https://doi.org/10.1016/j.janxdis.2012.09.002.
7. Van Ameringen M, Mancini C, Farvolden P. The impact of anxiety disorders on educational achievement. J Anxiety Disord. 2003;17(5):561–71. https://doi.org/10.1016/s0887-6185(02)00228-1.
8. Woodward LJ, Fergusson DM. Life course outcomes of young people with anxiety disorders in adolescence. J Am Acad Child Adolesc Psychiatry. 2001;40(9):1086–93. https://doi.org/10.1097/00004583-200109000-00018.
9. Kasteenpohja T, Marttunen M, Aalto-Setälä T, Perälä J, Saarni SI, Suvisaari J. Treatment adequacy of anxiety disorders among young adults in Finland. BMC Psychiatry. 2016;16:63. Published 2016 Mar 15. https://doi.org/10.1186/s12888-016-0766-0.
10. Stavropoulos V, Gomez R, Steen E, Beard C, Liew L, Griffiths MD. The longitudinal association between anxiety and internet addiction in adolescence: the moderating effect of classroom extraversion. J Behav Addict. 2017;6(2):237–47. https://doi.org/10.1556/2006.6.2017.026.
11. Lopez B, Turner RJ, Saavedra LM. Anxiety and risk for substance dependence among late adolescents/young adults. J Anxiety Disord. 2005;19(3):275–94. https://doi.org/10.1016/j.janxdis.2004.03.001.
12. Nelemans SA, Hale WW 3rd, Raaijmakers QA, Branje SJ, van Lier PA, Meeus WH. Longitudinal associations between social anxiety symptoms and cannabis use throughout adolescence: the role of peer involvement. Eur Child Adolesc Psychiatry. 2016;25(5):483–92. https://doi.org/10.1007/s00787-015-0747-8.
13. Dindo LN, Recober A, Haddad R, Calarge CA. Comorbidity of migraine, major depressive disorder, and generalized anxiety disorder in adolescents and young adults. Int J Behav Med. 2017;24(4):528–34. https://doi.org/10.1007/s12529-016-9620-5.
14. Bortoluzzi A, Salum GA, da Rosa ED, Chagas VS, Castro MAA, Manfro GG. DNA methylation in adolescents with anxiety disorder: a longitudinal study. Sci Rep. 2018;8(1):13800. https://doi.org/10.1038/s41598-018-32090-1.
15. Greenberg T, Bertocci MA, Chase HW, et al. Mediation by anxiety of the relationship between amygdala activity during emotion processing and poor quality of life in young adults. Transl Psychiatry. 2017;7(7):e1178. https://doi.org/10.1038/tp.2017.127.

16. Kraft JD, Grant DM, White EJ, Taylor DL, Frosio KE. Cognitive mechanisms influence the relationship between social anxiety and depression among college students. J Am Coll Heal. 2019:1–7. https://doi.org/10.1080/07448481.2019.1661844.
17. Lieb R, Miché M, Gloster AT, Beesdo-Baum K, Meyer AH, Wittchen HU. Impact of specific phobia on the risk of onset of mental disorders: a 10-year prospective-longitudinal community study of adolescents and young adults. Depress Anxiety. 2016;33(7):667–75. https://doi.org/10.1002/da.22487.
18. Stein MB, Fuetsch M, Müller N, Höfler M, Lieb R, Wittchen HU. Social anxiety disorder and the risk of depression: a prospective community study of adolescents and young adults. Arch Gen Psychiatry. 2001;58(3):251–6. https://doi.org/10.1001/archpsyc.58.3.251.
19. Gustavson K, Knudsen AK, Nesvåg R, Knudsen GP, Vollset SE, Reichborn-Kjennerud T. Prevalence and stability of mental disorders among young adults: findings from a longitudinal study. BMC Psychiatry. 2018;18(1):65. https://doi.org/10.1186/s12888-018-1647-5.
20. Boden JM, Fergusson DM, Horwood LJ. Anxiety disorders and suicidal behaviours in adolescence and young adulthood: findings from a longitudinal study. Psychol Med. 2007;37(3):431–40. https://doi.org/10.1017/S0033291706009147.
21. Miché M, Hofer PD, Voss C, Meyer AH, Gloster AT, Beesdo-Baum K, et al. Mental disorders and the risk for the subsequent first suicide attempt: results of a community study on adolescents and young adults. Eur Child Adolesc Psychiatry. 2018;27(7):839–48. https://doi.org/10.1007/s00787-017-1060-5.
22. Goldston DB, Daniel SS, Erkanli A, Reboussin BA, Mayfield A, Frazier PH, et al. Psychiatric diagnoses as contemporaneous risk factors for suicide attempts among adolescents and young adults: developmental changes. J Consult Clin Psychol. 2009;77(2):281–90. https://doi.org/10.1037/a0014732.
23. US Bureau of Labor Statistics. College enrollment and work activity of recent high school and college graduates summary. US Department of Labor. 2020. https://www.bls.gov/news.release/hsgec.htm. Accessed 1 July 2020.
24. Kessler RC, Chiu WT, Demler O, Merikangas KR, Walters EE. Prevalence, severity, and comorbidity of 12-month DSM-IV disorders in the National Comorbidity Survey Replication. Arch Gen Psychiatry. 2005;62(6):617–27. https://doi.org/10.1001/archpsyc.62.6.617.
25. American College Health Association. Hanover, MD, 2018. American College Health Association-National College Health Assessment II: Reference Group Executive Summary Fall 2017. https://www.acha.org/documents/ncha/NCHA-II_FALL_2017_REFERENCE_GROUP_EXECUTIVE_SUMMARY.pdf. Accessed 1 July 2020.
26. Wittchen HU, Lieb R, Schuster P, Oldehinkel AJ. When is onset? Investigations into early developmental stages of anxiety and depressive disorders. In: Rapoport JL, editor. Childhood onset of adult psychopathology: clinical and research advances. Washington, D.C.: American Psychiatric Press; 1999. p. 259–302.
27. Newman DL, Moffitt TE, Caspi A, Magdol L, Silva PA, Stanton WR. Psychiatric disorder in a birth cohort of young adults: prevalence, comorbidity, clinical significance, and new case incidence from ages 11 to 21. J Consult Clin Psychol. 1996;64(3):552.
28. Merikangas KR, He JP, Burstein M, Swanson SA, Avenevoli S, Cui L, et al. Lifetime prevalence of mental disorders in U.S. adolescents: results from the National Comorbidity Survey Replication--Adolescent Supplement (NCS-A). J Am Acad Child Adolesc Psychiatry. 2010;49(10):980–9. https://doi.org/10.1016/j.jaac.2010.05.017.
29. Hayward C, Wilson KA, Lagle K, Killen JD, Taylor CB. Parent-reported predictors of adolescent panic attacks. J Am Acad Child Adolesc Psychiatry. 2004;43(5):613–20. https://doi.org/10.1097/00004583-200405000-00015.
30. Biederman J, Petty C, Faraone SV, Henin A, Hirshfeld-Becker D, Pollack MH, et al. Effects of parental anxiety disorders in children at high risk for panic disorder: a controlled study. J Affect Disord. 2006;94(1–3):191–7. https://doi.org/10.1016/j.jad.2006.04.012.
31. Lieb R, Wittchen HU, Höfler M, Fuetsch M, Stein MB, Merikangas KR. Parental psychopathology, parenting styles, and the risk of social phobia in offspring: a prospective-longitudinal community study. Arch Gen Psychiatry. 2000;57(9):859–66. https://doi.org/10.1001/archpsyc.57.9.859.
32. Unnewehr S, Schneider S, Florin I, Margraf J. Psychopathology in children of patients with panic disorder or animal phobia. Psychopathology. 1998;31(2):69–84.
33. Hirshfeld-Becker DR, Micco JA, Simoes NA, Henin A. High risk studies and developmental antecedents of anxiety disorders. Am J Med Genet C Semin Med Genet. 2008;148C(2):99–117. https://doi.org/10.1002/ajmg.c.30170.
34. Weissman MM, Wickramaratne P, Nomura Y, Warner V, Pilowsky D, Verdeli H. Offspring of depressed parents: 20 years later. Am J Psychiatry. 2006;163(6):1001–8. https://doi.org/10.1176/ajp.2006.163.6.1001.
35. Yap MB, Pilkington PD, Ryan SM, Jorm AF. Parental factors associated with depression and anxiety in young people: a systematic review and meta-analysis. J Affect Disord. 2014;156:8–23. https://doi.org/10.1016/j.jad.2013.11.007.
36. Phillips NK, Hammen CL, Brennan PA, Najman JM, Bor W. Early adversity and the prospective prediction of depressive and anxiety disorders in adoles-

cents. J Abnorm Child Psychol. 2005;33(1):13–24. https://doi.org/10.1007/s10802-005-0930-3.
37. Pontillo M, Tata MC, Averna R, Demaria F, Gargiullo P, Guerrera S, et al. Peer victimization and onset of social anxiety disorder in children and adolescents. Brain Sci. 2019;9(6):132. https://doi.org/10.3390/brainsci9060132.
38. Hettema JM, Prescott CA, Myers JM, Neale MC, Kendler KS. The structure of genetic and environmental risk factors for anxiety disorders in men and women. Arch Gen Psychiatry. 2005;62(2):182–9. https://doi.org/10.1001/archpsyc.62.2.182.
39. Spatola CAM, Fagnani C, Pesenti-Gritti P, Ogliari A, Stazi MA, Battaglia M. A general population twin study of the CBCL/6-18 DSM-oriented scales. J Am Acad Child Adolesc Psychiatry. 2007;46(5):619–27. https://doi.org/10.1097/CHI.0b013e3180335b12.
40. Svihra M, Katzman MA. Behavioural inhibition: a predictor of anxiety. Paediatr Child Health. 2004;9(8):547–50. https://doi.org/10.1093/pch/9.8.547.
41. Schwartz CE, Snidman N, Kagan J. Adolescent social anxiety as an outcome of inhibited temperament in childhood. J Am Acad Child Adolesc Psychiatry. 1999;38(8):1008–15. https://doi.org/10.1097/00004583-199908000-00017.
42. Biederman J, Hirshfeld-Becker DR, Rosenbaum JF, Hérot C, Friedman D, Snidman N, et al. Further evidence of association between behavioral inhibition and social anxiety in children. Am J Psychiatry. 2001;158(10):1673–9. https://doi.org/10.1176/appi.ajp.158.10.1673.
43. McNally RJ. Anxiety sensitivity and panic disorder. Biol Psychiatry. 2002;52(10):938–46. https://doi.org/10.1016/s0006-3223(02)01475-0.
44. McLaughlin KA, Hatzenbuehler ML. Stressful life events, anxiety sensitivity, and internalizing symptoms in adolescents. J Abnorm Psychol. 2009;118(3):659–69. https://doi.org/10.1037/a0016499.
45. Schmidt NB, Zvolensky MJ, Maner JK. Anxiety sensitivity: prospective prediction of panic attacks and Axis I pathology. J Psychiatr Res. 2006;40(8):691–9. https://doi.org/10.1016/j.jpsychires.2006.07.009.
46. Nieto SJ, Patriquin MA, Nielsen DA, Kosten TA. Don't worry; be informed about the epigenetics of anxiety. Pharmacol Biochem Behav. 2016;146-147:60–72. https://doi.org/10.1016/j.pbb.2016.05.006.
47. Yang B, Wei J, Ju P, Chen J. Effects of regulating intestinal microbiota on anxiety symptoms: a systematic review. Gen Psychiatr. 2019;32(2):e100056. https://doi.org/10.1136/gpsych-2019-100056.
48. Devaux CA, Raoult D. The microbiological memory, an epigenetic regulator governing the balance between good health and metabolic disorders. Front Microbiol. 2018;9:1379. https://doi.org/10.3389/fmicb.2018.01379.
49. Beiter R, Nash R, McCrady M, et al. The prevalence and correlates of depression, anxiety, and stress in a sample of college students. J Affect Disord. 2015;173:90–6. https://doi.org/10.1016/j.jad.2014.10.054.
50. Cohen JM, Blasey C, Barr Taylor C, Weiss BJ, Newman MG. Anxiety and related disorders and concealment in sexual minority young adults. Behav Ther. 2016;47(1):91–101. https://doi.org/10.1016/j.beth.2015.09.006.
51. Safren SA, Pantalone DW. Social anxiety and barriers to resilience among lesbian, gay, and bisexual adolescents. In: Omoto AM, Kurtzman HS, editors. Contemporary perspectives on lesbian, gay, and bisexual psychology. Sexual orientation and mental health: examining identity and development in lesbian, gay, and bisexual people. Washington, D.C.: American Psychological Association; 2006. p. 55–71.
52. Pachankis JE, Goldfried MR. Social anxiety in young gay men. J Anxiety Disord. 2006;20(8):996–1015. https://doi.org/10.1016/j.janxdis.2006.01.001.
53. White SW, Oswald D, Ollendick T, Scahill L. Anxiety in children and adolescents with autism spectrum disorders. Clin Psychol Rev. 2009;29(3):216–29. https://doi.org/10.1016/j.cpr.2009.01.003.
54. Lever AG, Geurts HM. Psychiatric co-occurring symptoms and disorders in young, middle-aged, and older adults with autism spectrum disorder. J Autism Dev Disord. 2016;46(6):1916–30. https://doi.org/10.1007/s10803-016-2722-8.
55. Beidas RS, Stewart RE, Walsh L, Lucas S, Downey MM, Jackson K, et al. Free, brief, and validated: standardized instruments for low-resource mental health settings. Cogn Behav Pract. 2015;22(1):5–19. https://doi.org/10.1016/j.cbpra.2014.02.002.
56. Garcia-Lopez LJ, Salvador MC, De Los Reyes A. Assessment of social anxiety in adolescents. In: Ranta K, La Greca A, Garcia-Lopez LJ, Marttunen M, editors. Social anxiety and phobia in adolescents. Cham: Springer; 2015. https://doi.org/10.1007/978-3-319-16703-9_6.
57. Silverman WK, Saavedra LM, Pina AA. Test-retest reliability of anxiety symptoms and diagnoses with the anxiety disorders interview schedule for DSM-IV: child and parent versions. J Am Acad Child Adolesc Psychiatry. 2001;40(8):937–44. https://doi.org/10.1097/00004583-200108000-00016.
58. Kaufman J, Birmaher B, Axelson D, Perepletchikova F, Brent D, Ryan N. The kiddie schedule for affective disorders and schizophrenia for school-aged children (K-SADS-PL DSM-5). New Haven: Advanced Care for Intervention and Services Research (ACISR) for Early Onset Mood and Anxiety Disorders, Western Psychiatric Institute and Clinic, Child and Adolescent Research and Education (CARE) Program, Yale University; 2016.
59. Goldenring JM, Rosen DS. Getting into adolescent heads: an essential update. Contemp Pediatr. 2004;21(1):64–90.
60. Josephson AM, AACAP Work Group on Quality Issues. Practice parameter for the assessment of

the family. J Am Acad Child Adolesc Psychiatry. 2007;46(7):922–37. https://doi.org/10.1097/chi.0b013e318054e713.

61. Connolly SD, Bernstein GA, Work Group on Quality Issues. Practice parameter for the assessment and treatment of children and adolescents with anxiety disorders. J Am Acad Child Adolesc Psychiatry. 2007;46(2):267–83. https://doi.org/10.1097/01.chi.0000246070.23695.06.
62. Copeland W, Shanahan L, Costello EJ, Angold A. Cumulative prevalence of psychiatric disorders by young adulthood: a prospective cohort analysis from the Great Smoky Mountains Study. J Am Acad Child Adolesc Psychiatry. 2011;50(3):252–61. https://doi.org/10.1016/j.jaac.2010.12.014.
63. Singh SP. Transition of care from child to adult mental health services: the great divide. Curr Opin Psychiatry. 2009;22(4):386–90. https://doi.org/10.1097/YCO.0b013e32832c9221.
64. Kodish I, Rockhill C, Varley C. Pharmacotherapy for anxiety disorders in children and adolescents. Dialogues Clin Neurosci. 2011;13(4):439–52.
65. Patel DR, Feucht C, Brown K, Ramsay J. Pharmacological treatment of anxiety disorders in children and adolescents: a review for practitioners. Transl Pediatr. 2018;7(1):23–35. https://doi.org/10.21037/tp.2017.08.05.
66. Reivich K, Gillham JE, Chaplin TM, Seligman MEP. From helplessness to optimism: the role of resilience in treating and preventing depression in youth. In: Goldstein S, Brooks R, editors. Handbook of resilience in children. Boston: Springer; 2013. https://doi.org/10.1007/978-1-4614-3661-4_12.
67. Ng R, Ang RP, Ho MR. Coping with anxiety, depression, anger and aggression: the mediational role of resilience in adolescents. Child Youth Care Forum. 2012;41:529–46. https://doi.org/10.1007/s10566-012-9182-x.
68. Fry R. For first time in modern era, living with parents edges out other living arrangements for 18- to 34-year-olds. Washington, D.C.: Pew Research Center; 2016. https://www.pewsocialtrends.org/2016/05/24/for-first-time-in-modern-era-living-with-parents-edges-out-other-living-arrangements-for-18-to-34-year-olds. Accessed 1 July 2020.
69. Burstein M, Ginsburg GS, Tein JY. Parental anxiety and child symptomatology: an examination of additive and interactive effects of parent psychopathology. J Abnorm Child Psychol. 2010;38(7):897–909. https://doi.org/10.1007/s10802-010-9415-0.
70. Herbert JD, Gaudiano BA, Rheingold AA, Myers VH, Dalrymple K, Nolan EM. Social skills training augments the effectiveness of cognitive behavioral group therapy for social anxiety disorder. Behav Ther. 2005;36(2):125–38. https://doi.org/10.1016/S0005-7894(05)80061-9.
71. Landon TM, Barlow DH. Cognitive-behavioral treatment for panic disorder: current status. J Psychiatr Pract. 2004;10(4):211–26.
72. Walkup JT, Albano AM, Piacentini J, Birmaher B, Compton SN, Sherrill JT, et al. Cognitive behavioral therapy, sertraline, or a combination in childhood anxiety [published correction appears in N Engl J Med. 2013 Jan 31;368(5):490]. N Engl J Med. 2008;359(26):2753–66. https://doi.org/10.1056/NEJMoa0804633.
73. Kendall PC, Peterman JS. CBT for adolescents with anxiety: mature yet still developing. Am J Psychiatry. 2015;172(6):519–30. https://doi.org/10.1176/appi.ajp.2015.14081061.
74. Hoffman LJ, Guerry JD, Albano AM. Launching anxious young adults: a specialized cognitive-behavioral intervention for transitional aged youth. Curr Psychiatry Rep. 2018;20(4):25. Published 2018 Mar 27. https://doi.org/10.1007/s11920-018-0888-9.
75. Edlund NJ, Carlberg G. Psychodynamic psychotherapy with adolescents and young adults: outcome in routine practice. Clin Child Psychol Psychiatry. 2016;21(1):66–80. https://doi.org/10.1177/1359104514554311.
76. Markowitz JC, Lipsitz J, Milrod BL. Critical review of outcome research on interpersonal psychotherapy for anxiety disorders. Depress Anxiety. 2014;31(4):316–25. https://doi.org/10.1002/da.22238.
77. Hayes SC, Hofmann SG. The third wave of cognitive behavioral therapy and the rise of process-based care. World Psychiatry. 2017;16(3):245–6. https://doi.org/10.1002/wps.20442.
78. Lin J, Chadi N, Shrier L. Mindfulness-based interventions for adolescent health. Curr Opin Pediatr. 2019;31(4):469–75. https://doi.org/10.1097/MOP.0000000000000760.
79. Hjeltnes A, Molde H, Schanche E, Vøllestad J, Svendsen JL, Moltu C, et al. An open trial of mindfulness-based stress reduction for young adults with social anxiety disorder. Scand J Psychol. 2017;58(1):80–90. https://doi.org/10.1111/sjop.12342.
80. Evans S, Ferrando S, Findler M, Stowell C, Smart C, Haglin D. Mindfulness-based cognitive therapy for generalized anxiety disorder. J Anxiety Disord. 2008;22(4):716–21. https://doi.org/10.1016/j.janxdis.2007.07.005.
81. Hofmann SG, Gómez AF. Mindfulness-based interventions for anxiety and depression. Psychiatr Clin North Am. 2017;40(4):739–49. https://doi.org/10.1016/j.psc.2017.08.008.
82. Borquist-Conlon DS, Maynard BR, Brendel KE, Farina AS. Mindfulness-based interventions for youth with anxiety: a systematic review and meta-analysis. Res Soc Work Pract. 2019;29(2):195–205. https://doi.org/10.1177/1049731516684961.
83. Livheim F, Hayes L, Ghaderi A, Magnusdottir T, Högfeldt A, Rowse J, et al. The effectiveness of acceptance and commitment therapy for adolescent mental health: Swedish and Australian pilot outcomes. J Child Fam Stud. 2015;24:1016–33. https://doi.org/10.1007/s10826-014-9912-9.

84. Bluett EJ, Homan KJ, Morrison KL, Levin ME, Twohig MP. Acceptance and commitment therapy for anxiety and OCD spectrum disorders: an empirical review. J Anxiety Disord. 2014;28(6):612–24. https://doi.org/10.1016/j.janxdis.2014.06.008.
85. Swain J, Hancock K, Hainsworth C, Bowman J. Acceptance and commitment therapy in the treatment of anxiety: a systematic review. Clin Psychol Rev. 2013;33(8):965–78. https://doi.org/10.1016/j.cpr.2013.07.002.
86. Neacsiu AD, Rizvi SL, Linehan MM. Dialectical behavior therapy skills use as a mediator and outcome of treatment for borderline personality disorder. Behav Res Ther. 2010;48(9):832–9. https://doi.org/10.1016/j.brat.2010.05.017.
87. Marra T. Depressed and anxious: the dialectical behavior therapy workbook for overcoming depression and anxiety. New Harbinger Publications; 2004.
88. Welch SS, Osborne TL, Pryzgoda J. Augmenting exposure-based treatment for anxiety disorders with principles and skills from dialectical behavior therapy. In: Sookman D, Leahy RL, editors. Treatment resistant anxiety disorders: resolving impasses to symptom remission. Hoboken: Taylor & Francis; 2009.
89. U.S. Food and Drug Administration. 2005. "Class suicidality labeling language for antidepressants." https://www.accessdata.fda.gov/drugsatfda_docs/label/2005/20031s045,20936s020lbl.pdf. Accessed 8 July 2020.
90. Leslie LK, Newman TB, Chesney PJ, Perrin JM. The Food and Drug Administration's deliberations on antidepressant use in pediatric patients. Pediatrics. 2005;116(1):195–204. https://doi.org/10.1542/peds.2005-0074.
91. Ignaszewski MJ, Waslick B. Update on randomized placebo-controlled trials in the past decade for treatment of major depressive disorder in child and adolescent patients: a systematic review. J Child Adolesc Psychopharmacol. 2018;28(10):668–75. https://doi.org/10.1089/cap.2017.0174.
92. Leonte KG, Puliafico A, Na P, Rynn MA. Pharmacotherapy for anxiety disorders in children and adolescents. UpToDate. 2019. https://www.uptodate.com/contents/pharmacotherapy-for-anxiety-disorders-in-children-and-adolescents. Accessed 1 July 2020.
93. Barnett S, Riddle MA. Anxiolytics: benzodiazepines, buspirone and others. In: Martin A, Scahill L, Charney DS, et al., editors. Pediatric psychopharmacology: principles and practice. Oxford: Oxford Univ Press; 2003. p. 341–52.
94. Berney T, Kolvin I, Bhate SR, et al. School phobia: a therapeutic trial with clomipramine and short-term outcome. Br J Psychiatry. 1981;138:110–8. https://doi.org/10.1192/bjp.138.2.110.
95. Hazell P, O'Connell D, Heathcote D, Henry D. Tricyclic drugs for depression in children and adolescents. Cochrane Database Syst Rev. 2002;(2):CD002317. https://doi.org/10.1002/14651858.CD002317.
96. Patel DR, Brown KA, Greydanus DE. Anxiety disorders in children and adolescents. In: Greydanus DE, Calles L Jr, Patel DR, et al. editors. Clinical aspects of psychopharmacology in childhood and adolescence. New York: NOVA Science, 2017:117–128.
97. Blanco C, Okuda M, Wright C, Hasin DS, Grant BF, Liu S-M, et al. Mental health of college students and their non-college-attending peers: results from the National Epidemiologic Study on Alcohol and Related Conditions. Arch Gen Psychiatry. 2008;65(12):1429–37. https://doi.org/10.1001/archpsyc.65.12.1429.
98. Eisenberg D, Hunt J, Speer N, Zivin K. Mental health service utilization among college students in the United States. J Nerv Ment Dis. 2011;199(5):301–8. https://doi.org/10.1097/NMD.0b013e3182175123.
99. Findling RL, Stepanova E. The workforce shortage of child and adolescent psychiatrists: is it time for a different approach? J Am Acad Child Adolesc Psychiatry. 2018;57(5):300–1. https://doi.org/10.1016/j.jaac.2018.02.008.
100. DeNavas-Walt C, Proctor BD, Smith JC. Income, poverty, and health insurance coverage in the United States: 2012. Current Population Reports P60-245. US Census Bureau; 2013. https://files.eric.ed.gov/fulltext/ED575469.pdf. Accessed 1 July 2020.
101. Rowan K, McAlpine DD, Blewett LA. Access and cost barriers to mental health care, by insurance status, 1999–2010. Health Aff (Millwood). 2013;32(10):1723–30. https://doi.org/10.1377/hlthaff.2013.0133.
102. Chen JI, Romero GD, Karver MS. The relationship of perceived campus culture to mental health help-seeking intentions. J Couns Psychol. 2016;63(6):677–84. https://doi.org/10.1037/cou0000095.
103. Jivanjee P, Kruzich J, Gordon LJ. Community integration of transition-age individuals: views of young with mental health disorders. J Behav Health Serv Res. 2008;35(4):402–18. https://doi.org/10.1007/s11414-007-9062-6.
104. Edlund MJ, Wang PS, Berglund PA, Katz SJ, Lin E, Kessler RC. Dropping out of mental health treatment: patterns and predictors among epidemiological survey respondents in the United States and Ontario. Am J Psychiatry. 2002;159(5):845–51. https://doi.org/10.1176/appi.ajp.159.5.845.
105. Wang J. Mental health treatment dropout and its correlates in a general population sample. Med Care. 2007;45(3):224–9. https://doi.org/10.1097/01.mlr.0000244506.86885.a5.
106. Eisenberg D, Speer N, Hunt JB. Attitudes and beliefs about treatment among college students with untreated mental health problems. Psychiatr Serv. 2012;63(7):711–3. https://doi.org/10.1176/appi.ps.201100250.
107. English A, Lewis J. Privacy protection in billing and health insurance communications. AMA J Ethics.

2016;18(3):279–87. https://doi.org/10.1001/journalofethics.2016.18.3.pfor4-1603.
108. Society for Adolescent Health and Medicine; American Academy of Pediatrics. Confidentiality protections for adolescents and young adults in the health care billing and insurance claims process. J Adolesc Health. 2016;58(3):374–7. https://doi.org/10.1016/j.jadohealth.2015.12.009.
109. Rodríguez LF, Brown TM. From voice to agency: guiding principles for participatory action research with youth. New Dir Youth Dev. 2009;2009(123):19–1. https://doi.org/10.1002/yd.312.
110. Marker I, Norton PJ. The efficacy of incorporating motivational interviewing to cognitive behavior therapy for anxiety disorders: a review and meta-analysis. Clin Psychol Rev. 2018;62:1–10. https://doi.org/10.1016/j.cpr.2018.04.004.
111. Abramowitz JS, Deacon BJ, Whiteside SP. Exposure therapy for anxiety: principles and practice. New York: Guilford Publications; 2019.
112. McCabe SE, Boyd CJ, Teter CJ. Subtypes of nonmedical prescription drug misuse. Drug Alcohol Depend. 2009;102(1–3):63–70. https://doi.org/10.1016/j.drugalcdep.2009.01.007.
113. Higher Education Center for Alcohol and Drug Misuse Prevention and Recovery. 2015 College Prescription Drug Study Key Findings Report. The Ohio State University; 2015. http://hecaod.osu.edu/wp-content/uploads/2015/10/CPDS-Key-Findings-Report-1.pdf. Accessed 1 July 2020.
114. Bonn-Miller MO, Boden MT, Bucossi MM, Babson KA. Self-reported cannabis use characteristics, patterns and helpfulness among medical cannabis users. Am J Drug Alcohol Abuse. 2014;40(1):23–30. https://doi.org/10.3109/00952990.2013.821477.
115. Thomas SE, Randall CL, Carrigan MH. Drinking to cope in socially anxious individuals: a controlled study. Alcohol Clin Exp Res. 2003;27(12):1937–43. https://doi.org/10.1097/01.ALC.0000100942.30743.8C.
116. Hser YI, Mooney LJ, Huang D, Zhu Y, Tomko RL, McClure E, et al. Reductions in cannabis use are associated with improvements in anxiety, depression, and sleep quality, but not quality of life. J Subst Abus Treat. 2017;81:53–8. https://doi.org/10.1016/j.jsat.2017.07.012.
117. Crippa JA, Zuardi AW, Martín-Santos R, Bhattacharyya S, Atakan Z, McGuire P, et al. Cannabis and anxiety: a critical review of the evidence. Hum Psychopharmacol. 2009;24(7):515–23. https://doi.org/10.1002/hup.1048.
118. Martins SS, Fenton MC, Keyes KM, Blanco C, Zhu H, Storr CL. Mood and anxiety disorders and their association with non-medical prescription opioid use and prescription opioid-use disorder: longitudinal evidence from the National Epidemiologic Study on Alcohol and Related Conditions. Psychol Med. 2012;42(6):1261–72. https://doi.org/10.1017/S0033291711002145.
119. Lubman DI, Allen NB, Rogers N, Cementon E, Bonomo Y. The impact of co-occurring mood and anxiety disorders among substance-abusing youth. J Affect Disord. 2007;103(1–3):105–12. https://doi.org/10.1016/j.jad.2007.01.011.
120. Corrigan P. How stigma interferes with mental health care. Am Psychol. 2004;59(7):614–25. https://doi.org/10.1037/0003-066X.59.7.614.
121. Eisenberg D, Downs MF, Golberstein E, Zivin K. Stigma and help seeking for mental health among college students. Med Care Res Rev. 2009;66(5):522–41. https://doi.org/10.1177/1077558709335173.
122. Vogel DL, Wade NG, Haake S. Measuring the self-stigma associated with seeking psychological help. J Couns Psychol. 2006;53(3):325.
123. Rickwood D, Anile A, Telford N, Thomas K, Brown A, Parker A. Service innovation project component 1: best practice framework. headspace National Youth Mental Health Foundation. 2014. https://headspace.org.au/assets/Uploads/Corporate/Publications-and-research/headspace-best-practice-framework-april-2014.pdf. Accessed 1 July 2020.
124. Ginsburg GS, Becker-Haimes EM, Keeton C, Kendall PC, Iyengar S, Sakolsky D, et al. Results from the Child/Adolescent Anxiety Multimodal Extended Long-Term Study (CAMELS): primary anxiety outcomes. J Am Acad Child Adolesc Psychiatry. 2018;57(7):471–80. https://doi.org/10.1016/j.jaac.2018.03.017.
125. Kendall PC, Compton SN, Walkup JT, Birmaher B, Albano AM, Sherrill J, et al. Clinical characteristics of anxiety disordered youth. J Anxiety Disord. 2010;24(3):360–5. https://doi.org/10.1016/j.janxdis.2010.01.009.
126. Lawrence PJ, Rooke SM, Creswell C. Prevention of anxiety among at-risk children and adolescents–a systematic review and meta-analysis. Child Adolesc Mental Health. 2017;22(3):118–30. https://doi.org/10.1111/camh.12226.
127. Ginsburg GS, Drake KL, Tein JY, Teetsel R, Riddle MA. Preventing onset of anxiety disorders in offspring of anxious parents: a randomized controlled trial of a family-based intervention. Am J Psychiatry. 2015;172(12):1207–14. https://doi.org/10.1176/appi.ajp.2015.14091178.
128. Ginsburg GS. The Child Anxiety Prevention Study: intervention model and primary outcomes. J Consult Clin Psychol. 2009;77(3):580–7. https://doi.org/10.1037/a0014486.
129. Feiss R, Dolinger SB, Merritt M, Reiche E, Martin K, Yanes JA, et al. A systematic review and meta-analysis of school-based stress, anxiety, and depression prevention programs for adolescents. J Youth Adolesc. 2019;48(9):1668–85. https://doi.org/10.1007/s10964-019-01085-0.
130. Gopalan G, Lee SJ, Harris R, Acri MC, Munson MR. Utilization of peers in services for youth with emotional and behavioral challenges: a scoping review. J Adolesc. 2017;55:88–115. https://doi.org/10.1016/j.adolescence.2016.12.011.

131. Settipani CA, Hawke LD, Cleverley K, Chaim G, Cheung A, Mehra K, et al. Key attributes of integrated community-based youth service hubs for mental health: a scoping review. Int J Ment Health Syst. 2019;13:52. Published 2019 Jul 23. https://doi.org/10.1186/s13033-019-0306-7.
132. McGorry P, Trethowan J, Rickwood D. Creating headspace for integrated youth mental health care. World Psychiatry. 2019;18(2):140–1. https://doi.org/10.1002/wps.20619.
133. McGorry PD, Mei C. Unmet needs in youth mental health: transforming models of care to improve outcomes. In: Pompili M, McIntyre R, Fiorillo A, Sartorius N, editors. New directions in psychiatry. Cham: Springer; 2020. p. 181–91. https://doi.org/10.1007/978-3-030-42637-8_11.
134. Hilferty F, Cassells R, Muir K, Duncan A, Christensen D, Mitrou F, et al. Is headspace making a difference to young people's lives? Final report of the independent evaluation of the headspace program. Sydney: University of New South Wales; 2015. https://headspace.org.au/assets/Uploads/Evaluation-of-headspace-program.pdf. Accessed 1 July 2020.
135. Rickwood DJ, Telford NR, Parker AG, Tanti CJ, McGorry PD. Headspace – Australia's innovation in youth mental health: who are the clients and why are they presenting? Med J Aust. 2014;200(2):108–11. https://doi.org/10.5694/mja13.11235.
136. Rickwood DJ, Mazzer KR, Telford NR, Parker AG, Tanti CJ, McGorry PD. Changes in psychological distress and psychosocial functioning in young people visiting headspace centres for mental health problems. Med J Aust. 2015;202(10):537–42. https://doi.org/10.5694/mja14.01696.
137. McGorry PD, Mei C. Early intervention in youth mental health: progress and future directions. Evid Based Ment Health. 2018;21(4):182–4. https://doi.org/10.1136/ebmental-2018-300060.
138. Rickwood D, Van Dyke N, Telford N. Innovation in youth mental health services in Australia: common characteristics across the first headspace centres. Early Interv Psychiatry. 2015;9(1):29–37. https://doi.org/10.1111/eip.12071.
139. Fomby P, Goode JA, Truong-Vu KP, Mollborn S. Adolescent technology, sleep, and physical activity time in two us cohorts. Youth Soc. 2019:0044118X19868365. https://doi.org/10.1177/0044118X19868365.
140. Sedgwick R, Epstein S, Dutta R, Ougrin D. Social media, internet use and suicide attempts in adolescents. Curr Opin Psychiatry. 2019;32(6):534–41. https://doi.org/10.1097/YCO.0000000000000547.
141. Baiden P, Tadeo SK, Peters KE. The association between excessive screen-time behaviors and insufficient sleep among adolescents: findings from the 2017 youth risk behavior surveillance system. Psychiatry Res. 2019;281:112586. https://doi.org/10.1016/j.psychres.2019.112586.
142. Lee G, Lee J, Kwon S. Use of social-networking sites and subjective well-being: a study in South Korea. Cyberpsychol Behav Soc Netw. 2011;14(3):151–5. https://doi.org/10.1089/cyber.2009.0382.
143. Berry N, Lobban F, Belousov M, Emsley R, Nenadic G, Bucci S. #WhyWeTweetMH: understanding why people use twitter to discuss mental health problems. J Med Internet Res. 2017;19(4):e107. https://doi.org/10.2196/jmir.6173.
144. Robinson J, Cox G, Bailey E, et al. Social media and suicide prevention: a systematic review. Early Interv Psychiatry. 2016;10(2):103–21. https://doi.org/10.1111/eip.12229.
145. Sampogna G, Bakolis I, Evans-Lacko S, Robinson E, Thornicroft G, Henderson C. The impact of social marketing campaigns on reducing mental health stigma: results from the 2009-2014 time to change programme. Eur Psychiatry. 2017;40:116–22. https://doi.org/10.1016/j.eurpsy.2016.08.008.
146. Shen JH, Rudzicz F. Detecting anxiety through reddit. In: Proceedings of the fourth workshop on computational linguistics and clinical psychology—from linguistic signal to clinical reality. Vancouver: Association for Computational Linguistics; 2017. p. 58–65. https://doi.org/10.18653/v1/w17-3107.
147. Ponzini GT, Schofield CA. Randomized controlled trials evaluating the effectiveness of a direct-to-consumer marketing campaign for social anxiety disorder. Stigma Health. 2019;4(4):450. https://doi.org/10.1037/sah0000163.
148. Tay JL, Tay YF, Klainin-Yobas P. Effectiveness of information and communication technologies interventions to increase mental health literacy: a systematic review. Early Interv Psychiatry. 2018;12(6):1024–37. https://doi.org/10.1111/eip.12695.
149. Taylor-Rodgers E, Batterham PJ. Evaluation of an online psychoeducation intervention to promote mental health help seeking attitudes and intentions among young adults: randomised controlled trial. J Affect Disord. 2014;168:65–71. https://doi.org/10.1016/j.jad.2014.06.047.
150. Grist R, Croker A, Denne M, Stallard P. Technology delivered interventions for depression and anxiety in children and adolescents: a systematic review and meta-analysis. Clin Child Fam Psychol Rev. 2019;22(2):147–71. https://doi.org/10.1007/s10567-018-0271-8.
151. Arnberg A, Ost LG. CBT for children with depressive symptoms: a meta-analysis. Cogn Behav Ther. 2014;43(4):275–88. https://doi.org/10.1080/16506073.2014.947316.
152. Lebowitz ER. "Failure to launch": shaping intervention for highly dependent adult children. J Am Acad Child Adolesc Psychiatry. 2016;55(2):89–90. https://doi.org/10.1016/j.jaac.2015.10.014.

8 Trauma and Posttraumatic Stress in Transitional-Age Youth

Hilit Kletter, Evan Trager, Janice Kang, Marcelle Friedman, and Daryn Reicherter

Key Points

- No program or treatment geared toward TAY specifically exists despite this group having biological, psychological, and social factors increasing the potential impact of trauma.
- Several different evidence-based treatment programs, including trauma-focused cognitive-behavioral therapy, eye movement desensitization and reprocessing therapy, and cognitive processing, originating from adolescent or adult populations have been used with TAY; however, further research is needed to determine adaptability to this age group.
- The listed interventions as well as several other therapies utilize exposures to traumatic memories to decrease their psychological impact.
- Only two medications, sertraline and paroxetine, are Food and Drug Administration approved for the treatment of posttraumatic stress disorder (PTSD).
- A number of other medications have varying levels of evidence supporting their use.

Introduction

Transitional age youth (TAY) as a population has been defined as a heterogenous group of youth spanning older adolescence (15–18 years) to early adulthood (19–26 years) [1, 2]. Distinguished as the age of instability, self-focus, feeling "in-between," and, for some, a sense of newfound independence and possibility, the transition to adulthood ushers in an intensified period of self-exploration as young people negotiate this developmental task [3]. Among TAY impacted by economic, social, and/or psychological adversity in childhood and adolescence, the opportunities presented by this critical transition are often accompanied or overshadowed by significant risks [4]. An estimated 2.4 million (6.5%) of 18–26-year-olds in the United States have a serious mental health disorder according to national survey data [1, 2], and higher rates of mental health challenges have been documented in this

H. Kletter (✉) · E. Trager · J. Kang · D. Reicherter
Department of Psychiatry and Behavioral Sciences, Stanford School of Medicine, Stanford, CA, USA
e-mail: hkletter@stanford.edu; etrager1@stanford.edu; jhykang@stanford.edu; darynr@stanford.edu

M. Friedman
PGSP-Stanford PsyD Consortium, Palo Alto University, Palo Alto, CA, USA
e-mail: marcelle.friedman@stanford.edu

V. Chan, J. Derenne (eds.), *Transition-Age Youth Mental Health Care*,
https://doi.org/10.1007/978-3-030-62113-1_8

cohort relative to any other life stage [5, 6]. TAY between the ages of 18 and 25 years are also more likely to engage in substance use than any other demographic, and heavy alcohol consumption, illicit drug use, and nicotine use peak in their early 20s [7]. Not surprisingly, the prevalence of mental illness among TAY is even higher among the most marginalized subsets of this demographic. As many as one in three 17-year-olds in foster care, two thirds of 11–18-year-olds in the justice system, and half of homeless young adults ages 20–24 years are estimated to have a clinically significant mental health condition [8–10].

Lending greater complexity to the vulnerability of TAY, this time is a particularly sensitive developmental period with regard to the emergence of new major psychiatric disorders, with 50–75% of anxiety, mood, impulse control, and substance use disorders (per DSM-IV criteria) emerging between the ages of 14 and 24 years [11, 12]. These risks are further compounded by the temporal alignment of this developmental transition with institutional transitions between child and adult human service systems. Dictated by legal and bureaucratic factors rather than cultural or developmental concerns, research suggests that these systems of care are ill-equipped to buoy these vulnerable youth as their developmental stage catches up to their chronological age, leaving them without much-needed support [13–15]. A 2015 Institute of Medicine and National Research Council report exhorts improved medical and behavioral health transitions, improved preventive care, and developing evidence-based practices specifically for young adults [16].

This developmental period is defined by specific psychosocial transitions that are sensitive to cultural factors, contributing to the demographic's somewhat ambiguous age range [17]. While most adolescents in industrialized societies attend secondary school and reside with parents or primary caregivers, trajectories in TAY are less prescribed by social expectations and institutional constraints. Similarly, neurodevelopment and other aspects of physical maturation follow individualized trajectories during this period due to the variable influences of environmental and genetic factors [18]. Shaped by the unique interactions among evolving social roles, identities, and environmental circumstances, TAY navigate the developmental challenges of this transition in a similarly individualized manner [19–21]. Accordingly, life trajectories during the transition from adolescence to early adulthood have been found to vary as a function of socioeconomic status, gender, and ethnicity among other individual characteristics [12, 22–26].

Trauma can take a variety of forms in TAY and preceding developmental periods, ranging from acute traumatic experiences such as accidental injury, loss of a loved one, or natural disaster to more chronic forms of adversity, including exposure to domestic or community violence, or childhood maltreatment, which encompasses ongoing emotional, physical, or sexual abuse, neglect, assault (usually within the context of a caregiving system), as well as abandonment by, separation from, or impairment of caregivers [27, 28]. Among transitional age youth who have been exposed to trauma, development across one or multiple psychosocial domains may be delayed or otherwise undermined, leaving these individuals with a less stable repertoire of foundational skills to build upon when confronted with new challenges [29]. Trauma-exposed TAY reach chronological and legal adulthood, while their development of skills necessary to function successfully as adults often lags behind due to the pervasive impact of traumatic stress [13]. Further increasing this risk, cognitive maturation associated with risk-taking behavior, problem-solving, and emotion regulation skills continue to develop into the 20s, rendering TAY vulnerable to the neurobiological and behavioral sequelae of trauma [30, 31]. Given this context, a holistic approach to assessment and intervention that accounts for the biopsychosocial changes specific to TAY, alongside the enduring impact and developmental context of childhood trauma, is necessary to appropriately meet the needs of this vulnerable population [11, 12].

Epidemiology

The vast majority of epidemiological research related to trauma exposure and its sequelae has overlooked TAY as a distinct demographic, but what is known paints a somewhat grim picture. It appears that by the time individuals reach 18 years, many if not most have weathered potentially traumatic life events. Decades of research have revealed alarmingly high rates of trauma in childhood and adolescence, including direct exposure or witnessing of interpersonal violence or maltreatment (e.g., bullying or sexual or physical abuse), as well as accidental injury, natural disasters, traumatic loss, and severe family dysfunction [32–34]. By the age of 16 years, nearly two thirds of young people in the United States will have been exposed to at least one potentially traumatic event, including traumatic loss, sexual assault, child maltreatment, medical trauma, accidental injury, or witnessing domestic violence, according to a representative longitudinal study [35]. In a nonurban community sample of older adolescents, 43% reported exposure to at least one traumatic event, while more than a third reported experiencing multiple adverse events by the age of 18 years [36]. Lifetime exposure to potentially traumatic events fell slightly above 60% among 6400 adolescents surveyed in the US National Comorbidity Survey for Adolescents [37].

One increasingly popular research method for studying the impact of childhood trauma is the Adverse Childhood Experiences Scale (ACES), as defined in the Kaiser Foundation Study. This seminal joint study conducted by the Center for Disease Control and the Southern California Kaiser Foundation employing their HMO members' data revealed a dose-dependent relationship between self-reported ACEs and morbidity and mortality in later life (Fig. 8.1) [38, 39]. Moreover, such traumatic exposures (and childhood victimization, in particular) are disproportionately distributed within populations and are likely to co-occur or accumulate over time [28, 40, 41].

Other subsequent work supports a similar view; according to national survey data collected by Finkelhor, Ormrod, and Turner [42], nearly one-third of adolescents reported experiencing multiple forms of potentially traumatic victimization, and 57% of all child victimization nationally was accounted for by the 22% of youth who experienced at least four types of victimization in a single year. Vulnerability to such victimization is heightened by a variety of contextual factors,

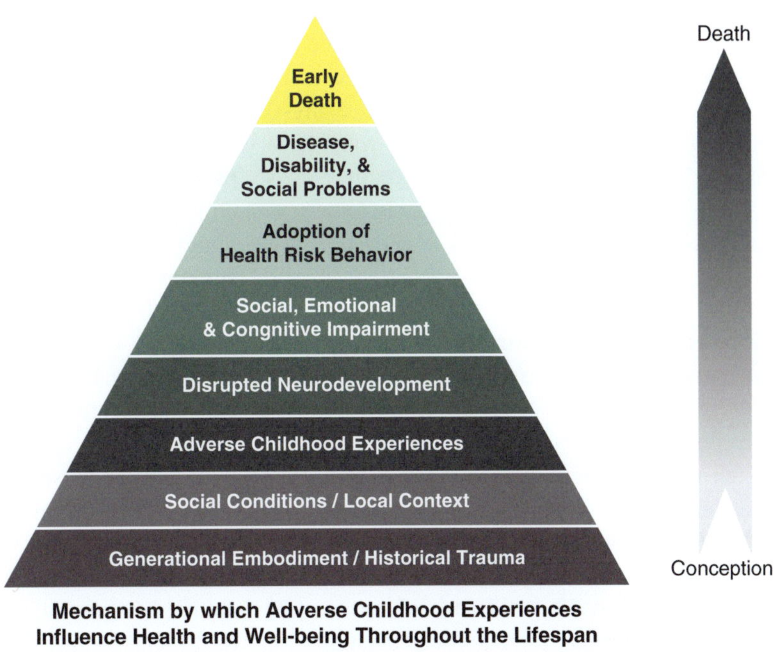

Fig. 8.1 ACE pyramid. (From CDC.gov)

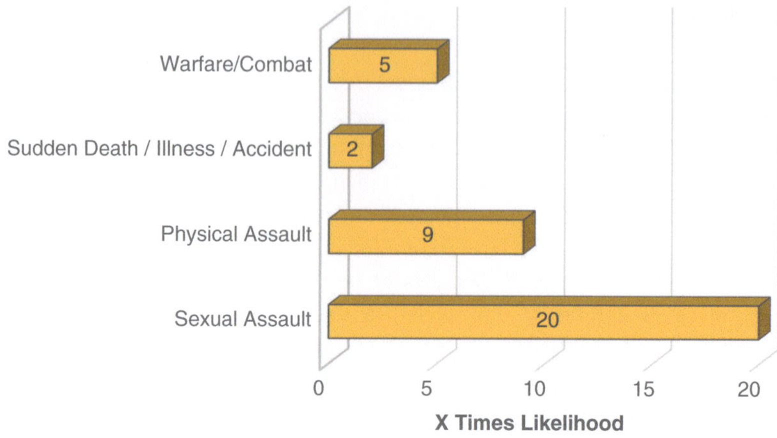

Fig. 8.2 Likelihood of trauma exposure in TAY relative to compared age groups

including poverty, out-of-home placement, involvement in the juvenile justice system, community disorder, ethnocultural disparities and political unrest, as well as home environments characterized by high conflict, instability, and low support [43–47].

TAY may also be more vulnerable to certain types of trauma exposure compared to other age groups (Fig. 8.2). When examining lifetime prevalence of potentially traumatic events as a function of age at exposure by cohort decade, young adults between the ages of 21 and 29 years were five times more likely to experience warfare or combat exposure than all other age groups combined; nearly twice as likely to experience the unexpected death, illness, or accident of a loved one; and nine times as likely to experience physical assault by a partner compared to youth ages 11–19 years. Furthermore, youth ages 11–29 years were 20 times more likely to be sexually assaulted than adults ages 31–60 years [48].

Consequences of Trauma in Transitional Age Youth

Psychosocial trajectories for trauma-exposed youth are heterogeneous and often evolve over the course of development and into adulthood as a function of individual patterns of vulnerability and risk factors. A majority of trauma-exposed youth are remarkably resilient and never meet criteria for a chronic-trauma-related disorder [35, 37, 49]. Some youth experience moderate to severe posttraumatic stress reactions that emerge within 3 months of trauma exposure but return to baseline levels of functioning with or without intervention [50]. Youth who are resilient in the wake of trauma may show comparatively few symptoms of distress, demonstrating adaptive coping processes that allow for normative development and preserved functioning [50].

Protective factors correlated with increased resilience include environmental factors such as socioeconomic resources, social support in the form of positive attachments to prosocial peers and supportive caregivers, residing in a safe community, and access to quality education. Strong emotion regulation and social cognition skills [51], problem-solving abilities, self-control, academic success, and an absence of preexisting psychiatric disorders or substance abuse in the child's personal and family history also moderate youth's risk and severity of adverse posttraumatic stress reactions [35, 52, 53]. Neurobiological factors, such as greater reward sensitivity and medial prefrontal cortex (mPFC)-amygdala functional connectivity, have also been experimentally associated with resilience among trauma-exposed youth [52, 54].

While the presence of such protective factors allows many trauma-exposed youth to continue along a normative developmental pathway, a larger share of young people with unique vulnerabilities (exposure to complex trauma, ethnic/racial and sexual minority identities, chronic illness, and involvement in the child welfare or juvenile justice systems) are at increased risk for an array of adverse outcomes across domains of biopsychosocial development and physical and emotional well-being with enduring, lifelong impact [21, 28, 55, 56]. Domains that can be affected include interpersonal relationship functioning, self-concept and identity formation, affect regulation, impulse control, physical illness, cognition, and learning [27, 57].

Differentiating Posttraumatic Stress Disorder (PTSD) from Adjustment Disorder

As mentioned above, TAY face many challenges both developmentally and socially as they transition from adolescence into adulthood. Common stressors include learning to manage their finances or living away from home and family and establishing more intimate and longer-lasting relationships. Differentiating a normal reaction to stress from disorder is important in diagnosis and treatment. A reaction to a stressor should be considered abnormal when the distress is beyond what is normally expected or culturally accepted, or if the reaction results in significant functional impairment [58].

The significant differences between adjustment disorder, acute stress disorder (ASD), and PTSD lie mainly in the type of stressor and the duration or course of symptoms. According to the Diagnostic and Statistical Manual of Mental Disorders, 5th Edition (DSM-5) criteria [58], a diagnosis of adjustment disorder requires an identifiable stressor—severity or type is not specified. However, with both ASD and PTSD, the traumatic event or stressor is defined in Criterion A, which requires exposure to actual or threatened death, serious injury, or sexual violence. The traumatic event needs to be either directly experienced, witnessed in person, discovered about a close friend or family member in which the experience was violent or accidental, or experienced repeatedly or with extreme exposure to details of the events, such as with first responders or police officers. Further criteria for both ASD and PTSD include symptoms related to intrusion, avoidance, negative cognition and mood, and alterations in arousal and reactivity. With ASD, symptoms related to dissociation are also included, whereas in PTSD dissociative symptoms are not a core criterion, but noted as a specifier if present.

The other major difference between adjustment disorder, ASD, and PTSD is symptom course and duration. For a diagnosis of adjustment disorder, the onset of symptoms must begin within 3 months of the identified stressor and last no longer than 6 months after the stressor and/or its consequences have resolved. For ASD, symptoms must last only between 3 days and 1 month; if symptoms resolve within 3 days, the criterion is not met. With PTSD, symptom onset may occur soon after the traumatic experience or many years later, also known as delayed onset. Symptom duration must continue beyond 1 month; otherwise, a diagnosis of ASD may be more appropriate. A comparison table (Table 8.1) and flow chart below help to highlight the similarities and differences (Fig. 8.3).

A thorough history, including any significant childhood events and timeline of symptoms, should be obtained to determine the most accurate diagnosis. The PTSD Checklist for DSM-5 (PCL-5) is a quick 20-item self-report screening tool that can be used with TAY to assess trauma symptoms [59]. This measure can also be used to track symptom progression. A more thorough measure for assessing PTSD diagnosis is the Clinician-Administered PTSD Scale for DSM-5 (CAPS-5), a 30-item structured interview [60], though it has mainly been validated in the military veteran population.

Vignette, Part 1

Sandy, a 21-year-old Latina female, enters your office and sits down. After introductions, she relates that 2 weeks ago she was in a serious car crash. While lucky to have emerged unscathed, she comments how she felt like she was going to die. Since the crash, she has been experiencing vivid flashbacks and vivid nightmares, has been

Table 8.1 Comparison of adjustment disorder, acute stress disorder, and PTSD diagnostic criteria adapted from the Diagnostic and Statistical Manual of Mental Disorders, 5th Edition (DSM-5)

	Adjustment disorder	Acute stress disorder	PTSD
Stressor	Identifiable stressor of *any* severity or type	Same as PTSD Criterion A	Criterion A trauma/ stressor
Diagnostic features	Development of emotional or behavioral symptoms in response to identifiable stressor Does not meet criteria for other mental disorders (including other trauma- or stressor-related disorders) or exacerbation of preexisting mental disorder Not normal bereavement Or meets Criterion A but not the other PTSD criteria Or does not meet Criterion A but meets the other PTSD criteria	Criterion B—need more than nine from any of the five categories of intrusion, negative mood, dissociation, avoidance, and arousal	Criteria B intrusion symptom (flashbacks, nightmares, triggers) Criteria C avoidance Criteria D negative alterations in cognition and mood Criteria E alterations in arousal and reactivity *Dissociation is not a core diagnostic feature of PTSD but should be specified if present*
Onset	Within 3 months (usually immediate)	Typically immediately after trauma	Can be years after the initial trauma
Duration	*Symptoms do not persist for more than 6 months* after the stressor, or its consequences have ended Can become *persistent/chronic* if stressor or its consequences persist	*3 days to 1 month* If symptoms resolve in <3 days, not acute stress disorder	*>1 month*
Impairment	Marked distress out of proportion to severity or the intensity of the stressor *AND/OR* Significant impairment in social, occupational, or other important areas of functioning	Must cause significant distress or impairment, and not due to substance use	Must cause significant distress or impairment, and not due to substance use
Specifiers	With depressed mood With anxiety With anxiety and depressed mood With disturbance of conduct With mixed disturbance of emotions and conduct Unspecified	–	With dissociative symptoms With delayed expression

avoiding thoughts and physical reminders of the event, finds herself with depressed mood, blames herself for the accident despite the police saying she was not at fault, is easily startled, and has been hypervigilant, always watching her surroundings.

While she meets all of the needed symptoms for PTSD, you diagnose her with acute stress disorder because the symptoms have been present for less than 1 month. You offer her a referral to a psychiatrist and discuss different types of psychotherapy she may find helpful, particularly if symptoms persist.

Vignette, Part 2

Six months later, Sandy returns to your office; she says that she was never able to see the psychiatrist due to issues with insurance, but she did attend some support sessions at a local church for a while. Her symptoms resolved after several months, but over the past few weeks she has had strong feelings of sadness and anxiety, although she states that she is sleeping well and does not feel troubled by memories or thoughts of the accident. In fact, she mentions how in another week she is planning to take her first long road

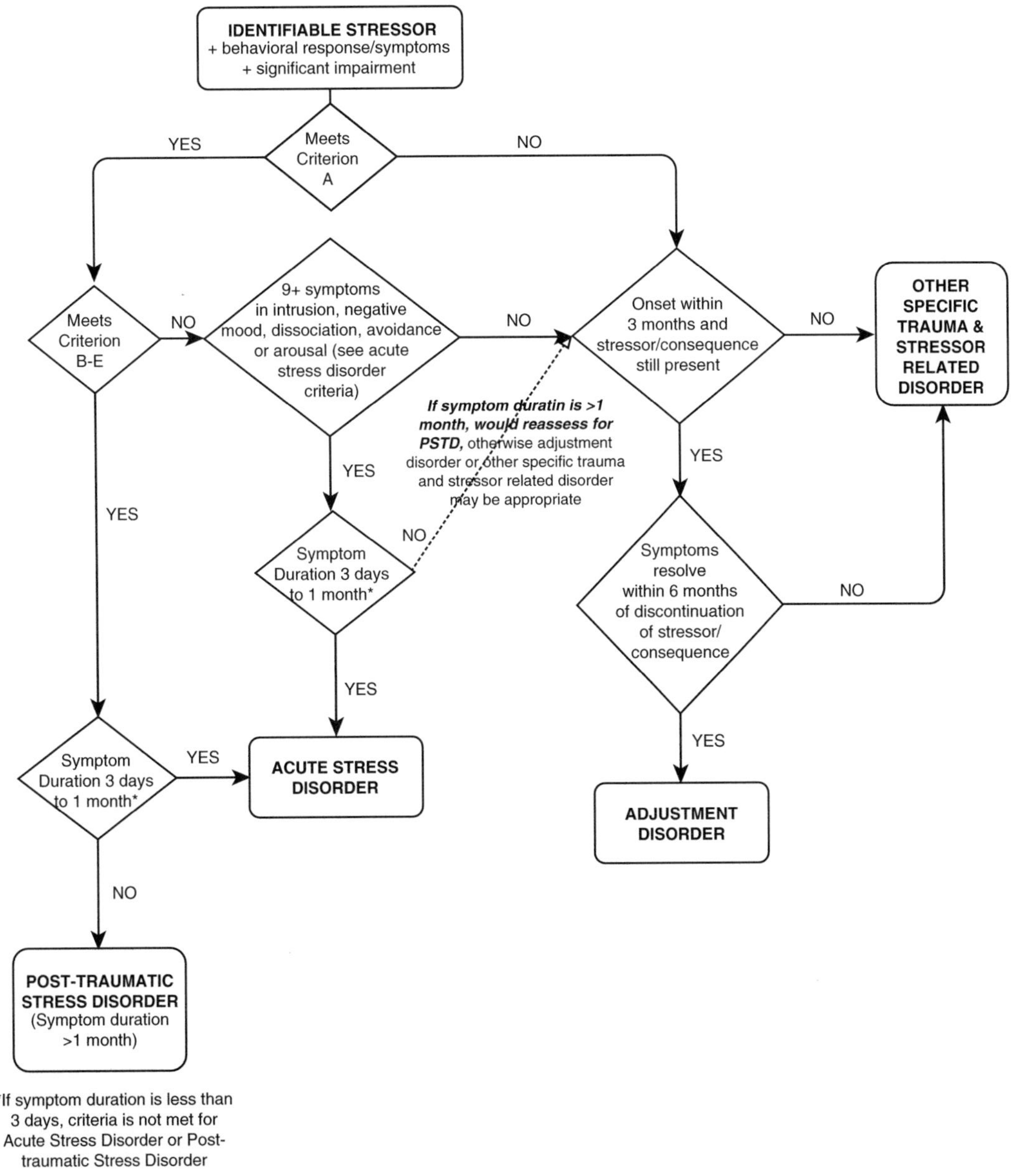

Fig. 8.3 Flowchart for assisting in differentiating various potential trauma sequelae

trip since the accident, but only after her final exams are over. Unfortunately, due to these new symptoms, she is worried that perhaps she should just stay home. After completing your assessment without identifying other relevant information, you provide reassurances and resources for stress reduction. You also ask that she check in after finals before the scheduled trip. At her check-in a week later, Sandy looks relaxed and carefree; she thinks it was all just related to her finals but asks you if it could have been related to the accident.

Given the symptoms, its relation to a known stressor, and the improvement following its resolution, you opine that an adjustment disorder seems more likely. Again, you reiterate the importance of self-care and wish her a fun journey.

Treatment for Trauma-Exposed Transitional Age Youth

Despite the proliferation of trauma-focused treatments developed in the last several decades, there remains a dearth of research examining the efficacy of trauma-focused treatments among TAY, and very few treatments have been specifically designed to address the unique sequelae of trauma and related psychosocial challenges in this particular population. Efforts to adapt existing clinical interventions designed for children, adolescents, or adults to address the particular needs and developmental concerns of TAY raise significant challenges. This is a heterogeneous population with regard to cognitive and developmental maturity, psychosocial context, and symptom presentation, not to mention the many systemic barriers that diminish TAY access to mental health care [13]. No known studies to date have indicated that TAY differentially respond to evidence-based treatments for trauma-related disorders compared to other age groups. However, it cannot be assumed that such treatments would be equally efficacious among TAY as minimal research has substantiated how unhealthy and unique this population can be [16]. Scholars have recommended that evidence-based practices for PTSD and other disorders associated with trauma exposure should be used while incorporating adaptations suited to the specific needs of young adults [12]. Evidence-based practices designed for children, adolescents, and adults may be appropriate for supporting trauma-exposed TAY if adjusted to reflect the developmental stage and presentation of each individual. Skehan and Davis [61] offer that cognitive-behavioral or behavioral therapeutic approaches with demonstrated efficacy among adolescents and adults are likely to be efficacious among TAY as their level of cognitive maturity presumably straddles both age groups.

While little is known about the comparative efficacy, feasibility, or acceptability of specific treatment protocols or interventions among trauma-exposed TAY, evidence suggests that transition-age youth are the most challenging age group to engage in ongoing treatment [61]. Identifying ways to mitigate attrition and promote their ongoing participation in treatment, such as implementing motivational enhancement interventions [62], may be the most important preliminary step toward facilitating treatment progress among TAY. Developing evidence-based interventions that are developmentally sensitive to the specific aspects of the transition from youth to adulthood is critical but insufficient to address the systemic and developmental obstacles at play. Intervention approaches targeting TAY must account for and address the array of barriers to service use in this population, including mistrust of authority, stigma regarding pursuing mental health treatment, lapses in insurance, and lack of sufficient social and financial resources to consistently engage in treatment [63].

Psychosocial Context of Trauma in TAY: Treatment Considerations

Various factors related to the psychosocial context of trauma in TAY are important to consider when evaluating the appropriateness of an intervention framework for trauma-exposed youth:

- Victimization may be ongoing due to the necessity to remain at home in the presence of abusing caregivers or in close proximity to other perpetrators, and youth in such circumstances may be dependent on family resources that constrain them to invalidating or dangerous social contexts. Furthermore, TAY exposed to trauma in environments characterized by social marginalization and/or socioeconomic disadvantage are unlikely to successfully remove themselves from these endangering circumstances, thus compounding the effects of previous trauma due to ongoing exposure to adversity.
- Findings substantiate the harsh reality that previous victimization itself may be the most significant risk factor for subsequent victimization, particularly among youth experiencing family violence or child maltreatment [42]. As such, adequately supporting trauma-

exposed TAY may often extend beyond the provision of efficacious psychotherapy to include additional systems intervention and infrastructure to protect against endangering environmental factors [64].

- TAY exposed to adversity, and especially those who have experienced complex trauma, are also more likely to engage in a wide range of self-endangering behaviors to externalize or cope with distress, including significant substance abuse, high-risk sexual behavior, excessive risk-taking, nonsuicidal self-injury, disordered eating, suicidal behavior, and physical aggression [65, 66].
- Other potentially self-endangering sequelae of posttraumatic stress among TAY can include involvement in problematic romantic relationships and difficulty defending oneself in dangerous situations due to dissociation or passivity [67].
- These considerations underscore the necessity for any treatment of trauma-exposed TAY to address issues of safety, and comorbidities bound to accompany trauma-related symptomatology, in tandem with targeted or adjunct interventions aimed at building adaptive skills [67].

Psychotherapeutic Interventions

Trauma-Focused Cognitive-Behavioral Therapy (TF-CBT)

TF-CBT is the most widely used and researched treatment for traumatized youth ages 3–21 years [68]. Originally developed for use with sexually abused youth, the intervention has since been expanded to include other forms of trauma and can be delivered in an individual or group format. The components of TF-CBT, used in some variation in most interventions for traumatized youth, are summarized by the acronym PRACTICE: psychoeducation and parenting skills, relaxation, affective regulation, cognitive coping, trauma narrative, in vivo exposure, conjoint session, and enhancing safety. Psychoeducation involves normalizing trauma reactions and providing statistics about the prevalence of trauma. Caregivers tend to be involved in every session of TF-CBT to learn parenting skills such as teaching praise, time out or taking space, selective attention and active ignoring, behavior charts, rewards, and modeling. Relaxation includes teaching of coping strategies such as deep breathing or progressive muscle relaxation to help the child tolerate distress related to his/her traumatic experience. Affective regulation includes identification and expression of emotions through techniques such as feelings lists or charts, charades, and an emotion thermometer. Cognitive coping teaches the connection between thoughts, emotions, and behaviors. The trauma narrative component involves creating a story for the traumatic experiences which can be done by having the child dictate the story to the therapist or having the therapist interview the child. In vivo exposure, which is optional, helps the child to gradually confront traumatic cues by developing more adaptive responses. TF-CBT also has conjoint sessions with the caregiver and child to share the trauma narrative, improve communication, and strengthen the relationship. The caregiver components of TF-CBT may need to be adapted for TAY as this is an age marked by increased independence and some may be already living away from home. Thus, it is recommended at the onset of therapy to determine with the individual how much involvement, if at all, they would like to have from their caregivers. Finally, the enhancing safety phase focuses on teaching body safety and healthy sexuality as well as problem-solving for the future. TF-CBT has proven efficacious in over 20 randomized controlled trials (RCTs) for the reduction of PTSD, depression, and other emotional and behavioral difficulties [69–71]. No research on the efficacy of TF-CBT specifically with TAY has been done; however, programs such as Cornerstone, described below, have used it with this population.

Cornerstone Program

While not specifically designed to address the effects of trauma among TAY, the psychosocial program Cornerstone was created to address the significant unmet mental health and psychosocial support needs during the developmental and systemic transition to adulthood for those with serious mental health concerns [72]. Piloted in Detroit, Michigan, and now being assessed in New York, the program aims to reduce the stigma of pursuing mental health services and increase trust, acceptance, and mental health service use among socioeconomically disadvantaged TAY with mental illness as they transition to adulthood. In doing so, the protocol-driven approach addresses both mental health concerns and logistical barriers (e.g., anxiety, depressed mood, anger, insufficient coping skills, adaptive life skills necessary to pursue necessary services, stable housing, etc.) that interfere with this critical transition.

The service components within this model include licensed master's level clinicians who serve as "boundary-spanning case managers" (BSCM); a peer mentor described as a "recovery role model;" a community-based practice; and groups that emphasize psychoeducation, mental health literacy, and skill building. Case managers help to promote two main goals, which include individuals' constructive ongoing involvement with mental health services as well as achievement of appropriate developmental milestones and general recovery, such as managing symptoms of mental illness, and securing employment and housing. Case managers work from community-based clinics that serve individuals across the life span, thus positioning them to support TAY as they bridge the gap between child and adult providers. Clinicians also provide trauma-focused cognitive-behavioral therapy (TF-CBT), making this program relevant to TAY who present primarily with trauma-related mental health concerns, and are trained in problem-solving interventions and person-centered treatment planning to help support TAY in navigating practical barriers to care and adjustment. Recovery role model mentors, another core component of the Cornerstone model, have lived experience related to living with serious mental health concerns and provide mentorship regarding consistent use of mental health services, negotiating issues of disclosure about mental health difficulties in the face of stigma, serving as models of a hopeful future, and supporting individuals' navigation of practical challenges (e.g., housing, employment, education) to pursue desired life outcomes.

Several dimensions of the Cornerstone intervention approach appear particularly applicable to the needs of TAY impacted by trauma, including but not limited to the incorporation of TF-CBT. In addition, Cornerstone's inclusion of recovery role models aims to mitigate feelings of shame, isolation, stigma, mistrust, and hopelessness surrounding individuals' mental health challenges and life circumstances, which are centrally relevant to the experience of victimization, particularly in childhood and adolescence. Such mentorship is also well suited to addressing relational challenges and issues with identity formation faced by trauma-exposed TAY. Mentors may model appropriate boundaries, help scaffold individuals' efforts to build social support, and model lives disencumbered by traumatic pasts. Furthermore, in providing both social workers and recovery role models who can support in vivo community-based exposures, Cornerstone addresses one of the glaring challenges of trauma-focused treatment for TAY who lack the familial support often utilized in TF-CBT and other interventions designed for youth to scaffold important treatment components outside of session. However, protocol materials do not explicitly outline how TF-CBT might be adapted for this population, and more work is necessary to elucidate and test such adaptations.

As of the time of this writing, results of the first randomized controlled trial evaluating the Cornerstone approach have yet to be published, but preliminary outcome data suggest that this mentoring approach within a mental health outpatient program is acceptable and feasible. Preliminary data also show promise regarding its potential to reduce mental health symptoms, promote life outcomes among TAY, and fill a critical gap in the service system for TAY impacted by mental illness [73]. However, further research is necessary to empirically evaluate its efficacy, feasibility, and acceptability among disadvantaged

TAY with serious mental health concerns broadly and for TAY impacted by posttraumatic stress more specifically.

Integrative Treatment of Complex Trauma in Adolescents (ITCT-A)

ITCT-A is a multicomponent, structured, and assessment-driven treatment model developed to address the sequelae of complex trauma in youth ages 12–21 years and has also been implemented with TAY through the age of 24 years [67, 74]. This approach is an adaptation of a treatment model initially developed for culturally diverse children exposed to a variety of stressors, including immigration and separation from primary caretakers, socioeconomic deprivation, minority stress, and community disorder [75]. A central feature of the treatment is its heavy utilization of multiinformant assessment in order to identify which treatment components are best suited to each person's presenting problems or symptoms. The treatment is described as "semi-structured" such that interventions should be adapted to address each individual's specific psychological functioning, developmental stage, cultural background, psychosocial context, and capacity for affect regulation. Accordingly, treatment length is not prescribed but, rather, based on the types and number of challenges faced by the affected person to reflect the complex symptomatology associated with complex trauma. Currently, training in ITCT-A originates at the University of Southern California.

Prolonged Exposure Therapy (PE)

PE has been empirically validated for adult populations over the past two decades in both research and clinical settings [76]. Grounded in emotional processing theory [77, 78], PE conceptualizes traumatic memory as a specific type of cognitive structure that contains representations of stimuli, responses, and meanings associated with traumatic experiences, which underlies posttraumatic stress responses. While trauma survivors are often inclined to avoid painful trauma-related emotions, thoughts, and situations, emotion processing theory posits that countering such avoidance through repeated activation of trauma memories allows unrealistic misperceptions of the world and the self to be disconfirmed. Accordingly, posttraumatic stress is treated in PE through confrontation of feared trauma-related stimuli, in tandem with new learning or emotional processing which allows for a corrective experience. As persons are encouraged to revisit and recount their traumatic memories (imaginal exposures), and safely and gradually confront situations that are trauma reminders through in vivo exposures, anxiety linked to previous traumatic experiences is expected to reduce over time as individuals enrich and clarify their understanding of past experiences, disrupt patterns of avoidance, and build self-efficacy in their ability to cope effectively [79].

While PE has not yet been formally adapted for TAY, it has been modified for use among trauma-exposed adolescents ages 12–18 years [79, 80]. PE-A is intended to be a flexible, individual psychotherapy treatment, allowing for varied session and treatment length, the addition of an optional pretreatment preparation phase, and the involvement of caregivers in sessions as needed to reflect the developmental and psychosocial needs of the client. Each of the four treatment phases, including pretreatment preparation, psychoeducation and treatment planning, exposures, and relapse prevention/termination, includes modules targeting specific therapy goals or tasks, and can be condensed or extended as indicated by the individuals' specific challenges.

In addition to significant reductions in PTSD symptoms associated with a variety of trauma types, PE has been shown to improve social functioning [81], feelings of guilt and anger [82, 83], and general anxiety and depression [84] when implemented among adults. Much less research has examined the efficacy of the adapted PE-A model; however, extant evidence in studies of adolescent populations supports its designation as "well-supported by research evidence." For example, when compared to time-limited dynamic psychotherapy, PE-A was linked to greater symptom reduction in PTSD and depression symptoms and improvement in global functioning among adolescents (n = 38, ages 12–18 years) with PTSD linked to a single index trauma. Gains were maintained at 6- and 17-month follow-up [85]. In a subsequent randomized controlled trial conducted in a community mental health clinic, adolescent females (n = 61, ages 13–18 years) with PTSD associated with sexual victimization demonstrated greater PTSD and depressive symptom reduction, greater functional improvement, and higher likelihood of no longer meeting criteria for PTSD posttreatment after receiving PE-A relative to those provided client-centered therapy [86]. Additional research is necessary to adapt and evaluate the utility of a prolonged exposure model in addressing the unique needs of TAY. However, given this treatment's demonstrated efficacy among adults and adolescents [86, 87], TAY would likely benefit from the protocol with the addition of developmentally sensitive adaptations.

To this end, there are a number of important factors to consider with regard to the adaptation of PE or PE-A for use among TAY. PE-A is generally inappropriate for adolescents experiencing active suicidal ideation, psychotic symptoms, or self-injurious behavior, or those living in environments that place them at high risk of victimization [80]. Given the vulnerability of trauma-exposed TAY to such comorbidities and environmental challenges, it is possible that the inclusion of an extended stabilization phase emphasizing safety and skill development prior to beginning psychoeducation would be an important adaptation when implementing prolonged exposure among emerging adults. Moreover, given that emerging adults between the ages of 18 and 25 years are more likely to engage in substance misuse than any other demographic, and heavy alcohol consumption, illicit drug use, and cigarette use peak during the early 20s [7], substance use may be a more prevalent obstacle to constructive engagement in prolonged exposure among TAY relative to other age groups. Substance-use screening upon intake, as well as interventions targeting substance use, may be necessary additions to the protocol to minimize emotional and cognitive avoidance of trauma-related stimuli through substance use both in and outside of session. The modular format and flexibility of PE-A is well suited to TAY's heterogeneous developmental trajectories and psychosocial circumstances, suggesting it might be readily tailored to the individual needs of trauma-exposed emerging adults. It is noteworthy, however, that while trauma processing is arguably critical in ameliorating posttraumatic stress, prolonged exposure does not directly address the immediate, daily needs of emerging adults struggling to negotiate practical challenges, such as securing housing and employment and developing other adaptive life skills essential for long-term self-sufficiency. As such, PE for TAY may be most useful as an adjunct to other case management, mentorship, and/or skill-building services, warranting further treatment development and empirical study.

Skills Training in Affective and Interpersonal Regulation (STAIR)

Much like PE, STAIR is a trauma-focused, cognitive-behavioral treatment designed originally for adults but has since been adapted for use among adolescents. STAIR specifically targets symptoms associated with complex trauma, defined as repeated or persistent exposure to interpersonal victimization, and accordingly addresses disruptions of attachment, emotion regulation, and interpersonal functioning commonly faced by survivors of chronic interpersonal violence [88]. In accordance with practice guidelines provided by the Complex Trauma Task Force of the International Society for Traumatic Stress Studies (ISTSS), the STAIR model is organized into two sequential phases, including an initial phase focused on developing affective regulation and interpersonal skills. The second phase focused on the review and reappraisal of traumatic experiences via narrative storytelling, the review of taped narratives to explore problematic interpersonal schemas about self and others, and the practice of affect modulation through grounding techniques [89, 90]. The

STAIR protocol is among the best-researched treatments designed specifically for complex trauma presentations in adults and has demonstrated efficacy in improving emotion regulation, interpersonal functioning, expression of anger, self-efficacy, PTSD and depressive symptoms, and perceived social support [88, 91].

Eye Movement Desensitization and Reprocessing (EMDR)

EMDR aims to reprocess traumatic memories and help to adaptively store them [92]. It has primarily been used for acute trauma experiences and used with children as young as 2 years up to adults. There are eight phases of treatment, including (1) history gathering and determination, if the individual is an appropriate candidate for EMDR; (2) preparation phase, in which the individual is taught strategies to manage distress during or in between treatment sessions; (3) assessment phase, to identify and access a target memory that will be processed; (4) desensitization phase, during which the target memory and stimuli that trigger the target memory are processed; (5) installation phase, in which the individual selects a positive cognition and bilateral stimulation is used to increase the connection between this positive cognition and existing positive cognitive networks; (6) body scan phase, during which residual physiological sensations are identified and processed; (7) closure phase, in which the individual's stability is assessed; and, finally, (8) reevaluation, to ensure that all target memories are in the closure phase; otherwise, a step may need to be repeated. EMDR has been effective in reducing PTSD, anxiety, depression, avoidance, and intrusive thoughts in a group of young women ages 16–25 years, over half of them with sexual trauma [93].

Cognitive Processing Therapy (CPT)

CPT helps traumatized individuals challenge and modify unhelpful trauma-related cognitive distortions. Treatment components include psychoeducation about trauma symptoms and the connection between emotions and thoughts, helping individuals identify automatic thoughts that developed as a result of the trauma, and formal processing of the traumatic experience by having the individual write the worst account of their trauma and using Socratic questioning and other techniques to challenge cognitive distortions and once the individual has developed the skills to identify and challenge these unhelpful thoughts, continuing to use these skills to evaluate and modify trauma-related thoughts [94]. Developmentally adapted cognitive processing therapy (D-CPT) has been developed for adolescents and young adults ages 14–21 years with sexual and/or physical abuse [87]. D-CPT makes four adjustments to CPT. The first is that the number of sessions devoted to the middle phase of treatment (i.e., processing of the trauma and cognitive distortions) is increased to improve motivation. Second, a commitment phase was added to further increase treatment motivation and therapeutic alliance. Third, behavior and emotion regulation techniques such as those used within dialectical behavior therapy (DBT) were incorporated, given that many survivors of child abuse lack these skills. Finally, D-CPT takes into consideration developmental tasks that impact the young adult's entire life, including vocational training, career choice, and romantic relationships. Results evaluating the efficacy of D-CPT found that compared to a waitlist group, individuals receiving D-CPT had greater reductions in PTSD severity, with gains maintained at follow-up. The D-CPT group also showed greater improvement in depression, borderline symptoms, behavior problems, and dissociation.

Psychopharmacology

General Principles

Pharmacotherapy for trauma in TAY may be helpful as an adjunct treatment to psychotherapy, especially if symptoms of the trauma disorder or any comorbidities result in functional impairment or safety concerns. While only two medications have been approved for the treatment of posttraumatic stress disorder (PTSD), other agents may be used for the treatment of comorbid illness such as major depressive disorder (MDD) or for targeting of symptoms such as hypervigilance and overactivation. Regardless of the agent used, evidence-based psychotherapy is the mainstay of PTSD treatment; as such, close collaboration with a patient's therapist is critical to better understand the patient's symptoms and progression of treatment.

Challenges in pharmacotherapy for trauma remain similar to treating TAY with pharmacotherapy in general. One concern is if the patient can adhere to medication treatment away from home, where until recently it was possible that a watchful concerned parent had been helping to administer medications. Furthermore, there may be a question regarding age of consent to take psychotropic medications, which varies depending on where one practices. It would be prudent to check the laws in the geographical area of practice.

Regardless of whether TAY have reached the age of majority, or the age when one is considered an adult legally, it is common for practitioners to consider involving parents or family in treatment. While obtaining consent and helping the TAY retain their agency is critical, family may be a significant source of support as they go through treatment for PTSD. This may include encouraging them to remain in treatment, improving adherence to medication, and providing collateral as to symptom changes over the course of therapy. These benefits should, of course, be weighed against the alternative, where involving family may be harmful in certain circumstances. One obvious exclusionary situation is when the perpetrator of the trauma may have originated from within the family structure. This underscores the need to obtain a full psychiatric history before starting treatment planning.

It is important to consider that while medications may help with symptoms of PTSD, patients will take time to heal and may continue to experience continued symptoms for a prolonged period of time. It should not be considered a failure if patients only show partial improvement and remain symptomatic but stable; medications may help but not treat all symptoms of trauma into remission. Medications provide the most benefit in conjunction with evidence-based psychotherapy in a stable, secure environment.

Current Guidelines

As of this writing, there are no guidelines specific to psychopharmacology in the conditions grouped under the DSM-5 category of trauma and stress-related disorder in TAY. This may reflect that there is no designated group studying only the transitional age population. The following are guidelines for children and adolescents with PTSD, followed by the guidelines for adults. When considering which medication to start, it would be advisable to first consider those listed in the guidelines with stronger evidence of efficacy.

Guidelines for Children and Adolescents

While in need of updating, given the time since publication, the American Academy of Child and Adolescent Psychiatry's Practice Parameter for the Assessment and Treatment of Children and Adolescents with Posttraumatic Stress Disorder in 2010 recommends that selective serotonin reuptake inhibitors (SSRIs) can be considered for the treatment of children and adolescents with PTSD (Recommendation 7) and that medications other than SSRIs may be considered for child and adolescents with PTSD (Recommendation 8). Both recommendations are considered "optional," indicating that they are acceptable based on emerging evidence or clinical opinion but lack strong empirical evidence and/or strong clinical consensus [95]. At the time of writing, there are no practice guidelines for medications for trauma in the pediatric population from the American Academy of Pediatrics.

Guidelines for Adults

In 2017, the American Psychological Association released the Clinical Practice Guideline for Treatment of PTSD, stating: "For medications, the panel suggests offering the following (in alphabetical order): *fluoxetine, paroxetine, sertraline, and venlafaxine*. There is insufficient evidence to recommend for or against offering risperidone and topiramate [96]."

While the American Psychiatric Association (APA) does not have a document on clinical guidelines for PTSD, on its website it references the guidelines provided by the Department of Veteran Affairs (VA) and the Department of Defense (DoD).

The VA/DoD Clinical Practice Guideline for the Management of PTSD and ASD, which was also released in 2017, provides perhaps the most robust recommendations regarding pharmacotherapy for adults with PTSD based on available evidence [97]. While extensive, well researched, and nuanced, the only recommendations with moderate to strong evidence are the following:

- Recommend *sertraline, paroxetine, fluoxetine, and venlafaxine* as monotherapy for PTSD for patients diagnosed with PTSD who choose not to engage in or are unable to access trauma-focused therapy (strong, evidence quality moderate, Rec 17)
- Recommend against treating PTSD with divalproex, tiagabine, guanfacine, risperidone, benzodiazepines, ketamine, hydrocortisone, or D-cycloserine as monotherapy due to lack of strong evidence for efficacy or due to adverse effects and associated risks (strong against, Rec 20)
- Recommend against treating PTSD with cannabis or cannabis derivatives due to lack of evidence for efficacy, known adverse effects, and associated risks (strong against, Rec 21)
- Recommend against using atypical antipsychotics, benzodiazepines, and divalproex as augmentation therapy due to low quality of evidence or absence of studies and their association with known adverse effects (strong against, Rec 25)

For a more in-depth review of the evidence, the practice parameters can be found online at https://www.healthquality.va.gov/guidelines/MH/ptsd/.

International guidelines also exist. Consistent with the VA/DoD recommendation, the Canadian Agency for Drugs and Technologies in Health (CADTH) also recommends sertraline, paroxetine, fluoxetine, and venlafaxine as first-line pharmacotherapy for PTSD [98]. The National Institute for Health and Care Excellence (NICE) in the United Kingdom recommends against benzodiazepines for the prevention of PTSD in adults and to consider venlafaxine or an SSRI such as sertraline for pharmacotherapy [99]. They also recommend against the use of medications for the treatment of PTSD in youth under 18 years of age. The NICE guidelines can be found at https://www.nice.org.uk/guidance/ng116, while the guidelines from CADTH, which also offers a quick comparison of other guidelines, may be reviewed at https://www.cadth.ca/sites/default/files/pdf/PTSD_Treatment_A_Summary_of_Clinical_Practice_Guidelines.pdf.

Specific Medications for the Treatment of PTSD

Expansive discussion of specific medications and evidence of efficacy for PTSD is outside the scope of this chapter. Important principles and safety concerns will be briefly elaborated on, and evidence for the most commonly used medications, namely antidepressants and alpha-2 agonists, will be reviewed.

Selective Serotonin Reuptake Inhibitors (SSRIs) and Other Antidepressants

Antidepressants, specifically SSRIs, are considered first-line pharmacotherapy for PTSD as they have the most evidence with a tolerable side-effect profile. Though only sertraline and paroxetine are approved by the US Food and Drug Administration (FDA) for the treatment of PTSD, *sertraline, paroxetine, fluoxetine and venlafaxine* are recommended by both the APA and VA in adults [97]. Antidepressants take some time for maximal effect, around 4–8 weeks; thus, caution

Table 8.2 FDA-approved indications for antidepressants in the pediatric population [111–113, 115, 116, 119–122]

Antidepressant	MDD	OCD	GAD	Nocturnal enuresis
Clomipramine	–	Age 10 years or more	–	–
Duloxetine	–	–	Age 7 years or more	–
Escitalopram	Age 12 years or more	–	–	–
Fluoxetine	Age 8 years or more	Age 7 years or more	–	–
Fluvoxamine	–	Age 8 years or more	–	–
Imipramine	–	–	–	Age 6 years or more
Sertraline	–	Age 6 years or more	–	–

is advised against increasing the dose too quickly and overmedicating.

There are no medications that are FDA approved for the treatment of PTSD in the pediatric population. Please refer to Table 8.2 for a summary of FDA-approved indications of antidepressants in the pediatric population.

Black Box Warning

Many clinicians are concerned about prescribing antidepressants to TAY due to the black box warning on SSRIs, selective norepinephrine reuptake inhibitors (SNRIs), and other similar medications. Even more so, they find it hard to talk to families about this warning. Below is the specific text of the US Food and Drug Administration (FDA) warning, followed by some general thoughts on how to frame the issue for clinicians in terms of safety monitoring and to discuss the issue with parents and patients.

Warning: Suicidal Thoughts and Behaviors

Antidepressants increased the risk of suicidal thoughts and behavior in children, adolescents, and young adults in short-term studies. These studies did not show an increase in the risk of suicidal thoughts and behavior with antidepressant use in patients over age 24; there was a reduction in risk with antidepressant use in patients aged 65 and older [see Warnings and Precautions (5.1)].

In patients of all ages who are started on antidepressant therapy, monitor closely for worsening and for emergence of suicidal thoughts and behaviors. Advise families and caregivers of the need for close observation and communication with the prescriber [see Warnings and Precautions (5.1)].

While the above language is vague as to "monitor closely," many clinicians take this to mean having at least once weekly clinical check-ins during the time period while medication is being started or when dose adjustments occur. This can be by the primary prescriber or a proxy such as a primary therapist or support staff with experience in mental health and safety assessments.

When framing the issue for parents, it can be good to first provide a background on the origin of the black box warning. In brief, the FDA became aware in the early 2000s that among youth enrolled in placebo-controlled trials of antidepressants, there was a small discrepancy in suicidal thoughts. Specifically, approximately 2% of youth in placebo groups versus approximately 4% of youth in the treatment groups reported or recorded in diaries (provided for part of the study) suicidal ideation. Of note, of the approximately 2000 youth included in the analysis, there was not one suicide attributed to the effects of SSRIs. It may also be helpful to note to families that in the period after the publication of this warning, antidepressant prescription rates went down in numerous jurisdictions [100–102] while attempted or completed suicides went up. While this, of course, is not direct proof, this association is seen to support the idea that antidepressants overall are protective against suicide.

Sertraline

Sertraline is FDA approved for PTSD in adults and as such is the recommended first-line medication for PTSD for both treatment and prevention of relapse. In available data from clinical trials, sertraline was generally well tolerated by both pediatric and adult populations. The most common side effects include headache, nausea, and gastrointestinal disturbance [97].

Multiple studies have been conducted supporting sertraline's efficacy in treatment and relapse prevention in adults. A 12-week, double-blind, placebo-controlled trial of 187 outpatients with a diagnosis of PTSD showed a statistically significant improvement vs. placebo with decreased avoidance/numbing, with decreased arousal, but not with experiencing/intrusion symptoms [103]. A 28-week study with a 12-week double-blind, placebo-controlled acute treatment phase followed by a 24-week open-label continued treatment resulted in a lower PTSD relapse rate of 5% vs. 26% [104]. A 64-week study assessing quality of life and functional impairment associated with PTSD showed that with sertraline, there was a rapid improvement in quality of life, which was progressive and sustained over the course of 1 year of treatment [105]. When sertraline was discontinued, there was a recurrence of PTSD and a worsening of quality of life.

Complicating matters, a 10-week double-blind trial of sertraline vs. placebo in children and adolescents (ages 6–17 years) showed that sertraline was generally well tolerated but was not more effective than placebo [105, 106]. Also, a randomized control trial of TF-CBT with sertraline only showed minimal benefit vs. TF-CBT alone in a group of female children and adolescents aged 10–17 years, suggesting that a trial of TF-CBT alone should be considered first prior to adding medication [107].

These opposing findings make it challenging to provide a clear recommendation for treating TAY with PTSD. While FDA approval specific to sertraline use in PTSD is for those 18 years and older, given what is known about brain growth and development, it is entirely plausible that TAY may be similar to either children and adolescents or adults in how they respond to treatment. Or they may represent a third distinct state with different patterns or response altogether. In general, it seems reasonable to attempt and treat either comorbid MDD or the severe depressive mood, anxiety symptoms, and anhedonia that frequently occur in PTSD with sertraline but to be prepared if a suboptimal response occurs.

Paroxetine

Paroxetine is also FDA approved for PTSD in adults, with a similar side-effect profile to sertraline. There is an increased risk of discontinuation syndrome due to paroxetine's short half-life. Two double-blind, placebo-controlled 12-week trials in adults saw statistically significant improvement in all three symptom clusters of PTSD (reexperiencing, avoidance/numbing, and hyperarousal) with reduction in disability with overall good tolerance to the medication [108, 109].

Paroxetine is not FDA approved for use in children and adolescents, and is generally not recommended for use in this population, given the black box warning and adverse side effects [110, 111].

Fluoxetine, Fluvoxamine, and Venlafaxine

While not FDA approved, all three of these medications have recommendations for the treatment of PTSD in adults from either the APA in the case of fluoxetine or the VA/DoD for all three. Evidence for their efficacy is fairly characterized as inconclusive but can be reviewed at the link provided above previously.

In children and adolescents, fluoxetine is approved for major depressive disorder (MDD) beginning from 8 years of age and for obsessive compulsive disorder (OCD) starting from 7 years of age [112]. Fluvoxamine is only approved for OCD beginning at 8 years of age [113]. Neither fluoxetine nor fluvoxamine is approved for PTSD in children and adolescents but may be used to treat comorbidities. Venlafaxine is not approved for use in the pediatric population [114].

Tricyclic Antidepressants (TCAs) and Monoamine Oxidase Inhibitors (MAOIs)

Overall, TCAs and MAOIs are often less prescribed than SSRIs for a number of reasons. TCAs are poorly tolerated by many patients, may require blood level monitoring, and are extremely deadly in overdose. MAOIs require adherence to a strict dietary protocol to avoid a potential deadly hypertensive crisis. It is strongly recommended that these are only started and monitored by or with close supervision by a practitioner well familiar with the nuances of these medications.

In the pediatric population, clomipramine is FDA approved beginning at 10 years of age for OCD [115], and imipramine is approved for nocturnal enuresis beginning at 6 years of age [116]. MAOIs are generally not prescribed in the pediatric population.

Other Antidepressants: Mirtazapine

Mirtazapine is a noradrenergic and specific serotonergic antidepressant that is generally well tolerated with some potential for treatment in PTSD. Its main side effects include appetite increase and sedation, both of which may be desired in patients with depression and PTSD, though weight gain may be a concern. One small 29-patient double-blind RCT of mirtazapine for PTSD showed improvement in some measures with mirtazapine compared to placebo and was well tolerated [117].

Mirtazapine is not FDA approved for use in the pediatric population [118].

Anxiolytics

While commonly used (and many would argue overused) in anxiety disorders, benzodiazepines have strong evidence against their use in PTSD [123]. Biologically, it is well known that PTSD is associated with hypoactivity of the prefrontal structures of the brain; this and other changes can contribute to increase disinhibition with benzodiazepine use, as well as increased risk for dissociative events with their use [123].

Anticonvulsants

No clear and convincing evidence exists for the use of anticonvulsant agents in the treatment of PTSD. Various trials of carbamazepine, valproate, topiramate, tiagabine, and lamotrigine have all been largely negative or of low quality due to sample size or experimental design [124–132]. As with the antipsychotics, discussed later, there are significant considerations when contemplating prescribing these agents; it is recommended that practitioners familiarize themselves with specific side-effect profiles. Of particular note, carbamazepine has a small risk of blood dyscrasia and hyponatremia, and lamotrigine has elevated risk for Steven-Johnson syndrome, as well as hemophagocytic lymphohistiocytosis (HLH) in certain populations, or when it is titrated too rapidly [133].

Alpha-Adrenergic Modifying Medications

While evidence in the form of large, well-designed clinical trials is weak for this category of medications [134, 135], they are often used clinically off-label to decrease the sympathetic overactivation seen in patients with PTSD. Clonidine and guanfacine are both FDA approved for use in children and adolescents as an alternative or adjunct to stimulants for attention deficit hyperactivity disorder (ADHD) [136, 137], especially in the hyperactive subtype, making their use in younger children relatively common. Clinical tips and notes for these agents and prazosin would include the need for vital sign monitoring, cautioning the patient to remain well hydrated to potentially reduce hypotension and to avoid standing up quickly or engaging in significant physical activity until the effect of the medication is known. Autonomic rebound can happen with rapid discontinuation of any of the three, but clonidine is regarded as being slightly more prone to this effect.

Prazosin

Prazosin is an alpha-1 adrenergic antagonist with mixed evidence regarding efficacy for PTSD symptoms. Historically, prazosin was recommended for the treatment of PTSD-related nightmares, and there are several small studies with evidence of efficacy for improving sleep disturbances and trauma-related nightmares. Recently, though, a large, well-run randomized control trial was decisively negative in terms of efficacy between prazosin and placebo, raising significant questions and leading the VA to change its recommendation to "insufficient evidence" to recommend for or against prazosin for nightmares related to PTSD [138–141].

There is limited data on prazosin in children and adolescents for treating PTSD. A systematic review of nine studies for the treatment of nightmares with prazosin highlighted promising outcomes, but six of the nine studies were case reports. Further research is needed as in most of the clinical questions discussed here [142].

Guanfacine and Clonidine

Guanfacine and clonidine reduce sympathetic tone and response through activation of alpha-2 presynaptic autoreceptors on adrenergic neurons. No strong data exist supporting either of their efficacy, but clinical experience and mechanistic overlap with prazosin have led to use in treating PTSD.

Antipsychotics

No antipsychotic medications are approved for the treatment of PTSD. Due to their risk for metabolic syndrome and movement disorders, it is generally recommended that, if prescribed, these are used near the end of the treatment algorithm and ideally in coordination with a provider experienced in their use. Laboratory monitoring, which includes a lipid panel, hgbA1c, comprehensive metabolic panel, and CBC, should occur at baseline. Additional recommendations are detailed in the table below (Table 8.3), adapted from the Center for Quality Assessment and Improvement in Mental Health's guide to metabolic monitoring in using antipsychotic medications [143] (http://www.cqaimh.org/pdf/tool_metabolic.pdf), which represents a reasonable schedule of metrics to monitor over time. As in the case of all medications mentioned in this chapter, clinicians should be aware of the monitoring recommendations and requirements before prescribing any medication.

Chapter Summary

At baseline, TAY represent a heterogeneous grouping of individuals navigating a complex biologic and societal transition point, leaving them at increased risk to traumatic events and their sequelae. While a vast majority are resilient, for those that develop long-term trauma-related illnesses, certain general principles can assist in supporting them in treatment. These include gathering as much developmental history and context as possible and working, when appropriate, to include family members and support systems in the treatment. In terms of specific interventions, using evidenced-based treatments is best, but due to the dearth of research specific to this population, no clear best practice exists. In general, referral to or consultation with experienced providers, when available, is ideal. Though medication may provide significant symptomatic relief, remission of symptoms is likely best accomplished when taken in conjunction with therapy.

Table 8.3 Recommended schedule for monitoring patients on second-generation antipsychotics

	Initial screening				Continued screening		
	baseline	4 weeks	8 weeks	12 weeks	Quarterly	Annually	Every 5 years
Personal and family history	X	–	–	–	–	X	–
Weight (BMI)	X	X	X	X	X	–	–
Waist circumference	X	–	–	–	–	X	–
Blood pressure	X	–	–	X	–	X	–
Fasting plasma glucose (or hgbA1c)	X	–	–	X	–	X	–
Fasting lipid profile	X	–	–	X	–	–	X

Adapted from the Center for Quality Assessment and Improvement in Mental Health STABLE Resource Toolkit

References

1. Wilens TE, Rosenbaum JF. Transitional aged youth: a new frontier in child and adolescent psychiatry. J Am Acad Child Adolesc Psychiatry. 2013;52(9):887–90.
2. Frounfelker R, Klodnick VV, Mueser KT, Todd S. Trauma and posttraumatic stress disorder among transition-age youth with serious mental health conditions. J Trauma Stress. 2013;26(3):409–12.
3. Arnett JJ. Emerging adulthood: Oxford University Press New York, NY; 2014.
4. Côté JE. The dangerous myth of emerging adulthood: an evidence-based critique of a flawed developmental theory. Appl Dev Sci. 2014;18(4):177–88.
5. Turner RJ, Jay Turner R, Lloyd DA. The stress process and the social distribution of depression. J Health Soc Behav. 1999;40(4):374.
6. Kessler RC, McGonagle KA, Zhao S, Nelson CB, Hughes M, Eshleman S, et al. Lifetime and 12-month prevalence of DSM-III-R psychiatric disorders in the United States: results from the National Comorbidity Survey. Arch Gen Psychiatry. 1994;51(1):8–19.
7. Park MJ, Jane Park M, Mulye TP, Adams SH, Brindis CD, Irwin CE. The health status of young adults in the United States. J Adolesc Health. 2006;39(3):305–17.
8. Underwood LA, Washington A. Mental illness and juvenile offenders. In: The encyclopedia of juvenile delinquency and justice; John Wiley & Sons, Inc: Hoboken, NJ; 2017. p. 1–8.
9. Kozloff N, Stergiopoulos V, Adair CE, Cheung AH, Misir V, Townley G, et al. The unique needs of homeless youths with mental illness: baseline findings from a housing first trial. Psychiatr Serv. 2016;67(10):1083–90.
10. Havlicek JR, Garcia AR, Smith DC. Mental health and substance use disorders among foster youth transitioning to adulthood: past research and future directions. Child Youth Serv Rev. 2013;35(1):194–203.
11. Kessler RC, Berglund P, Demler O, Jin R, Merikangas KR, Walters EE. Lifetime prevalence and age-of-onset distributions of DSM-IV disorders in the national comorbidity survey replication. Arch Gen Psychiatry. 2005;62(6):593.
12. Price M, Arditi R, Olezeski C, McMahon TJ. Psychological assessment and treatment of emerging adults exposed to complex trauma. Evidence-Based Practice in Child and Adolescent Mental Health. 2019;4(3):273–95.
13. Blaustein ME, Kinniburgh KM. When age doesn't match stage: challenges and considerations in services for transition-age youth with histories of developmental trauma. Focal Point: Youth, Young Adults, & Mental Health. 2015;(29):17–20.
14. Osgood DW, Wayne Osgood D, Michael Foster E, Flanagan C, Ruth GR, editors. On your own without a net: the transition to adulthood for vulnerable populations. Chicago: University of Chicago Press; 2005.
15. Davis M. Addressing the needs of youth in transition to adulthood. Admin Pol Ment Health. 2003;30(6):495–509.
16. Stroud C, Walker LR, Davis M, Irwin CE. Investing in the health and well-being of young adults. J Adolesc Health. 2015;56(2):127–9.
17. Oesterle S. Background paper: pathways to young adulthood and preventive interventions targeting young adults. In: IOM (Institute of Medicine), NRC (National Research Council), editor. Improving the health, safety, and well-being of young adults: workshop summary. Washington, DC: The National Academies Press; 2013. p. 147–76.
18. Martel A, Catherine FD. Transitional age youth and mental illness – influences on young adult outcomes. Child Adolesc Psychiatr Clin N Am. 2017;26(2):xiii–vii.
19. Osgood DW, Wayne Osgood D, Ruth G, Eccles JS, Jacobs JE, Barber BL. Six paths to adulthood. In: Settersten Jr RA, Furstenberg FF, Rumbaut RG, editors. On the frontier of adulthood: theory, research, and public policy: Chicago Scholarship Online; 2005. p. 320–55.
20. Schulenberg JE, Sameroff AJ, Cicchetti D. The transition to adulthood as a critical juncture in the course of psychopathology and mental health. Dev Psychopathol [Internet]. 2004;16(4). Available from: https://doi.org/10.1017/s0954579404040015.
21. McMahon TJ. Child maltreatment and emerging adulthood: past, present, and future. Child Maltreat. 2014;19(3–4):135–44.
22. Cohen P, Kasen S, Chen H, Hartmark C, Gordon K. Variations in patterns of developmental transmissions in the emerging adulthood period. Dev Psychol. 2003;39(4):657–69.
23. Landberg M, Lee B, Noack P. What alters the experience of emerging adulthood? How the experience of emerging adulthood differs according to socioeconomic status and critical life events. Emerg Adulthood. 2019;7(3):208–22.
24. du Bois-Reymond M, du Bois-Reymond M. Emerging adulthood theory under scrutiny. Emerg Adulthood. 2016;4(4):242–3.
25. Norona JC, Preddy TM, Welsh DP. How gender shapes emerging adulthood. In: Arnett JJ, editor. The Oxford handbook of emerging adulthood. Oxford: Oxford University Press; 2014.
26. Syed M, Mitchell LL. How race and ethnicity shape emerging adulthood. In: Arnett JJ, editor. The Oxford handbook of emerging adulthood. Oxford: Oxford University Press; 2014.
27. Musicaro RM, Spinazzola J, Arvidson J, Swaroop SR, Grace LG, Yarrow A, et al. The complexity of adaptation to childhood polyvictimization in youth and young adults: recommendations for multidisciplinary responders. Trauma Violence Abuse. 2019;20(1):81–98.
28. Ford JD, Courtois CA, editors. Treating complex traumatic stress disorders in children and adoles-

cents: Scientific foundations and therapeutic models: Guilford Press New York, NY; 2013.
29. Davis M, Stoep A. The transition to adulthood for youth who have serious emotional disturbance: developmental transition and young adult outcomes. J Behav Health Serv Res. 1997;24(4):400–27.
30. Taber-Thomas B, Pérez-Edgar K. Emerging adulthood brain development. In: Arnett JJ, editor. The Oxford handbook of emerging adulthood. Oxford: Oxford University Press; 2014.
31. Hiser J, Koenigs M. The multifaceted role of the ventromedial prefrontal cortex in emotion, decision making, social cognition, and psychopathology. Biol Psychiatry. 2018;83(8):638–47.
32. Finkelhor D, Ormrod R, Turner H, Hamby SL. The victimization of children and youth: a comprehensive, national survey. Child Maltreat. 2005;10(1):5–25.
33. Finkelhor D, Turner HA, Shattuck A, Hamby SL. Prevalence of childhood exposure to violence, crime, and abuse. JAMA Pediatr. 2015;169(8):746.
34. Finkelhor D, Turner H, Ormrod R, Hamby SL. Violence, abuse, and crime exposure in a national sample of children and youth. Pediatrics. 2009;124(5):1411–23.
35. Copeland WE, Keeler G, Angold A, Costello EJ. Traumatic events and posttraumatic stress in childhood. Arch Gen Psychiatry. 2007;64(5):577–84.
36. Giaconia RM, Reinherz HZ, Silverman AB, Pakiz B, Frost AK, Cohen E. Traumas and posttraumatic stress disorder in a community population of older adolescents. J Am Acad Child Adolesc Psychiatry. 1995;34(10):1369–80.
37. McLaughlin KA, Koenen KC, Hill ED, Petukhova M, Sampson NA, Zaslavsky AM, et al. Trauma exposure and posttraumatic stress disorder in a national sample of adolescents. J Am Acad Child Adolesc Psychiatry. 2013;52(8):815–30.e14.
38. Felitti VJ, Anda RF, Nordenberg D, Williamson DF, Spitz AM, Edwards V, et al. Relationship of childhood abuse and household dysfunction to many of the leading causes of death in adults. Am J Prev Med. 1998;14(4):245–58.
39. National Center for Injury Prevention and Control, Division of Violence Prevention. About the CDC-Kaiser ACE study [Internet]. CDC; 2019. Available from: https://www.cdc.gov/violenceprevention/childabuseandneglect/acestudy/about.html
40. Finkelhor D, Turner H, Shattuck A, Hamby S, Kracke K. Children's exposure to violence, crime, and abuse: an update. Laurel: Office of Juvenile Justice and Delinquency Prevention; 2015. (Juvenile Justice Bulletin: National Survey of Children's Exposure to Violence).
41. Ford JD, Elhai JD, Connor DF, Christopher FB. Poly-victimization and risk of posttraumatic, depressive, and substance use disorders and involvement in delinquency in a national sample of adolescents. J Adolesc Health. 2010;46(6):545–52.
42. Finkelhor D, Ormrod RK, Turner HA. Poly-victimization: a neglected component in child victimization. Child Abuse Negl. 2007;31(1):7–26.
43. Harris WW, Putnam FW, Fairbank JA. Mobilizing trauma resources for children. In: Lieberman AF, DeMartino R, editors. Shaping the future of children's health. Calverton: Johnson & Johnson Pediatric Institute; 2006. p. 311–39.
44. Atwoli L, Stein DJ, Williams DR, Mclaughlin KA, Petukhova M, Kessler RC, et al. Trauma and posttraumatic stress disorder in South Africa: analysis from the South African Stress and Health Study. BMC Psychiatry [Internet]. 2013;13(182). Available from: https://doi.org/10.1186/1471-244x-13-182.
45. Turner HA, Finkelhor D, Ormrod R, Hamby S, Leeb RT, Mercy JA, et al. Family context, victimization, and child trauma symptoms: variations in safe, stable, and nurturing relationships during early and middle childhood. Am J Orthopsychiatry. 2012;82(2):209–19.
46. Turner H, Shattuck A, Hamby S, Finkelhor D. Community disorder, victimization exposure, and mental health in a national sample of youth. J Health Soc Behav. 2013;54(2):258–75.
47. Turner HA, Shattuck A, Finkelhor D, Hamby S. Polyvictimization and youth violence exposure across contexts. J Adolesc Health. 2016;58(2):208–14.
48. Ogle CM, Rubin DC, Berntsen D, Siegler IC. The frequency and impact of exposure to potentially traumatic events over the life course. Clin Psychol Sci. 2013;1(4):426–34.
49. Sugar J, Ford JD. Peritraumatic reactions and posttraumatic stress disorder in psychiatrically impaired youth. J Trauma Stress. 2012;25(1):41–9.
50. Layne CM, Beck C, Rimmasch H, Southwick J, Moreno MA, Hobfoll S. Promoting "resilient" posttraumatic adjustment in childhood and beyond: "unpacking" life events, adjustment trajectories, resources, and interventions. In: Brom D, Pat-Horencyzk R, Ford JD, editors. Treating traumatized children: risk, resilience, and recovery. London: Routledge; 2008. p. 13–47.
51. Schwartz D, Proctor LJ. Community violence exposure and children's social adjustment in the school peer group: the mediating roles of emotion regulation and social cognition. J Consult Clin Psychol. 2000;68(4):670–83.
52. McLaughlin KA, Lambert HK. Child trauma exposure and psychopathology: mechanisms of risk and resilience. Curr Opin Psychol. 2017;14:29–34.
53. Milan S, Zona K, Acker J, Turcios-Cotto V. Prospective risk factors for adolescent PTSD: sources of differential exposure and differential vulnerability. J Abnorm Child Psychol. 2013;41(2):339–53.
54. Herringa RJ, Burghy CA, Stodola DE, Fox ME, Davidson RJ, Essex MJ. Enhanced prefrontal-amygdala connectivity following childhood adversity as a protective mechanism against internal-

izing in adolescence. Biol Psychiatry Cogn Neurosci Neuroimaging. 2016;1(4):326–34.
55. Schilling EA, Aseltine RH, Gore S. Adverse childhood experiences and mental health in young adults: a longitudinal survey. BMC Public Health [Internet]. 2007;7(1). Available from: https://doi.org/10.1186/1471-2458-7-30.
56. Shonkoff JP, Garner AS, Siegel BS, Dobbins MI, Earls MF, Garner AS, et al. The lifelong effects of early childhood adversity and toxic stress. Pediatrics. 2012;129(1):e232–46.
57. Anda RF, Felitti VJ, Bremner JD, Walker JD, Whitfield C, Perry BD, et al. The enduring effects of abuse and related adverse experiences in childhood. A convergence of evidence from neurobiology and epidemiology. Eur Arch Psychiatry Clin Neurosci. 2006;256(3):174–86.
58. American Psychiatric Association. Diagnostic and statistical manual of mental disorders (DSM-5®): American Psychiatric Pub Washington DC; 2013. 991 p.
59. Blevins CA, Weathers FW, Davis MT, Witte TK, Domino JL. The Posttraumatic Stress Disorder Checklist for DSM-5 (PCL-5): development and initial psychometric evaluation. J Trauma Stress. 2015;28(6):489–98.
60. Weathers FW, Bovin MJ, Lee DJ, Sloan DM, Schnurr PP, Kaloupek DG, et al. The Clinician-Administered PTSD Scale for DSM–5 (CAPS-5): development and initial psychometric evaluation in military veterans. Psychol Assess. 2018;30(3):383–95.
61. Skehan B, Davis M. Aligning mental health treatments with the developmental stage and needs of late adolescents and young adults. Child Adolesc Psychiatr Clin N Am. 2017;26(2):177–90.
62. Mistler LA, Sheidow AJ, Davis M. Transdiagnostic motivational enhancement therapy to reduce treatment attrition: use in emerging adults. Cogn Behav Pract. 2016;23(3):368–84.
63. Munson MR, Jaccard J, Smalling SE, Kim H, Werner JJ, Scott LD. Static, dynamic, integrated, and contextualized: a framework for understanding mental health service utilization among young adults. Soc Sci Med. 2012;75(8):1441–9.
64. Saxe GN, Ellis BH, Kaplow JB. Collaborative treatment of traumatized children and teens: the trauma systems therapy approach. New York: Guilford Publications; 2007. 338 p.
65. Cook A, Spinazzola J, Ford J, Lanktree C, Blaustein M, Cloitre M, et al. Complex trauma in children and adolescents. Psychiatr Ann. 2005;35(5):390–8.
66. Briere J, Spinazzola J. Phenomenology and psychological assessment of complex posttraumatic states. J Trauma Stress. 2005;18(5):401–12.
67. Lanktree C, Briere J. Integrative treatment of complex trauma. In: Ford JD, Courtois CA, editors. Treating complex traumatic stress disorders in children and adolescents: scientific foundations and therapeutic models Guilford Press, New York, NY; 2013. p. 143–61.
68. Cohen JA, Mannarino AP. Trauma-focused cognitive behavioural therapy for children and parents. Child Adolesc Mental Health. 2008;13(4):158–62.
69. Cohen JA, Deblinger E, Mannarino AP, Steer RA. A multisite, randomized controlled trial for children with sexual abuse–related PTSD symptoms. J Am Acad Child Adolesc Psychiatry. 2004;43(4):393–402.
70. Cohen JA, Mannarino AP, Knudsen K. Treating sexually abused children: 1 year follow-up of a randomized controlled trial. Child Abuse Negl. 2005;29(2):135–45.
71. Scheeringa MS, Weems CF, Cohen JA, Amaya-Jackson L, Guthrie D. Trauma-focused cognitive-behavioral therapy for posttraumatic stress disorder in three-through six year-old children: a randomized clinical trial. J Child Psychol Psychiatry. 2011;52(8):853–60.
72. Munson MR, Cole A, Stanhope V, Marcus SC, McKay M, Jaccard J, et al. Cornerstone program for transition-age youth with serious mental illness: study protocol for a randomized controlled trial. Trials [Internet]. 2016;17(1). Available from: https://doi.org/10.1186/s13063-016-1654-0.
73. Cole A, Munson M, Ben-David S, Sapiro B, Railey J, Stanhope V. Feasibility, acceptability, and preliminary impact of the cornerstone mentoring program. Implement Sci. 2018;13:1–67.
74. Chen K, Lanktree CB, Semple RJ, Briere J, Maida C. Integrative treatment of complex trauma for adolescents (ITCT-A): an implementation guide for organizations [Internet]. USC Adolescent Trauma Training Center (USC-ATTC); 2019. Available from: https://keck.usc.edu/adolescent-trauma-training-center/wp-content/uploads/sites/169/2019/09/ITCT-A_Implementation_Guide_20190904.pdf.
75. Lanktree C, Briere J. Integrative treatment of complex trauma for children (ITCT-C): a guide for the treatment of multiply-traumatized children aged eight to twelve years. Long Beach: Miller Children's Abuse and Violence Intervention Center-USC; 2008.
76. Foa EB, Hembree E, Rothbaum BO. Prolonged exposure therapy for PTSD: emotional processing of traumatic experiences, therapist guide. Oxford/New York: Oxford University Press; 2007.
77. Foa EB, Kozak MJ. Emotional processing of fear: exposure to corrective information. Psychol Bull. 1986;99(1):20–35.
78. Foa EB, Huppert JD, Cahill SP. Emotional processing theory: an update. In: Rothbaum B, editor. Pathological anxiety: emotional processing in etiology and treatment. New York: The Guilford Press; 2006. p. 3–24.
79. Foa EB, Chrestman KR, Gilboa-Schechtman E. Prolonged exposure therapy for adolescents with PTSD therapist guide: emotional processing of traumatic experiences: Oxford University Press New York, NY; 2008.
80. Capaldi S, Zandberg LJ, Foa EB. Prolonged exposure therapy for adolescents with PTSD: emotional

processing of traumatic experiences. In: Landolt M, Cloitre M, Schnyder U, editors. Evidence-based treatments for trauma related disorders in children and adolescents. Cham: Springer; 2017. p. 209–26.
81. Markowitz JC, Petkova E, Neria Y, Van Meter PE, Zhao Y, Hembree E, et al. Is exposure necessary? A randomized clinical trial of interpersonal psychotherapy for PTSD. Am J Psychiatry. 2015;172(5):430–40.
82. Resick PA, Williams LF, Suvak MK, Monson CM, Gradus JL. Long-term outcomes of cognitive-behavioral treatments for posttraumatic stress disorder among female rape survivors. J Consult Clin Psychol. 2012;80(2):201–10.
83. Cahill SP, Rauch SA, Hembree EA, Foa EB. Effect of cognitive-behavioral treatments for PTSD on anger. J Cogn Psychother. 2003;17(2):113–31.
84. Powers MB, Halpern JM, Ferenschak MP, Gillihan SJ, Foa EB. A meta-analytic review of prolonged exposure for posttraumatic stress disorder. Clin Psychol Rev. 2010;30(6):635–41.
85. Gilboa-Schechtman E, Foa EB, Shafran N, Aderka IM, Powers MB, Rachamim L, et al. Prolonged exposure versus dynamic therapy for adolescent PTSD: a pilot randomized controlled trial. J Am Acad Child Adolesc Psychiatry. 2010;49(10):1034–42.
86. Foa EB, McLean CP, Capaldi S, Rosenfield D. Prolonged exposure vs supportive counseling for sexual abuse-related PTSD in adolescent girls: a randomized clinical trial. JAMA. 2013;310(24):2650–7.
87. Rosner R, Rimane E, Frick U, Gutermann J, Hagl M, Renneberg B, et al. Effect of developmentally adapted cognitive processing therapy for youth with symptoms of posttraumatic stress disorder after childhood sexual and physical abuse. JAMA Psychiat. 2019;76(5):484.
88. Cloitre M, Koenen KC, Cohen LR, Han H. Skills training in affective and interpersonal regulation followed by exposure: a phase-based treatment for PTSD related to childhood abuse. J Consult Clin Psychol. 2002;70(5):1067–74.
89. Cloitre M, Courtois CA, Charuvastra A, Carapezza R, Stolbach BC, Green BL. Treatment of complex PTSD: results of the ISTSS expert clinician survey on best practices. J Trauma Stress. 2011;24(6):615–27.
90. Cloitre M, Courtois C, Ford J, Green B, Alexander P, Briere J, et al. The ISTSS expert consensus treatment guidelines for complex PTSD in adults. https://www.istss.org/ISTSS_Main/media/Documents/ISTSS-Expert-Concesnsus-Guidelines-for-Complex-PTSD-Updated-060315.pdf. 2012.
91. Levitt JT, Malta LS, Martin A, Davis L, Cloitre M. The flexible application of a manualized treatment for PTSD symptoms and functional impairment related to the 9/11 World Trade Center attack. Behav Res Ther. 2007;45(7):1419–33.
92. Shapiro F. Efficacy of the eye movement desensitization procedure in the treatment of traumatic memories. J Trauma Stress. 1989;2(2):199–223.
93. Scheck MM, Schaeffer JA, Gillette C. Brief psychological intervention with traumatized young women: the efficacy of eye movement desensitization and reprocessing. J Trauma Stress. 1998;11(1):25–44.
94. Resick PA, Monson CM, Chard KM. Cognitive processing therapy for PTSD: a comprehensive manual: Guilford Publications New York, NY; 2016. 312 p.
95. Cohen JA, Bukstein O, Walter H, Benson SR, Chrisman A, Farchione TR, et al. Practice parameter for the assessment and treatment of children and adolescents with posttraumatic stress disorder. J Am Acad Child Adolesc Psychiatry. 2010;49(4):414–30.
96. American Psychological Association. Clinical practice guideline for the treatment of posttraumatic stress disorder (PTSD) in adults [Internet]. 2017. Available from: https://www.apa.org/ptsd-guideline/ptsd.pdf
97. VA/DOD clinical practice guideline for the management of posttraumatic stress disorder and acute stress disorder [Internet]. {The US Department of Veterans Affairs and Department of Defense}; 2017. Available from: healthquality.va.gov/guidelines/MH/ptsd/VADoDPTSDCPGFinal.pdf.
98. Canadian Agency for Drugs & Technologies in Health. Treatment for post-traumatic stress disorder, operational stress injury, or critical incident stress: a summary of clinical practice guidelines. Canadian Agency for Drugs & Technologies in Health; 2015.
99. National Institute for Health and Care Excellence. Post-traumatic stress disorder - NICE guideline [NG116] [Internet]. National Institute for Health and Care Excellence. 2018 [cited 2020 Feb 29]. Available from: https://www.nice.org.uk/guidance/ng116.
100. Pozzi M, Radice S, Clementi E, Molteni M, Nobile M. Antidepressants and, suicide and self-injury: causal or casual association? Int J Psychiatry Clin Pract. 2016;20(1):47–51.
101. Bachmann CJ, Aagaard L, Burcu M, Glaeske G, Kalverdijk LJ, Petersen I, et al. Trends and patterns of antidepressant use in children and adolescents from five western countries, 2005-2012. Eur Neuropsychopharmacol. 2016;26(3):411–9.
102. Friedman RA. Antidepressants' black-box warning — 10 years later. N Engl J Med. 2014;371(18):1666–8.
103. Brady K, Pearlstein T, Asnis GM, Baker D, Rothbaum B, Sikes CR, et al. Efficacy and safety of sertraline treatment of posttraumatic stress disorder. JAMA. 2000;283(14):1837.
104. Davidson J, Pearlstein T, Londborg P, Brady KT, Rothbaum B, Bell J, et al. Efficacy of sertraline in preventing relapse of posttraumatic stress disorder: results of a 28-week double-blind, placebo-controlled study. Am J Psychiatry. 2001;158(12):1974–81.

105. Rapaport MH, Endicott J, Clary CM. Posttraumatic stress disorder and quality of life: results across 64 weeks of sertraline treatment. J Clin Psychiatry. 2002;63(1):59–65.
106. Robb AS, Cueva JE, Sporn J, Yang R, Vanderburg DG. Sertraline treatment of children and adolescents with posttraumatic stress disorder: a double-blind, placebo-controlled trial. J Child Adolesc Psychopharmacol. 2010;20(6):463–71.
107. Cohen JA, Mannarino AP, Perel JM, Staron V. A pilot randomized controlled trial of combined trauma-focused CBT and sertraline for childhood PTSD symptoms. J Am Acad Child Adolesc Psychiatry. 2007;46(7):811–9.
108. Tucker P, Zaninelli R, Yehuda R, Ruggiero L, Dillingham K, Pitts CD. Paroxetine in the treatment of chronic posttraumatic stress disorder. J Clin Psychiatry. 2001;62(11):860–8.
109. Marshall RD, Beebe KL, Oldham M, Zaninelli R. Efficacy and safety of paroxetine treatment for chronic PTSD: a fixed-dose, placebo-controlled study. Am J Psychiatry. 2001;158(12):1982–8.
110. Paxil® (paroxetine hydrochloride) prescribing information [Internet]. GlaxoSmithKline; 2012. Available from: https://www.accessdata.fda.gov/drugsatfda_docs/label/2012/020031s067,020710s031.pdf.
111. Education Medicaid Integrity Contractor for the CMS Medicaid Program Integrity Education (MPIE). Antidepressant medications: use in pediatric patients [Internet]. CMS; 2015. Available from: https://www.cms.gov/Medicare-Medicaid-Coordination/Fraud-Prevention/Medicaid-Integrity-Education/Pharmacy-Education-Materials/Downloads/ad-pediatric-factsheet11-14.pdf
112. Prozac® (fluoxetine) prescribing information [Internet]. Lilly USA, LLC; 2017. Available from: https://www.accessdata.fda.gov/drugsatfda_docs/label/2017/018936s108lbl.pdf.
113. Luvox® (fluvoxamine maleate) prescribing information [Internet]. Jazz Pharmaceuticals; 2007. Available from: https://www.accessdata.fda.gov/drugsatfda_docs/label/2007/021519lbl.pdf.
114. Venlafaxine hydrochloride prescribing information [Internet]. Teva Pharmaceuticals USA; 2014. Available from: https://www.accessdata.fda.gov/drugsatfda_docs/label/2014/076690s020lbl.pdf
115. Anafranil TM (clomipramine hydrochloride) prescribing information [Internet]. Patheon; 2019. Available from: https://www.accessdata.fda.gov/drugsatfda_docs/label/2019/019906s043lbl.pdf.
116. Imipramine hydrochloride prescribing information [Internet]. Excellium Pharmaceutical, Inc.; Available from: https://www.accessdata.fda.gov/drugsatfda_docs/label/2012/040903lbl.pdf.
117. Davidson JRT, Weisler RH, Butterfield MI, Casat CD, Connor KM, Barnett S, et al. Mirtazapine vs. placebo in posttraumatic stress disorder: a pilot trial. Biol Psychiatry. 2003;53(2):188–91.
118. Remeron® (mirtazapine) prescribing information [Internet]. Merck Sharp & Dohme B.V.; 2019. Available from: https://www.accessdata.fda.gov/drugsatfda_docs/label/2019/020415s035lbl.pdf.
119. Education Medicaid Integrity Contractor for the CMS Medicaid Program Integrity Education (MPIE). Antidepressant medications: U.S. Food and Drug Administration-approved indications and dosages for use in pediatric patients [Internet]. CMS; 2015. Available from: https://www.cms.gov/Medicare-Medicaid-Coordination/Fraud-Prevention/Medicaid-Integrity-Education/Pharmacy-Education-Materials/Downloads/ad-pediatric-dosingchart11-14.pdf.
120. Cymbalta® (duloxetine) prescribing information [Internet]. Lilly USA, LLC; 2017. Available from: https://www.accessdata.fda.gov/drugsatfda_docs/label/2017/021427s049lbl.pdf.
121. Lexapro® (escitalopram) prescribing information [Internet]. Allergan; 2017. Available from: https://www.accessdata.fda.gov/drugsatfda_docs/label/2017/021323s047lbl.pdf.
122. Zoloft® (sertraline hydrochloride) prescribing information [Internet]. Roerig; 2016 Dec. Available from: https://www.accessdata.fda.gov/drugsatfda_docs/label/2016/019839S74S86S87_20990S35S44S45lbl.pdf
123. Guina J, Rossetter SR, DeRhodes BJ, Nahhas RW, Welton RS. Benzodiazepines for PTSD: a systematic review and meta-analysis. J Psychiatr Pract. 2015;21(4):281–303.
124. Lipper S, Davidson JRT, Grady TA, Edinger JD, Hammett EB, Mahorney SL, et al. Preliminary study of carbamazepine in post-traumatic stress disorder. Psychosomatics. 1986;27(12):849–54.
125. Clark RD, Cañive JM, Calais LA, Qualls CR, Tuason VB. Divalproex in posttraumatic stress disorder: an open-label clinical trial. J Trauma Stress. 1999;12(2):395–401.
126. Davis LL, Davidson JRT, Ward LC, Bartolucci A, Bowden CL, Petty F. Divalproex in the treatment of posttraumatic stress disorder: a randomized, double-blind, placebo-controlled trial in a veteran population. J Clin Psychopharmacol. 2008;28(1):84–8.
127. Tucker P, Trautman RP, Wyatt DB, Thompson J, Wu S-C, Capece JA, et al. Efficacy and safety of topiramate monotherapy in civilian posttraumatic stress disorder: a randomized, double-blind, placebo-controlled study. J Clin Psychiatry. 2007;68(2):201–6.
128. Fesler FA. Valproate in combat-related posttraumatic stress disorder. J Clin Psychiatry. 1991;52(9):361–4.
129. Yeh MSL, Mari JJ, Costa MCP, Andreoli SB, Bressan RA, Mello MF. A double-blind randomized controlled trial to study the efficacy of topiramate in a civilian sample of PTSD. CNS Neurosci Ther. 2011;17(5):305–10.
130. Hertzberg MA, Butterfield MI, Feldman ME, Beckham JC, Sutherland SM, Connor KM, et al. A

preliminary study of lamotrigine for the treatment of posttraumatic stress disorder. Biol Psychiatry. 1999;45(9):1226–9.
131. Davidson JRT, Brady K, Mellman TA, Stein MB, Pollack MH. The efficacy and tolerability of tiagabine in adult patients with post-traumatic stress disorder. J Clin Psychopharmacol. 2007;27(1):85–8.
132. Berlant J, van Kammen DP. Open-label topiramate as primary or adjunctive therapy in chronic civilian posttraumatic stress disorder: a preliminary report. J Clin Psychiatry. 2002;63(1):15–20.
133. Deng Y, Li S, Zhang L, Jin H, Zou X. Association between HLA alleles and lamotrigine-induced cutaneous adverse drug reactions in Asian populations: a meta-analysis. Seizure. 2018;60:163–71.
134. Neylan TCMD, Lenoci MMA, Samuelson KWPD, Metzler TJMA, Henn-Haase C, Psy D, Hierholzer RWMD, et al. No improvement of posttraumatic stress disorder symptoms with guanfacine treatment. AJP. 2006;163(12):2186–8.
135. Connor DF, Grasso DJ, Slivinsky MD, Pearson GS, Banga A. An open-label study of guanfacine extended release for traumatic stress related symptoms in children and adolescents. J Child Adolesc Psychopharmacol. 2013;23(4):244–51.
136. Chiu S, Campbell K. Clonidine for the treatment of psychiatric conditions and symptoms: a review of clinical effectiveness, safety, and guidelines. Ottawa: Canadian Agency for Drugs and Technologies in Health; 2018.
137. Intuniv® (guanfacine) prescribing information [Internet]. Shire US Inc.; 2013. Available from: https://www.accessdata.fda.gov/drugsatfda_docs/label/2013/022037s009lbl.pdf.
138. Raskind MA, Peskind ER, Hoff DJ, Hart KL, Holmes HA, Warren D, et al. A parallel group placebo controlled study of prazosin for trauma nightmares and sleep disturbance in combat veterans with post-traumatic stress disorder. Biol Psychiatry. 2007;61(8):928–34.
139. Raskind MA, Peskind ER, Chow B, Harris C, Davis-Karim A, Holmes HA, et al. Trial of prazosin for post-traumatic stress disorder in military veterans. N Engl J Med. 2018;378(6):507–17.
140. George KC, Kebejian L, Ruth LJ, Miller CWT, Himelhoch S. Meta-analysis of the efficacy and safety of prazosin versus placebo for the treatment of nightmares and sleep disturbances in adults with posttraumatic stress disorder. J Trauma Dissociation. 2016;17(4):494–510.
141. Byers MG, Allison KM, Wendel CS, Lee JK. Prazosin versus quetiapine for nighttime posttraumatic stress disorder symptoms in veterans: an assessment of long-term comparative effectiveness and safety. J Clin Psychopharmacol. 2010;30(3):225–9.
142. Akinsanya A, Marwaha R, Tampi RR. Prazosin in children and adolescents with posttraumatic stress disorder who have nightmares: a systematic review. J Clin Psychopharmacol. 2017;37(1):84–8.
143. Metabolic monitoring [Internet]. Center for Quality Assessment and Improvement in Mental Health. Available from: http://www.cqaimh.org/pdf/tool_metabolic.pdf.

9 Obsessive-Compulsive and Related Disorders in Transitional-Age Youth

Nnenna Kalaya Okereke

Key Points

- TAY with OCRD are at risk of worsening symptoms due to the stresses of living independently, taking responsibility for medical treatment, and making the transition from pediatric to adult care.
- The assessment and treatment of TAY with OCRD is similar to that of children and adults. With permission, clinicians may be able to involve parents and other collateral supports in treatment.
- Cognitive behavioral therapy (CBT) and selective serotonin reuptake inhibitors (SSRIs) are recommended as safe, evidence-based, and effective first-line treatments for obsessive-compulsive disorder (OCD) and body dysmorphic disorder (BDD). Cognitive behavioral therapy, particularly habit reversal training, is the recommended treatment for hoarding disorder, trichotillomania, and excoriation (skin picking) disorder.
- Acute residential treatment, deep brain stimulation, and transcranial direct current stimulation are available for treatment-resistant cases of OCRD.
- Careful planning when transitioning to college or starting a job can help transitional age youth (TAY) avoid common pitfalls leading to deterioration in symptoms.

Introduction

TAY may be at higher risk of developing common mental illnesses because they are often under significant stress as they transition from adolescence to adulthood [1]. In addition, these same developmental stressors occur at the chronological age when mental health problems first occur [2]. Obsessive-compulsive disorder (OCD) was previously categorized as an anxiety disorder in the DSM-IV-TR [3, 4], but now is classified as one of the obsessive-compulsive spectrum disorders (OCSDs). This diagnostic category also includes body dysmorphic disorder, hoarding disorder, trichotillomania (hair-pulling), and excoriation (skin-picking) disorder [5]. This change in categorization resulted from the body of evidence from genetic studies, neurological studies, and treatment outcome research that suggested nosological associations among those disorders. Thus, obsessive-compulsive disorder (OCD) is not currently categorized as an anxiety disorder in the DSM-5 [5]. Although OCD

N. K. Okereke (✉)
Greater Metro NYC Psychiatric, White Plains, NY, USA

V. Chan, J. Derenne (eds.), *Transition-Age Youth Mental Health Care*,
https://doi.org/10.1007/978-3-030-62113-1_9

spectrum disorders are related to one another in terms of their range of diagnostically validated risk, it is noted that there are close relationships between them and the anxiety disorders [5].

Obsessive-compulsive disorder (OCD) is characterized by the presence of obsessive thoughts and/or compulsions. It is common, emerges early in life (most cases arise before age 18 years), and tends to run a chronic, impairing course. OCD in children shows high rates of persistence despite treatment. Reasons for the chronic, impairing course of OCD are varied, but include overall earlier age of onset and longer duration of untreated illness. The duration of untreated illness is attributed to various individual reasons such as shame and secretiveness [6], as well as family factors such as parental anxiety or psychopathology leading to limited insight into need for treatment. Environmental and psychosocial factors such as limited availability of appropriate treatment may also play a role [7]. An early onset of illness and subsequent lag in initial OCD treatment is associated with poor outcomes. In addition, the duration of untreated illness for OCD can be up to 10 years in adults [7]. This is one of the highest for any serious mental disorder with the availability of effective treatments. Delays in treatment are associated with considerable suffering for the individual and the family [8], and various studies have documented a negative impact on clinical outcomes [6]. A longer duration of untreated OCD is associated with increased clinical comorbidity and functional disability, as well as significantly poor treatment-related clinical outcomes including treatment response and remission [7]. With regard to neurobiology, children and adolescents with OCD have similar altered functional activations in brain regions with affective and cognitive cortico-striatal thalamic circuits as compared to adult OCD patients [9]. This suggests that OCD is underpinned by complex, nonlinear neurodevelopmental mechanisms [10, 11].

Table 9.1 compares and contrasts the symptoms of obsessions versus compulsions.

Table 9.1 Obsessions vs. compulsions

Obsessions	Compulsions
Recurrent and persistent *thoughts, urges, or images* that are experienced as *intrusive and unwanted*	Repetitive *behaviors or mental acts* that a person feels ***driven to perform in response to an obsession*** *or according to rules that must be rigidly applied*
Not pleasurable	Not pleasurable, although many experience relief from anxiety or distress after completion
Not experienced voluntarily	Aim is to reduce distress triggered by obsessions or to prevent a third event from occurring
Cause marked distress or anxiety in most individuals	

[a](American Psychiatric Assn, DSM5) [5]

Individuals with body dysmorphic disorder (BDD) become preoccupied with perceived bodily flaws and become convinced that other people are focused on these flaws. Preoccupations are unwanted and time-consuming and lead to various feelings of shame and overly critical self-evaluation which, in turn, leads to distress or impairment in functioning [5, 12]. In one study of adolescents with BDD, 18% of students with BDD dropped out of school entirely due to severe BDD symptoms that interfered with their ability to maintain certain academic standards [12]. In hoarding disorder, affected people have such difficulty parting with possessions that they accumulate and clutter living areas to the point of compromising their activities of daily life [5].

Hoarding often begins before adulthood, but hoarding symptoms are more often mild during childhood and adolescence [13]. This may be because parents can prevent clutter and children do not have the same financial means as adults to acquire items [14, 15]. Trichotillomania is characterized by recurrent pulling out of one's hair at various body sites leading to alopecia. It is also associated with marked distress and functional impairment [5, 16]. If hair is swallowed (a phenomenon called trichophagia), there can be a resultant formation of gastrointestinal hair balls, which are called trichobezoars [16]. Excoriation disorder, or skin picking, is a type of body-focused repetitive behavior that is similar to trichotillomania, in which individuals engage in repetitive, habitual, picking at the skin [5, 17].

Symptoms of OCRDs can worsen during times of stress. Life transitions, such as, from high school to college or from high school to employment, are common times for symptom exacerbation. Novel environments with new people may trigger new worries about how one is being perceived by others. There may be an increase in appearance-related preoccupations and an increase in related repetitive behaviors, rituals, or mental acts aimed at neutralizing these preoccupations. TAY experience increasing independence, assuming new responsibilities upon attaining the age of legal adulthood, adjusting to new physical environments, and navigating academic and learning pressures. These TAY also often have suboptimal physical health habits that can impact their psychiatric symptoms, such as poor nutrition, lack of sleep and exercise, increased use of caffeine and tobacco, and abuse of substances, such as alcohol and illicit drugs [1].

Epidemiology

Historically, likely due to underreporting, many held the erroneous assumption that OCD is rare. It is now more commonly recognized that OCD is, in fact, the fourth most common mental disorder following substance abuse, phobias, and major depression [18]. The 12-month prevalence of OCD in the United States (US) is 1.2%, with a similar prevalence internationally (1.1% to 1.8%). Females are affected at a slightly higher rate in males in adulthood, although males are more commonly affected in childhood [5]. OCD has an estimated lifetime prevalence of 2 to 3% under DSM-III, DSM-III-R, and DSM-5 criteria [18–20]. The most common age of onset of OCD was historically reported to occur around 20–30 years of age. However, there appears to be two peaks of incidence, one with a pre-adolescent onset (mean age 11 years) and another in adulthood (mean age 23 years) [21].

Whereas OCD is overrepresented in females in community studies, males with OCD are overrepresented in those with early onset of the illness. Early-onset OCD is associated with a number of distinguishing features, of relevance for clinical intervention, including comorbidity with neurodevelopmental disorders, such as tic disorder and attention-deficit/hyperactivity disorder and familial clustering which suggests a greater genetic contribution in early-onset OCD (see Fig. 9.1) [21]. There is also a specific gene variant that supports this notion [22, 23].

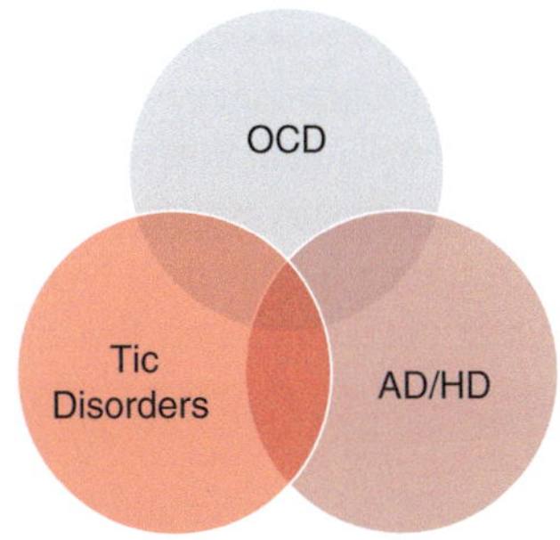

Fig. 9.1 Comorbid disorders associated with early-onset OCD

For 80% of people with OCD, other symptoms began in childhood, with the first peak of onset being reported around age 11 years [21, 24]. Early life factors including physical abuse, negative emotionality, prenatal insults, poor motor development, and personality or conduct problems have been reported to predict the incidence of OCD [25]. The 12-month prevalence of OCD and related disorders among adults in the United States is 1.2% [19]. Although it is also important to note that many people with OCD may have a positive, loving upbringing, the presence of such early life factors has made the study of childhood environmental factors a potential target area of investigation. As noted with other adult studies, many patients with this disorder do not seek treatment and do not confide in others about their symptoms due to high levels of associated shame.

The point prevalence of body dysmorphic disorder (BDD) in the United States among adults is 2.4%, with a slightly higher female prevalence. There are notable higher prevalence rates of BDD among dermatology and cosmetic surgery patients. The mean age of onset for BDD is 16–17 years, most commonly starting age 12–13 years, with two-thirds having an onset of

BDD prior to age 18 years old [5, 26]. Hoarding disorder has a point prevalence of about 2–6% of individuals in the United States and in Europe based on community surveys [5, 27]. However, it should note that the prevalence of hoarding disorder in youth is not known and that lack of data could be due hoarding disorder's relatively new recognition as a DSM disorder and to difficulty in ascertaining its presence in youth due to parental compensatory behaviors which may contain hoarding symptoms in children and adolescents [27, 14]. The 12-month prevalence for trichotillomania in adults and adolescents is 1–2%, with females being more frequently affected than males at about a 10:1 ratio [28]. The lifetime prevalence of excoriation disorder in adults in the general population is about 1.4%, with female to male gender ratio of about 3:1 [17].

Sulkowski et al. [29] conducted a recent epidemiological study of obsessive-compulsive spectrum disorder symptoms in college students. In this study, about 358 undergraduate students were given the obsessive-compulsive inventory questionnaire revised version (OCI-R), and about 5% scored 27 or above, which is usually clinically significant. Other similar research suggests that about 6% of college students may have pathological skin picking, 3% may have trichotillomania, 5% may have body dysmorphic disorder, 5% may have obsessive-compulsive disorder, and 7% may have elevated health anxiety symptoms [29].

OCD occurs across the world. There are no differences in rates of OCD related to race, socioeconomic status, marital status, intelligence, or educational level which is based on data from large epidemiological studies in the United States, Canada, Puerto Rico, Germany, Taiwan, Korea, and New Zealand, as well as the Epidemiological Catchment Area study from five US communities [18, 19, 30]. However, there may be disparities with regard to access to treatment and involvement of minority group members as subjects in OCD research. For example, epidemiological studies have shown that the number of African Americans who are suffering with OCD is the same as in the overall US population, but African Americans have been less likely to receive treatment. Among those who did receive treatment, few received specialized treatment, and only 20% were using an SRI medication [31]. Under-represented minorities are not fully represented in research studies on OCD as compared to their corresponding percentage numbers in the overall US population [32–34]. This may be, in part, due to barriers in providing culturally sensitive research recruitment efforts and a lack of research clinicians who are members of the target research communities [35].

There are also a variety of reports on body dysmorphic disorder (BDD) from different parts of the world, including Germany, South America, Turkey, Africa, and the Indian subcontinent which suggests that BDD contains similar clinical features [36]. Similarly, the clinical characteristics of skin picking disorder are the same across many cultures—in various international countries throughout the world [17].

Course of Illness

In the United States, the mean age of onset of OCD is 19.5 years, and 25% of cases develop by age 14 years. Onset after 35 years is unusual but does occur. Males have an earlier age of onset than females; nearly 25% of males of onset before age 10 years. The onset of symptoms is typically gradual. Without treatment, remission rates in adults are low (about 20% for those reevaluated 40 years later). Onset in childhood or adolescence can lead to a lifetime of OCD symptoms. However, 40% of individuals with onset of OCD in childhood or adolescence may experience remission by early adulthood without treatment [5].

Assessment

The assessment and diagnosis of OCD and related disorders in TAY, as with any adult, is approached in a multimodal fashion including clinical and diagnostic interviews with the patient and relevant informants (including family members, if possible) and review of collateral information. Symptoms described in the DSM-5 criteria should be explored completely. The clinical interview may also identify internal and external symptom triggers which would be essential for the development and implementation of a treatment plan. Internal triggers, such as thoughts or images, can evoke obsessions or rituals. External triggers are environmental situations that may lead to intrusive thoughts or behaviors and may be easier for patients to identify. Given the secretiveness and shame that can be associated with OCD symptoms, the clinician needs to ask about symptoms in a neutral, non-judgmental, and non-shaming manner. There are a number of areas in which people tend to experience OCD symptoms, and these should be explored in detail. These include those of cleaning (contamination obsessions and cleaning compulsions); symmetry (symmetry obsessions and repeating, ordering, and counting compulsions); and forbidden or taboo thoughts (e.g., aggressive, sexual, and religious obsessions and compulsions) [5]. Assessing avoidance behaviors is essential in providing a clear picture of compulsive behavior. Involving family members may be helpful, especially as parents or other family members may have been accommodating or providing reassurance. Active reassurance seeking behavior is truly itself a compulsion and should be interpreted and treated as such. Family members and others involved in the patient's avoidance behaviors can help with this [37].

Interviewing and eliciting information from transitional age youth (TAY) patients can differ somewhat from doing so with adults. For example, the elicited chief complaint for TAY patients may be filled with general statements such as "feeling stressed" or "having relationship problems." These complaints are general and often imply underlying anxiety or depression. Often collateral informants (e.g., parents, college instructors, etc.) can assist with the assessment of symptoms, with the provision of informed consent by the patient to obtain this information. It is important to also complete a safety assessment and to inquire about aggressive behavior. As previously mentioned, suicidal behavior has been reported in all the OCRDs [5]. Although assaultive urges in OCD patients are usually part of their obsessional thinking and expressed inwardly, anger and rage expressed externally to others have been reported in OCD patients [38].

A complete standard medical and psychiatric assessment is essential for identifying comorbid conditions and excluding other possibilities of the differential diagnoses, including tics, psychosis, or eating disorders. Medical assessments should be considered for the individual patient symptoms that are elicited. For example, in trichotillomania, stomach pains and various gastrointestinal complaints may lead one to consider hair-pulling with trichophagia. Thus, an appropriate physical exam and possibly GI studies may be warranted [16]. If obsessive-compulsive symptoms developed abruptly in the setting of an illness, further work-up to rule out pediatric autoimmune neuropsychiatric syndrome (PANS) should be considered.

Rating Scales and Structured Interviews

Rating scales can be used to aid in making a diagnosis and to follow progress through treatment. Rating the baseline severity of OCD symptoms and co-occurring conditions is recommended to assess the patient's functioning. If a rating scale is not used for diagnostic purposes, it is helpful to document the patient's estimate of the number of hours per day spent obsessing and performing compulsive behaviors, as well as the degree of effort needed to resist the behaviors [3].

The Yale-Brown Obsessive-Compulsive Scale (Y-BOCS) is a symptom checklist that provides an efficient structure for gathering information about obsessive-compulsive disorder [39]. This checklist covers the various areas of obsessions and compulsions. The Y-BOCS can be used as a diagnostic tool for OCD indicating a continuum of impairment from within normal limits to impaired or severe based on the total score [40, 41]. There is also a computerized version available with good correlation with a clinically administered version, making the task of repeated measures of treatment effectiveness more convenient [42].

The Obsessive-Compulsive Inventory-Revised (OCI-R) is a self-report measure that uses a Likert scale that provides both scores on subscales of OCD symptoms and also a score on total OCD symptoms. It has been shown to have good internal consistency, convergent validity, and test-retest reliability [43] and has been similarly validated and found reliable in nonclinical college samples [44]. It has been translated into many non-English languages. It is relatively brief, as it only has 18 items. It can be used as an efficient screening tool, while it still assesses a broad range of symptoms that are most common in patients with OCD.

The Anxiety Disorders Interview Schedule-R (ADIS-R) is a semi-structured diagnostic interview which requires the diagnostician to make a severity rating for each diagnosis given. The severity rating is made on a 0 through 8 scale and indicates a level of distress and/or functional impairment associated with a diagnosis in the diagnostician's judgment. It has been found reliable and has been validated in previous studies [45].

Treatment Considerations in TAY

After reaching the age of maturity, many TAY with pre-existing OCD and related disorders must now make the transition from pediatric to adult care settings. It can be helpful for TAY who are college students to establish medical and psychiatric care with their campus student counseling center and/or student health center prior to their college enrollment and on-campus orientation [46]. In those settings without on-campus access to subspecialty care, families may need to make appointments with psychiatrists and psychotherapists in their surrounding area. Bringing copies of past treatment records and any past psychological testing or evidence of past school accommodations can also be helpful to secure needed services. On-campus and local community support groups can be helpful for college students with OCD and related disorders, but they should not replace evidence-based psychotherapy [47].

Parental involvement can be helpful, but TAY must consent to have their parents involved in treatment. Also, parental mental health may play a factor, as many TAY with OCD and related disorders also have family histories of OCD or other mental health issues that may make it harder for their parents to support their children. For TAY who are enrolled in college, increased unstructured time in college can worsen their psychiatric symptoms. Many find psychotherapy helpful in learning coping skills, including the ability to relinquish the need for tight control over their life circumstances and learn the value of "letting go and embracing uncertainty" [48].

As with all patients with OCD and related disorders, establishing the goals for treatment of those disorders in TAY should include decreasing symptom frequency and severity, improving the patient's functioning, and helping the patient to improve his or her quality of life [49]. The appropriate treatment setting typically is usually an outpatient level of care although symptom severity may dictate the need for a higher level of care [3].

College accessibility (or disability services) offices may be able to help students access classroom and campus accommodations. These services typically require records that document past psychiatric diagnosis and treatment or past secondary school accommodations for support at the collegiate level. Title II of the American with Disabilities Act (ADA) and Section 504 of the Rehabilitation Act of 1973 both enable college students to access reasonable accommodations for OCD and related disorders at college. These laws also protect students from any discrimination on the basis of any disability (i.e., the student's psychiatric disorder). Some students find it helpful to be open with their college professors or their college Dean's office about their condition in an aim to obtain more support, but disclosure of one's psychiatric diagnosis and treatment is not required. One's health information is protected from disclosure to others without express, written consent from the college student as by federal and state law, with certain exceptions [50]. For college students without a prior diagnosis who are experiencing symptoms of OCD or related disorders, getting an evaluation through their college's student counseling center or college student health center is important.

In addition, some TAY, including college students, do not have health insurance and the costs of an evaluation and any recommended psychotherapy and medications for OCD and related disorders may be prohibitive for them. The Partnership for Prescription Assistance (www.pparx.org) or NeedyMeds (www.needymeds.org) are two programs that may be of financial assistance for TAY who cannot afford to pay for prescription their psychiatric medications (see resources).

Evidence-based Treatment of OCD

Cognitive behavioral therapy (CBT) and selective serotonin reuptake inhibitors (SSRIs) are recommended as safe and effective first-line treatments for OCD. Whether to utilize CBT, an SSRI, or combined treatment will depend on many factors. These include the nature and severity of the patient's symptoms, any co-occurring psychiatric and medical conditions and their treatments, and the patient's past treatment history. Additional considerations include the availability of CBT, current medications, and the patient's treatment preferences [3].

Psychotherapy

Cognitive behavioral therapy alone is recommended as an initial treatment for OCD [51]. It may be best suited for a patient who is not too depressed, anxious, or severely ill to cooperate with this treatment modality or who prefers not to take medications and is willing to do the work that CBT requires [3]. Exposure and response prevention (ERP) is an effective behavioral therapy for patients with obsessive-compulsive disorder [51]. In exposure, the patient is asked to confront the feared situation or thought. In response prevention, the patient is asked to delay or prevent the compulsion that assuages that feared situation or thought. There is consensus agreement that exposure and response prevention is considered a first-line treatment for obsessive-compulsive disorder [52].

Conducting psychotherapy for transitional age youth and college students with OCD using CBT with an exposure-based therapy involves using a Subjective Units of Distress Scale (SUDS) to make a hierarchy of intensity of their OCD symptoms to address in therapy. SUDS is based on each individual OCD symptom's subjective distress, as rated by the patient. Some psychotherapists have more recently favored simultaneously conducting CBT with exposure-based therapy for OCD from an Acceptance and Commitment Therapy (ACT) framework, using value-based exposure exercises and using a Willingness Scale instead of a traditional SUD scale [53]. This is thought to emphasize willingness, or acceptance, toward uncomfortable OCD thoughts and feelings rather than emphasize the more traditional reduction in discomfort, or habituation [53, 54].

Habit reversal training (HRT) is a behavioral therapy that has, for decades, been used for the treatment of nervous habits like skin-picking, hair-pulling, and tics. Habit reversal therapy consists of several components, including awareness training with self-monitoring, relaxation training, and competing response training [55]. Awareness training and competing response training are widely accepted to be the two key components of this intervention [56].

Psychopharmacology: First Line

The medications mostly commonly used in the treatment of OCD include tricyclic antidepressants (TCAs), selective serotonin reuptake inhibitors (SSRIs), and selective serotonin-norepinephrine reuptake inhibitors (SNRIs). Other medications and augmentation strategies are sometimes implemented, as warranted. Clinicians using medication treatments must be aware of possible medication side effects and must discuss these with the patient prior to and throughout treatment. Only antidepressants that potently inhibit presynaptic reuptake of serotonin appear to be effective in treating obsessive-compulsive disorder (OCD). Clomipramine (Anafranil) is the only tricyclic antidepressant (TCA) with this property [36, 57, 58].

Tricyclic Antidepressants (TCAs) Clomipramine is FDA approved to treat in OCD. It is a dibenzazepine compound that inhibits the membrane pump mechanism responsible for uptake of norepinephrine and serotonin in adrenergic and serotonergic neurons. Clomipramine affects serotonin uptake, and it affects norepinephrine uptake when converted into its metabolite desmethylclomipramine [57].

Selective Serotonin Reuptake Inhibitors (SSRIs) These medications selectively inhibit the reuptake of serotonin at the presynaptic region of the neural membrane. SSRIs have the advantages of ease of dosing and low toxicity in overdose. Available SSRIs include fluoxetine (Prozac), fluvoxamine (Luvox), paroxetine (Paxil), citalopram (Celexa), escitalopram (Lexapro), and sertraline (Zoloft). Only fluoxetine, fluvoxamine, and sertraline are FDA approved for the treatment of OCD [59].

SSRIs or clomipramine should be advanced as tolerated to a therapeutic dose. Clinical response may take 6–10 weeks to become apparent. The clinician should review adequacy of dose, duration of therapy, and compliance before deciding that a medication is ineffective. The SSRIs are generally preferred over clomipramine in treating OCD. The adverse effect profiles of SSRIs are less prominent, so improved compliance is promoted. SSRIs do not have the cardiac arrhythmia risk associated with TCAs; however, citalopram causes dose-dependent QT prolongation [60, 61]. Arrhythmia risk is especially pertinent in overdose, and suicide risk must always be considered when treating youth or a young adult up to age 25 years with a mood disorder.

Serotonin-Norepinephrine Reuptake Inhibitors (SNRIs) The dual serotonin-norepinephrine reuptake inhibitors (SNRIs) venlafaxine (Effexor) and duloxetine (Cymbalta) may also have efficacy in OCD, and they have safety and tolerability profiles comparable to those of the SSRIs. However, neither medication has yet been FDA approved specifically for the treatment of OCD.

The FDA issued a public health advisory in October of 2004 [62] mandating a black box warning for antidepressants. Antidepressant treatment of children and adolescents with depression then significantly decreased over the next 2 years, although apparently so did suicides for this population. In 2007, the FDA extended its warning to young adults up to age 24 years [63].

Currently, evidence does not exist to associate an increased risk of suicide in patients with OCD and/or other anxiety disorders being treated with SSRIs. However, physicians should closely attend to whether treated patients have unusual, uncomfortable adverse reactions (e.g., akathisia) or if they might have comorbid bipolar disorder and may have related kindling effects from the SSRI medication [57]. Caution may also be considered with use of SSRI medications for OCD in patients with comorbid major depressive disorder (MDD). The increased risk of suicidality in adolescents with MDD treated with antidepressants, compared to adults, is small, but consistent across most studies, although epidemiological studies do not support a clear relationship between use of antidepressants and the completed suicide rate [64, 65]. Close monitoring is needed, and adequate follow-up care should be provided for patients after initiation of a new antidepressant [64].

The starting dose recommended for pharmacological treatment is that which is recommended by the medication manufacturer. For patients who are worried about medication side effects, one may consider starting at a much lower dose. Most patients will not experience substantial improvement until 4–6 weeks after starting medication, and some who will ultimately significantly respond may experience little improvement for as many as 10–12 weeks. Medication doses may be titrated up weekly in increments recommended by the manufacturer during the first month of treatment. When little or no symptom improvement is seen within 4 weeks of starting medication, the dose may be increased weekly or biweekly to the maximum dose comfortably tolerated and indicated. The treatment trial is to be continued at the dosage for at least 6 weeks [3].

Successful medication treatment should be continued for 1–2 years before considering a gradual taper by decrements of 10–25% every 1–2 months while observing for symptom return or exacerbation. In medication discontinuation trials, risks of relapse for medication trial discontinuation for insufficient, but partial, clinical response are substantial, but vary widely because of major demographic differences across studies. Thus, discontinuation of pharmacotherapy should be carefully considered, and for most patients, some form of continued treatment is recommended. Uncontrolled follow-up studies of OCD treatment trials suggest that CBT may delay or mitigate the risk of relapse when SSRI treatment is discontinued [3].

Psychopharmacology-Augmentation Strategies

Antipsychotics Medications such as haloperidol, olanzapine, and risperidone have been used with some success in augmenting SSRIs in patients with OCD, particularly in patients with comorbid Tourette disorder or other tic disorders [66]. A Cochrane review found some evidence of efficacy for quetiapine or risperidone as a general augmentation strategy (not specifically for those with comorbid tics) [67]. However, heterogeneity was noted in doses used and in response, and the number of subjects in these studies was generally small. Antipsychotic agents are not FDA approved for the treatment of OCD but may be beneficial.

Antianxiety Agents Augmentation with antianxiety agents such as buspirone may be beneficial in patients with OCD. Buspirone is a 5-HT1 agonist with serotonergic neurotransmission and some dopaminergic effects in the CNS. Buspirone is not FDA approved for the treatment of OCD [57].

Lithium While lithium is indicated for bipolar disorder, it also influences the reuptake of serotonin and/or norepinephrine at cell membranes. It has been used in the treatment of OCD; however, it is not FDA approved for this indication [57].

Methylphenidate In one recent study, combined treatment with methylphenidate ER demonstrated an enhanced clinical rate of response compared to placebo when given with SSRI treatment with fluvoxamine in treatment-refractory OCD [68].

D-Cycloserine This may be a promising CBT augmentation strategy, but only in antidepressant-free patients with OCD. Research findings suggest that antidepressants may interact with DCS to block its facilitating effect on fear extinction [69].

Combined Psychotherapy and Psychopharmacology

Combined treatment should be considered for (a) patients with an unsatisfactory response to monotherapy; (b) those with co-occurring psychiatric conditions (e.g., major depressive or anxiety disorders) for which treatment with traditional medications, such as SSRIs, has been shown to be effective; and (c) those who wish to limit the duration of SSRI treatment by attempting to get a quick treatment response first with a medication and then continue treatment later on with psychotherapy alone [3]. Combined treatment has historically been considered in patients with severe OCD symptoms, especially since medication treatment may diminish their OCD symptom severity sufficiently to allow the patient to engage in psychotherapy with CBT [3]. However, recent evidence has questioned the added value of pharmacological interventions to psychotherapy [70].

Despite the availability of effective treatments for OCD, the treatment gap (the difference between individuals with OCD needing treatment and those actually receiving treatment) was estimated, in Europe, to stand at 25% of cases in 2004 [71]. The proportion of subjects not being treated worldwide in more recent epidemiological studies was estimated to vary between 22% and up to 92%, with 30 to 90% of individuals not even seeking treatment or advice [72].

Recovery can be a realistic goal for subgroups of the OCD population, but the real-world clinical outcomes are often disappointing.

Relapse rates are high; fewer than 40% of treatment seeking adults with OCD are reported to achieve a sustained remission when followed in long-term follow-up studies. The median duration of OCD symptoms was 16 years in one study [73]. Roughly one-third of OCD cases did not remit, and a poor prognosis for remission was seen in those with more severe or longer duration of illness and psychiatric comorbidity, although seeking professional help [8, 74]. Even with the best available treatments, about 10% of patients remain severely affected and experience treatment refractory OCD [75].

Treatment-Resistant OCD

Short-Term Residential Treatment A higher level of care is considered when someone is not able to make any significant gains in an outpatient setting. Patients may have a decrease in their basic functioning such that they are unable to meet basic needs like activities of daily living, nutrition, or hydration. They may struggle with taking medication or completing the recommended outpatient behavioral therapy/ERP homework. Patients who live in underserved areas may be unable to access specialized OCD treatment. Still others may wish to work more intensively on ameliorating their OCD symptoms even after they have made some gains in treatment in an outpatient setting [76].

Osgood-Hynes et al. [76] studied short-term residential treatment in three different residential treatment programs for OCD across the United States (McLean Hospital, Rogers Memorial Hospital, and Menninger Clinic). All three programs used an approach based on ERP CBT and medication to reduce OCD symptoms. However, in contrast to more traditional once a week outpatient management, all the residential programs studied offered more structured opportunities for repeat and prolonged ERP sessions in order to increase the probability of anxiety habituation. The average length of stay across the programs was between 1.5 and 2 months. Sometimes the duration of treatment was longer for adolescents. In addition to reducing OCD symptoms, all three residential programs emphasized the importance of discharge planning and follow-up for each patient [76].

Transcranial Direct Current Stimulation tDCS is a noninvasive neuromodulation technique which delivers low amplitude direct currents to the brain between two large surface electrodes (anode and cathode) positioned on distinct areas of the scalp with a rubber headband which reportedly causes cortical excitability in relevant brain areas postulated to treat OCD symptoms [77, 78]. This technique may be efficacious in the treatment of OCD, but future studies need to be conducted to further elucidate its utility and role in treatment-resistant OCD [78].

Deep Brain Stimulation DBS is a treatment involving implantation of electrodes, which send electrical impulses to specific brain locations with the aim of attenuating altered activity in affected circuits. Stimulation targets for DBS in patients with OCD include the ventral anterior limb of the internal capsule, ventral striatum, subthalamic nucleus, and nucleus accumbens [79]. Despite the overall efficacy and tolerability of DBS and its potential to improve the lives of many patients with refractory OCD, the evidence for the effectiveness and deep of DBS and OCD patient remains limited due to the small total number of OCD patients who have been treated with DBS worldwide (probably not exceeding 250 total patients) [79].

Treatment of OCD-Related Disorders

Body Dysmorphic Disorder

The treatments of choice in BDD are cognitive behavioral therapy (CBT), the selective serotonin reuptake inhibitor (SSRI) medications, and clomipramine, which is a potent selective serotonin reuptake inhibitor (SRI) [36, 51, 80]. The evidence for the use of SSRIs and clomipramine in BDD is based on three randomized controlled trials [81–83].

Hoarding Disorder

Hoarding disorder is treated primarily with psychotherapy, mainly cognitive behavioral therapy [84]. A theory of the development of hoarding disorder posits that early experiences and cognitive challenges in affected individuals result in mistaken beliefs about and attachments to possessions, with resulting negative emotions that lead to difficulty with letting go of items due to avoidance behavior and subsequent accumulation of clutter [85]. The elements of mental health treatment for hoarding are based on the theoretical model for this multidimensional problem. The protocol uses a manualized cognitive behavioral therapy (CBT) approach that incorporates assessment and goal setting, organizing and problem-solving skills training, exposure practice methods to reduce acquiring and remove clutter, and motivational interviewing to address patient resistance when it arises during treatment [85–87].

Trichotillomania

There is a small evidence base for psychotherapy for trichotillomania, and it suggests that behavioral therapy is the most promising. Habit reversal therapy is the most commonly used treatment, but acceptance and commitment therapy and dialectical-behavioral therapy have also been explored [16]. Although no pharmacotherapies are considered first-line treatments [16], there is recent evidence to support efficacy for the treatment of trichotillomania with clomipramine, olanzapine, and N-acetylcysteine [88]. N-Acetylcysteine in one study was given successfully at a dose of 1200 mg twice a day, taking about 9 weeks to work [89].

Excoriation Disorder

Treatment options for excoriation disorder are largely focused on cognitive behavioral therapy, with evidence for habit reversal or acceptance-enhanced behavioral therapy. Psychopharmacological treatments are largely focused on SSRI medications, naltrexone, and N-acetylcysteine [17].

Summary

Obsessive-compulsive and related disorders are common and life-impairing in transitional age youth (TAY). Obsessive-compulsive disorder (OCD), in particular, is common, has a chronic course, and tends to emerge early in life. Symptoms of these disorders can worsen in transitional age youth (TAY) as they begin to take on newfound independence, responsibilities, surroundings, and circumstances. Knowledge of evidence-based diagnosis, assessment, and treatment of OCD and related disorders in TAY is useful to provide symptom stabilization in these young adult patients and to avoid many of the common pitfalls of managing these disorders in this age group.

Resources for OCD and Related Disorders in TAY

- Mental Health America
  - http://www.mentalhealthamerica.net/conditions/ocd
- National Alliance on Mental Illness
  - https://www.nami.org/Learn-More/Mental-Health-Conditions/Obsessive-Compulsive-Disorder
- International OCD foundation
  - https://iocdf.org
- Paying for treatment
  - Partnership for Prescription Assistance www.pparx.org
  - NeedyMeds www.needymeds.org

References

1. Huang J, Nigatu YT, Smail-Crevier R, Zhang X, Wang J. Interventions for common mental health problems among university and college students: a systematic review and meta-analysis of randomized controlled trials. J Psychiatr Res. 2018;107:1–10.

2. Cuijpers P, Cristea IA, Ebert DD, Koot HM, Auerbach RP, Bruffaerts R, Kessler KC. Psychological treatment of depression in college students: a meta-analysis. Depress Anxiety. 2016;33(5):400–14.
3. American Psychiatric Association. Practice guidelines for the treatment of patients with obsessive-compulsive disorder, American Psychiatric Association; 2010.
4. American Psychiatric Association. Diagnostic and Statistical Manual of Mental Disorders. 4th Edition, Text Revision (DSM-IV-TR). Washington, DC: American Psychiatric Association; 2000.
5. American Psychiatric Association. Diagnostic and statistical manual of mental disorders, 5th edition (DSM-5). Arlington: American Psychiatric Association; 2013.
6. Fineberg NA, Dell'Osso B, Albert U, Maina G, Geller D, Carmi L, Sireau N, Walitza S, Grassi G, Pallanti S, Hollander E, Brakoulias V, Menchon JM, Marazziti D, Ioannidis K, Apergis-Schoute A, Stein DJ, Cath DC, Veltman DJ, Van Ameringen M, Fontenelle LF, Shavitt RG, Costa D, Diniz JB, Zohar J. Early intervention for obsessive-compulsive disorder: an expert consensus statement. Eur Neuropsychopharmacol. 2019;29:549–65.
7. Altamura AC, Buoli M, Albano A, Dell'Osso B. Age at onset and latency to treatment (duration of untreated illness) in patients with mood and anxiety disorders: a naturalistic study. Int Clin Psychopharmacol. 2010;25:172–9.
8. Fineberg NA, Hengartner MP, Bergbaum CE, Gale T, Rossler W, Angst J. A prospective population-based cohort study of the prevalence, incidence and impact of obsessive-compulsive symptomatology. Int J Psychiatry Clin Pract. 2013a;17(3):170–8.
9. Brem S, Hauser TU, Iannaccone R, Brandeis D, Drechsler R, Walitza S. Neuroimaging of cognitive brain function in paediatric obsessive compulsive disorder: a review of literature and preliminary meta-analysis. J Neural Transm (Vienna). 2012;119:1425–48.
10. Boedhoe PSW, Schmaal L, Abe Y, Alonso P, Ameis SH, Anticevic A, Arnold PD, Batistuzzo MC, Benedetti F, Beucke JC, Bollettini I, Bose A, Brem S, Calvo A, Calvo R, Cheng Y, Cho KIK, Ciullo V, Dallaspezia S, Denys D, Feusner JD, Fitzgerald KD, Fouche JP, Fridgeirsson EA, Gruner P, Hanna GL, Hibar DP, Hoexter MQ, Hu H, Huyser C, Jahanshad N, James A, Kathmann N, Kaufmann C, Koch K, Kwon JS, Lazaro L, Lochner C, Marsh R, Martínez-Zalacaín I, Mataix-Cols D, Menchón JM, Minuzzi L, Morer A, Nakamae T, Nakao T, Narayanaswamy JC, Nishida S, Nurmi E, O'Neill J, Piacentini J, Piras F, Reddy YCJ, Reess TJ, Sakai Y, Sato JR, Simpson HB, Soreni N, Soriano-Mas C, Spalletta G, Stevens MC, Szeszko PR, Tolin DF, van Wingen GA, Venkatasubramanian G, Walitza S, Wang Z, Yun JY, Thompson PM, Stein DJ, van den Heuvel OA. Cortical abnormalities associated with pediatric and adult obsessive-compulsive disorder: findings from the enigma obsessive-compulsive disorder working group. Am J Psychiatr. 2018;175:453–62.
11. Boedhoe PSW, Schmaal L, Abe Y, Ameis SH, Arnold PD, Batistuzzo MC, Benedetti F, Beucke JC, Bollettini I, Bose A, Brem S, Calvo A, Calvo R, Cheng Y, Cho KIK, Dallaspezia S, Denys D, Fitzgerald KD, Fouche JP, Giménez M, Gruner P, Hanna GL, Hibar DP, Hoexter MQ, Hu H, Huyser C, Ikari K, Jahanshad N, Kathmann N, Kaufmann C, Koch K, Kwon JS, Lazaro L, Lochner C, Marsh R, Martínez-Zalacaín I, Mataix-Cols D, Menchón JM, Minuzzi L, Nakamae T, Nakao T, Narayanaswamy JC, Piras F, Pittenger C, Reddy YC, Sato JR, Simpson HB, Soreni N, Soriano-Mas C, Spalletta G, Stevens MC, Szeszko PR, Tolin DF, van Wingen GA, Venkatasubramanian G, Walitza S, Wang Z, Xu J, Xu X, Yun JY, Zhao Q, Thompson PM, Stein DJ, van den Heuvel OA. Distinct subcortical volume alterations in pediatric and adult OCD: a worldwide meta- and mega-analysis. Am J Psychiatr. 2017;174:60–9.
12. Phillips KA, Didie ER, Menard W, Pagano ME, Fay C, Weisberg RB. Clinical features of body dysmorphic disorder in adolescents and adults. Psychiatry Res. 2006;141:305–14.
13. Tolin DF, Meunier SA, Frost RO, Steketee G. Course of compulsive hoarding and its relationship to life events. Depress Anxiety. 2010;27(9):829–38.
14. Burton CL, Arnold PD, Soreni N. Three reasons why studying hoarding in children and adolescents is important. J Can Acad Child Adolesc Psychiatry. 2015;24(2):128–30.
15. Storch EA, Rahman O, Park JM, Reid J, Murphy TK, Lewin AB. Compulsive hoarding in children. J Clin Psychol. 2011;67(5):507–16.
16. Grant JE, Chamberlain SR. Treatment in psychiatry: trichotillomania. Am J Psychiatr. 2016;173(9):868–74.
17. Grant JE, Odlaug BL, Chamberlain SR, Keuthen NJ, Lochner C, Stein DJ. Skin picking disorder. Am J Psychiatr. 2012;169:1143–9.
18. Robins LN, Helzer JE, Weissman MM, Orvaschel H, Gruenberg E, Burke JD, Regier DA. Lifetime prevalence of specific psychiatric disorders in three sites. Arch Gen Psychiatry. 1984;41:949–58.
19. Ruscio AM, Stein DJ, Chiu WT, Kessler RC. The epidemiology of obsessive-compulsive disorder in the National Comorbidity Survey Replication. Mol Psychiatry. 2010;15:53–63.
20. Weissman MM, Bland RC, Canino GJ, Greenwald S, Hwu HG, Lee CK, Newman SC, Oakley-Browne MA, Rubio-Stipec M, Wickramaratne PJ. The cross-national epidemiology of obsessive-compulsive disorder. Cross National Collaborative Group. J Clin Psychiatry. 1994;55:5–10.
21. Taylor S. Early versus late onset obsessive-compulsive disorder: evidence for distinct subtypes. Clin Psychol Rev. 2011;31:1083–100.
22. Walitza S, Marinova Z, Grünblatt E, Lazic SE, Remschmidt H, Vloet TD, Wendland JR. Trio study and meta-analysis support the association of genetic

variation at the serotonin transporter with early-onset obsessive-compulsive disorder. Neurosci Lett. 2014;580:100–3.

23. Grünblatt E, Oneda B, Ekici AB, Ball J, Geissler J, Uebe S, Romanos M, Rauch A, Walitza S. High resolution chromosomal microarray analysis in paediatric obsessive-compulsive disorder. BMC Medicine Genom. 2017;10:68.
24. Goodman W, Rasmussen S, Leckman JF. A family study of obsessive-compulsive disorder. Am J Psychiatr. 1995;152:76–84.
25. Grisham JR, Fullana MA, Mataix-Cols D, Moffitt TE, Caspi A, Poulton R. Risk factors prospectively associated with adult obsessive-compulsive symptom dimensions and obsessive-compulsive disorder. Psychiatr Med. 2011;15:1–12.
26. Koran L, Abujaoude E, Large M, et al. The prevalence of body dysmorphic disorder in the US adult population. CNS Spectr. 2008;13:316–22.
27. Pertus A, Frost R, Fullana M, et al. Refining the diagnostic boundaries of compulsive hoarding. Clinical Psychological Reviews. 2010;30:371–86.
28. Stein D, Grant J, et al. Trichotillomania, skin picking disorder, and stereotypic movement disorder: toward DSM-V. Depression & Anxiety. 2010;27:611–26.
29. Sulkowski MI, Mariaskin A, Storch EA. Obsessive-compulsive spectrum disorder symptoms in college students. J Am Coll Health. 2011;59(5):342–8.
30. Karno M, Golding JM, Sorenson SB, Burnam MA. The epidemiology of obsessive-compulsive disorder in five US communities. Arch Gen Psychiatry. 1988;45:1094–9.
31. Himle JA, Muroff JR, Taylor RJ, Baser RE, Abelson JM, Hanna GL, Jackson JS. Obsessive-compulsive disorder among African Americans and blacks of Caribbean descent: results from the national survey of American life. Depress Anxiety. 2008;2(12):993–1005.
32. Williams MT, Domanico J, Marques L, Leblanc N, Turkheimer E. Barriers to treatment among African Americans with obsessive-compulsive disorder. J Anxiety Disord. 2012;26(4):555–63.
33. Wetterneck C, Little T, Rinehart K, Cervantes ME, Hyde E, Williams MT. Latinos with obsessive-compulsive disorder: mental healthcare utilization and inclusion in clinical trials. J Obsessive Compuls Relat Disord. 2012;1(2):85–97.
34. Williams MT, Powers M, Yun YG, Foa EB. Minority participation in randomized controlled trials for obsessive-compulsive disorder. J Anxiety Disord. 2010;24(2):171–7.
35. Williams MT, Tellawi G, Wetterneck CT, Chapman LK. Recruitment of ethnoracial minorities for mental health research. Behav Ther. 2013;36(6):151–6.
36. Singh AR, Veale D. Understanding and treating body dysmorphic disorder. Indian J Psychiatry. 2019;61(Suppl 1):S131–5.
37. Hallion LS, Sockol LE, Wilhelm S. Obsessive compulsive disorder. In: Stein DJ, Vythilingum B, editors. Anxiety disorders and gender. Cham: Springer International Publishing; 2015.
38. Whiteside SP, Abramowitz JS. The expression of anger and its relationship to symptoms and cognitions in obsessive-compulsive disorder. Depress Anxiety. 2005;21:106–11.
39. Goodman WK, Price LH, Rasmussen SA, Mazure C, Fleischmann RL, Hill CL, et al. The Yale-Brown obsessive compulsive scale. I. Development, use, and reliability. Arch Gen Psychiatry. 1989;46: 1006–11.
40. Demal U, Lenz G, Mayrhofer A, Zapotoczky HG, Zitterl W. Obsessive compulsive disorder and depression: a retrospective study on course and interaction. Psychopathology. 1993;26:145–50.
41. Kim SW, Dysken MW, Kuskowski M. The Yale-Brown obsessive-compulsive scale: a reliability and validity study. Psychiatry Res. 1990;34:96–106.
42. Rosenfeld R, Dar R, Anderson D, Kobak K, Greist J. A computer-administered version of the Yale-Brown obsessive-compulsive scale. Psychol Assess. 1992;4:329–32.
43. Foa EB, Huppert JD, Leiberg S, Langner R, Kichic R, Hajcak G, et al. The obsessive-compulsive inventory: development and validation of a short version. Psychol Assess. 2002;14:485–95.
44. Hajcak G, Huppert JD, Simons RF, Foa EB. Psychometric properties of the OCI-R in a college sample. Behav Res Ther. 2004;42:115–23.
45. DiNardo, et al. Reliability of DSM–III–R anxiety disorder categories: using the anxiety disorders interview schedule, revised (ADIS–R). Arch Gen Psychiatry. 1993;50:251–6.
46. Chan V, Rasminsky S, Viesselman JO. A primer for working in campus mental health: a system of care. Acad Psychiatry. 2015;39(5):533–40.
47. American Academy of Child & Adolescent Psychiatry. Starting College with a Psychiatric Illness. Facts for Families. 1994. https://www.aacap.org/AACAP/AACAP/Families_and_Youth/Facts_for_Families/FFF-Guide/Starting-College-with-a-Psychiatric-Illness-115.aspx. Accessed 2019.
48. Pasalowicz PR. Navigating college with OCD. International OCD Foundation. 2018. https://iocdf.org/blog/2018/11/26/navigating-college-with-ocd/. Accessed 2019.
49. Weiss Roberts L, editor. Student mental health: a guide for psychiatrists, psychologists, and leaders serving in higher education. Washington, DC: American Psychiatric Association Publishing; 2018.
50. Department of Justice, US, 1973. https://www.dol.gov/agencies/oasam/centers-offices/civil-rights-center/statutes/section-504-rehabilitation-act-of-1973. Accessed 2019.
51. National Institute for Health and Clinical Excellence (NICE). Obsessive-compulsive disorder: core interventions in the treatment of obsessive-compulsive disorder and body dysmorphic disorder: National Institute for Health and Clinical Excellence. London, England; 2005.

52. McKay D, Sookman D, Neziroglu F, Wilhelm S, Stein DJ, Kyrios M, Matthews K, Veale D. Efficacy of cognitive-behavioral therapy for obsessive-compulsive disorder. Psychiatry Res. 2015;225(3):236–46.
53. Twohig MP, Hayes SC, Plumb LD, Collins AB, Hazelett-Stevens H, Woindeck MR. A randomized clinical trial of acceptance and commitment therapy verses progressive relaxation training for obsessive-compulsive disorder. J Consult Clin Psychol. 2010;78:705–16.
54. Twohig MP, Abramowitz JS, Bluetta LE, Fabricant RJ, Morrision LR, Smith BM. Exposure therapy for OCD from an acceptance and commitment therapy (ACT) framework. J Obsessive Compuls Relat Disord. 2015;6:167–73.
55. Azrin NH, Peterson AL. Habit reversal for the treatment of Tourette syndrome. Behav Res Therapy. 1988;26:347–51.
56. Azrin NH, Nunn RG. Habit reversal: a method of eliminating nervous habits and tics. Behav Res Therapy. 1973;11:619–28.
57. Greenberg WM. Obsessive-compulsive disorder medication. Medscape article, May 17, 2018. Accessed: 2/26/2020.
58. Griest JH, Jefferson JW, Kobak KA, Katzelnick DJ, Serlin RC. Efficacy and tolerability of serotonin transport inhibitors in obsessive-compulsive disorder. A meta-analysis. Arch Gen Psychiatry. 1995;52(1):53–60.
59. Antidepressant medications: U.S. Food and Drug Administration-approved indications and dosages for use in pediatric patients. https://www.cms.gov/Medicare-Medicaid-Coordination/Fraud-Prevention/Medicaid-Integrity-Education/Pharmacy-Education-Materials/pharmacy-ed-materials.html. Accessed 7/2020.
60. Celexa (citalopram hydrobromide) [package insert]. St. Louis, Missouri: Forest Pharmaceuticals, Inc. August 2011.
61. US Food and Drug Administration (FDA). Celexa (citalopram hydrobromide): Drug safety communication – abnormal heart rhythms associated with high doses. Available at: http://www.fda.gov/Safety/MedWatch/SafetyInformation/SafetyAlertsforHumanMedicalProducts/ucm269481.htm. Accessed 2/26/2020.
62. FDA (2004). Public health advisory: suicidality in children and adolescents being treated with antidepressant medications. FDA Website. October 15, 2004, pp. 1–3.
63. FDA (2007). FDA proposes new warnings about suicidal thinking, behavior in young adults who take antidepressant medications. FDA Website. May 2, 2007, pp. 1–3.
64. Pompili M, Serafini G, Innamorati M, Ambrosi E, Giordano G, Girardi P, Tatarelli R, Lester D. Antidepressants and suicide risk: a comprehensive overview. Pharmaceuticals (Basel). 2010;3(9):2861–83.
65. Masi G, Liboni F, Brovedani P. Pharmacotherapy of major depressive disorder in adolescents. Expert Opin Pharmacother. 2010;11(3):375–86.
66. Bloch MH, Landeros-Weisenberger A, Kelmendi B, Coric V, Bracken MB, Leckman JF. A systematic review: antipsychotic augmentation with treatment refractory obsessive-compulsive disorder. Mol Psychiatry. 2006;11(7):622–32.
67. Komossa K, Depping AM, Meyer M, Kissling W, Leucht S. Second-generation antipsychotics for obsessive compulsive disorder. Cochrane Database Syst Rev. 2010. https://doi.org/10/1002/14651858.CD008141.pub2.
68. Zheng H, Jia F, Han H, Wang S, Guo G, Quan D, Li G, Huang H. Combined fluvoxamine and extended-release methylphenidate improved treatment response compared to fluvoxamine alone in patients with treatment-refractory obsessive-compulsive disorder: a randomized double-blind, placebo-controlled study. Eur Neuropsychopharmacol. 2019;29:397–404.
69. Andersson E, Hedman E, Enander J, Djurfeldt DR, Ljotsson B, Cervenka S, Isung J, Svanborg C, Matais-Cols D, Kaldo V, Andersson G, Lindefors N, Ruck C. D-Cycloserine vs placebo as adjunct to cognitive behavioral therapy for obsessive-compulsive disorder and interaction with antidepressants: a randomized clinical trial. JAMA Psychiat. 2015;72(7):659–67.
70. Torp NC, Dahl, Skarphedinsson G, Thomsen PH, Valderhaug R, Weidle B, et al. Effectiveness of cognitive behavior treatment for pediatric obsessive-compulsive disorder: acute outcomes from the Nordic long-term OCD treatment study (NordLOTS). Behav Res Therapy. 2015;64:15–23.
71. Kohn R, Saxena S, Levav I, Saraceno B. The treatment gap in mental health care. Bull World Health Organ. 2004;82:858–66.
72. García-Soriano G, Rufer M, Delsignore A, Weidt S. Factors associated with non-treatment or delayed treatment seeking in OCD sufferers: a review of the literature. Psychiatry Res. 2014;220:1–10.
73. Skoog G, Skoog I. A 40-year follow-up of patients with obsessive-compulsive disorder. Arch Gen Psychiatry. 1999;56(2):121–7.
74. Fineberg NA, Hengartner MP, Bergbaum CE, Gale T, Rossler W, Angst J. Lifetime comorbidity of obsessive-compulsive disorder and sub-threshold obsessive-compulsive symptomatology in the community: impact, prevalence, socio-demographic and clinical characteristics. Int J Psychiatry Clin Pract. 2013b;17(3):186–96.
75. Denys D, Fineberg N, Carey PD, Stein DJ. Quetiapine addition in obsessive-compulsive disorder: is treatment outcome affected by type and dose of serotonin reuptake inhibitors. Biological Psychiatry, 2007;61:412–14.
76. Osgood-Hynes, et al. Short-term residential treatment for obsessive-compulsive disorder. Brief Treat Crisis Interv. 2003;3:413–35.
77. Wagner T, Valero-Cabre A, Pascual-Leone A. Noninvasive human brain stimulation. Annu Rev Biomed Eng. 2007;9:527–65.

78. Rachid F. Transcranial direct current stimulation for the treatment of obsessive-compulsive disorder? A qualitative review of safety and efficacy. Psychiatry Res. 2019;271:259–64.
79. Denys, D, et al. (2020). Efficacy of deep brain stimulation of the ventral anterior limb of the internal capsule for refractory obsessive-compulsive disorder: And clinical cohort of 70 patients. Am J Psychiatry. AJP in Advance. Accessed 29 Jan 2020.
80. Greenberg JL, Markowitz S, Petronko MR, Taylor CE, Wilhelm S, Wilson GT. Cognitive behavioral therapy for adolescent body dysmorphic disorder. Cognit Behav Pract. 2010;17(3):248–58.
81. Phillips KA, Albertini RS, Rasmussen SA. A randomized placebo-controlled trial of fluoxetine in body dysmorphic disorder. Arch Gen Psychiatry. 2002;59:381–8.
82. Hollander E, Allen A, Kwon J, Aronowitz B, Schmeidler J, Wong C, et al. Clomipramine vs desipramine crossover trial in body dysmorphic disorder: selective efficacy of a serotonin reuptake inhibitor in imagined ugliness. Arch Gen Psychiatry. 1999;56:1033–9.
83. Phillips KA, Keshaviah A, Dougherty DD, Stout RL, Menard W, Wilhelm S, et al. Pharmacotherapy relapse prevention in body dysmorphic disorder: a double-blind, placebo-controlled trial. Am J Psychiatr. 2016;173:887–95.
84. Grisham JR, Norberg MM. Compulsive hoarding: current controversies and new directions. Dialogues Clin Neurosci. 2010;12(2):233–40.
85. Steketee G, Frost RO. Compulsive hoarding and acquiring: a therapist guide. New York: Oxford University Press; 2007.
86. Muroff, J., Bratiotis, C., & Steketee, G. (2011). Treatment for Hoarding Behaviors: A Review of the Evidence. *Clinical Social Work Journal*. 39:406–23.
87. Steketee G, Frost RO. Compulsive hoarding and acquiring: workbook. New York: Oxford University Press; 2007.
88. Rothbart R, Amos T, Siegfried N, et al. Pharmacotherapy for trichotillomania. Cochrane Database Syst Rev. 2013. https://doi.org/10.1002/14651858.CD007662.pub2.
89. Grant JE, Odlaug BL, Kim SW. N-acetylcysteine: a glutamine modulator in the treatment of trichotillomania: a double-blind, placebo-controlled study. Arch Gen Psychiatry. 2009;66:756–63.

Eating Disorders Among Transition-Age Youth

10

Danielle Colborn and Hope Levin

Key Points

- Eating disorders are serious psychiatric illnesses, and their prevalence is high in transition-age youth who face particular challenges around increased autonomy, decreased familial involvement, and increased external demands.
- Screening tools can be important in identifying individuals of concern, especially among transition-age youth where parental involvement is decreasing and autonomy is increasing. Appropriate assessment and accurate diagnosis by a multidisciplinary team are essential, as is intervention by providers specialized in the treatment of eating disorders.
- Eating disorders do not discriminate and affect a wide variety of individuals regardless of gender, race, sexual orientation, and socioeconomic background. Clinicians working with this population are encouraged to be sensitive to their own biases and to support access to care for all those affected by eating disorders.
- For those individuals previously diagnosed with an eating disorder, advance planning regarding where to attend college and the type of support available is strongly recommended and can help mitigate many of the difficulties experienced by patients and families during this transitional period.
- Respecting the increased autonomy of transition-age youth is essential, and they should always be informed about confidentiality and their rights as legal adults. At the same time, parents remain an important resource, and most young adults value the support of their family, especially when familial involvement is appropriately coordinated and planned.

D. Colborn (✉)
Department of Child and Adolescent Psychiatry, Stanford University School of Medicine, Palo Alto, CA, USA
e-mail: dcolborn@stanford.edu

H. Levin
Counseling and Psychological Services, University of California, Los Angeles, Los Angeles, CA, USA
e-mail: hlevin@caps.ucla.edu

Introduction

Eating disorders (ED) are serious psychiatric illnesses with mental, emotional, and physical implications. ED typically have their onset during early adolescence and early adulthood. For this latter group of transition-age youth (TAY),

V. Chan, J. Derenne (eds.), *Transition-Age Youth Mental Health Care*,
https://doi.org/10.1007/978-3-030-62113-1_10

navigating the developmental challenges of increased independence and less parental involvement makes them particularly vulnerable to the development of ED and can complicate issues around intervention and treatment. TAY are typically moving away from familiar familial environments, taking on more personal responsibility, and frequently entering IHE with new demands and higher workloads. It is not surprising that the rates of ED are high in this population, and it stands to reason that navigating assessment, diagnosis, and connection to treatment requires unique consideration. In this chapter, we describe the types of ED that may present in TAY and their prevalence in this population; provide information on assessment and treatment, including considerations for newly versus previously diagnosed individuals; discuss issues related to medication; and provide guidelines for coordinating care.

Overview of ED in TAY

There are five main types of ED that may present among TAY: anorexia nervosa, bulimia nervosa, binge eating disorder, avoidant restrictive food intake disorder, and other specified feeding or eating disorder. We describe each of them in more detail.

Anorexia Nervosa According to the *Diagnostic and Statistical Manual of Mental Disorders 5th Edition* (DSM-5), anorexia nervosa (AN) is characterized by a restriction of intake leading to weight loss significantly below what is expected, an intense fear of gaining weight, a distortion in their perception of themselves, and/or a failure to recognize the seriousness of their condition [1]. Individuals with AN often engage in rigid, bizarre eating rituals; exercise excessively; become socially isolated; and may develop secondary symptoms of depression, lethargy, and co-occurring medical complications. The latter may include loss of menses or failure to start menstruation, low heart rate and blood pressure, and loss of bone density leading to osteoporosis or osteopenia.

DSM-5 recognizes two subcategories of AN: restricting type and binge-purge type. Individuals with restricting-type AN primarily engage in restriction, while those with binge-purge subtype will also have episodes of binge eating, followed by compensatory behaviors such as self-induced vomiting or abuse of laxatives. Although it is the least common type of ED, AN is the most medically serious and has the highest mortality rate of any mental illness.

Bulimia Nervosa Bulimia nervosa (BN) involves restriction of intake in order to lose weight, along with episodes of binge eating, followed by compensatory measures to prevent weight gain, such as self-induced vomiting, excessive exercise, or use of diuretics and laxatives [1]. Binge eating is characterized by consuming an excessively large amount of food (more than what would be considered typical given the circumstances) in a relatively short amount of time (less than 2 hours) and experiencing a loss of control while doing so. It is this loss of control that separates binge eating from common overeating.

Individuals with BN have a distorted image of their bodies and place undue value on shape and weight. There are many medical complications involved with BN, including heart rate abnormalities, electrolyte imbalances, and eroding of tooth enamel due to frequent vomiting-type purging episodes. Individuals with BN tend to be normal weight, which can make detection of their illness difficult and lead the individual to feel that they are suffering in isolation.

Binge Eating Disorder Binge eating disorder (BED) is the most common type of eating disorder and is characterized by recurrent episodes of binge eating but without the compensatory behaviors seen in BN. Binge episodes often occur in secret and can involve eating rapidly, eating in the absence of physiological hunger, and eating past the point of fullness. These episodes are followed by negative feelings, including guilt, shame, regret, and significant distress about the episode [1].

Avoidant Restrictive Food Intake Disorder Avoidant restrictive food intake disorder (ARFID) is an illness characterized by restricted food intake or lack of interest in eating due to sensory qualities of the food and/or anxiety about negative consequences of eating, such as fear of vomiting or choking [1]. These issues with eating lead to significant impairment in the individual's life and physical health. ARFID typically has onset during infancy or early childhood but may continue into adulthood and can be exacerbated during times of increased stress, such as the transition into young adulthood.

Other Specified Feeding or Eating Disorder Other specified feeding or eating disorder (OSFED), previously known as eating disorder not otherwise specified, is the category for disorders in which issues related to feeding and eating cause significant distress and impairment but do not meet the full criteria for any of the above categories. Individuals with OSFED may present with subclinical symptoms of one or more of the above illnesses or have a disorder that is not captured by the above categories, such as someone who purges in the absence of binge episodes.

Vulnerabilities of TAY

Before we move into our discussion of how eating disorders present in TAY, we would like to discuss the unique vulnerabilities faced by TAY that make them susceptible to the development and exacerbation of ED. Transitions are, by their nature, times of uncertainty, excitement, vulnerability, and loss. Transitions involve leaving something that is familiar and moving toward something that is not yet known. We see this in a pronounced way in youth who are transitioning from adolescence into young adulthood, often leaving the familiarity of a home environment to move toward a future that is uncertain and still unfolding, and experiencing a significant increase in their level of independence. Youth in this developmental stage are leaving an environment that, ideally, has been fairly structured and familiar and moving toward one that is typically more amorphous, with an increased degree of autonomy. The decrease in the level of support and increase in the level of expected personal responsibility during this time period are exponential. This is true for individuals who go on to IHE as well as those who pursue other paths. This unique period of transition puts youth at risk of developing ED while also presenting challenges for continuity of care and exacerbation of symptoms in those previously diagnosed with ED.

For TAY who go on to university settings, the academic environment can bring added stress and pressure that can exacerbate preexisting ED and contribute to the development and onset of disordered eating. Rates of ED are higher on college campuses compared to the general population [2]. In addition to academic challenges, students entering college face new eating environments, with many students finding themselves responsible for managing their own meals for the first time. The array of cafeteria food options can be overwhelming and may promote binging or overeating, while irregular schedules do not facilitate consistent meals. Schedules and class times may conflict with dining service hours [3]. A heightened body image culture on many college campuses emphasizes an unrealistic thin ideal. Internalization of this thin ideal can lead to body-image dissatisfaction, increased dietary restraint, and negative affect, all of which can put individuals at an increased risk of development of ED [4].

Although there are many challenges to attending IHE, universities often have embedded support systems that can help detect students of concern and connect them to resources both on campus and in the surrounding community. Resident advisors in student housing are trained to recognize worrisome behavior in students as are academic advisors, and both can refer students to on-campus student health and counseling centers for assessment and treatment. While many universities are not fully equipped to treat the level of ED that can present in students, they are a good resource for identification and connection to broader community providers.

Not all TAY attend IHE after high school. Many opt to take a gap year and travel or volunteer. Some choose to enter the military, and many decide to directly enter the workforce [3]. For TAY who do not elect to attend college, detection and engagement in treatment can be more challenging without the built-in support of an academic setting. Youth in this category still face the challenges of increased independence, change in lifestyle structure impacting eating and meal times, and the inherent uncertainty present in this transitional period. However, they do not have the same institutional support that is typically found in IHE that can allow for the detection of mental health challenges and connection to treatment sources. Parents may struggle with how to enforce engagement in treatment without the motivation of being able to remain in school. Additionally, without the built-in social network that is found in university and college settings, TAY in other environments, particularly those taking a gap year or going directly into the workforce, are at risk of isolation, which can further impact disordered eating.

Some youth with histories of ED may end up delaying entrance into higher education and other developmental tasks of young adulthood in order to recover from an eating disorder. They may opt to attend community college, work part time while engaging in outpatient treatment, or participate in higher levels of care, such as intensive outpatient programs, partial-hospitalization programs, or residential treatment. While delaying matriculation to a university has the benefit of addressing eating disorder symptoms and thus increasing the likelihood of success in higher education, it does put individuals on a different developmental trajectory compared to their peers. It also requires thoughtful consideration by the youth, parents, and treatment team providers about how to support the individual and what factors determine when someone is ready to advance to a full-time academic setting.

Prevalence of ED in TAY

Epidemiology

Eating disorders have two time periods of typical onset: onset of puberty (ages 11–14 years) and transition from adolescence to young adulthood (ages 17–20 years). According to the DSM-5, 12-month prevalence rates for EDs in females is 0.40% for AN, 1–1.5% for BN, and 1.6% for BED. Less is known about the rates of AN and BN in males, but there is an approximate 10:1 female-to-male ratio for both illnesses. BED has a prevalence of 0.8% in males. It is noteworthy that with the publication of DSM-5 in 2013, the rates of eating disorders shifted, with a significant increase in the rates of AN, a decrease in the rates of ED-NOS/OSFED, and rates of BN staying the same [5]. This is likely reflective of the new diagnostic criteria for AN that capture individuals who previously would have received a diagnosis of OSFED.

In the TAY population, prevalence rates of ED suggest a higher percentage of BN and BED and a slightly lower prevalence of AN, which typically appear in earlier adolescence. A recent study looking at the prevalence rates of ED among adults using DSM-5 criteria found that 18- to 29-year-olds had 12-month prevalence rates of 0.08%, 0.23%, and 0.45% for AN, BN, and BED, respectively [6] (Fig. 10.1). A longitudinal study examining the natural history of eat-

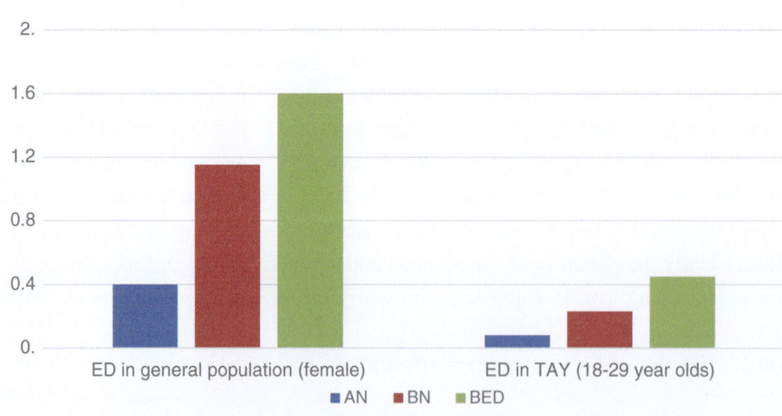

Fig. 10.1 Eating disorder 12-month prevalence rates (Data source: DSM-5; Udo and Grilo [6])

ing disorders found, by age 20 years, a 0.6% lifetime prevalence for AN, 1.6% for BN, and 1% for BED [7]. This study also suggested a peak age of onset of 17–18 years for BN and BED.

Among college students, rates of ED are high, with some studies suggesting rates of 8–17% [2] and subclinical rates as high as 34–67% [8]. Research using the SCOFF, a very simple and easy-to-use screening questionnaire that follows an acronym (S – do you make yourself **S**ick; C – do you worry about losing **C**ontrol over eating; O – have you recently lost **O**ne stone, i.e., 14 lbs., or more; F – do you worry you are **F**at when others think you are thin; F – does **F**ood dominate your life), found 13.5% of females and 3.6% of males screening positively for disordered eating among a sample of college students [2]. There is also evidence that rates of ED among college students are increasing over time in both females and males [9].

Given that most of the research on ED in young adults is done with college students, due to the convenience in sampling this population, there is limited information on ED prevalence specifically in non-college-bound TAY. However, there is reason to believe that youth going through this transitional time period are at risk of ED similarly to those entering IHE.

Underserved Groups

At one time thought to primarily affect affluent, heterosexual white females, there is now extensive data showing that eating disorders do not discriminate. ED affect a wide range of individuals across gender spectrum, racial and socioeconomic backgrounds, and sexual orientation identification. Clinicians working with individuals with ED are encouraged to be sensitive to the presentation of ED in underserved groups and to promote access to care for all individuals impacted by ED.

Males There is increasing data to suggest that ED are more prevalent among young adult males than previously thought. Previously, it was thought that ED affected males at a 10:1 ratio compared to females; more recent data suggest that this ratio is much smaller, and in particular on college campuses may be closer to 3:1 [2]. Another study found smaller gender differences in reported eating disorder symptoms than previously thought, with males reporting similar rates of compensatory behaviors compared with females (29% and 31%, respectively). Weight status (i.e., being overweight or obese) is the most significant predictor of eating disorder risk regardless of gender [10]. Males are less likely to seek treatment for ED, given the shame and stigma about what has historically been considered a female illness. Males may be missed on screening measures that have been normed on females. Further, the reported shape and weight concerns presented by males are often different than females, with males more likely to express a desire for a lean, muscular shape rather than a drive for thinness. However, the result can be the same in that efforts designed to achieve the desired physique can lead to excessive exercise, restriction, excessive weight loss, body image disturbance, and compensatory behaviors.

LGBTQ ED can affect individuals across the spectrum of sexual orientation and gender identity. There is evidence that gay men are at greater risk for ED compared to straight men and lesbian females [11]. The reasons for this are likely complex, with some studies suggesting that physical appearance may be central to sense of self in gay men. Transgender youth may be particularly vulnerable to disordered eating, with a recent literature review finding that the rates of ED were significantly higher in transgender compared to cisgender youth [12]. A consistent finding across studies in this review was that transgender youth often engage in restriction and weight loss attempts in order to delay the onset of puberty and the development of secondary sex characteristics, suggesting that for these youth, ED symptoms may be a way to manage distress related to gender identity rather than the body image concern that is typically seen in more traditional forms of ED.

Ethnic Minorities Although some data suggest that AN and BN occur less frequently in African American women compared with Caucasian women, there is growing evidence that ED affect individuals regardless of ethnic background. A study found that symptoms of restriction, binging, purging, and amenorrhea did not differ significantly across a wide variety of ethnic groups across college campuses [13]. Additionally, research has shown that ethnic minorities are less likely to seek treatment for ED, are less likely to be diagnosed with an ED, and are less likely to be referred for treatment compared to their Caucasian counterparts [14].

Treatment for ED Among TAY

Although individuals presenting with ED symptoms may vary in their level of clinical severity, it is ideal that treatment be provided by clinicians specializing in the treatment of ED. Additionally, ED treatment requires thorough assessment by a multidisciplinary team involving psychological, medical, and nutritional consultation to ensure accurate assessment, diagnosis, and ongoing care. For practitioners working with students in university settings, we recommend a stepped-care approach that involves screening, prevention, guided self-help, and treatment when indicated [4].

Considerations for Newly Diagnosed Versus Already Diagnosed

There are unique considerations when addressing treatment needs for TAY previously diagnosed with ED versus those who have been newly diagnosed. For youth who have been previously diagnosed with ED, families and patients have the advantage of establishing appropriate care and creating new treatment teams prior to the individual leaving home. We recommend as much advance planning as possible during this transition, including researching university treatment options for those TAY going on to IHE. Planning should start with a consideration of the institution itself—how far away from home is feasible for the individual? What is the campus setting and surrounding environment? What sort of treatment options are available? These are all important considerations when supporting people with ED in transitioning to college. While some universities have counseling centers and student health centers with multidisciplinary teams that can coordinate care among providers and may have specialists in ED on staff, many universities are limited in the amount of ongoing care they can provide for ED. The resources at counseling centers and student health centers vary significantly, often depending on the size of the school, geographic location, whether there is a medical center on campus, and whether the school is privately or publicly funded; additionally, many counseling centers do not have therapists with the level of specialty training necessary to treat ED [15]. Also, some schools offer unlimited therapy sessions on campus, while others have session limits, which can typically range from 3 to 12 sessions per year. For this reason, families are encouraged to become informed about treatment options in the surrounding areas and often need to factor in this cost when planning for college. Families should also explore whether it is beneficial to obtain the student health insurance instead of or in addition to the family's health insurance plan.

For TAY who are not college bound, whether it is to focus on continued recovery from ED or because they have chosen a different path, treatment planning can still be complicated. Determining the level of support versus the level of autonomy is central to this decision-making process. Important considerations for patients and families include the person's level of independence with eating and feeding, their medical status, and how physically demanding their daily tasks will be, whether working or traveling.

For individuals newly diagnosed with ED, the primary concerns are identification and connection to treatment. As we discuss below, appropriate screening measures are essential to identifying individuals of concern and connecting them to care. We recommend that IHEs make screening a regular process, particularly with incoming freshmen, to identify potential students in need of care.

Screening and Assessment

Because individuals with ED often do not think their difficulties warrant intervention or they do not desire help (as is often the case with AN), we recommend that clinicians implement screening tools to identify individuals of concern and connect them to appropriate resources. This is particularly true for clinicians working in university settings, but screenings can also be implemented in community clinics or offered by individual practitioners or groups who advocate for intervention and awareness of ED. There are many widely available and easy-to-use screening tools, such as the SCOFF, that are brief, easy to administer, and well validated [16] (Table 10.1).

In addition to screening, ED require thorough assessment by a multidisciplinary team, which includes psychological evaluation, medical assessment, and registered dietitian consultation.

Table 10.1 Eating disorder screening tools

Screening tool	Reference/resource
SCOFF	Morgan JF, Reid F, Lacey JH. The SCOFF questionnaire: assessment of a new screening tool for eating disorders. BMJ. 1999;04;319(7223):1467–8
Eating Disorder Examination Questionnaire (EDE-Q)	Fairburn CG, Beglin SJ. Assessment of eating disorders: interview or self-report questionnaire. Int J Eat Disord. 1994;16:363–70
Eating Attitudes Test (EAT)	Garner DM, Garfinkel PE. The eating attitudes test: an index of the symptoms of anorexia nervosa. Psych Med. 1979;9:273–79
EAT-26 (abbreviated version of the EAT)	https://www.eat-26.com/
Eating Disorder Inventory (EDI)	Garner DM, Olmsted MP, Plivy J. Development and validation of a multidimensional eating disorder inventory for anorexia nervosa and bulimia. Int J Eat Disord. 1983;2:15–34
Female Athlete Screening Tool (FAST)	McNulty KY, Adams CH, Anderson JM, Affenito SG. Development and validation of a screening tool to identify eating disorders in female athletes. J Am Diet Assoc. 2001;101:886–92; quiz 893–4

The treatment team ideally together makes recommendations for ongoing care. Some universities, community clinics, and practitioners in private practice may not have access to a multidisciplinary team. When working with patients who have eating disorders, it is essential to collaborate with other necessary specialties and/or know when to refer out.

Outpatient Clinical Treatment

Most patients with eating disorders are able to be treated on an outpatient basis. The following are outpatient psychotherapy interventions for each ED as specified.

Anorexia Nervosa As of this writing, there are limited evidence-based psychotherapeutic interventions for adults with AN. Family-based therapy (FBT) is the treatment intervention with the most evidence base for adolescent AN and has been modified for use with young adults. Principle tenets of FBT include agnosticism to the cause of AN and seeing the illness as something separate from the patient. FBT puts primary focus on recovery through renourishment by charging parents with the task of refeeding. In young adult adaptations of FBT, the patient is typically allowed to choose whom to have as a supportive adult. The young person is more involved in the decision-making about food and meal times and is allowed more individual time with the therapist [17, 18]. Although dropout rates were high in two recent studies of FBT for TAY, those participants who did complete treatment had good outcomes: participants were able to restore weight, and the treatment intervention was found feasible and acceptable [17, 18].

Adolescent-focused psychotherapy (AFT), also known as ego-oriented individual therapy (EOIT) in earlier versions, has been found to be effective for adolescents with AN. There is reason to extrapolate that AFT can be effective for work with TAY when the level of parental involvement required for FBT may not be feasible or indicated. With its origins in psychodynamic and developmental theories, AFT conceptualizes AN as occurring in the context of developmental challenges that are overwhelming to the individual. Thus, AN serves as a maladaptive protectant against perceived psychological and emotional threats [19]. AFT treatment is based on collaborative case formulation, and the therapeutic relationship becomes a vehicle for developing a stronger sense of self. Increasingly, tolerance of varied affective states occurs, resulting in reduced reliance on AN behaviors [19]. Two randomized controlled trials of AFT have found improvement in weight and psychological variables comparable to FBT [20, 21].

Finally, cognitive behavior therapy (CBT) has been used with adults with AN, with mixed results. A recent study of enhanced cognitive behavior therapy (CBT-E) that used body mass index (BMI) as its primary outcome found statistically significant weight improvement after 12-month follow up, although the treatment had a high attrition rate (50%) that is common with this population [22]. Another study of CBT for adults with underweight ED found improvement in weight and psychological symptoms in subjects who completed the protocol, although this study again had a high dropout rate (46%) [23].

Bulimia Nervosa Cognitive behavior therapy remains the gold standard of care for adults with BN with a significant evidence base to support its effectiveness [24]. CBT for BN involves creating a model of how thoughts, feelings, and behaviors maintain the eating disorder; implementation of strategies to regulate eating and decrease bingeing and purging behaviors; and development of skills to restructure cognitions and regulate emotions. Enhancements to CBT for eating disorders (CBT-E) have helped deepen our understanding of the core psychopathology of eating disorders and seem to be effective for patients with more severe comorbidity [24].

Interpersonal psychotherapy (IPT) has been shown to be an effective intervention for BN. IPT assesses interpersonal relationship patterns and their association with the development and maintenance of ED. IPT for BN has been found to have similar long-term outcomes to CBT, although results tend to happen more slowly [24].

Dialectical behavior therapy (DBT) is a treatment with promising results for BN that combines behavioral therapeutic techniques with concepts rooted in eastern mindfulness. DBT targets specific behaviors and uses skills related to distress tolerance, emotion regulation, and interpersonal effectiveness to promote behavior change. A version of DBT specifically modified for BN has led to a significant reduction in binge-purge symptoms with a rapid response rate [25]. DBT may be particularly effective for individuals with comorbid substance abuse and/or self-harm behaviors, and it has been found highly effective for these diagnoses as well [26].

Binge Eating Disorder Similar to bulimia nervosa, CBT, IPT, and DBT appear to be effective interventions for BED. Treatment should focus on the establishment of regular eating patterns to reduce vulnerability to bingeing, along with tools to address contributing stressors and negative emotions. It is worth noting that treatments for BED do not typically lead to weight loss.

Avoidant Restrictive Food Intake Disorder Although research on adults with ARFID is lacking, CBT (which is effective for younger children) appears to be the most practical and viable intervention, and it has been applied across age groups [27]. CBT for ARFID involves working to create a ranking of foods that the individual finds easy, moderate, or difficult to consume. Then shaping and chaining techniques are engaged to gradually increase exposure to a greater variety of foods and decrease anxious and aversive reactions to food.

Other Specified Feeding or Eating Disorder Because the presentation of OSFED can vary greatly from patient to patient, clinicians are advised to use their judgment about the most effective intervention in a given case. It can be reasonably concluded that OSFED may respond to specific interventions when presentations resemble subclinical variants of other ED. In general, therapies that focus on nutrition, skills to address emotions and cognitive distortions, and relapse prevention are recommended.

Novel Treatments There are several novel psychotherapeutic interventions being developed for use with ED that show promise when working with TAY. Three are described here. Cognitive remediation therapy (CRT) is a treatment that targets neurocognitive processes using exercises that aim to improve cognitive flexibility, global processing, and metacognition. Although not recommended as a stand-alone treatment, CRT has been shown to reduce attrition rates and improve cognitive flexibility when used in conjunction with other therapies [28]. Acceptance and commitment therapy (ACT), which advocates for the acceptance of one's thoughts, feelings, and adherence to values as motivation for change, has been found to be effective for young adults with ED. In one study, a group format of ACT led to decreased eating disorder pathology and lower risk of rehospitalization compared to treatment as usual [29]. Finally, motivational interviewing (MI) has been used as an effective adjunct to a variety of therapies and has been found particularly effective for the treatment of ED. MI seeks to augment individual engagement in treatment and motivation for recovery by having the therapist validate and empathize with reasons not to change, thus freeing the patient to explore the potential benefits of therapy. MI has been found useful in the treatment of ED, particularly in regard to enhancing readiness and motivation to change [30].

Higher Levels of Care

Whenever possible, we recommend treatments that allow patients to stay in their normative environment and involve the least disruption to daily life. This is particularly true for TAY who are navigating the transition to young adulthood. However, ED are serious illnesses with medical complications that may require participation in higher levels of care for a period of time. Additionally, some patients with ED do not respond to outpatient treatment and may need more intensive support.

Medical Hospitalization For some individuals with ED, their illness progresses to the point that they require admission to a hospital or other medical facilities in order to stabilize their physical symptoms and prevent cardiac arrest or other life-threatening complications. There are a number of signs that may indicate hospitalization due to ED, including bradycardia (heart rate less than 50 beats per minute (BPM) during waking hours), orthostatic vital signs (an increase of pulse 20 bpm or decrease of systolic blood pressure 20 mmHg from lying to standing), hypotension (blood pressure below 90/60 mmHg), extremely low body weight (less than 75% median body mass index (mBMI)), and electrolyte abnormalities [31]. Being medically hospitalized because of ED constitutes a medical emergency. Academic institutions and employers are required to work with individuals in this situation so that they are not unduly penalized for absences due to hospitalization.

Residential Treatment For individuals needing continuous support, residential treatment programs have participants live on-site for weeks or months at a time in order to receive intensive psychotherapy, nutritional support, and medical monitoring. We typically recommend residential treatment after an individual has not been successful at lower levels of care and strongly recommend treatment programs with solid discharge planning to help reorient and integrate the patient back into daily life. In some cases, a step-down approach may be indicated where patients move from residential to partial hospitalizations, intensive outpatient care (PHP/IOP), and then outpatient care.

Partial Hospitalization (PHP) and Intensive Outpatient (IOP) Care PHP typically involves attending a treatment center 4–7 days per week for a full day up to 12 hours. While there, patients participate in individual and group therapy, receive mealtime and nutritional support, and have access to real-time intervention for eating-disorder-related distress. IOP is similar but shorter in duration, with patients typically staying for several hours rather than a full day. PHP and IOP can be beneficial for individuals who need more consistent support than weekly outpatient sessions in order to recover from ED.

Psychopharmacology and Eating Disorders

General Principles In patients with eating disorders, medication is considered an adjunctive treatment to psychotherapy and nutritional rehabilitation or is used for the treatment of comorbidities. Prior to starting medication, patients need a thorough diagnostic assessment. Eating disorders can cause, exacerbate, or mask symptoms of anxiety and depression. History is crucial to determining if anxiety and mood symptoms are secondary to malnourishment or separate; carefully assessing the chronology of symptoms and psychiatric family history is recommended. Patients with eating disorders are often very concerned about potential weight gain from medications, so this should be directly discussed.

It should be noted that almost all medications are off-label for eating disorders. The two exceptions to this are fluoxetine, which is US Food and Drug Administration (FDA)-approved for BN in adults, and lisdexamfetamine, which is FDA-approved for BED in adults. In the literature, there are very few randomized controlled trials of psychopharmacology, especially in AN, due to low enrollment and high dropout rates.

Anorexia Nervosa As previously stated, medication is not the initial or primary treatment for AN. Medication should be considered only for patients who do not respond to nutritional rehabilitation and psychotherapy. Most treatment approaches use a "food is medicine" philosophy for anorexia nervosa, in which weight restoration is the initial primary goal since many symptoms will improve once a patient is no longer malnourished. Energy, mood, and anxiety often improve with adequate nutrition. Pharmacotherapy has limited efficacy in AN and should be considered adjunctive [32]. The reasons for this are not fully known, but it is theorized that starvation may alter neurotransmitter function and lower the levels of available serotonin which may impact medication response [33]. Also, restrictive eating behavior may become so neurobiologically entrenched that medications have minimal impact [34]. Often, obsessionality and depression only improve with weight gain [35]. Due to a higher risk of side effects in low-weight patients, any medication, if considered, should be started at low dosages [35]. In the literature, there are few randomized controlled trials of medication in AN due to difficulty with recruitment and medical fragility of these patients [36].

Second-generation antipsychotics (SGAs), also commonly referred to as atypical antipsychotics, have been studied in patients with AN and refractory symptoms that have not responded to psychotherapy and nutritional rehabilitation, with the rationale that they may help to promote weight gain, address rumination, perseveration, anxiety and near-delusional thinking in anorexia [36]. There are several randomized studies which concluded that olanzapine is modestly effective for weight gain [35, 37–39]. Olanzapine may also help with obsessions and concerns about eating and body shape. However, a recent 2019 randomized controlled trial of olanzapine in adult outpatients with AN did not show benefits in obsessionality or cognitive symptoms of AN despite improvement in weight [35]. Patients with very intense and rigid eating disorder cognitions who have trouble tolerating or progressing with weight restoration may be appropriate candidates for olanzapine. Dosages of 2.5 mg to 10 mg daily are commonly used [37, 38, 40]. Studies of other SGAs have shown limited efficacy in AN. One retrospective study of aripiprazole showed some benefit [41], but no benefit was found in randomized trials of risperidone and quetiapine [42, 43]. Patients are often reluctant to take SGAs due to fear of weight gain, low insight into the illness, and ambivalence about recovery. The risk of adverse metabolic effects of SGAs may be less pronounced in patients with AN compared to other psychiatric illnesses. However, in medically fragile patients, there is greater potential for QTc prolongation, which increases the risk of *torsades des pointes* and cardiac arrest, so cardiac monitoring is indicated with SGA use.

In the literature, there is a lack of evidence that selective serotonin reuptake inhibitors (SSRIs) are effective for the treatment of the core symptoms of AN [44, 45]. SSRIs may be used to treat co-occurring moderate or severe anxiety and depression that does not improve with weight restoration. While this class of medication is used to treat obsessive-compulsive disorder, unfortunately, studies have not shown SSRIs to help with the obsessive thoughts in AN. Similarly, they do not help with weight restoration. It was initially shown that this class of medication could help to prevent relapse in adults with AN [46], but this was not supported by a larger study [47]. QTc prolongation can also be a concern with SSRI use.

Benzodiazepines are sometimes used prior to meals to reduce anticipatory anxiety, but there is no evidence in the literature to support this practice. A 2014 study did not show benefit of alprazolam in reducing premeal anxiety in adults with AN but found that it did increase fatigue [48].

Bulimia Nervosa In contrast to AN, antidepressants may be used as a first-line treatment in BN, in combination with therapy and nutritional rehabilitation. The neurobiology of bulimia and the mechanism of action for pharmacotherapy are not known, but it is theorized that central nervous system serotonin pathways are disturbed in patients with BN [49].

Fluoxetine, an SSRI, is FDA approved for adults with BN. It is the most studied and most effective medication for reducing urges to binge and purge, drive for thinness, and other psychological symptoms. These benefits are seen regardless of baseline mood status. Dosages of 60 mg daily are more effective than lower dosages, an early response in the first 3 weeks is predictive of treatment response, and a significant improvement is expected by 4–8 weeks after starting fluoxetine [50, 51]. Fluoxetine is often continued for 6–12 months after symptom response or remission [52]. Other SSRIs are considered second line to fluoxetine as they have shown symptom improvement in small studies [53–56]. When considering SSRIs other than fluoxetine, a family history of positive response and potential for side effects guide the medication selection since they are considered interchangeable in terms of efficacy. Paroxetine is usually avoided due to the common adverse effect of weight gain, which tends to make it less tolerable for eating disorder patients. Citalopram is generally avoided or used cautiously due to concern for the cardiac adverse effect of QTc prolongation since electrolyte disturbances may occur in patients with BN.

Topiramate has also been shown to reduce binge-purge episodes in adults with BN. Its use is limited by sedation and cognitive side effects. Also, topiramate may cause a side effect of weight loss, so it should be avoided in patients in low or low-normal weight ranges [57–59]. Tricyclic antidepressants and monoamine oxidase (MAO) inhibitors are usually avoided due to adverse side effects but may be used as third- or fourth-line medications with caution. Bupropion is contraindicated in BN due to increased risk of seizures found in a 1988 study and is generally not recommended in any formulation for eating disorder patients [60].

Binge Eating Disorder In BED, medications are a second-line treatment after psychotherapy since they are generally considered to be less effective. Medication may be preferred due to lower cost and less time requirement or if therapy is inaccessible. Medication can help with short-term reduction in binge eating but not necessarily weight loss. Most studies are short term in duration. Targets of medication treatment may include reduction of binge eating episodes, eating disorder cognitions, and weight loss [61].

SSRIs are recommended as a first-line medication (but are used off FDA label) due to demonstrated efficacy and tolerability [62]. The stimulant medication lisdexamfetamine was FDA approved in 2015 for severe BED (four or more episodes/week.) It is a second-line medication option after failure of 1–2 SSRI trials. Studies showed weight loss and increased abstinence from binges over placebo. It carries a potential for misuse, abuse, and diversion [63, 64].

Topiramate is another second-line medication option after failure of 1–2 SSRI trials. Like lisdexamfetamine, studies showed increased abstinence from binges over placebo. It may enhance outcomes in combination with cognitive behavioral therapy. Possible side effects include paresthesias, cognitive impairment, and sedation [65]. Other medications that have demonstrated some efficacy for BED in trials include zonisamide, orlistat, acamprosate, atomoxetine, and duloxetine [61].

Involving Family

Although TAY are often legally adults, they are usually still embedded in their families of origin. Families are often an essential source of support for individuals with ED. When working with TAY, it is important to balance their need for increased autonomy and independence with appropriate familial support. It is also important as a provider to be clear with the individual from the outset about confidentiality and its limits. With the exception of emergency situations when individuals have become so medically or psychologically compromised that they are in grave danger, adults typically must authorize permission for caregivers to communicate with parents or other family members through signed consent prior to any contact. It is recommended that institutions and private practitioners working with TAY with ED have open communication from the beginning about when and how it may be beneficial for parents to be involved in treatment. Many providers in collaboration with TAY patients find it quite helpful to involve parents in treatment, and often, young adults are more open to this than expected. In both studies on FBT for TAY described in the treatment section, the majority of participants chose a parent as their supportive adult, suggesting TAY value support from concerned family members [16, 17].

Many concerned parents struggle with how to support their adult children who are struggling with ED, especially when the patient is reluctant to engage in treatment or even acknowledge the need for intervention. While the autonomy needs and rights of young adults are different from those of children and adolescents, we often remind parents that they still have leverage in many areas—most TAY are still financially dependent on parents to some degree and often continue to live at home for several years after reaching the age of majority. Given the serious, often life-threatening nature of ED, parents have the option of making financial support and/or the ability to remain at home contingent on the youth getting treatment. It is worth noting that research studies on ED in TAY have found that youth often desire to have parents involved in their treatment and care and respond positively to limits that are coming from a source of deep concern and care [17, 18].

Summary and Conclusions

TAY are a population particularly vulnerable to ED, given the complicated nature of transitions in general and the intricacies of transitioning from adolescence to young adulthood in particular. For those individuals previously diagnosed with ED, families are encouraged to plan well in advance for this transition and educate themselves as much as possible on the most appropriate course of action and available resources for those TAY going onto university. Many IHE are not equipped to address the full range of ED that may present on campus, and families often have to seek resources outside of campus. For TAY not attending universities, special coordination and planning by parents and care providers can help determine the most appropriate course of action and set them up for success while mitigating challenges. Screening and assessment are essential to identifying individuals of concern who present at universities and community clinics. Once identified, assessment and diagnosis by multidisciplinary teams specialized in the treatment of eating disorders is essential for accurate diagnosis and treatment recommendations. Institutions and community providers working with ED are encouraged to collaborate with appropriate resources in order to provide comprehensive care. When attending to the adult autonomy and legal rights of TAY, it is important to remember that families remain an essential source of support, and most TAY value their input and involvement when appropriately coordinated.

References

1. American Psychiatric Association. Diagnostic and statistical manual of mental disorders. 5th ed. Washington, D.C.: American Psychiatric Publishing; 2013.
2. Eisenberg D, Nicklett EJ, Roeder K, Kirz N. Eating disorder symptoms among college students: prevalence, persistence, correlates, and treatment-seeking. J Am Coll Heal. 2011;59(8):700–7.
3. Derenne J. Eating disorders in transitional age youth. Child Adolesc Psychiatric Clin N Am. 2019;28(4):567–72.
4. Colborn D, Robinson A. Eating disorders and body image concerns. In: Roberts LW, editor. Student mental health: a guide for psychiatrists, psychologists and leaders serving in higher education. Washington, D.C.: American Psychiatric Association Press; 2018. p. 231–48.
5. Mancuso SG, Newton JR, Bosanac P, Rossell SL, Nesci JB, Castle DJ. Classification of eating disorders: comparison of relative prevalence rates using DSM-IV and DSM-5 criteria. Br J Psychiatry. 2015;206(6):519–20.
6. Udo T, Grilo CM. Prevalence and correlates of DSM-5-defined eating disorders in a nationally representative sample of US adults. Biol Psychiatry. 2018;84(5):345–54.
7. Stice E, Marti CN, Shaw H, Jaconis M. An 8-year longitudinal study of the natural history of threshold, subthreshold, and partial eating disorders from a community sample of adolescents. J Abnorm Psychol. 2009;118(3):587–97.
8. Fitzsimmons-Craft EE, Harney MB, Koehler LG, et al. Explaining the relation between thin ideal internalization and body dissatisfaction among college women: the roles of social comparison and body surveillance. Body Image. 2012;9(1):43–9.
9. White S, Reynolds-Malear JB, Cordero E. Disordered eating and the use of unhealthy weight control methods in college students: 1995, 2002, and 2008. Eat Disord. 2011;19(4):323–34. https://doi.org/10.1080/10640266.2011.584805.
10. Lipson SK, Sonneville KR. Eating disorder symptoms among undergraduate and graduate students at 12 U.S. colleges and universities. Eat Behav. 2017;24:81–8.
11. McClain Z, Peebles R. Body image and eating disorders among lesbian, gay, bisexual, and transgender youth. Pediatr Clin N Am. 2016;63(6):1079–90.
12. Coelho JS, Suen J, Clark BA, Marshall SK, Geller J, Lam P. Eating disorder diagnoses and symptom presentation in transgender youth: a scoping review. Curr Psychiatry Rep. 2019;21:107. https://doi.org/10.1007/s11920-019-1097-x.
13. Franco DL, Becker AE, Thomas JJ, Herzog DB. Cross-ethnic differences in eating disorder symptoms and related distress. Int J Eat Disord. 2007;40(2):156–64.
14. Sinha S, Warfa N. Treatment of eating disorders among ethnic minorities in western settings: a systematic review. Psychiatr Danub. 2013;25(2):295–9.
15. Wilfley DE, Agras WS, Taylor CB. Reducing the burden of eating disorders: a model for population-based prevention and treatment for university and college campuses. Int J Eat Disord. 2013;46(5):529–32.
16. Morgan JF, Reid F, Lacey JH. The SCOFF questionnaire: assessment of a new screening tool for eating disorders. BMJ. 1999;319(7223):1467–8.
17. Chen EY, Weissman JA, Zeffiro TA, Yui A, Eneva KT, et al. Family-based therapy for young adults with anorexia nervosa. Int J Eat Disord. 2016;49(7):701–7.
18. Dimitropoulos G, Landers AL, Freeman V, Novick J, Garber A, Le Grange D. Open trial of family-based treatment for anorexia nervosa for transition age youth. J Can Acad Adolesc Psychiatry. 2018;27:50–61.
19. Lock J Adolescent focused therapy: a developmental approach. Guilford Press (in press due out spring 2020).
20. Robin A, Siegal P, Moye A, Gilroy M, Daniels A, Sikand A. A controlled comparison of family versus individual therapy for adolescents with anorexia nervosa. J Am Acad Child Adolesc Psychiatry. 1999;38(12):1482–9.
21. Lock J, Le Grange D, Agras WS, Moye A, Bryson S, Jo BA. Randomized controlled clinical trial comparing family based treatment to adolescent focused individual therapy for adolescents with anorexia nervosa. Arch Gen Psychiatry. 2010;67(10):1025–32.
22. Frostad S, Danielsen YS, Rekkedal GA, Jevene C, Dalle Grave R, Rø Ø, et al. Implementation of enhanced cognitive behavior therapy (CBT-E) for adults with anorexia nervosa in an outpatient eating-disorder unit at a public hospital. J Eat Disord. 2018;6:12.
23. Jenkins PE, Morgan C, Houlihan C. Outpatient CBT for underweight patients with eating disorders: effectiveness within a national health service (NHS) eating disorders service. Behav Cogn Psychother. 2019;47(2):217–29.
24. Agras WS, Walsh BT, Fairburn CG, Wilson GT, Kraemer HC. A multicenter comparison of cognitive-behavioral therapy and interpersonal psychotherapy for bulimia nervosa. Arch Gen Psychiatry. 2000;57(5):459–6.
25. Hill DM, Craighead LW, Safer DL. Appetite-focused dialectical behavior therapy for the treatment of binge eating with purging: a preliminary trial. Int J Eat Disord. 2011;44(3):249–61.
26. Fischer S, Peterson C. Dialectical behavior therapy for adolescent binge eating, purging, suicidal

behavior, and non-suicidal self-injury: a pilot study. Psychotherapy. 2015;52(1):78–92.
27. Thomas JJ, Eddy KT. Cognitive-behavioral therapy for avoidant/restrictive food intake disorder : children, adolescents, and adults: Cambridge University Press; 2018.
28. Dalgren C, Øyvind R. A systematic review of cognitive remediation therapy for anorexia nervosa—development, current state and implications for future research and clinical practice. J Eat Disord. 2014;2(1):26.
29. Juarascio A, Shaw J, Forman E, Timko CA, Herbert J, Butryn M, et al. Acceptance and commitment therapy as a novel treatment for eating disorders: an initial test of efficacy and mediation. Behav Modif. 2013;37(4):459–89.
30. Macdonald P, Hibbs R, Corfield F, Treasure J. The use of motivational interviewing in eating disorders: a systematic review. Psychiatry Res. 2012;200(1):1–11.
31. Derenne J. The role of higher levels of care for eating disorders in youth. Child Adolesc Psychiatr Clin N Am. 2019;28(4):573–82.
32. Halmi K. Pharmacotherapy and physiological intervention for eating disorders. Focus. 2014;12(4):388–93.
33. Phillipou A, Russelll SK, Castle DJ. The neurobiology of anorexia nervosa: a systematic review. Aust N Z J Psychiatry. 2014;48:128–52.
34. Walsh BT. The enigmatic persistence of anorexia nervosa. Am J Psychiatry. 2013;170:477–84.
35. Attia E, Steinglass JE, Walsh BT, et al. Olanzapine versus placebo in adult outpatients with anorexia nervosa: a randomized clinical trial. Am J Psychiatry. 2019;176:449–56.
36. Dold M, Aigner M, Klabunde M, et al. Second-generation antipsychotic drugs in anorexia nervosa: a meta-analysis of randomized controlled trials. Psychother Psychosom. 2015;84:110–6.
37. Attia A, Kaplan AS, Walsh BT, Gershkovich M, Yilmaz Z, Musante D, Wang Y. Olanzapine versus placebo for outpatients with anorexia nervosa. Psychol Med. 2011;41(10):2177–82.
38. Bissada H, Tasca G, Barber A, Bradwejn J. Olanzapine in the treatment of low body weight and obsessive thinking in women with anorexia nervosa: a randomized, double-blind, placebo-controlled trial. Am J Psychiatr. 2008;165:1281–8.
39. Brambilla F, Garcia CS, Fassino S, et al. Olanzapine therapy in anorexia nervosa: psychobiological effects. Int Clin Psychopharmacol. 2007;22:197–204.
40. Mondraty N, Birmingham CL, Touyz S, Sundakov V, Chapman L, Beumont P. Randomized controlled trial of olanzapine in the treatment of cognitions in anorexia nervosa. Australas Psychiatry. 2005;13(1):72–5.
41. Hagman J, Gralla J, Sigel E, Ellert S, Dodge M, Gardner R, O'Lonergan T, Frank G, Wamboldt MZ. A double-blind, placebo-controlled study of risperidone for the treatment of adolescents and young adults with anorexia nervosa: a pilot study. J Am Acad Child Adolesc Psychiatry. 2011;50(9):915–24.
42. Frank G, Shott M, Hagman J, Schiel M, DeGuzman M, Rossi B. The partial dopamine D2 receptor agonist aripiprazole is associated with weight gain in adolescent anorexia nervosa. Int J Eat Disord. 2017;50:447–50.
43. Powers PS, Klabunde M, Kaye W. Double-blind placebo-controlled trial of quetiapine in anorexia nervosa. Eur Eat Disord Rev. 2012;20(4):331–4. Epub 2012 April 26
44. Attia E, Schroeder L. Pharmacologic treatment of anorexia nervosa: where do we go from here? Int J Eat Disord. 2005;37:S60–3.
45. Aigner M, Treasure J, Kaye W, Walter S, World Federation of Societies of Biological Psychiatry Task Force on Eating Disorders. World Federation of Societies of Biological Psychiatry guidelines for the pharmacological treatment of eating disorders. World J Biol Psychiatry. 2011;12(6):400–43.
46. Kaye WH, Nagata T, Weltzin TE, Hsu LK, Sokol MS, McConaha C, Deep D, et al. Double-blind placebo-controlled administration of fluoxetine in restricting- and restricting-purging-type anorexia nervosa. Biol Psychiatry. 2001;49(7):644–52.
47. Walsh BT, Kaplan AS, Attia E, Olmsted M, Parides M, Carter JC, et al. Fluoxetine after weight restoration in anorexia nervosa: a randomized controlled trial. JAMA. 2006;295(22):2605–12.
48. Steinglass JE, Kaplan SC, Liu Y, Wang Y, Walsh BT. The (lack of) effect of alprazolam on eating behavior in anorexia nervosa: a preliminary report. Int J Eat Disord. 2014;47(8):901–4. Epub 2014 Aug 19.
49. Kaye WH, Bailer UF, Frank GK, et al. Brain imaging of serotonin after recovery from anorexia and bulimia nervosa. Physio Behav. 2005;86(1–2):15–7.
50. Goldstein DJ, Wilson MG, Thompson VL, Potvin JH, Rampey AH Jr, Fluoxetine Bulimia Nervosa Research Group. Long-term fluoxetine treatment of bulimia nervosa. Br J Psychiatry. 1995;166(5):660–6.
51. Fluoxetine Bulimia Nervosa Collaborative Study Group. Fluoxetine in the treatment of bulimia nervosa. A multicenter, placebo-controlled, double-blind trial. Arch Gen Psychiatry. 1992;49(2):139–47.
52. Romano SJ, Halmi KA, Sarkar NP, Koke SC, Lee JS. A placebo-controlled study of fluoxetine in continued treatment of bulimia nervosa after successful acute fluoxetine treatment. Am J Psychiatry. 2002;159(1):96–102.
53. Milano W, Petrella C, Sabatino C, Capasso A. Treatment of bulimia nervosa with sertraline: a randomized controlled trial. Adv Ther. 2004;21(4):232–7.
54. Milano W, Siano C, Putrella C, Capasso A. Treatment of bulimia nervosa with fluvoxamine: a randomized controlled trial. Adv Ther. 2005;22:278–83.
55. Fichter MM, Leibl C, Krüger R, et al. Effects of fluvoxamine on depression, anxiety, and other areas of general psychopathology in bulimia nervosa. Pharmacopsychiatry. 1997;30(3):85–92.
56. Leombruni P, Amianto F, Delsedime N, et al. Citalopram versus fluoxetine for the treat-

ment of patients with bulimia nervosa: a single-blind randomized controlled trial. Adv Ther. 2006;23(3):481–94.
57. Hedges DW, Reimherr FW, Hoopes SP, Rosenthal NR, Kamin M, Karim R, et al. Treatment of bulimia nervosa with topiramate in a randomized, double-blind, placebo-controlled trial, part 2: improvement in psychiatric measures. J Clin Psychiatry. 2003;64(12):1449–54.
58. Hoopes SP, Reimherr FW, Hedges DW, Rosenthal NR, Kamin M, Karim R, Capece JA, Karvois D. Treatment of bulimia nervosa with topiramate in a randomized, double-blind, placebo-controlled trial, part 1: improvement in binge and purge measures. J Clin Psychiatry. 2003;64(11):1335–41.
59. Nickel C, Tritt K, Muehlbacher M, Pedrosa Gil F, Mitterlehner FO, Kaplan P, et al. Topiramate treatment in bulimia nervosa patients: a randomized, double-blind, placebo-controlled trial. Int J Eat Disord. 2005;38(4):295–300.
60. Horne RL, Ferguson JM, Pope HG Jr, Hudson JI, Lineberry CG, Ascher J, et al. Treatment of bulimia with bupropion: a multicenter controlled trial. J Clin Psychiatry. 1988;49(7):262–6.
61. Crow S. Treatment of binge eating disorder. Curr Treat Options Psychiatry. 2014;1(4):307–14.
62. Flament MF, Bissada H, Spettigue W. Evidence-based pharmacotherapy of eating disorders. Int J Neuropsychopharmacol. 2012;15(2):189–207.
63. Hudson J, McElroy S, Ferreira-Cornwell C, Radewonuk J, Gasior M. Efficacy of Lisdexamfetamine in adults with moderate to severe binge-eating disorder. JAMA Psychiat. 2017;74(9):903–10.
64. McElroy SL, Hudson JI, Mitchell JE, Wilfley D, Ferreira-Cornwell MC, Gao J, et al. Efficacy and safety of lisdexamfetamine for treatment of adults with moderate to severe binge-eating disorder: a randomized clinical trial. JAMA Psychiat. 2015;72(3):235–46.
65. McElroy SL, Hudson JI, Capece JA, Beyers K, Fisher AC, Rosenthal NR. Topiramate for the treatment of binge eating disorder associated with obesity: a placebo-controlled study. Biol Psychiatry. 2007;61:1039–48.

11 Transition-Age Youth with Autism Spectrum Disorder

McLeod Frampton Gwynette, Natasha Marrus, and Roma A. Vasa

Key Points

- Transition-age youth with autism spectrum disorder (TAYASD) face challenges in health care, adaptive functioning, and quality of life. Psychiatrists can guide families in implementing highly individualized treatment interventions, thereby optimizing clinical outcomes.
- The severity of co-occurring psychiatric and behavioral conditions is a major factor in determining an individual's living arrangements and daily activities.
- Medical conditions impact TAYASD to a greater extent than typically developing individuals, contributing to decreased life expectancy. Advocacy and appropriate medical care can have a significant positive impact for patients.
- Psychiatrists can guide TAYASD and their families during the transition process by connecting them to resources in the areas of postsecondary education, living arrangements, finances, vocational options, and decision-making.

Introduction

Autism spectrum disorder (ASD) is a lifelong neurodevelopmental disorder characterized by social and communication deficits, along with restricted/repetitive interests, behaviors, and activities [1]. Symptoms can vary considerably across individuals with ASD; for example, some individuals may have relative strengths in social motivation, whereas others may be socially indifferent. Additionally, ASD is associated with varying cognitive and language abilities, as well as high rates of co-occurring psychiatric and medical disorders [2–4], which together with the core features of ASD create a heterogenous profile of symptoms. Indeed, one common expression in the field that reflects this heterogeneity is, "If you have seen one person with ASD, you have seen one person with ASD."

The prevalence of ASD has soared over the last several decades, with recent estimates indicating that 1 in 59 children are affected by this

M. F. Gwynette (✉)
Medical University of South Carolina, Department of Psychiatry and Behavioral Sciences, Charleston, SC, USA
e-mail: gwynette@musc.edu

N. Marrus
Washington University School of Medicine, Department of Psychiatry, St. Louis, MO, USA

R. A. Vasa
Kennedy Krieger Institute, Johns Hopkins University School of Medicine, Baltimore, MD, USA

V. Chan, J. Derenne (eds.), *Transition-Age Youth Mental Health Care*,
https://doi.org/10.1007/978-3-030-62113-1_11

disorder [5]. This rising prevalence has resulted in a growing population of adults with ASD, with recent data indicating that approximately 50,000 adolescents with ASD will transition into adulthood every year [6]. It is therefore important for psychiatrists to become familiar with how to help individuals with ASD and their families successfully navigate the transition process from adolescence to adulthood. According to the Individuals with Disabilities Education Act (IDEA), transition planning should be incorporated within the IEP starting no later than age 16 years [7]. Nevertheless, since individuals with ASD have many complex and changing needs, it can be beneficial for transition planning to begin even earlier (e.g., age 13 years) and extend into young adulthood (e.g., age 30 years) to allow ample time for repeating developmental assessments, determining appropriate educational and residential placement, and identifying necessary multidisciplinary supports in each setting.

This chapter highlights key biopsychosocial factors (Table 11.1), including co-occurring psychiatric and medical conditions, education and

Table 11.1 Biopsychosocial factors to consider during transition planning for individuals with ASD

Factors	Considerations for management
Co-occurring psychiatric/ behavioral conditions	Regularly assess current and emerging symptoms and disorders Refer for specialized behavioral treatment or psychotherapies Prescribe psychotropic medications judiciously as part of a larger multidisciplinary plan that addresses educational, medical, developmental, psychosocial factors
Medical conditions	Identify an adult primary care provider Refer to appropriate medical specialists Regularly assess medical risks when prescribing psychotropic medications (e.g., metabolic syndrome, obesity) Encourage compliance with medical treatments Recognize the interplay between medical and psychiatric disorders
Planning for socialization	Clarify social interests, as well as social strengths and weaknesses Pursue developmentally appropriate socialization opportunities Identify potential barriers to socialization (e.g., fixation on electronic screen media, social anxiety)
Educational options	Obtain appropriate assessments, including repeat neuropsychological testing, to assess interests, strengths, and weaknesses Weigh formal postsecondary education (e.g., college, technical school) versus community-based education (e.g., day programs) Evaluate fit of each option relative to needs of the TAYASD (e.g., local versus long-distance, 2-year versus 4-year programs) Advocate for educational supports in college
Vocational options	Pursue day programs for individuals with intellectual disability Assess the need for vocational assessment, training, or job search assistance.
Living arrangements	Evaluate independent, family-based, or residential living options based on the needs and interests of the TAYASD and family Consider residential placement for those with more severe behavioral and developmental challenges Provide support (e.g., necessary documentation) to access local resources and funding needed to coordinate housing Implement structured activities and safety planning for the TAYASD at home
Decision-making options	Determine TAYASD's capacity to make medical, legal, financial, and other business decisions Pursue legal planning (e.g., power of attorney) to ensure family's input in medical/legal decision-making
Developmental considerations	Determine TAYASD's ability to drive Implement supports needed for transportation Evaluate TAYASD's judgment related to romantic relationships, interpersonal boundaries, social norms, and risks for victimization Review importance of medication adherence

vocational programs, living arrangements, and determination of decision-making capacities, which should be considered during the planning period facing transition-age youth with ASD (TAYASD) and their families (Table 11.1). Clinicians often receive suboptimal training in ASD during psychiatric residency and fellowship [8], and currently, there is very little research in this age group to guide their clinical practice [9, 10]. This chapter is therefore intended to review what is known about transition planning for individuals with ASD both with and without intellectual disability (ID). Information in this chapter is derived from the available literature as well as the authors' extensive experience in working with this age group. It is our hope that this chapter provides a framework for clinicians to assist patients in achieving productive and meaningful lives in adulthood.

Co-occurring Psychiatric/Behavioral Conditions

Individuals with ASD have high rates of co-occurring psychiatric conditions [11], which impact daily functioning above and beyond the core symptoms of ASD [12]. The presence of psychiatric disorders in TAYASD can impact decisions about work, postsecondary education, and independent living. Very few studies focus exclusively on the TAYASD population, and therefore most data on the prevalence and types of psychopathology in this age group are gleaned from studies of children that include older adolescents or studies of adults that include TAYASD. Research suggests that 70% of children and adolescents (up to age 18 years) [13] and 79% of adults (ages 19–79 years) with ASD have a co-occurring psychiatric disorder [2]. Although longitudinal studies are lacking, these data suggest that psychopathology in ASD appears to be prevalent in TAYASD and, as noted in the sections below, can manifest with classic or atypical presentations of DSM-based disorders [14].

Accurate diagnosis of psychiatric disorders in individuals with ASD can be challenging and requires attention to several special considerations in order to avoid overdiagnosis and unnecessary exposure to medication trials or underdiagnosis which can lead to persistent impairments. The first challenge is realizing that some TAYASD may have compromised self-report due to cognitive and language impairments associated with ASD, which can make it particularly difficult to assess internalizing symptoms, such as depression and anxiety. Second, core symptoms of ASD can overlap with those of psychiatric disorders, which can result in diagnostic overshadowing [15], whereby the clinician misattributes the patient's symptoms to ASD rather than a separate psychiatric disorder. Misdiagnosis, a second diagnostic pitfall, can also occur and refers to incorrectly attributing certain behaviors to a psychiatric disorder rather than ASD [3]. For example, symptoms of increased social withdrawal in a young adult with ASD could be attributed to their social/communication deficits, rather than an emerging depressive or social anxiety disorder. Conversely, mood lability or behavioral outbursts may lead a clinician to diagnose bipolar disorder, even though this presentation actually stems from inflexibility in routines, which is a core symptom of ASD [16].

The third factor to consider when conducting a psychiatric evaluation is that many factors can contribute to psychopathology in TAYASD including medical illness, inability to communicate, and lack of educational supports, among others. It is therefore critical that clinicians take the time to carefully query and recognize the context and precipitating factors related to emotional or behavioral symptoms. Last, it is important to remember that other psychiatric conditions can exacerbate ASD symptoms. Hence, it is important to understand the baseline profile of ASD symptoms (e.g., the individual has always been socially disinterested) and what constitutes an acute change in baseline (e.g., the individual now will not leave their room), as the latter can signal the presence of an emerging psychiatric disorder. In this regard, multi-informant collateral and handoff of any childhood psychiatric records to adult mental health providers is important, as is planning for this step in advance.

Treatment of psychiatric disorders in TAYASD requires a multidisciplinary approach that includes pharmacotherapy, psychotherapy, environmental modifications, treatment of medical conditions, and other engagements in developmentally appropriate activities. Here, it is important to remember that psychotropic medications are considered one part of the treatment of psychopathology in TAYASD. As noted below, there is a limited evidence base for the use of psychotropic medications in TAYASD, and the existing literature in children indicates high rates of side effects. Hence, decisions about medications are often based on evidence of their use in children with ASD or from typically developing (TD) adults. In each case, the risks and benefits of medications need to be weighed carefully in the context of the overall health and level of supports available for each individual.

Attention-Deficit/Hyperactivity Disorder

Until publication of the *Diagnostic and Statistical Manual of Mental Disorders-5* (DSM-5) [14], attention-deficit/hyperactivity disorder (ADHD) could not be co-diagnosed in patients with ASD, who frequently display overlapping ADHD symptomatology. ADHD is now recognized as a highly prevalent co-occurring condition in approximately 41–78% of children with ASD [13, 17]. The only known study of ADHD co-occurrence in TAYASD found a 15% prevalence rate [18]. While longitudinal studies in adults with ASD have not been published, cross-sectional data from several adult studies found varying ADHD prevalence rates (11–68%) [18–21], suggesting a prevalence similar to children with ASD. The presence of co-occurring ADHD in TAYASD has a profound effect on social functioning, communication, adaptive functioning, and executive functioning, which are all critical skills for navigating employment, relationships, and possibly independent living during the transition period. Therefore, optimizing ADHD treatment is crucial for TAYASD to improve both ADHD symptoms and overall developmental functioning [22].

Establishing an ADHD diagnosis in individuals with ASD can be challenging because symptoms of inattention, hyperactivity, emotional impulsivity, and decreased executive function can also arise from ASD [23]. For example, inattention in individuals with ASD could be due to preoccupation with internal thoughts rather than difficulties with sustained focus. Similarly, hyperactivity could reflect the need for sensory input rather than primary difficulties with motor inhibition. Guidelines for diagnosing and treating ASD have been developed in children and can be applied to TAYASD. Key principles emphasized include the importance of conducting a multi-informant assessment that includes information obtained from teachers, parents, and other providers. If ADHD-focused questionnaires, such as the Conners scale [24] and Vanderbilt scale [25], are to be used, they must be interpreted in the context of an individual's developmental level and ASD symptoms. Another important diagnostic pearl is to first rule out whether other factors could be contributing to ADHD symptoms such as medical problems, sleep disorders, or other co-occurring psychiatric conditions (e.g., anxiety). Symptoms of ADHD must also be present across two settings to support the diagnosis.

In terms of treatment, there are very few published pharmacological trials for TAYASD with ASD/ADHD. The few trials that exist in adults indicate efficacy and good tolerability in adults with ASD/ADHD [22]. Data on methylphenidate for children with ASD/ADHD indicate lower response rates (49% in children with ASD versus 69% in children without ASD) and higher rates of discontinuation due to side effects, with emotional lability (18%) being the most common reason for study dropout [26–28]. Given the limited research base and concern for potential side effects, it is recommended that physicians prescribe stimulants carefully for ADHD, starting at low doses and titrating slowly with close monitoring of side effects. Potential side effects include irritability, insomnia, and anxiety, all of which are often associated with ASD itself; thus, careful monitoring is needed to avoid aggravating any pre-existing comorbid symptoms. Non-stimulants, including guanfacine [29], clonidine [30, 31], and atomoxetine [32], have significant evidence in children with ASD/ADHD, but no published trials in adults with ASD/ADHD.

Evidence for non-pharmacological interventions in adults with ASD/ADHD is scarce. Internet-based coaching and physical exercise may be beneficial for adolescents and adults with ASD/ADHD [33, 34]. While cognitive behavioral therapy [35] and neurofeedback [36] have moderate effect size in children with ADHD without ASD, at this time they are not well-studied in patients with ASD/ADHD. Physicians and families therefore need to weigh the low likelihood of side effects with the modest evidence for treatment response.

Irritability/Aggression

Irritability can be defined as an increased proneness to anger relative to peers at the same developmental level [37]. Irritability can result in aggressive and self-injurious behaviors; in some studies, this trio of irritability, aggression, and self-injury are often clustered together and referred to as irritability/aggression (IA). Although the exact prevalence of IA in adults with ASD is unknown, rates of IA in children with ASD are significant, with up to 65% exhibiting some aggression toward parents or peers [38], 45% having high levels of angry mood and tantrums [39], and 20% having moderate to severe IA [40]. Based on one prospective study, IA does not appear to decrease in TAYASD [41] but may wane later in adulthood [42].

IA has a profound impact on daily functioning in TAYASD because it can result in behaviors that pose a danger to self and others. This constant concern about safety places tremendous stress on the family, particularly for parents who are older and have health problems. For this reason, the presence of severe IA may necessitate discussions about out-of-home placement.

IA in ASD can stem from many factors, and hence it is critical that the clinician first address potential underlying contributors [43]. Guidelines for treatment of IA emphasize the importance of evaluating five contributing factors: medical problems, functional communication deficits, psychosocial stressors, maladaptive reinforcement stressors, and co-occurring psychiatric disorders [43]. If IA is acute, medical problems are always the first to consider in the differential diagnosis. Individuals with ASD may have difficulty reporting bodily experiences, and therefore medical symptoms may lead to IA. Common conditions that can trigger IA include headaches, dental pain, constipation, upper respiratory infections, and musculoskeletal pain. Second, children with ASD often struggle with changes to daily routines or surroundings. Therefore, unexpected changes such as weather-related school closures, a substitute teacher, or even changes in one's personal appearance can trigger IA. Additionally, psychosocial stressors such as divorce, death of a loved one, or new members in the household can contribute to IA. Operant factors are also important to consider, including the desire to escape from a non-preferred activity, engage in a preferred activity (such as screen time), gain attention, self-stimulate, or attain other goals. Simultaneous, multifactorial etiologies can often contribute to IA. Explaining this formulation to the family can enable their engagement in developing an individualized multidisciplinary treatment plan. Safety monitoring throughout the process is critical.

Once underlying precipitators have been addressed, the next step in treatment for IA due to operant factors is behavioral therapy [43–45]. This includes applied behavioral analysis (ABA) and ABA-derived behavioral modification interventions designed to identify the function of problem behaviors and reinforce more appropriate behaviors through intense practice. While ABA in ASD is often thought of as only for young children, ABA can also be prescribed for older individuals with ASD to target maladaptive behaviors, adaptive functioning, and core ASD symptoms [46]. ABA and ABA-based therapies can be intensive and costly. Clinicians may therefore need to advocate (e.g., write letters to insurance companies) on behalf of their patients in order to secure access to these services.

When behavioral therapies alone do not result in substantial improvement, psychotropic medications should be considered (see guidelines put forth by Fung et al. [47]). Risperidone and aripiprazole are both US Food and Drug Administration (FDA)-approved medications for the treatment of irritability in children with ASD ages 6–17 years and have moderate to large effect sizes [47]. These medications, however, are associated with significant weight gain in both short- and longer-term trials (e.g. risperidone and aripiprazole caused a 1.6 kg and 1.1 kg weight gain in short-term studies up to a maximum of 8 weeks, respectively) [47]. Therefore, their use requires careful consideration in individuals with ASD who have pre-existing obesity and metabolic problems [48]. Other first- and second-line antipsychotic medications can also be considered for the treatment of IA although formal studies in TAYASD have not been conducted. Similarly, stimulants, alpha-agonists, mood stabilizers, and N-acetylcysteine (NAC) could also be considered for the treatment of IA. Given the scarcity of evidence for pharmacological treatment of IA in TAYASD, physicians should use medications judiciously and only after detailed review with the family of the limited data on risks and benefits. Close follow-up is required to establish any signs of improvement and potential adverse effects, and such monitoring is also key for avoiding unnecessary polypharmacy.

Anxiety and Obsessive-Compulsive Disorders

Anxiety disorders are one of the most common co-occurring conditions in ASD. A meta-analysis of studies of adults with ASD indicates that the current and lifetime prevalence of any anxiety disorder was 27% and 42%, respectively [49]. These studies included adults with and without ID who were assessed in community and clinical settings; most studies relied on self-report except when ID was present, in which case clinician interviews were conducted to ascertain diagnosis. This prevalence of anxiety disorders in adults with ASD is considerably higher than in adults in the general population, which is estimated to be between 1% and 12% [50]. Precise reasons for this heightened prevalence of anxiety disorders in adults with ASD remain unknown; however, preliminary data indicate that younger age and greater ASD severity may confer increased risk [2].

A wide variety of anxiety disorders can present in adults with ASD, with specific phobia and social anxiety disorder being the most common current disorders and generalized anxiety disorder and specific phobia being the most common lifetime disorders [49]. Other disorders that can manifest in this population include separation anxiety, panic disorder, agoraphobia, and post-traumatic stress disorder, although these are less prevalent. Finally, obsessive-compulsive disorder has been reported in adults with ASD with evidence showing that individuals with ASD exhibit the same types of compulsions as TD individuals (e.g., cleaning, checking, hoarding, ordering).

Diagnosing anxiety in individuals with ASD requires careful attention to two factors. First, it is important to assess an individual's self-report capacity of fear and worry, which can vary according to developmental level. Some individuals with ASD are self-aware of their emotions and can report worry and internalizing experiences [51]. When self-report capacity is compromised, however, behavioral information from sources such as parents, teachers, employers, or loved ones is needed to establish an anxiety disorder diagnosis. Signs of anxiety can include irritability, aggression, fearful affect, avoidance of the anxiety-provoking stimulus, withdrawal, and sleep disturbances [52, 53]. Another factor to consider in the evaluation process is the overlapping symptomatology between anxiety and ASD [54]. Symptoms such as social avoidance, poor eye contact, and need for sameness can be features of both anxiety and ASD. Repetitive behaviors are also common to both anxiety and obsessive-compulsive disorder (OCD). An increase in severity of these overlapping symptoms can suggest the presence of an anxiety disorder. One particular disorder that deserves close attention in the diagnostic process is OCD, which can be difficult to diagnose, as obsessions are hard to elicit in individuals with ASD. Some caregivers may express concern that preoccupation with overfocused interests, which are a sign of ASD, are obsessions. Education about the egodystonic nature of obsessions versus the egosyntonic nature of overfocused interests is therefore important [55]. Repetitive behaviors are likely compulsions when they appear ego dystonic and have an anxious quality (i.e., the individual appears distressed until the compulsion has been completed) and anticipatory anxiety prior to the compulsion is present [64]. Repetitive behaviors in ASD, in contrast, are pleasurable and not associated with anticipatory anxiety, but may cause disruption if interrupted. Uncontrolled worry due to stressors, which also has a repetitive quality, is more consistent with anxiety versus the repetitive behaviors in ASD.

Case Vignette 1 *Peter graduated high school and within 1 year obtained a job at a manufacturing plant. His duties included working a specific section of the products as they passed through the assembly line. Peter was performing at a high level for several months, until the procedure at his workstation was altered significantly. He struggled to accommodate to the new procedure and began to fall behind on his work, resulting in a slowdown for the entire assembly line. Peter received some modest support from his employer, but he developed significant anxiety about his competence on the job, fearing he would fall behind and get fired. He worried excessively about his ability to live independently and be successful in relationships, always feeling that he would never be good enough. After several weeks of experiencing persistent job anxiety, Peter decided to quit his job and has not worked since. His parents are very eager for him to find another job soon, but he is demoralized and does not want to fail again.*

As seen in the above vignette, anxiety disorders have a profound impact on a young adult's ability to socialize, develop mature relationships, and be successful at work or in day programs. Promptly recognizing and treating these conditions is therefore imperative. Research on psychotherapies for anxiety in adults with ASD is slowly growing and has primarily focused on treatments for individuals with average or above-average cognitive functioning [56]. These data indicate that modified cognitive behavioral therapy, which refers to therapies that focus more heavily on behavioral exposures and relaxation versus cognitive restructuring, may be helpful for some adults with ASD [57–59]. In Peter's case, modified cognitive behavior therapy could be implemented to decrease his anticipatory anxiety about falling behind during his workday. Mindfulness-based interventions also show promise and provide symptom relief through guided meditation and focus on awareness of emotions and bodily sensations without active efforts to reduce symptoms [60]. Research on treatments for anxiety in TAYASD with ID are lagging; however, findings from case studies indicate that behaviorally-based interventions including exposure therapies combined with modeling and behavioral reinforcement may be effective [61–63].

Few psychotropic medication trials for anxiety have been conducted in the ASD population. Medication choices are therefore based on evidence in TD children and adults. SSRIs, which have proven efficacy in TD individuals, can be tried in individuals with ASD, particularly if anxiety is severe and psychotherapy is ineffective or unavailable [64]. Titrating slowly and close monitoring of side effects is warranted given data on high rates of SSRI-induced behavioral activation in the ASD population [65]. Medications to address specific anxiety symptoms can also be used, including alpha-agonists for hyperarousal, melatonin for sleep problems, and, if necessary, atypical antipsychotics for severe behavioral disturbances that are triggered by anxiety [66].

Mood Disorders

Major Depressive Disorder

Patients with ASD are four times more likely to develop major depressive disorder (MDD) in their lifetime compared to TD individuals [67]. MDD impacts an estimated 26–70% of adults with ASD [21, 68, 69] and is associated with increased rates of suicidal ideation and attempts compared to TD individuals [70, 71]. While studies of risk factors for suicide in adults with ASD are limited, data in children and adolescents indicate that lower ASD severity and average to above-average cognitive functioning can increase risk for depressive symptoms and suicidality [67, 71, 72]. One reason for these findings may be that individuals with higher cognitive functioning are potentially more aware of their disability [73] and may be interested in friendships but feel socially isolated. Other identified risk factors for depression are similar to those in TD adults, i.e., a family history of depression, recent losses, or family stressors [72].

Individuals with ASD can exhibit the typical syndrome of MDD as defined by the DSM-5 diagnostic criteria [14]. Some individuals are capable of reporting low mood and anhedonia, and therefore it is important to ask these questions. Behavioral symptoms such as avoidance of activities can also signal a depressive episode in patients with ASD. In some cases, including in individuals with ID, atypical presentations of depression have been reported. These symptoms include increased irritability and aggression, self-injury, increased social isolation, and a regression in adaptive skills such as personal hygiene [70, 74].

Diagnosing MDD can be challenging because of similarities in symptom presentations between MDD and ASD. For example, isolative behaviors and blunted affect may be attributed to core ASD symptoms rather than depression. Similarly, diminished appetite and poor sleep may be attributed to food selectivity and primary insomnia, respectively, which are both common in individuals with ASD who do not have a depressive disorder.

In patients with ASD, rates of suicidal ideation are up to nine times that of the general population, with increased risk for suicide attempts [21, 69, 75, 76] and use of lethal means to attempt suicide [77]. One study of adults with ASD presenting to a specialty diagnostic clinic found that 66% reported suicidal ideation, plan, or attempt [75]. Loneliness and lack of social supports are major risk factors for both major depressive disorder and suicidal ideation [69]. In adults with ASD, unmet social needs, non-suicidal self-injury, and social camouflaging, the latter defined as the use of strategies by autistic individuals to minimize the visibility of their autism in social situations [78], are associated with suicidality [79]. Suicidality is therefore a crucial area of assessment and intervention in the care of TAYASD.

Case Vignette 2 *Tammy is a 24-year-old woman with ASD and moderate ID. She graduated from a public high school with a certificate of attendance at age 21 years and currently lives with her parents who are in their early 60 years of age. Tammy has some interest in being with others but struggles with reciprocal relationships. She often blurts out inappropriate statements or engages in perseverate self-talk. She is very preoccupied with animals, particularly dogs. Since completing high school, Tammy has struggled to make friends and is quite isolated socially. Her parents have noticed that she is increasingly irritable and reactive when events do not go as expected. Tammy seems more distracted in recent months and has had more trouble keeping up with aspects of her self-care routine, including bathing. She sleeps after coming home from her day program and does not want to join her parents on weekend outings, which she previously enjoyed. Her self-talk has decreased, and she seems less interested in dogs. Recently, her verbalizations are often dwelling on animals dying.*

In the case above, Tammy's depressive episode may be triggered by difficulty adapting to life after high school and having fewer structured opportunities to engage in activities that can provide enjoyment and a possible source of friends. Her depressive symptoms should be treated using either individual or group therapy or a combination of modalities. Tammy is also a good candidate for a half-day community college program where she can participate in life skills workshops, community service, and physical activity (e.g., dance class). This could alleviate her social isolation, a major risk factor for depressive symptoms in adults with ASD. Antidepressant medication may be considered, although evidence for adults with ASD and MDD is limited.

Research on psychotherapy for depression in adults with ASD is limited but slowly growing. Group cognitive behavioral therapy (CBT) can be useful for depressive symptoms in high-functioning TAYASD [57]. Preliminary evidence suggests that social skills training and vocational training could also be potentially effective in decreasing depressive symptoms in young adults with ASD [80].

There is limited evidence investigating the efficacy and safety of antidepressant medication in adults with ASD [81]. Some studies suggest that anti-depressant medication may cause irritability or even exacerbate core symptoms of ASD [82]. Clinicians should therefore use caution when prescribing antidepressants for MDD in adults with ASD.

Brain stimulation, including repetitive transcranial magnetic stimulation (rTMS) and electroconvulsive therapy (ECT) may also be an option for TAYASD with MDD, since these treatments have both been cleared by the FDA for adults. Preliminary evidence indicates that rTMS is feasible and well tolerated in depressed adults with ASD [83], although more definitive trials are needed to establish efficacy.

Bipolar Disorder

Patients with ASD also have an elevated risk for bipolar disorder, which has a point prevalence of approximately 6–9% in adults with ASD [19, 68] and an estimated lifetime prevalence of 20% or more [19, 84]. As in TD individuals, the core features of mania, including decreased need for sleep with resulting increased goal-directed and/or pleasurable activities with risky consequences, are required for diagnosis of bipolar disorder (BD) and ASD. Compared to youth with BD alone, youth with bipolar disorder and ASD (BD/ASD) more frequently present with distractibility, racing thoughts, depressed mood, social withdrawal, and a lack of improved mood in response to pleasant activities [85]. Patients with BD/ASD are also less likely to exhibit euphoric mood and more likely to appear irritable, anxious, and agitated while in a manic state [84].

ASD and bipolar disorder can be very challenging to differentiate, as ASD can overshadow symptoms of bipolar disorder. For example, episodes of irritability, insomnia, impulsivity, or other manic symptoms consistent with bipolar disorder may be inaccurately attributed to ASD. Conversely, patients with ASD exhibiting intermittent irritability triggered by changes in routine may be incorrectly diagnosed with bipolar disorder [3]. Clinicians can differentiate ASD from bipolar disorder by keeping in mind that apparent mood symptoms stemming from ASD are likely to be chronic, while those attributable to bipolar disorder are episodic [3]. Gathering a thorough family history can be highly informative, as relatives of patients with BD/ASD have significant elevated prevalence of BD.

Non-pharmacological interventions, including individual therapy and family therapy are logical approaches, given the minimal risk of harm, but studies on non-pharmacological treatment of BD/ASD are lacking. From a pharmacological standpoint, there are no controlled trials for adults with BD/ASD. It is reasonable for clinicians to use medications that have been shown to be effective in case series and open trials for BD/ASD, including risperidone, aripiprazole, and mood stabilizers [84]. Antidepressants may be effective in treating depressive episodes in patients with BD/ASD, but carry a high risk of activation and/or manic switch [81, 82, 84], and therefore warrant cautious usage in collaboration with the family and other providers.

Schizophrenia/Psychotic Disorders

Schizophrenia (SCZ), a disorder which most commonly emerges in adolescence and young adulthood, has a prevalence of approximately 1% in the general population [86]. Cohort studies of children with childhood onset schizophrenia (COS), which is highly rare (estimated prevalence of 1 in 40,000) [87], have shown that 28–55% children with COS have a pre-existing or co-occurring ASD diagnosis. A recent meta-analysis involving almost 15,000 individuals with ASD indicated that SCZ occurs in an estimated 3–4% of individuals with ASD [88]. Another recent meta-analysis of studies of adults with ASD and average IQ showed a pooled prevalence of 6.4% for schizophrenia spectrum disorders, which includes SCZ as well as schizophreniform disorder, schizoaffective disorder, and schizotypal personality disorder [89].

The assessment of SCZ in ASD is complicated by the phenotypic overlap of these neurodevelopmental disorders, which also share some common genetic risk factors and underlying neurobiology [90]. Both ASD and SCZ are associated with social cognitive deficits, social withdrawal, impaired emotional expression and recognition, executive function deficits, and elements of thought disorder [91–94]. Additionally, correlations between ASD and schizotypal traits (e.g., paranoid thinking, constricted affect, atypical speech, and eccentricities) have been observed in individuals with ASD [95] as well as in nonclinical control populations [96]. These behavioral similarities increase the likelihood of both diagnostic overshadowing and misdiagnosis. For example, in the case of diagnostic overshadowing, psychosis in an individual with ASD could be missed due to misattributing social withdrawal, paranoid ideation regarding others, responding to internal stimuli, and disorganized speech to core ASD-related social communication deficits or because descriptions suggestive of hallucinations are misattributed to sensory atypicality. The same set of symptoms could alternatively lead to misdiagnosis if unusual social behavior, including perseverative self-talk and sensory experiences representative of ASD, are misconstrued as a separate psychotic disorder.

To differentiate psychotic symptoms from manifestations of core ASD symptoms in TAYASD, it is critical to understand an individual's functional baseline by obtaining a thorough and careful developmental history that clarifies the TAYASD's level of cognition and adaptive functioning. The clinician should also inquire about any deviations from baseline and, whenever possible, gather information through collateral sources. Longitudinal mental status examinations are also helpful, as well as repeat neuropsychological testing if cognitive decline is suspected. Of note, lower baseline verbal function has been associated with features suggestive of thought disorder [97], and functional decline, i.e., regression in adaptive, social, and communication skills, has been noted to precede the emergence of psychosis in adults with ASD [98]. Evaluating the progression and context of any behaviors concerning for psychosis, i.e., whether such behaviors reflect emotional or sensory reactivity secondary to ASD, new and acutely progressing psychotic symptoms, or another emerging diagnosis (e.g., mood disorder), is also important for diagnostic clarification. A stable behavioral pattern featuring preoccupation with unusual ideas, perseverative self-talk, and concrete speech, with exacerbation of these behaviors in the context of transitions or changes in routine, would be more consistent with ASD than psychosis [99]. However, new onset or rapid escalation of these behaviors, associated with increasing agitation, vague or illogical speech, impaired reality testing, and cognitive decline, would be more concerning for a schizophrenia spectrum condition. The development of negative symptoms is another possible presentation, with some work reporting this may be more common in individuals with ID [100].

The use of atypical antipsychotics, the mainstay of current treatment in SCZ, has not been examined empirically in individuals with ASD and SCZ, although these medications are commonly used in clinical practice. Some literature has noted concerns for a greater likelihood of suboptimal response to antipsychotics in individuals with psychosis and ASD, including an increased risk of motor side effects in adults with SCZ and ASD [101] and multiple antipsychotic treatment failures in first-episode psychosis among children and adolescents with ASD [102, 103]. Psychotherapeutic interventions for SCZ spectrum conditions, such as CBT, have also not been formally tested in individuals with ASD and SCZ spectrum disorders, although it is reasonable to consider these interventions in TAYASD, as increasing evidence supports the effectiveness of modified CBT in individuals with ASD and anxiety and depression [104]. Generally, practitioners should recognize the increased likelihood of SCZ spectrum conditions in TAYASD versus the general population and that characterizing the patient's baseline, including the period prior to adulthood, will be key for diagnostic clarification and assessing treatment response.

Substance Abuse Disorders

Substance use disorder (SUD) has recently started to receive increased recognition and attention in the ASD population. The prevalence of co-occurring SUD in ASD (SUD/ASD) has been estimated to range from 0.7% to 36% based on the few studies that exist. The largest study, which reviewed nearly 27,000 individuals with ASD, found a prevalence of approximately 4% [105] and a twofold elevation in risk compared to TD individuals [105]. Similar to data in TD individuals, adults with SUD/ASD have a high prevalence of psychiatric comorbidities including anxiety, depression, and ADHD; these conditions are independently associated with higher rates of SUD [105, 106]. Other risk factors for SUD include social isolation, reduced insight secondary to theory of mind deficits, lack of motivation in the context of impaired executive functioning, and a sense of feeling overwhelmed by emotions [107]. Despite these risk factors, clinicians may overlook SUD while focusing on other clinical symptoms associated with ASD [108].

Research is needed to establish treatment recommendations that are customized for TAYASD with SUD [106].Treatment of SUD/ASD can be particularly challenging, since patients with ASD may not be amenable to traditional interventions, such as group therapy and 12-step interventions. Barriers may include social communication difficulties, diminished capacity for motivation and insight, and other obstacles to treatment engagement, e.g., social anxiety symptoms that may interfere with participation in group therapy [108]. Reviewing objective facts about the patient's substance use and criteria for SUD in concrete language, such as the number of alcoholic beverages used per occasion or the number of days per week using other substances, during sessions can be beneficial [108]. Depending on the patient's communication abilities, parents or family members can be immensely important in gathering a history [105, 109]. Extra care should be taken to identify emotional or physiological triggers for SUD [108], keeping in mind how these are related to stress reactivity in the context of ASD. These patients may require more tangible reinforcers in order to stay abstinent [108], and finding healthier peers who are less likely to expose the TAYASD to substance use can be a significant help to overcoming SUD in patients with ASD. Individuals with SUD/ASD may require more supervision and monitoring of activities by family members in order to maximize the chances of recovery from SUD. Preliminary evidence suggests that modified CBT can be effective in the treatment of adults with SUD/ASD [110]. The field of SUD/ASD is just emerging, and more comprehensive and customized treatment options are needed.

Sleep Disorders

Patients with ASD are at significant risk for sleep disorders across the lifespan [111–114]. Forty to 80% of children and adolescents with ASD suffer from sleep problems, particularly insomnia, a higher rate than TD children [115]. Up to 80% of adults with ASD have sleep problems [116], including insomnia, low sleep efficiency, short sleep duration, long sleep latency, frequent nighttime awakenings, poorer refreshment scores on awakening, and daytime sleepiness [111, 113, 117, 118].

Sleep disorders can have a cascading effect on core ASD symptoms [117] and other comorbid conditions in patients of all ages. In children with ASD, sleep problems are associated with behavioral problems, social and cognitive difficulties, and increased parental stress [119–121]. In adults with ASD, sleep problems are one of the most important predictors of quality of life [122]. Risk factors for insomnia in children with ASD include ASD symptom severity, gastrointestinal problems, sensory sensitivities, epilepsy, depression, and anxiety [123–126]. Social, school, and vocational challenges, along with sensory sensitivities, can all contribute to the risk of insomnia in adults with ASD, as the lack of daily social interactions, school or work routines, and avoidance of bright light can disrupt circadian rhythms [127–129]. Furthermore, core ASD symptoms and sleep problems appear to impact one another in a bidirectional manner, as ASD symptoms can cause and exacerbate sleep problems, while sleep problems can exacerbate ASD symptom severity [130].

When evaluating and treating sleep problems in ASD, clinicians should use a multidisciplinary approach. A comprehensive assessment is recommended including a sleep log and actigraphy, the latter being a recording of activity via a wearable device while awake and/or asleep [131]. Cognitive behavioral therapy is the first-line treatment for insomnia in patients with ASD [132]. Research on pharmacological treatments for sleep in adults with ASD is limited. Melatonin can be combined with behavioral therapy [132] or used alone and appears to be very well tolerated, with minimal, if any, side effects in children and adults with ASD [133, 134]. In children with ASD, numerous studies have demonstrated that exogenous melatonin given at bedtime leads to improved sleep and decreased ASD severity [126]. For children needing to advance timing of sleep onset, low doses (300 μg) of melatonin given 3–5 hours before bedtime can be used as a chronobiotic [135]. Although melatonin has not been studied sufficiently in adults [136], available evidence of its benefit and tolerability make it a reasonable adjunct to a multidisciplinary treatment approach [134].

Co-occurring Medical Conditions

Individuals with ASD have higher rates of medical morbidity and mortality and a life expectancy 16 years shorter than TD individuals [4, 137–140]. Reasons for this disparity may include differential funding of child and adult services, differing eligibility criteria for care, and limited awareness of adult neurodevelopmental disorders [141]. Medical problems are often underrecognized in individuals with ASD, particularly those with limited communication abilities, and as such can present as a worsening of ASD symptoms or new onset anxiety, irritability, and behavioral problems. For example, problems such as dental pain, constipation, and headaches can manifest as irritability and aggression. It is therefore especially important for clinicians to assess for medical problems when there is a sudden change in behavior in an individual with ASD.

Chronic medical conditions occurring at higher rates in patients with ASD include epilepsy, obesity, hypertension, diabetes mellitus, inflammatory bowel disease, and numerous others. It is therefore immensely important for the family to find an adult primary care physician (PCP) who can assess for and manage medical problems in close collaboration with the psychiatrist. Evaluation of TAYASD in the transition to an adult provider should include a full medical history, physical examination, and consideration of known genetic associations with ASD [141], which may be useful for informing risk for co-occurring conditions and family planning [142].

Physicians should also be aware of medication-induced medical sequelae. A significant number (60%) of adolescents and adults with ASD take psychotropic medications, with antipsychotics being the most commonly prescribed medication class (39%) [143]. Antipsychotics pose significant risks for metabolic syndrome and/or extrapyramidal side effects, a particular concern for younger adults who potentially accumulate risk of side effects over many years. It is therefore important for clinicians to provide informed consent, continuously weigh the risks and benefits of medications, and consider tapering medications if symptoms have remitted.

Psychosocial Planning for Transition Age Youth with Autism Spectrum Disorder

Planning for Socialization

Social deficits are a major challenge facing individuals with ASD of any age. They are particularly impactful when an individual with ASD is interested in friendships but unsuccessful in having friends [144]. These deficits tend to become more apparent during adolescence [145] and adulthood [146] as social demands increase at this stage of life, e.g., in terms of recognizing and following more sophisticated social conventions or interacting in situations that entail more accountability. Major life events such as prom and high school graduation, which are symbolic of growing independence in TD individuals, can be extremely stressful or avoided altogether by TAYASD. Bullying, either overtly or exclusionary, can peak during adolescence and also carry over into adulthood [147, 148]. Experiences of bullying can contribute to social isolation in late adolescence and early adulthood, which can in turn compromise psychological and adaptive functioning.

Case Vignette 3 *Thomas is a 17-year-old male who is in 11th grade. He was diagnosed with ASD at age 4 years. Thomas is verbal, with intellectual functioning in the average range. He attends mostly general education classes at school, with two class periods each day in a self-contained/resource classroom. Thomas has expressed interest in friends; however, he has virtually no friends at school, and he mostly keeps to himself during recess and lunch time, preferring to draw quietly alone rather than interact with peers. Thomas reports that he can feel overwhelmed in social gatherings due to the noise level and how close people stand to each other. He also reports feeling confused about what to say when talking to other teenagers. Thomas has a diagnosis of ADHD which has responded well to stimulants without complication. Thomas has recently articulated that he wants to go the Junior Prom at school, but "he doesn't know how to go the prom." His mother notes that there are some major obstacles, including Thomas's lack of a date or friends to accompany him to the event and that he has no information about any pre- or post-prom events.*

For TAYASD such as Thomas, who are motivated to have friendships, social skills training (SST) can be effective in treating social and communication deficits, enhancing adaptive functioning, and decreasing social anxiety [149–152]. For example, the UCLA Program for Education and Enrichment of Relational Skills (PEERS®) program is a well-studied form of SST for 12- to 24-year-olds with ASD utilizing a standardized, published treatment protocol and parent coaching. Research on PEERS has shown improvement in social skills, social anxiety, and feelings of parental effectiveness, with gains lasting as long as 5 years posttreatment and generalizing outside the clinical setting [149, 151].

SST focuses on making and keeping friends by teaching basic social and conversational skills, finding common interests with peers through the exchange of information, and frequent practice of emerging social skills through social get-togethers. One mainstay of SST for TAYASD is joining peer activities, such as sports teams, video game clubs, or robotics teams. With encouragement through SST, a TAYASD may find and join clubs of interest (e.g., Dungeons and Dragons role playing game, anime) to enjoy an activity while simultaneously establishing peer connections. In the case of Thomas, SST could help him find a friend group, ask a date to the prom, and successfully navigate the prom event itself. When local social skills groups are unavailable, clinicians are advised to encourage TAYASD to increase and maintain their engagement with peers who have common interests.

The use of electronic screen media (ESM) is an important topic for TAYASD. Data shows that children with ASD spend more time on ESM than TD peers [153, 154] and have difficulty disengaging from ESM. Social skills deficits cause youth with ASD to be vulnerable to cyberbullying and social isolation while online [155]. Most youth with ASD do not use ESM in a social way, preferring to play video games alone or with strangers online [156]. This pattern begins during childhood and continues into adulthood. Data shows that individuals with ASD appear more engaged and motivated when using ESM [157]. This affinity for ESM makes technology a potentially powerful interventional tool for TAYASD. While data show that ESM poses some risks and challenges, target symptoms in ASD, including social skills, executive functioning skills, academic skills, and even restricted/repetitive behaviors, can be positively impacted by technology-based interventions [155].

There are no evidence-based medications targeting social and communication deficits in patients with ASD. Several agents such as intranasal oxytocin, memantine, and intranasal vasopressin have demonstrated potential in treating social skills deficits in patients with ASD, but require further study [158–160]. Overall, although social deficits make up a significant portion of core ASD symptoms, evidence-based treatments are currently quite limited, and no proven biological treatments exist.

Planning for Postsecondary Education

Although transition planning for postsecondary education ideally begins years before the end of high school, the coordination of educational goals continues through adulthood [161]. TAYASD have several postsecondary education options including traditional college programs, specialized transitional college programs geared for students with ASD, and vocational or technical school. For individuals requiring more hands-on supervision, such as those with ID, ongoing education may be pursued through day programs or job training in a supportive employment setting. Effective transition plans should reflect the TAYASD's cognitive level, unique interests, current skills, and areas for growth, to ensure that the TAYASD participates in an educational environment that is a good fit for their abilities and needs. Prior academic experiences (e.g., general education settings or homeschooling) and current levels of academic and adaptive functioning are thus important factors to consider in the planning process [162].

IEPs are common (but not necessarily universal) among TAYASD and provide an important platform for transition planning. Under the Individuals with Disabilities Education Act [7], part of the IEP includes creating a transition plan by the age of 16 years, as well as annual review of this plan until the end of high school, which for TAYASD with IEPs may continue through the age of 21 years. The transition plan is created based on a review of the student's current performance, use of services, community experiences, and objectives for employment or other aspects of postsecondary living, with the aim of aligning schooling with the student's goals and aspirations [163]. TAYASD require updated developmental evaluations to inform the transition plan. This includes neuropsychological testing of cognition and adaptive function, vocational assessments, and if necessary physical therapy, occupational therapy, or speech therapy evaluations for students with ongoing deficits in these areas. Transition planning under an IEP should ensure that coursework fulfills college prerequisites for a TAYASD who is college-bound, and document eligibility for programs designed for TAYASD requiring more extensive support. The TAYASD's active participation in transition planning should be strongly encouraged to enhance self-advocacy skills and self-determination as part of evidence-based practice [164].

For TAYASD without an IEP, there is a need for greater initiative and resourcefulness to identify appropriate postsecondary programs and resources, as well as to collect any necessary documentation of eligibility. In these cases, clinicians can recommend transition practices that have been linked to greater likelihood for postsecondary success, such as inclusion in general education settings, paid work experience while in school, training in self-care and independent living skills, and family and peer social support [165]. Clinicians can direct TAYASD and their families to several online transition planning toolkits that are available from organizations including agencies focused on ASD, such as Autism Speaks, as well as governmental agencies including the US Department of Education and the Office of Disability Employment [166–168]. Clinicians should also be prepared to provide documentation supporting the TAYASD's disability and recommended supports or accommodations.

College and vocational training are frequent choices among TAYASD. In one study of data from the National Longitudinal Transition Study-2 (NTLS-2) [169], 6 years post-high school, 28.0% and 12.1% of TAYASD had attended a 2- or 4-year college, respectively, and 9.3% had attended a technical school. For TAYASD with comorbid ID, some states have "Transition Postsecondary Education Programs for Students with Intellectual Disabilities," through which students may engage in educational and social experiences within the college environment. In some cases, students may have options for course credit, to promote inclusion and increased employment opportunities.

Figure 11.1 illustrates the various factors to consider when selecting a postsecondary school. Factors such as program location and duration strongly influence the degree of adjustment required as part of the college transition. The absence of local family support and longer, more intensive degree programs demand more maturity, persistence, and flexibility from the TAYASD. Local community college offers the advantages of exposure to college-level coursework, greater access to family support, and reduced educational expenses. According to data from the NTLS-2, 2-year college programs were more commonly attended by TAYASD than 4-year programs [167]. The level of institutional support for disabilities is also a key consideration, since this may vary across institutions. After high school, educational accommodations within institutions receiving federal funding are no longer regulated under IDEA, but rather under the less well-specified guidelines of the Americans with Disabilities Act [170] and Section 504 of the Rehabilitation Act of 1973 [171]. TAYASD must therefore self-identify to the school's office of disability services to establish eligibility for accommodations. This is a potential barrier, as described below.

Case Vignette 4 *Sandra is a 19-year-old female with ASD and social anxiety disorder. In high school, she had a 504 plan and demonstrated consistently strong academic performance. Sandra is enrolled in full-time in a 4-year college and is taking 12 credit hours during her first semester. She considered letting her college know about accommodations she received under her prior 504 plan, but because she previously had good grades and was nervous about self-disclosing her diagnosis, she decided not to pursue accommodations. One of her classes was a marketing class in which the entire grade for the course was based on a small group project that required working with four other students. As the*

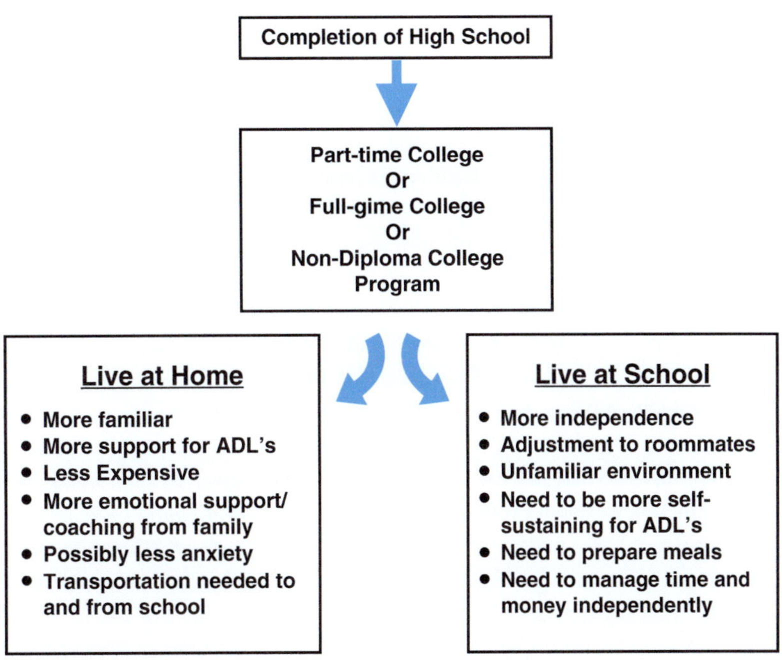

Fig. 11.1 Diagram illustrating challenges of living at home versus living at school for transition-age youth with ASD who take college classes

other students all formed groups, Sandra was embarrassed that no one chose her to be in their group. She hesitated to reach out to her professor because she felt like an outcast for not being selected. As the semester progressed, Sandra realized that she was inevitably going to fail her marketing class and became increasingly anxious and depressed. Her performance in other classes suffered. Sandra ultimately failed the marketing course and multiple other courses that semester. She withdrew from school and has not returned in 2 years since.

College students with ASD have been reported to feel confident academically [172], but those with additional diagnoses are at risk for poor psychological outcomes [173]. College coursework is generally more complex and time-consuming. Co-occurring ADHD or executive function deficits associated with ASD may compromise TAYASD's time management, leading to falling behind and feeling overwhelmed. Social communication deficits associated with ASD can make it challenging to interact effectively with professors or negotiate group assignments [174, 175]. In Sandra's case, informing her school's Office of Disability Services about her diagnosis could have facilitated accommodations like promoting communication with professors, more distributed pacing of her coursework, and assistance with finding a study group. Sandra would have benefited from hands-on guidance, ideally before college, about the process for obtaining accommodations. She also could have learned how to effectively communicate with her school's disability services office, and process with family and clinicians any distress associated with disclosing her learning needs. Sandra's story also illustrates the importance of continuing mental health care during the transition process [176]. By regularly discussing self-advocacy, problem-solving, and resources as part of clinical care, providers can guide TAYASD in obtaining the services needed to manage setbacks during the postsecondary transition.

Vocational Options

Adults with ASD have very low rates of employment, with only 55% holding paid jobs during the first 6 years after high school [169]. This is due to a wide range of challenges, including intellectual and functional impairment, organizational and motivational difficulties, difficulty coping with the interview process, and lack of on-site job coaching. It is important for the clinician and family to bear in mind that a job need not be long-term to be a positive experience for TAYASD. As with educational options, it is important for the TAYASD to consider factors that promote a good fit when seeking employment. These include not only the type of job, for example, a clerical or manual job, but also the day-to-day pace, total number of hours, physical environment, and task complexity. Features such as the physical setting (e.g., indoors and climate-controlled or outdoors with varying temperature), the social demands (e.g., people-intensive, such as a cashier, or more independent, such as filing books at the local library), and the extent to which duties are straightforward or repetitive versus multistep and administrative (e.g., data entry versus project coordinator) can influence the TAYASD's likelihood of success. Most importantly, the TAYASD should be aware of how much support geared to adults with ASD will be available in the work environment. Many of the social communication deficits that are at the core of ASD can potentially alienate TAYASD from work teams, requiring significant coaching and education of the other employees.

Case Vignette 5 *David is a 20-year-old male who recently started working at a radio station. His work includes event planning and marketing for the station. David has been performing well overall at his job, although he often requires redirection from his supervisors in order to stay on task and complete projects. David is well-liked by everyone at the radio station and brings a cheerful attitude to work each day. David struggles with social boundaries. Sometimes, he will ask co-workers about personal information that is not welcomed or appropriate. One day, David interrupted a large team meeting to tell a co-worker that he had romantic feelings for her in front of the entire group. Feeling embarrassed, David's co-worker immediately left the room. It took several months for David to understand the inappropriate nature and timing of his comments. David* *was ultimately able to keep his job and is now on good terms with the female co-worker he had previously embarrassed. Without the coaching, support, and redirection available to him in this work setting, David would otherwise have likely been dismissed. David has steadily learned appropriate boundaries in the work setting and has even started to mentor other peers in this area.*

As illustrated in David's example, successful vocational approaches offer support for TAYASD, where they are given feedback, coaching, and opportunities to practice emerging skills in an environment that is autism friendly. There are numerous local programs that offer vocational training for TAYASD that have used this model successfully. One national program, the nonPareil Institute (npitx.org), provides work opportunities for adults with ASD to build digital products such as video games. Several online listings of disability-friendly employers, including from the US Department of Labor's Office of Disability Employment Policy (www.dol.gov), are also available.

Living Arrangements

The majority of adults with ASD live either with their family of origin (47%) or in a group home (27%) [177]. Only approximately 9% live independently without support [177]. The family's decision regarding whether the TAYASD will live at home or away from family is a crucial one and is based on the patient's functional skills, financial resources, and the ability of family members to provide in-home support for the patient. Significant challenging behaviors, such as IA, elopement, and severe impulsivity, may lead to safety risks, particularly as the TAYASD's parents are aging. Residential placement may be a consideration in this case. Many residential homes are associated with vocational programs, which can be beneficial.

One complex aspect of residential placement is availability. Obtaining placement in a residential facility can be an arduous and time-consuming task, taking up to a year or even longer, even in cases of severe and dangerous behaviors. Therefore, if a family is considering residential placement, starting the application process early and involving a case manager or care coordinator are paramount. In the event of a critical need, involving a state or county case worker with the disabilities board can help expedite placement. Even for acute cases requiring hospitalization, the patient is not likely to be maintained on an inpatient psychiatric unit indefinitely pending placement, since insurance carriers are likely to deny funding for an extended inpatient stay. This underscores the importance of advanced planning for residential placement.

If a TAYASD is transitioned to residential placement, it is important to clarify who will be making medical decisions on behalf of the patient. In most cases of residential placement, the family will maintain medical decision-making power given the TAYASD's higher need for support. With respect to the treatment plan in residential care, the wishes of the family must be balanced with the safety needs of the staff and other patients within the facility. For example, families may wish to minimize their loved one's psychotropic medication dosages, whereas residential home staff note aggression that has been refractory to behavioral interventions. This is an opportunity for the psychiatrist to help build a consensus between the family and the residential facility staff and to adjust psychotropic medications to maximize benefit and minimize adverse side effects. Reminding all parties of the common goal to maximize the patient's quality of life, by combining behavioral interventions and psychotropics, is a reasonable first step for the psychiatrist during treatment team discussions.

Decision-Making

When a youth with ASD turns 18 years old, they will by default gain decision-making power. The family needs to carefully consider the child's capacity for medical, legal, and financial decision-making. The adaptive functioning difficulties associated with TAYASD mean that even with normal intelligence, TAYASD may not have the necessary judgment to integrate information needed for making sound decisions related to personal care involving health, finances, and housing. If this is the case, TAYASD may not be capable of full independence, and guardianship or other legal arrangements to support decision-making are indicated. While guardianship allows broadest coverage for decision-making, the family can consult with a special needs attorney over other arrangements (e.g., power of attorney, limited guardianship, conservatorship) that are more specific to a particular aspect of decision-making.

Parents should plan well in advance if they wish to retain decision-making authority for the TAYASD after age 18 years, given the time needed to put legal guardianship in place. Some parents may overlook the importance of maintaining decision-making for their child, including being able to assist with educational planning or medical care, as parents no longer have automatic access to educational or health records after the age of majority. Others may overestimate their child's cognitive capacity and believe their child is capable of making medical decisions. Providing families with an understanding of what medical decision-making entails, i.e., with an example of a medical emergency (such as an appendectomy), can be useful to illustrate the point that they will likely want to be involved by law in any of their TAYASD's decision-making even after age 18 years. The family should also name a backup decision-maker in the event that the parents are unavailable or deceased. In cases where patients clearly do not have the capacity to make decisions, psychiatrists may elect to help the family complete the requisite evaluation documents from the court. In more subtle cases, deferring to a court-appointed evaluator for neuropsychiatric testing may be appropriate.

Financial decision-making is another topic that will need to be discussed with the family. For example, a TAYASD may or may not be able to manage their own finances when they receive income from a job or disability benefits. In such cases, parents will ideally have a written, legal plan in place to ensure that the TAYASD patient's finances are within their purview and that their child is not able to make large purchases (such as vehicles or houses) without their parents' or trustee's consent. TAYASD may be vulnerable to financial scams, so parents maintaining financial decision-making can be protective. In the event that the TAYASD will be managing their finances independently, encouraging the patient to maintain an open and supportive relationship with parents is generally advisable. Families may consider opening a tax-advantaged savings account for individuals with eligible disabilities to help pay for certain qualified expenses while not negatively impacting public benefit eligibility, in accordance with the Achieving a Better Life Experience (ABLE) Act of 2014 [178].

Case Vignette 6 *Violet is a 21-year-old female with ASD and ADHD. She is currently taking two college classes and living at home with her parents. She drives herself to and from classes using her parents' car. Violet's parents gave her a credit card for incidental expenses at school, such as meals and parking while she is on campus. One day after classes, a group of classmates asked Violet to attend a dinner at a nearby restaurant. Violet was very excited to be invited, since she previously had only minimal interaction with college classmates. At the conclusion of the dinner, several of Violet's classmates suggested that she pay for the dinner. Violet agreed and paid for the meal, totaling almost $500. On another occasion, Violet went to a car dealership to have her car repaired and ended up being sold a new vehicle because she had good credit. Violet's parents are extremely concerned about her financial decision-making, and the car purchase caused tremendous financial strain on the family.*

In the case above, the family may consider financial coaching or money management classes for the patient. It may also be beneficial to create a special needs trust for the TAYASD. This will ensure that assets left to their child will be placed in the special needs trust and not given personally to the child. If assets are passed on to the TAYASD, this could disqualify them from critical resources such as Medicaid health insurance and disability income. Within the trust, the family should name a trustee in the event that the parents pass away. This trustee would make medical, legal, and financial decisions on the patient's behalf.

Developmental Considerations

Many TAYASD strive to meet milestones in concert with their TD peers. These include driving and dating. With support, TAYASD can meet these desired goals in many cases. However, many patients with ASD exhibit a discrepancy between cognitive functioning and adaptive functioning, especially in cognitively-able individuals. Social deficits are a major driver of this disconnect [179], impairing the TAYASD's ability to effectively access activities and exercise judgment expected for adults, which can affect mobility, intimate relationships, and management of their mental health care.

Transportation and driving are major components of independence and significant barriers for many TAYASD. The decision about whether a TAYASD drives is ideally a consensus between the clinician and the family weighing the risks and benefits. A low percentage of TAYASD actually drive, and this is due to a variety of factors, including deficits in attention, high levels of anxiety, sensory processing difficulties, and financial barriers. Technology interventions may be useful in this area, as there is a significant amount of research underway aimed at assisting TAYASD in learning to drive through the use of virtual reality training [180, 181]. Ride-hailing mobile applications (e.g., Uber, Lyft) can alleviate some of the burden of transportation, but these services are not available in all areas and require financial resources for their utilization. Public transportation in the United States can require significant executive skills to navigate, so hands-on teaching and opportunities to practice can significantly reduce stress and promote more efficient use.

Sexuality is another topic that often requires attention during care of TAYASD, who may need guidance from family and clinicians as they seek to enter into romantic relationships either online or in person [182]. Patients may require coaching regarding safe sexual practices and appropriate sexual boundaries, as TAYASD are at risk to be both victimized sexually and potentially accused of inappropriate or illegal behaviors, largely due to a lack of understanding of social norms, expectations, and laws. Psychiatrists should encourage and facilitate these discussions between TAYASD and their families. TAYASD can be highly vulnerable to sexual predators either online or in person and require significant supervision. Online tools can be useful for sexual education and maximizing safety while using social media [183].

Gender dysphoria (GD) (or gender variance) appears to be more common in individuals with ASD compared to TD individuals [184]. GD symptoms can pose an additional layer of challenges to clinicians, and attempts to transition outwardly can contribute to social isolation, bullying, and family conflict. As a result, patients with GD and ASD (GD/ASD) are potentially at elevated risk for depressive symptoms, anxiety symptoms, and suicidality. Ideally, clinicians are able to assist individuals in understanding their gender identity and facilitate an exploration of gender roles [185]. Consultation and ongoing follow-up with endocrinology is recommended for individuals with GD/ASD in order to discuss options for puberty suppression or other hormone therapies. In clinical practice, community programs with multidisciplinary teams to support individuals with GD can be helpful for TAYASD with GD.

As young adults, TAYASD often have the opportunity to assume more autonomy managing their medications, which can result in poor compliance, particularly if family members or the school were very involved in administration of medications during childhood. It is therefore important for providers to engage TAYASD in being aware of the benefits and risks of their medications, how to take them appropriately, and the need for regular follow-up with treatment providers. Providers also need to plan in advance, transfer records, and closely communicate to ensure a smooth hand-off between clinicians at transition age.

Conclusion

Individuals with ASD require intensive transition planning as they approach adulthood. Multiple factors need to be considered in the planning process including the individual's developmental level, severity of psychiatric and behavioral disorders, living arrangements, capacity for postsecondary education, and plans for guardianship. It is important for psychiatrists working with individuals with ASD to begin the conversation with families about the transition process as early as possible to ensure that individuals with ASD have the best possible outcomes in adulthood.

References

1. American Psychiatric Association. Diagnostic and statistical manual of mental disorders. 5th ed. Arlington: American Psychiatric Association; 2013.
2. Lever AG, Geurts HM. Psychiatric co-occurring symptoms and disorders in young, middle-aged, and older adults with autism spectrum disorder. J Autism Dev Disord. 2016;46(6):1916–30.
3. Rosen TE, et al. Co-occurring psychiatric conditions in autism spectrum disorder. Int Rev Psychiatry. 2018;30(1):40–61.
4. Cashin A, et al. A scoping review of what is known of the physical health of adults with autism spectrum disorder. J Intellect Disabil. 2018;22(1):96–108.
5. Baio J, et al. Prevalence of autism spectrum disorder among children aged 8 years - autism and developmental disabilities monitoring network, 11 Sites, United States, 2014. MMWR Surveill Summ. 2018;67(6):1–23.
6. 12/05/2019. Available from: https://www.autismspeaks.org/adults-autism.
7. Individuals with Disabilities Education Act, in 20 U.S.C. § 1400 2004.
8. Marrus N, et al. Training of child and adolescent psychiatry fellows in autism and intellectual disability. Autism. 2014;18(4):471–5.
9. Anderson C, Lupfer A, Shattuck PT. Barriers to receipt of services for young adults with autism. Pediatrics. 2018;141(Suppl 4):S300–s305.
10. Anderson KA, et al. Social-ecological correlates in adult autism outcome studies: a scoping review. Pediatrics. 2018;141(Suppl 4):S306–s317.
11. Houghton R, Liu C, Bolognani F. Psychiatric comorbidities and psychotropic medication use in autism: a matched cohort study with ADHD and general population comparator groups in the United Kingdom. Autism Res. 2018;11(12):1690–700.
12. Kraper CK, et al. The gap between adaptive behavior and intelligence in autism persists into young adulthood and is linked to psychiatric co-morbidities. J Autism Dev Disord. 2017;47(10):3007–17.
13. Simonoff E, et al. Psychiatric disorders in children with autism spectrum disorders: prevalence, comorbidity, and associated factors in a population-derived sample. J Am Acad Child Adolesc Psychiatry. 2008;47(8):921–9.
14. APA. Diagnostic and statistical manual of mental disorders: DSM-5. 5th ed. Washington, DC: American Psychiatric Association; 2013. xliv, 947 p
15. Reiss S, Levitan GW, Szyszko J. Emotional disturbance and mental retardation: diagnostic overshadowing. Am J Ment Defic. 1982;86(6):567–74.
16. Mazefsky CA, et al. ASD, a psychiatric disorder, or both? Psychiatric diagnoses in adolescents with high-functioning ASD. J Clin Child Adolesc Psychol. 2012;41(4):516–23.
17. Murray MJ. Attention-deficit/hyperactivity disorder in the context of autism spectrum disorders. Curr Psychiatry Rep. 2010;12(5):382–8.
18. Davignon MN, et al. Psychiatric and medical conditions in transition-aged individuals with ASD. Pediatrics. 2018;141(Suppl 4):S335–s345.
19. Joshi G, et al. Psychiatric comorbidity and functioning in a clinically referred population of adults with autism spectrum disorders: a comparative study. J Autism Dev Disord. 2013;43(6):1314–25.
20. Stahlberg O, et al. Bipolar disorder, schizophrenia, and other psychotic disorders in adults with childhood onset AD/HD and/or autism spectrum disorders. J Neural Transm (Vienna). 2004;111(7):891–902.
21. Croen LA, et al. The health status of adults on the autism spectrum. Autism. 2015;19(7):814–23.
22. Joshi G, et al. A prospective open-label trial of long-acting liquid methylphenidate for the treatment of attention deficit/hyperactivity disorder in intellectually capable adults with autism spectrum disorder. World J Biol Psychiatry. 2020;21(4):274–90.
23. Craig F, et al. Overlap between autism spectrum disorders and attention deficit hyperactivity disorder: searching for distinctive/common clinical features. Autism Res. 2015;8(3):328–37.
24. Conners CK, et al. The revised Conners' Parent Rating Scale (CPRS-R): factor structure, reliability, and criterion validity. J Abnorm Child Psychol. 1998;26(4):257–68.
25. Wolraich ML, et al. Psychometric properties of the Vanderbilt ADHD diagnostic parent rating scale in a referred population. J Pediatr Psychol. 2003;28(8):559–67.
26. Mahajan R, et al. Clinical practice pathways for evaluation and medication choice for attention-deficit/hyperactivity disorder symptoms in autism spectrum disorders. Pediatrics. 2012;130(Suppl 2):S125–38.
27. Autism, Psychopharmacology. Randomized, controlled, crossover trial of methylphenidate in pervasive developmental disorders with hyperactivity. Arch Gen Psychiatry. 2005;62(11):1266–74.

28. Jensen PS. A 14-month randomized clinical trial of treatment strategies for attention-deficit/hyperactivity disorder. The MTA Cooperative Group. Multimodal treatment study of children with ADHD. Arch Gen Psychiatry. 1999;56(12):1073–86.
29. Scahill L, et al. Extended-release guanfacine for hyperactivity in children with autism spectrum disorder. Am J Psychiatry. 2015;172(12):1197–206.
30. Ming X, et al. Use of clonidine in children with autism spectrum disorders. Brain Dev. 2008;30(7):454–60.
31. Fankhauser MP, et al. A double-blind, placebo-controlled study of the efficacy of transdermal clonidine in autism. J Clin Psychiatry. 1992;53(3):77–82.
32. Patra S, et al. Atomoxetine for attention deficit hyperactivity disorder in children and adolescents with autism: a systematic review and meta-analysis. Autism Res. 2019;12(4):542–52.
33. Wentz E, Nyden A, Krevers B. Development of an internet-based support and coaching model for adolescents and young adults with ADHD and autism spectrum disorders: a pilot study. Eur Child Adolesc Psychiatry. 2012;21(11):611–22.
34. Tan BW, Pooley JA, Speelman CP. A meta-analytic review of the efficacy of physical exercise interventions on cognition in individuals with autism spectrum disorder and ADHD. J Autism Dev Disord. 2016;46(9):3126–43.
35. Pan MR, et al. A comparison of efficacy between cognitive behavioral therapy (CBT) and CBT combined with medication in adults with attention-deficit/hyperactivity disorder (ADHD). Psychiatry Res. 2019;279:23–33.
36. Lambez B, et al. Non-pharmacological interventions for cognitive difficulties in ADHD: a systematic review and meta-analysis. J Psychiatr Res. 2020;120:40–55.
37. Brotman MA, et al. Irritability in youths: a translational model. Am J Psychiatry. 2017;174(6):520–32.
38. Kanne SM, Mazurek MO. Aggression in children and adolescents with ASD: prevalence and risk factors. J Autism Dev Disord. 2011;41(7):926–37.
39. Mayes SD, et al. Disruptive mood dysregulation disorder symptoms by age in autism, ADHD, and general population samples. J Ment Health Res Intellect Disabil. 2017;10(4):345–59.
40. Lecavalier L. Behavioral and emotional problems in young people with pervasive developmental disorders: relative prevalence, effects of subject characteristics, and empirical classification. J Autism Dev Disord. 2006;36(8):1101–14.
41. Rattaz C, et al. Challenging behaviours at early adulthood in autism spectrum disorders: topography, risk factors and evolution. J Intellect Disabil Res. 2018;62(7):637–49.
42. Shattuck PT, et al. Change in autism symptoms and maladaptive behaviors in adolescents and adults with an autism spectrum disorder. J Autism Dev Disord. 2007;37(9):1735–47.
43. McGuire K, et al. Irritability and problem behavior in autism spectrum disorder: a practice pathway for pediatric primary care. Pediatrics. 2016;137(Suppl 2):S136–48.
44. Brosnan J, Healy O. A review of behavioral interventions for the treatment of aggression in individuals with developmental disabilities. Res Dev Disabil. 2011;32(2):437–46.
45. Doehring P, et al. Behavioral approaches to managing severe problem behaviors in children with autism spectrum and related developmental disorders: a descriptive analysis. Child Adolesc Psychiatr Clin N Am. 2014;23(1):25–40.
46. Bishop-Fitzpatrick L, Minshew NJ, Eack SM. A systematic review of psychosocial interventions for adults with autism spectrum disorders. J Autism Dev Disord. 2013;43(3):687–94.
47. Fung LK, et al. Pharmacologic treatment of severe irritability and problem behaviors in autism: a systematic review and meta-analysis. Pediatrics. 2016;137(Suppl 2):S124–35.
48. Yoon Y, et al. Weight gain effects of second-generation antipsychotic treatment in autism spectrum disorder. J Child Adolesc Psychopharmacol. 2016;26(9):822–7.
49. Hollocks MJ, et al. Anxiety and depression in adults with autism spectrum disorder: a systematic review and meta-analysis. Psychol Med. 2019;49(4):559–72.
50. Kessler RC, et al. The epidemiology of panic attacks, panic disorder, and agoraphobia in the National Comorbidity Survey Replication. Arch Gen Psychiatry. 2006;63(4):415–24.
51. Ung D, et al. A systematic review and meta-analysis of cognitive-behavioral therapy for anxiety in youth with high-functioning autism spectrum disorders. Child Psychiatry Hum Dev. 2015;46(4):533–47.
52. Jennett H, Vasa R, Hagopian L. Anxiety in autism spectrum disorders, in pediatric anxiety disorders, a clinical guide. New York: Humana Press; 2013.
53. Weisbrot DM, et al. The presentation of anxiety in children with pervasive developmental disorders. J Child Adolesc Psychopharmacol. 2005;15(3):477–96.
54. Kerns CM, et al. Traditional and atypical presentations of anxiety in youth with autism spectrum disorder. J Autism Dev Disord. 2014;44(11):2851–61.
55. Postorino V, et al. Anxiety disorders and obsessive-compulsive disorder in individuals with autism spectrum disorder. Curr Psychiatry Rep. 2017;19(12):92.
56. Keefer A, et al. Psychosocial interventions for internalizing disorders in youth and adults with ASD. Int Rev Psychiatry. 2018;30(1):62–77.
57. McGillivray JA, Evert HT. Group cognitive behavioural therapy program shows potential in reducing symptoms of depression and stress among young people with ASD. J Autism Dev Disord. 2014;44(8):2041–51.
58. Murray K, et al. Outcomes of cognitive behaviour therapy for obsessive-compulsive disorder in young people with and without autism spectrum

disorders: a case controlled study. Psychiatry Res. 2015;228(1):8–13.
59. Wise JM, et al. Open trial of modular cognitive-behavioral therapy in the treatment of anxiety among late adolescents with autism spectrum disorder. Child Psychiatry Hum Dev. 2019;50(1):27–34.
60. Spek AA, van Ham NC, Nyklicek I. Mindfulness-based therapy in adults with an autism spectrum disorder: a randomized controlled trial. Res Dev Disabil. 2013;34(1):246–53.
61. Cooney P, Tunney C, O'Reilly G. A systematic review of the evidence regarding cognitive therapy skills that assist cognitive behavioural therapy in adults who have an intellectual disability. J Appl Res Intellect Disabil. 2018;31(1):23–42.
62. Lydon S, et al. A systematic review of the treatment of fears and phobias among children with autism spectrum disorders. Rev J Autism Dev Disord. 2015;2(2):141–54.
63. Rosen TE, Connell JE, Kerns CM. A review of behavioral interventions for anxiety-related behaviors in lower-functioning individuals with autism. Behav Interv. 2016;31(2):120–43.
64. Vasa RA, et al. A systematic review of treatments for anxiety in youth with autism spectrum disorders. J Autism Dev Disord. 2014;44(12):3215–29.
65. King BH, et al. Lack of efficacy of citalopram in children with autism spectrum disorders and high levels of repetitive behavior: citalopram ineffective in children with autism. Arch Gen Psychiatry. 2009;66(6):583–90.
66. Vasa RA, et al. Assessment and treatment of anxiety in youth with autism spectrum disorders. Pediatrics. 2016;137(Suppl 2):S115–23.
67. Hudson CC, Hall L, Harkness KL. Prevalence of depressive disorders in individuals with autism spectrum disorder: a meta-analysis. J Abnorm Child Psychol. 2019;47(1):165–75.
68. Lugnegard T, Hallerback MU, Gillberg C. Psychiatric comorbidity in young adults with a clinical diagnosis of Asperger syndrome. Res Dev Disabil. 2011;32(5):1910–7.
69. Hedley D, et al. Risk and protective factors underlying depression and suicidal ideation in autism spectrum disorder. Depress Anxiety. 2018;35(7):648–57.
70. Charlot L, et al. Mood and anxiety symptoms in psychiatric inpatients with autism spectrum disorder and depression. J Ment Health Res Intellect Disabil. 2008;1(4):238–53.
71. De-la-Iglesia M, Olivar JS. Risk factors for depression in children and adolescents with high functioning autism spectrum disorders. Scientific World Journal. 2015;2015:127853.
72. Pezzimenti F, et al. Depression in youth with autism spectrum disorder. Child Adolesc Psychiatr Clin N Am. 2019;28(3):397–409.
73. Wing L. Asperger's syndrome: a clinical account. Psychol Med. 1981;11(1):115–29.
74. Lainhart JE, Folstein SE. Affective disorders in people with autism: a review of published cases. J Autism Dev Disord. 1994;24(5):587–601.
75. Cassidy S, et al. Suicidal ideation and suicide plans or attempts in adults with Asperger's syndrome attending a specialist diagnostic clinic: a clinical cohort study. Lancet Psychiatry. 2014;1(2):142–7.
76. Zahid S, Upthegrove R. Suicidality in autistic spectrum disorders. Crisis. 2017;38(4):237–46.
77. Kato K, et al. Clinical features of suicide attempts in adults with autism spectrum disorders. Gen Hosp Psychiatry. 2013;35(1):50–3.
78. Lai M-C, et al. Quantifying and exploring camouflaging in men and women with autism. Autism. 2017;21(6):690–702.
79. Cassidy S, et al. Risk markers for suicidality in autistic adults. Mol Autism. 2018;9:42.
80. Hillier AJ, et al. Social and vocational skills training reduces self-reported anxiety and depression among young adults on the autism spectrum. J Dev Phys Disabil. 2011;23(3):267–76.
81. Williams K, et al. Selective serotonin reuptake inhibitors (SSRIs) for autism spectrum disorders (ASD). Cochrane Database Syst Rev. 2013;(8):Cd004677.
82. Kolevzon A, Mathewson KA, Hollander E. Selective serotonin reuptake inhibitors in autism: a review of efficacy and tolerability. J Clin Psychiatry. 2006;67(3):407–14.
83. Gwynette MF, et al. Treatment of adults with autism and major depressive disorder using transcranial magnetic stimulation: an open label pilot study. Autism Res. 2020;13:346–51.
84. Vannucchi G, et al. Bipolar disorder in adults with aspergers syndrome: a systematic review. J Affect Disord. 2014;168:151–60.
85. Borue X, et al. Longitudinal course of bipolar disorder in youth with high-functioning autism spectrum disorder. J Am Acad Child Adolesc Psychiatry. 2016;55(12):1064–1072.e6.
86. McGrath J, et al. Schizophrenia: a concise overview of incidence, prevalence, and mortality. Epidemiol Rev. 2008;30:67–76.
87. Gochman P, Miller R, Rapoport JL. Childhood-onset schizophrenia: the challenge of diagnosis. Curr Psychiatry Rep. 2011;13(5):321–2.
88. Zheng Z, Zheng P, Zou X. Association between schizophrenia and autism spectrum disorder: a systematic review and meta-analysis. Autism Res. 2018;11(8):1110–9.
89. Lugo Marin J, et al. Prevalence of schizophrenia spectrum disorders in average-IQ adults with autism spectrum disorders: a meta-analysis. J Autism Dev Disord. 2018;48(1):239–50.
90. Chisholm K, et al. The association between autism and schizophrenia spectrum disorders: a review of eight alternate models of co-occurrence. Neurosci Biobehav Rev. 2015;55:173–83.
91. Eack SM, et al. Commonalities in social and non-social cognitive impairments in adults with autism

spectrum disorder and schizophrenia. Schizophr Res. 2013;148(1–3):24–8.

92. Couture SM, et al. Comparison of social cognitive functioning in schizophrenia and high functioning autism: more convergence than divergence. Psychol Med. 2010;40(4):569–79.
93. Ziermans T, et al. Formal thought disorder and executive functioning in children and adolescents with autism spectrum disorder: old leads and new avenues. J Autism Dev Disord. 2017;47(6):1756–68.
94. Konstantareas MM, Hewitt T. Autistic disorder and schizophrenia: diagnostic overlaps. J Autism Dev Disord. 2001;31(1):19–28.
95. Spek AA, Wouters SGM. Autism and schizophrenia in high functioning adults: behavioral differences and overlap. Res Autism Spectr Disord. 2010;4(4):709–17.
96. Hurst RM, et al. The relationship of Asperger's characteristics and schizotypal personality traits in a non-clinical adult sample. J Autism Dev Disord. 2007;37(9):1711–20.
97. van der Gaag RJ, et al. A controlled study of formal thought disorder in children with autism and multiple complex developmental disorders. J Child Adolesc Psychopharmacol. 2005;15(3):465–76.
98. Larson FV, et al. Psychosis in autism: comparison of the features of both conditions in a dually affected cohort. Br J Psychiatry. 2017;210(4):269–75.
99. Lai MC, Baron-Cohen S. Identifying the lost generation of adults with autism spectrum conditions. Lancet Psychiatry. 2015;2(11):1013–27.
100. Bouras N, et al. Schizophrenia-spectrum psychoses in people with and without intellectual disability. J Intellect Disabil Res. 2004;48(Pt 6):548–55.
101. Raja M, Azzoni A. Autistic spectrum disorders and schizophrenia in the adult psychiatric setting: diagnosis and comorbidity. Psychiatr Danub. 2010;22(4):514–21.
102. Foss-Feig JH, et al. Clinical profiles and conversion rates among young individuals with autism spectrum disorder who present to clinical high risk for psychosis services. J Am Acad Child Adolesc Psychiatry. 2019;58(6):582–8.
103. Downs JM, et al. The association between comorbid autism spectrum disorders and antipsychotic treatment failure in early-onset psychosis: a historical cohort study using electronic health records. J Clin Psychiatry. 2017;78(9):e1233–41.
104. Sizoo BB, Kuiper E. Cognitive behavioural therapy and mindfulness based stress reduction may be equally effective in reducing anxiety and depression in adults with autism spectrum disorders. Res Dev Disabil. 2017;64:47–55.
105. Butwicka A, et al. Increased risk for substance use-related problems in autism spectrum disorders: a population-based cohort study. J Autism Dev Disord. 2017;47(1):80–9.
106. Arnevik EA, Helverschou SB. Autism spectrum disorder and co-occurring substance use disorder - a systematic review. Subst Abus. 2016;10:69–75.
107. Kronenberg LM, et al. Everyday life consequences of substance use in adult patients with a substance use disorder (SUD) and co-occurring attention deficit/hyperactivity disorder (ADHD) or autism spectrum disorder (ASD): a patient's perspective. BMC Psychiatry. 2014;14:264.
108. Isenberg BM, et al. Considerations for treating young people with comorbid autism spectrum disorder and substance use disorder. J Am Acad Child Adolesc Psychiatry. 2019;58(12):1139–41.
109. Merikangas KR, et al. Lifetime prevalence of mental disorders in U.S. adolescents: results from the National Comorbidity Survey Replication--Adolescent Supplement (NCS-A). J Am Acad Child Adolesc Psychiatry. 2010;49(10):980–9.
110. Helverschou SB, Brunvold AR, Arnevik EA. Treating patients with co-occurring autism spectrum disorder and substance use disorder: a clinical explorative study. Subst Abus. 2019;13:1178221819843291.
111. Baker EK, Richdale AL. Sleep patterns in adults with a diagnosis of high-functioning autism spectrum disorder. Sleep. 2015;38(11):1765–74.
112. Goldman SE, et al. Sleep is associated with problem behaviors in children and adolescents with autism spectrum disorders. Res Autism Spectr Disord. 2011;5(3):1223–9.
113. Limoges É, et al. Atypical sleep architecture and the autism phenotype. Brain. 2005;128(Pt 5):1049–61.
114. Tani P, et al. Insomnia is a frequent finding in adults with Asperger syndrome. BMC Psychiatry. 2003;3(1):12.
115. Asano M, et al. Ramelteon monotherapy for insomnia and impulsive behavior in high-functioning autistic disorder. J Clin Psychopharmacol. 2014;34(3):402–3.
116. Oyane NM, Bjorvatn B. Sleep disturbances in adolescents and young adults with autism and Asperger syndrome. Autism. 2005;9(1):83–94.
117. Carmassi C, et al. Systematic review of sleep disturbances and circadian sleep desynchronization in autism spectrum disorder: toward an integrative model of a self-reinforcing loop. Front Psych. 2019;10:366.
118. Goldman SE, et al. Characterizing sleep in adolescents and adults with autism spectrum disorders. J Autism Dev Disord. 2017;47(6):1682–95.
119. Klukowski M, Wasilewska J, Lebensztejn D. Sleep and gastrointestinal disturbances in autism spectrum disorder in children. Dev Period Med. 2015;19(2):157–61.
120. Mazurek MO, Sohl K. Sleep and behavioral problems in children with autism spectrum disorder. J Autism Dev Disord. 2016;46(6):1906–15.
121. Blackmer AB, Feinstein JA. Management of sleep disorders in children with neurodevelopmental disorders: a review. Pharmacotherapy. 2016;36(1):84–98.
122. Deserno MK, et al. Sleep determines quality of life in autistic adults: a longitudinal study. Autism Res. 2019;12(5):794–801.

123. Mazurek MO, Petroski GF. Sleep problems in children with autism spectrum disorder: examining the contributions of sensory over-responsivity and anxiety. Sleep Med. 2015;16(2):270–9.
124. Hollway JA, Aman MG, Butter E. Correlates and risk markers for sleep disturbance in participants of the autism treatment network. J Autism Dev Disord. 2013;43(12):2830–43.
125. Robinson-Shelton A, Malow BA. Sleep disturbances in neurodevelopmental disorders. Curr Psychiatry Rep. 2016;18(1):6.
126. Rossignol DA, Frye RE. Melatonin in autism spectrum disorders. Curr Clin Pharmacol. 2014;9(4):326–34.
127. Baker EK, Richdale AL, Hazi A. Employment status is related to sleep problems in adults with autism spectrum disorder and no comorbid intellectual impairment. Autism. 2019;23(2):531–6.
128. Hohn VD, et al. Insomnia severity in adults with autism spectrum disorder is associated with sensory hyper-reactivity and social skill impairment. J Autism Dev Disord. 2019;49(5):2146–55.
129. Grandin LD, Alloy LB, Abramson LY. The social zeitgeber theory, circadian rhythms, and mood disorders: review and evaluation. Clin Psychol Rev. 2006;26(6):679–94.
130. Adams HL, et al. The relationship between autism symptom severity and sleep problems: should bidirectionality be considered? Res Autism Spectr Disord. 2014;8(3):193–9.
131. Autism spectrum disorder in under 19s: support and management. [cited 2019 12/31/2019]. Available from: www.nice.org.uk/guidance/cg170.
132. Cortesi F, et al. Controlled-release melatonin, singly and combined with cognitive behavioural therapy, for persistent insomnia in children with autism spectrum disorders: a randomized placebo-controlled trial. J Sleep Res. 2012;21(6):700–9.
133. Schwichtenberg AJ, Malow BA. Melatonin treatment in children with developmental disabilities. Sleep Med Clin. 2015;10(2):181–7.
134. Galli-Carminati G, Deriaz N, Bertschy G. Melatonin in treatment of chronic sleep disorders in adults with autism: a retrospective study. Swiss Med Wkly. 2009;139(19–20):293–6.
135. Reynolds AM, Malow BA. Sleep and autism spectrum disorders. Pediatr Clin North Am. 2011;58(3):685–98.
136. Guenole F, et al. Melatonin for disordered sleep in individuals with autism spectrum disorders: systematic review and discussion. Sleep Med Rev. 2011;15(6):379–87.
137. Jones KB, et al. A description of medical conditions in adults with autism spectrum disorder: a follow-up of the 1980s Utah/UCLA autism epidemiologic study. Autism. 2016;20:551–61.
138. Hirvikoski T, et al. Premature mortality in autism spectrum disorder. Br J Psychiatry. 2016;208(3):232–8.
139. Nicolaidis C, et al. Comparison of healthcare experiences in autistic and non-autistic adults: a cross-sectional online survey facilitated by an academic-community partnership. J Gen Intern Med. 2013;28(6):761–9.
140. Akobirshoev I, et al. In-hospital mortality among adults with autism spectrum disorder in the United States: A retrospective analysis of US hospital discharge data. Autism. 2020;24(1):177–89.
141. Murphy CM, et al. Autism spectrum disorder in adults: diagnosis, management, and health services development. Neuropsychiatr Dis Treat. 2016;12:1669–86.
142. Muhle RA, et al. Clinical diagnostic genetic testing for individuals with developmental disorders. J Am Acad Child Adolesc Psychiatry. 2017;56(11):910–3.
143. Khanna R, Jariwala K, West-Strum D. Use and cost of psychotropic drugs among recipients with autism in a state Medicaid fee-for-service programme. J Intellect Disabil Res. 2013;57(2):161–71.
144. Laushey KM, Heflin LJ. Enhancing social skills of kindergarten children with autism through the training of multiple peers as tutors. J Autism Dev Disord. 2000;30(3):183–93.
145. Tantam D. The challenge of adolescents and adults with Asperger syndrome. Child Adolesc Psychiatr Clin N Am. 2003;12(1):143–63, vii–viii.
146. Klin A, Volkmar FR. Asperger syndrome: diagnosis and external validity. Child Adolesc Psychiatr Clin N Am. 2003;12(1):1–13, v.
147. McLeod JD, Meanwell E, Hawbaker A. The experiences of college students on the autism spectrum: a comparison to their neurotypical peers. J Autism Dev Disord. 2019;49(6):2320–36.
148. Fink E, et al. Bullying-related behaviour in adolescents with autism: links with autism severity and emotional and behavioural problems. Autism. 2018;22(6):684–92.
149. Laugeson EA, et al. Evidence-based social skills training for adolescents with autism spectrum disorders: the UCLA PEERS program. J Autism Dev Disord. 2012;42(6):1025–36.
150. Oswald TM, et al. A pilot randomized controlled trial of the ACCESS program: a group intervention to improve social, adaptive functioning, stress coping, and self-determination outcomes in young adults with autism spectrum disorder. J Autism Dev Disord. 2018;48(5):1742–60.
151. Laugeson EA, et al. A randomized controlled trial to improve social skills in young adults with autism spectrum disorder: the UCLA PEERS((R)) program. J Autism Dev Disord. 2015;45(12):3978–89.
152. Beidel DC, et al. The impact of social skills training for social anxiety disorder: a randomized controlled trial. J Anxiety Disord. 2014;28(8):908–18.
153. Healy S, et al. Physical activity, screen-time behavior, and obesity among 13-year olds in Ireland with and without autism spectrum disorder. J Autism Dev Disord. 2017;47(1):49–57.
154. Mazurek MO, Engelhardt CR. Video game use in boys with autism spectrum disorder, ADHD, or typical development. Pediatrics. 2013;132(2):260–6.
155. Gwynette MF, Sidhu SS, Ceranoglu TA. Electronic screen media use in youth with autism spectrum

disorder. Child Adolesc Psychiatr Clin N Am. 2018;27(2):203–19.
156. Mazurek MO, et al. Prevalence and correlates of screen-based media use among youths with autism spectrum disorders. J Autism Dev Disord. 2012;42(8):1757–67.
157. Whalen C, et al. Behavioral improvements associated with computer-assisted instruction for children with developmental disabilities. J Speech Lang Pathol Appl Behav Anal. 2006;1(1):11–26.
158. Joshi G, et al. A prospective open-label trial of memantine hydrochloride for the treatment of social deficits in intellectually capable adults with autism spectrum disorder. J Clin Psychopharmacol. 2016;36(3):262–71.
159. Parker KJ, et al. A randomized placebo-controlled pilot trial shows that intranasal vasopressin improves social deficits in children with autism. Sci Transl Med. 2019;11(491):eaau7356.
160. Keech B, Crowe S, Hocking DR. Intranasal oxytocin, social cognition and neurodevelopmental disorders: a meta-analysis. Psychoneuroendocrinology. 2018;87:9–19.
161. Chan V. Special needs: scholastic disability accommodations from K-12 and transitions to higher education. Curr Psychiatry Rep. 2016;18(2):21.
162. Test DW, Smith LE, Carter EW. Equipping youth with autism spectrum disorders for adulthood: promoting rigor, relevance, and relationships. Remedial Spec Educ. 2014;35(2):80–90.
163. Roberts KD. Topic areas to consider when planning transition from high school to postsecondary education for students with autism spectrum disorders. Focus Autism Other Dev Disabil. 2010;25(3):158–62.
164. Francis GL, Duke JM, Chiu C. The college road trip: supporting college success for students with autism. Div Autism Dev Disabil Online J. 2017;4:20–35.
165. Test DW, et al. Evidence-based secondary transition predictors for improving postschool outcomes for students with disabilities. Career Dev Except Individ. 2009;32(3):160–81.
166. Transition tool kit for families on the journey from adolescence to adulthood. 2018. Available from: https://www.autismspeaks.org/sites/default/files/2018-08/Transition%20Tool%20Kit.pdf.
167. A transition guide to postsecondary education and employment for students and youth with disabilities. 3/10/2020. Available from: https://www2.ed.gov/about/offices/list/osers/transition/products/postsecondary-transition-guide-may-2017.pdf.
168. What to know about youth transition service for students and youth with disabilities. 3/10/2020. Available from: https://www.dol.gov/odep/categories/youth/Federal-Partners-in-Transition.htm.
169. Shattuck PT, et al. Postsecondary education and employment among youth with an autism spectrum disorder. Pediatrics. 2012;129(6):1042–9.
170. Americans With Disabilities Act of 1990. 1990, Pub. L. No. 101-336, 104 Stat. 328.
171. Department of Health, E., and Welfare, Office of the Secretary, Office for Civil Rights., Section 504 of the Rehabilitation act of 1973. Fact sheet : handicapped persons rights under Federal law. Section 504 of the Rehabilitation act of 1973. 1978: United States.
172. Paul T. Shattuck, et al. Disability Identification and Self-Efficacy among College Students on the Autism Spectrum. Autism Research and Treatment, vol. 2014, Article ID 924182, 7 pages, 2014. https://doi.org/10.1155/2014/924182.
173. Sturm A, Kasari C. Academic and psychosocial characteristics of incoming college freshmen with autism spectrum disorder: the role of comorbidity and gender. Autism Res. 2019;12(6):931–40.
174. Cai RY, Richdale AL. Educational experiences and needs of higher education students with autism spectrum disorder. J Autism Dev Disord. 2016;46(1):31–41.
175. Cullen JA. The needs of college students with autism spectrum disorders and Asperger's syndrome. J Postsecond Educ Disabil. 2015;28(1):89–101.
176. Zukerman G, Yahav G, Ben-Itzchak E. Increased psychiatric symptoms in university students with autism spectrum disorder are associated with reduced adaptive behavior. Psychiatry Res. 2019;273:732–8.
177. Farley M, et al. Mid-life social outcomes for a population-based sample of adults with ASD. Autism Res. 2018;11(1):142–52.
178. About ABLE accounts. [cited 2020 03/02/2020]. Available from: https://www.ablenrc.org/what-is-able/what-are-able-acounts/.
179. Tillmann J, et al. Investigating the factors underlying adaptive functioning in autism in the EU-AIMS Longitudinal European Autism Project. Autism Res. 2019;12(4):645–57.
180. Cox DJ, et al. Can youth with autism spectrum disorder use virtual reality driving simulation training to evaluate and improve driving performance? An exploratory study. J Autism Dev Disord. 2017;47(8):2544–55.
181. Zhang L, et al. Cognitive load measurement in a virtual reality-based driving system for autism intervention. IEEE Trans Affect Comput. 2017;8(2):176–89.
182. Cheak-Zamora NC, et al. Sexual and relationship interest, knowledge, and experiences among adolescents and young adults with autism spectrum disorder. Arch Sex Behav. 2019;48(8):2605–15.
183. Ambitious about autism. 03/02/2020. Available from: https://www.ambitiousaboutautism.org.uk/understanding-autism/independence/sex-education.
184. Hisle-Gorman E, et al. Gender dysphoria in children with autism spectrum disorder. LGBT Health. 2019;6:95–100.
185. van Schalkwyk GI, Klingensmith K, Volkmar FR. Gender identity and autism spectrum disorders. Yale J Biol Med. 2015;88(1):81–3.

AD/HD & Learning Disorders 12

Lisa Jacobs and Anthony Rostain

Key Points

- Untreated ADHD is dangerous. ADHD is associated with early mortality, obesity, and hypertension [1]. It is correlated with more police contacts, arrests, car accidents, substance abuse problems, and a greater risk of teen pregnancy [2]. Life expectancy of children with combined-type ADHD is shortened by more than 8 years [3].
- ADHD and learning disorders (LD) are correlated with low educational attainment. Adults with LD are much less likely to attend 4-year colleges, and adults with ADHD are seven times less likely to earn a bachelor's degree [2].
- ADHD and LD are common, with one in ten school-aged children affected [4, 5]. Up to 40% of individuals with ADHD also have an LD diagnosis [6]. Among college students, 2–8% have been diagnosed with ADHD and 3% with LD [7].
- ADHD most often persists into adulthood. Three in four children with ADHD continue to have impairing symptoms in young adulthood, with about half still meeting full diagnostic criteria [8, 9]. Therefore, treatment is often required into adulthood.
- Young adults with ADHD and LD may struggle starting college or joining the workforce when existing deficits related to self-regulation, planning, and task completion become magnified in the setting of increased independence and decreased support and scaffolding from families and schools.

L. Jacobs (✉)
Department of Psychiatry and Behavioral Sciences, Stanford University School of Medicine, Palo Alto, CA, USA

A. Rostain
Cooper University Medical School of Rowan University, Camden, NJ, USA

Perelman School of Medicine, Philadelphia, PA, USA
e-mail: Rostain@pennmedicine.upenn.edu

Introduction

Attention-deficit/hyperactivity disorder (ADHD) is a chronic, disabling neurodevelopmental condition that is highly treatable across the lifespan. Functional impairments associated with ADHD go far beyond school performance. Adults with ADHD have more financial stress compared to matched controls, get fired and quit jobs more

V. Chan, J. Derenne (eds.), *Transition-Age Youth Mental Health Care*,
https://doi.org/10.1007/978-3-030-62113-1_12

often, have shorter durations of employment, and experience a higher likelihood of needing public assistance.

Treating young adults with ADHD and LD presents unique challenges. Symptoms of ADHD often change over time, with inattention persisting as hyperactivity lessens. School, work, and relationships may become unmanageable in the setting of significant symptoms of inattention such as getting distracted, making careless errors, not listening when spoken to, and procrastinating on tasks requiring high levels of cognitive control. As the organization and instrumental support provided by secondary school and family lessens, many young adults with ADHD realize for the first time during their transition to adulthood that their deficits in planning, attention, and organization are more significant. College students with ADHD are at increased risk of failing, withdrawing from classes, and not graduating because of underdeveloped self-management skills [7].

Unfortunately, there are not enough psychiatrists in the USA to meet the demand for treatment of this high-risk population. In fact, most ADHD treatment is delivered by primary care providers. In 2007, 49% of ADHD medications were prescribed by primary care physicians and pediatricians, whereas psychiatrists oversaw 30% of ADHD medication management [10].

Increasingly, general practitioners, family doctors, nurse practitioners, and physician assistants are tasked along with adult psychiatrists with assuming the care of young adults with ADHD and LD as they seek to gain greater independence and autonomy. With the rise in rates of ADHD seen in this population, practitioners are faced with new clinical challenges: Can new ADHD be legitimately diagnosed in young adults? How is the diagnosis made for a 20-year-old? What else could account for similar symptoms? What if they are seeking to misuse amphetamines? Where is a good place to start when prescribing medications and what are the options? How effective are cognitive behavioral therapy (CBT), coaching, cognitive training, and mindfulness?

This chapter will explore the research behind these questions. While the treatment of ADHD and LD in adulthood is supported by far less data than treatment in childhood, there are now many effective evidence-based interventions that may help modify risks and improve quality of life for adults with ADHD and LD. This chapter will provide an overview of diagnosis, treatment, and important considerations in providing treatment to this age group.

New Diagnosis in Young Adulthood

Longitudinal Case, part 1: Tina is an 18-year-old female college freshman living away from home for the first time. She is afraid of failing her first semester classes and is struggling to focus for long enough to finish her reading and assignments. She earned straight As in high school without studying much but now reports unfinished assignments, procrastination, feeling overwhelmed, and poor-mediocre grades. She is convinced her problems are due to ADHD and is seeking an evaluation and help.

If someone makes it through childhood with excellent grades and no clear academic problems, could ADHD be the issue? Tina presents a common scenario: a young adult seeking treatment after environmental demands have changed. Her abilities may have been sufficient to meet the demands of high school, when school assignments were less challenging, and her teachers and parents likely reminded her of tests and assignments and helped her to organize her studying. But now, in college, with less oversight, increased academic demands, and more distractions, she is falling further and further behind.

Why might ADHD be missed in childhood? There are many reasons. Bias is one. As a girl, Tina is less likely to be referred for ADHD evaluation or treatment. Less is known about how ADHD presents and impairs girls and women most likely because of gender bias in prior research [6]. Moreover, girls have fewer behavioral problems than boys. As a result, they are referred less frequently for being disruptive or misbehaving.

Tina's intelligence is another barrier to getting diagnosed with ADHD. Excellent grades make it difficult for teachers or parents to recognize that there is a problem that may warrant treatment. When academic demands were easier and teachers would go over the same concepts repeatedly, Tina's inattention and forgetfulness didn't affect her grades because her intelligence was high and expectations were relatively low. Now, expectations are higher, and help and structure have decreased. While intelligence may partially compensate for ADHD, there often comes a time when demands rise to the point where this is no longer possible. Research has shown that while teachers are less likely to note attentional concerns in students with high intelligence, issues with attention may be noted more frequently and be more impairing in other environments, like at home. There is a particularly large discrepancy between what teachers and parents observe in both low and high intelligence students, which creates a risk for delayed identification and treatment of ADHD [11]. Transitions to grade school, high school, college, graduate school, and the workplace are typical times when expectations shift and previously masked inefficiencies and deficiencies suddenly become visible and impairing.

Misunderstandings about ADHD might also delay the diagnosis. Many people falsely believe that hyperactivity and disruptive behavior are required for an ADHD diagnosis and don't realize that quiet inattention can be equally impairing. Another common misunderstanding is that the ability to concentrate on certain things rules out ADHD. Parents often think their child cannot have ADHD if they can focus on video games or fun tasks. However, intense focus and difficulty shifting attention are consistent with an ADHD diagnosis. In fact, hyper-focus in specific areas can be a feature of ADHD [12]. Tina's parents and teachers may not have realized there was a problem due to not knowing about the inattentive symptoms of ADHD or, more generally, not understanding or believing in mental health treatment.

Because ADHD requires symptoms to have been present since childhood, these long-standing tendencies may be misattributed to personality characteristics or oppositionality rather than seen as an impairment arising from a neurodevelopmental disorder. Tina's parents might have seen her as lackadaisical, absent-minded, or even lazy. They might have told her to "grow up" or "get her act together" when she said or did things impulsively, forgot obligations, missed deadlines, or lost her license, keys, or cell phone repeatedly.

Despite these valid reasons why Tina's presumptive ADHD might have been missed in the past, it is also possible that her symptoms are *not* due to ADHD. She might be depressed, anxious, using illicit drugs, or seeking to misuse prescription drugs. Or she might simply be unprepared for college due to "immaturity" or to insufficient self-management skills. These are seen in individuals with ADHD but are not unique to the disorder. There are many disagreements about the validity of the new diagnosis of adult ADHD with delayed presentation as arguably reflecting a misdiagnosis of other complex comorbidities [13].

Mood disorders, anxiety, learning disabilities, and substance use disorders occur frequently with ADHD, further confusing the diagnostic picture when attention, organization, and learning difficulties are the presenting complaints [14]. Depression can mimic ADHD, with memory impairment, poor concentration, and decreased interest. By the same token, ADHD can create symptoms of depression, especially in the setting of poor self-esteem and guilt about being a failure or a disappointment. Similarly, anxiety may impair attention and memory and cause symptoms of restlessness that mimic ADHD, but ADHD can also cause performance anxiety from anticipating making errors and disappointing others. Malnutrition secondary to disordered eating can lead to poor concentration and focus. Someone using marijuana may seem forgetful, and someone using cocaine may be hyperactive, but pre-existing undiagnosed ADHD is associated with increased likelihood of illicit and prescription drug abuse. Because of this diagnostic complexity and confusion between cause and effect, conducting a full psychiatric and medical evaluation is essential and is explained in detail below.

Diagnosis

ADHD is a heterogeneous disorder. A wide constellation of symptoms may appear in different combinations over time. The quality and degree of resulting impairments may also change in response to environmental triggers and expectations. While the most well-recognized symptoms of ADHD are hyperactivity and impulsivity, a combined presentation including both hyperactive-impulsive and inattentive symptoms is the most common.

The fifth edition of the *Diagnostic and Statistical Manual of Mental Disorders* (DSM-5) includes the symptoms, which must occur often and have been present for at least 6 months [15]:

Symptoms of hyperactivity and impulsivity	Symptoms of inattention
Fidgets or squirms in seat	Doesn't pay attention to details, makes careless errors
Doesn't stay seated	Can't hold attention to tasks or play, easily distracted
Runs or climbs inappropriately (teens and adults may only feel restless)	Does not listen when spoken to
Can't play or do leisure activities quietly	Does not finish things, poor follow-through
Always on the go, moves excessively	Avoids, dislikes, or procrastinates difficult activities requiring focus and concentration
Talks excessively	Loses things
Blurts out answers too soon	Easily distracted
Interrupts or intrudes impulsively	Forgetful
Struggles to wait their turn	Difficulty organizing

Hyperactive children may run, climb, or leave their seats inappropriately. They do not like to sit still or engage in quiet activities. They talk a lot, blurt things out, do not wait for their turns, and interrupt others. These symptoms of impulsivity and the resulting disruption often prompt an ADHD evaluation in children.

Symptoms of hyperactivity often lessen as children age. Running, jumping, and climbing may turn into fidgeting by young adulthood. However, impulsivity can remain and is very dangerous in adulthood, related to the higher rates of car accidents, sexual partners, and substance use disorders in adults with ADHD.

The inattentive symptoms of ADHD may be more subtle and harder to recognize. Symptoms of inattention are quiet. Diagnosis may be delayed because daydreaming and forgetfulness do not disrupt homes and classrooms as do running, jumping, and interrupting. Inattentiveness is harder to recognize because the deficits lie in what is missing, rather than what is present. In this case, what is *not* done is the problem. Distraction results in careless errors and not understanding, remembering, or being able to follow through on expectations. Complex or detail-oriented tasks are avoided, delayed, completed with errors, or never finished. Poor organization results in things being frequently lost and forgotten.

Daydreaming may be noticed, but this alone is often insufficient to prompt medical evaluation if grades are decent or behavior is not disruptive. Teenagers and adults may have irritable moods, anxiety, frustration, and low self-esteem, as they struggle to meet the demands of school and work environments. When they achieve less than their peers despite putting in more effort and working longer hours to achieve the same results, they may blame themselves and wonder why they are not "living up to their potential." Adolescents and young adults may have car accidents due to lapses in attention. They may experience relationship or marital issues from not listening or for failing to follow through on obligations. They may encounter performance issues in the workplace due to excessive procrastination or poor attention to detail.

The DSM-5 requires six symptoms from either cluster up to age 16 years and five symptoms for ages 17 years and older to meet criteria for the diagnosis. Several symptoms must have been present before age 12 years because ADHD is a neurodevelopmental disorder, related to how the brain is "wired." Symptoms should persist across multiple settings, including school, work, home, and leisure activities, and must interfere with functioning. DSM-5 stipulates "presentation" (i.e., primary symptom constellation) at the time of diagnosis: inattentive, hyperactive-impulsive, or combined.

For the diagnosis to be made, ADHD must be the best explanation for the presenting symptoms as many other disorders can mimic ADHD. If someone is often distracted, forgetful, and avoidant because they are having flashbacks from trauma, PTSD is the more likely diagnosis. If a top student suddenly loses interest in school, sports, and friends, and cannot concentrate in ways they were able to do before, depression is a more likely diagnosis. If a person's behavior becomes erratic, they cannot sustain focus on their work, and they are less motivated to engage in their usual activities, a substance use disorder should be suspected. If someone starts losing and forgetting things for the first time in old age, cognitive impairment or dementia is a more likely diagnosis.

While ADHD is a clinical diagnosis and does not require formal psychological testing, it should always be confirmed with information detailing the presence, scope, and impairments related to relevant symptoms in different environments, including home, school, or work. Data must be collected from others who observe deficits that may not be visible during the examination. Parents, teachers, family, romantic partners, bosses, and co-workers can often provide relevant details and vignettes that may help to confirm the diagnosis, or bring other concerns like depression or substance use to light.

In evaluating Tina, some questions to ask her parents might include the following: How messy was her room growing up? How often did she lose things? How often did you have to remind her to do things like homework or chores? How hard was school for her? What did she have trouble focusing on and what held her focus? Did she seem to have to work harder than her peers, or harder than she should have, considering her intelligence? What things did you do to help her organize? How did she manage when this support was reduced? How much risk taking did she engage in? How was her driving record? How many car or bicycle accidents has she had?

Relevant questions for teachers might include the following: Do her grades match her intelligence? Where are points being lost? Does she struggle to finish assignments? Does she lose credit from careless errors or unfinished assignments? How does she act during class? Is she on time for class and with assignments? Information from past teachers can be gathered via report cards and behavior cards. A serial examination of past report cards or changes in grade point averages over time may highlight when difficulties arose. Symptom scales sent to relevant parties and returned electronically or by mail, or interviews conducted by phone or in person, may help clarify the frequency and extent, as well as the longevity, of the impairments.

All interviews should explore present functioning as it relates to performance, health, and mood. Some questions might include the following: What is an average day like for you? How hard is it to get things done? Who helps you? How do you remember what you need to do? How many reminders are needed and how do you get them? How are your grades (if in school) or performance reviews (if working)? What do your teachers or bosses criticize you for? What obligations are not being met now?

A complete medical history should be gathered to rule out potential medical causes for symptoms like inattention, impulsivity, and academic and social difficulties. Hearing impairments, head trauma, in utero exposure to drugs or alcohol, dementia, and seizures are just a few examples of the many medical conditions that can mimic ADHD.

Sleep, diet, exercise, mood, and anxiety should be assessed as they may be contributing to impaired functioning. Insufficient sleep can make it difficult to focus on or retain information. Insufficient caloric intake can impair attention and focus. Insufficient exercise can cause restlessness and difficulty sitting still. Relevant questions might include the following: Do you get angry at yourself or feel down when you struggle to get things done? Do you get nervous that you'll make mistakes? Do you beat yourself up for the errors you've made? Do you ever lose sleep or get tense from worrying that you'll mess up or forget something? Do you feel your mood has been more negative than usual?

As already stated, ADHD is a clinical diagnosis that does not require psychological testing. However, in cases that are complicated by medical factors, physical disabilities, or psychiatric comorbidities, psychoeducational testing can be a useful reference point. In any case, validated symptom rating scales are standard tools to help clinicians confirm a diagnosis of ADHD. There are currently 14 adult ADHD rating scales available for use. The Conner's Adult ADHD Rating Scale (CAARS), the Barkley Scales (Symptoms and Impairment), and the Wender Utah Rating Scale (short version) are preferred, based on data from analyses of 35 validation studies [16].

Learning disabilities (LD) are distinct from ADHD in that formal psychoeducational testing is required as an integral part of the diagnosis. Testing is used to detect learning differences and to compare intelligence to performance to demonstrate that a significant discrepancy exists.

The DSM-5 characterizes "specific learning disorders" as struggling with reading, understanding what is read, spelling, written expression, math, or mathematical reasoning for at least 6 months despite interventions being made. Academic skills must be substantially below what is expected for a child's age and intelligence, and the difficulties must have started at school age and caused problems at home, school, or work. As with ADHD, there are many other things that can mimic LD, which must be excluded. Intellectual disability is a common cause of difficulty in learning that must be excluded. Head trauma resulting in concussions or traumatic brain injuries can impair learning, but these are considered *acquired* rather than *innate* (i.e., developmental) learning disorders. Language barriers, poor vision, and hearing are other potential confounders for LD. Insufficient instruction (such as can be seen in under-resourced schools) may also cause underperformance or difficulties with learning that are correctable but not related to LD.

A diagnosis must be based on a "comprehensive evaluation," which may have variable components and can be performed by multiple specialists including teachers, psychologists, social workers, school nurses, school administrators, guidance counselors, speech pathologists, physical therapists, and occupational therapists [17]. Educational history, classroom observations, and diagnostic testing should be included in this evaluation.

For both ADHD and LD, neuropsychological and educational testing is critical to access learning and testing accommodations. This entails a battery of validated measures and examinations using scales, surveys, as well as tests of intelligence, attention, and problem-solving abilities. Testing is usually performed over several days with an in-depth report that describes the individual's academic performance in comparison to their intelligence and to the general population. This report normally outlines diagnoses, specific areas of deficits, and suggested learning accommodations. Colleges often require such a report to grant academic accommodations.

While school districts often provide and fund testing for younger children as part of an evaluation for special education, getting testing as an adult can be expensive and difficult to obtain. While testing is commonly available at universities and major medical centers, as well as via private practitioners in individual and group practices, there may be obstacles to obtaining this testing including long wait times, limited personnel, and high fees.

Medication Treatment

Why do we use medications to treat children with ADHD? Is it worth treating into adulthood? While there is sparse data on the long-term efficacy of treatment with stimulants for ADHD, and resulting debate about the appropriate length of treatment, far more robust data exists supporting short-term outcomes [18].

Medications for ADHD treatment go beyond mitigating present distress with a goal of protecting the future. Children treated with stimulants for ADHD are less likely to later develop mood, anxiety, or disruptive behavior disorders or to start smoking or develop other addictions, according to longitudinal studies [9, 19]. ADHD treatment may also be lifesaving. Stimulants reduce the risk of car accidents by about 40% [20]. Medication also lowers social risk factors, including criminality, in young adults with ADHD [21, 22].

ADHD responds robustly, and often rapidly, to evidence-based treatments. There is a growing body of evidence that suggests adults benefit from the same ADHD medications as children, albeit with slightly smaller effect sizes [21]. However, the data is less robust, with meta-analyses including a maximum of 2204 participants, 10% of the size of the studies described above related to childhood ADHD [23].

A meta-analysis of 26,114 children with ADHD from 190 randomized controlled trials investigating 52 interventions established basic treatment principles. Efficacious treatments include stimulants (i.e., methylphenidate, amphetamine), non-stimulants (i.e., atomoxetine, guanfacine, and clonidine), and behavioral therapy. The most effective treatment for children with ADHD is combined stimulants and behavior therapy, which also has superior treatment retention. Stimulants are the most effective single intervention, superior to non-stimulants, behavioral therapy, or cognitive training [19].

For adults, stimulants are also the most effective treatment, with some meta-analyses citing a 75% response rate. Non-stimulants are also highly effective in treating adults with ADHD, with a 60% response rate, and bupropion is nearly as effective as stimulants. Patients can be assured there is an excellent chance that pharmacotherapy can greatly improve their ADHD symptoms.

Longitudinal Case, part 2: Tina goes for testing since her primary care doctor is not comfortable making the diagnosis of ADHD in an adult. She returns with a 22-page report with the diagnosis ADHD, inattentive type, asking to start a medication that will help her with final examinations.

With so many effective options for treating ADHD, it can be difficult to know where to start. A practical, stepwise approach to starting medication treatment for ADHD is described here.

ADHD Medication Prescribing Guide

This is a simplified approach for prescribing medications for ADHD. Both amphetamine and methylphenidate preparations (steps 1 and 2) come in liquids, in transdermal patches, and in pills using "beaded technology" to combine immediate and extended-release formulations. They are less likely to be covered by insurance, so it is most reasonable to try them only after identifying specific issues with compliance or tolerability in steps 1 and 2.

Step	Medication	Starting dose	Max. dose	Increase by	Notes
1	Extended-release mixed amphetamine salts (amphetamine-dextroamphetamine)	10 mg	30 mg	5 mg	
2	Methylphenidate extended osmotic release	18 mg	72 mg	5 mg	Skip to step 4 if step 2 was favorable to step 1
3	Lisdexamfetamine	20 mg	70 mg	10 mg	
4	Dexmethylphenidate extended release	10 mg	40 mg	5 mg	
5	Atomoxetine	40 mg	100 mg	10 mg	Not abusable
6	Bupropion (SR or XL)	150 mg	450 mg	150 mg	Off-label for ADHD. Also used for depression and smoking cessation

Question 1 Is there a relative contraindication to using a stimulant?

With robust data supporting stimulants as the single most efficacious treatment for ADHD in both adults and children, treatment with long-acting methylphenidate or amphetamine should be considered first. In addition to being less effective, non-stimulants have the disadvantage of being slower to take effect, generally requiring weeks or months for clinically observable effects as compared with hours or days for stimulants. While there are no absolute contraindications to stimulants, non-stimulants should be considered in the setting of substance use disorders, eating disorders, or psychotic disorders to minimize the potential harm caused by stimulants. The risks and benefits of choosing a stimulant or non-stimulant medication should be discussed with patients and the treatment decision made collaboratively.

Question 2 Are short-acting or long-acting formulations preferable?

Long-acting formulations have multiple advantages in that they are less likely to be misused and can be given once daily, which is more convenient and may improve adherence [25]. Psychiatrists prescribe long-acting stimulants about twice as frequently as short-acting stimulants, whereas the reverse is true among primary care providers [10].

Question 3 Should an amphetamine or methylphenidate compound be tried first?

All stimulants are derived from two-parent compounds: amphetamine and methylphenidate. Amphetamines are slightly more effective than methylphenidate for adults, but evidence is limited [24]. Individuals may have a more robust response or fewer side effects to amphetamine or methylphenidate formulations. This is generally clarified through trial and error. During medication titrations, it is important to monitor for side effects and for changes in weight, blood pressure, and heart rate during titration.

Longitudinal Case, part 3: Tina reports increased focus and productivity after increasing extended-release mixed amphetamine salts to 15 mg but lost 8 pounds due to decreased appetite. She also had some benefit from methylphenidate 36 mg, but it took her hours to fall asleep. She wants to know about other options.

Question 4 What are next steps if the first stimulant trials fail or are not tolerated?

Tina experienced common side effects of stimulants, appetite suppression, and insomnia. Since Tina benefitted from an amphetamine preparation with fewer side effects, it would make sense to try another amphetamine derivative to see if the positive benefit can be maintained with reduced adverse effects.

If subsequent trials are also not tolerated, there are three non-stimulants with proven efficacy in adults with ADHD that may be reasonable alternatives: atomoxetine, bupropion, and desipramine [26–29]. Of the non-stimulants, atomoxetine has the most significant data supporting its efficacy in adults, but the results are still modest. About one in three adults with ADHD treated with atomoxetine has a response after 12 weeks [30]. It has no potential for abuse, so it may be an appropriate choice for patients with substance use disorders.

Medications for LD

Compared with ADHD, medications for LD have far less demonstrated efficacy and markedly less data supporting their use, particularly for adults. In a randomized controlled trial of 209 children and adolescents (10–16 years) with dyslexia only, combined ADHD and dyslexia, and ADHD only, atomoxetine (ATX) treatment had positive effects on reading performance. The dyslexia-only subjects treated with ATX showed strong improvements in word attack, reading skills, and reading vocabulary with effect sizes ranging from 0.48 to 0.73 ($p \leq 0.02$). Similar results were seen in subjects with combined dyslexia and ADHD [31]. There are no comparable studies of ATX in adults with dyslexia.

Studies have shown some benefit from stimulant medications for children with LD and ADHD in terms of attention, concentration, and academic performance, but it is unclear if this is solely due to improvement in ADHD symptoms or if this finding translates to adults. Other agents that have been investigated for LD, like piracetam, have limited data supporting their use and no demonstrated efficacy in adults [32].

Medication Adherence

As with other chronic conditions, medication adherence in patients with ADHD is a major clinical challenge. Estimates of non-adherence in published reviews of clinical trials range from 13 to 64%, although these are likely underestimates of actual incidence since many studies relied on patient reports [33, 34]. With respect to stimulants, adherence to regimens with short-acting medications was worse than with longer-acting agents. Stated reasons for discontinuation of treatment include adverse effects, ineffective symptom control, or suboptimal response, costs, dosing inconvenience, social stigma, negative perceptions of medication, insufficient physician-patient communication, and assessment that ADHD symptoms were not of sufficient importance to warrant medication.

Symptoms of ADHD, like forgetfulness, disorganization, and executive functioning deficits, also contribute to difficulties with adherence. Patients who stopped their treatment most often decided that the negatives outweigh the positives. In addition to stopping, a sizeable proportion of adult patients with ADHD modify the dosing schedule, taking the medication "as needed" rather than daily [34].

College students with ADHD are especially selective about taking medications as recommended. In general, they take half the medication doses they are prescribed, which can cause these individuals to underperform in school and which contributes to the nonmedical use of stimulants via "sharing" (see next section) [35]. Often, such modifications of treatment reflect a developmentally appropriate attempt to take charge of their lives and to assert their autonomy.

Case Vignette: Charlie is an 18-year-old college freshman with combined presentation ADHD and mild dyslexia. From elementary through high school, he took medications and had learning and testing accommodations. In college, he did not make use of his assigned ADHD coach, his academic accommodations, or the learning center, and he "adjusted" his medications as he saw fit. He also admitted to excessive online gaming, staying up late, and missing morning classes. As a result, he failed two classes and was put on academic probation. When asked why he did not take advantage of his available help, Charlie replied, "I wanted to see if I could make it on my own" [36].

Charlie's statement of wanting to see if he could succeed without reliance on either medication or academic accommodations is an effort to normalize himself by minimizing the impact of ADHD on his chances for success in college. His "positive attributional bias" (i.e., believing he could manage without help) led him to underestimate the importance of treatment adherence. With ongoing conversations and the use of motivational interviewing techniques, Charlie eventually chose to restart his medication and sought academic help from the learning center.

Strategies for improving treatment adherence include (1) enhancing clinician-patient communication and focusing on alliance-building; (2) creating a collaborative framework for working together on "issues"; (3) defining realistic goals, expectations, and time frame for treatment; (4) addressing predictable sources of treatment resistance (e.g., side effects, forgetfulness, desire to do it on one's own); (5) staying ever mindful about new or persistent barriers to adherence; (6) sustaining a focus on patterns of avoidance underlying non-adherence; (7) adopting a non-judgmental, compassionate, hopeful engagement in the change process; and (8) re-evaluating treatment practices to foster realistic outcomes. With respect to the use of motivational interviewing techniques, clinicians should always "roll with the resistance," express empathy, avoid argumentation, point out discrepancies in the patient's goals and behaviors, and support self-efficacy and self-management in whatever forms the patient is most likely to accept. It is also important to maintain frequent and regular contact with the patient and family in order to support whatever steps the patient is willing to take toward engaging with treatment in a sustained and meaningful way [37].

Nonmedical Use of Prescription Stimulants

Nonmedical use (NMU) refers to the use of a medication without a prescription or in a way other than prescribed [38]. NMU includes both medication misuse and abuse [36].

The NMU of prescription stimulants is highly prevalent in the USA and has been increasing recently with especially high rates among college students. A review of 111 studies providing empirical data about NMU of stimulants in adolescents and adults found rates varying from 2.1% to 58.7% with highest levels seen among college students, 17–31%, primarily because of easier access and greater acceptance of NMU in this population [39].

Factors contributing to the rise of NMU over the past two decades include pre-college access to prescription drugs, greater availability of prescription drugs, higher rates of ADHD diagnosis in young adults, increased pressures to achieve in college, the perception that "everybody does it," peer culture, and marketing/media messages suggesting that stimulants are safe to use. The most cited reasons for prescription NMU among college students include performance enhancement, euphoria seeking, self-medication of suspected ADHD, curiosity, weight control, and reducing sleep need or fatigue. The most common means of obtaining stimulants include obtaining them from friends and family members, purchasing them from others, and engaging in fraudulent behavior (e.g., "faking ADHD") to obtain a prescription from a healthcare provider [39].

The medical consequences of prescription stimulant NMU can range from mild symptoms (appetite suppression, heartburn, diarrhea, vomiting, sleep disturbance) to severe ones (including seizures, agitation, psychosis, tachycardia, chest pain, hypertension) and even death. Life-threatening symptoms are most often associated with non-oral route of administration (e.g., insufflation or intravenous) but can also be seen with chronic and excessive oral dosing [39]. In addition to medical risks, there are legal and ethical risks of NMU of stimulants. It is against the law to share one's medications with others, and there is a risk of suspension/expulsion from school and dismissal from work. Moreover, there is liability associated with sharing one's prescriptions if harm results.

Clinicians should always be mindful of the potential risk of their patients engaging in NMU or participating in stimulant diversion (i.e., sharing or selling their medication). Red flags that might indicate a patient is at risk for NMU include demands for immediate release rather than extended-release preparations, repeatedly discordant pill counts, frequently lost prescriptions, requests to increase dosage, and attempts to secure prescriptions from more than one healthcare provider. Controlled substance prescribing databases have been adopted in some states to address these concerns.

Patient education is the first line of intervention in confronting NMU. Explaining the medical, ethical, and legal risks of NMU and insisting that patients agree to refrain from misusing, abusing, or diverting their medication are essential steps. Prevention strategies such as not letting others know about the prescription, keeping the medication in a lock box or safe, and refraining from leaving loose pills in plain view of others should be emphasized. Asking patients to sign an "appropriate medication use contract" can reinforce the message that NMU is seen as a serious issue and that violating the contract is enough to terminate the doctor-patient relationship. Last but not least, clinicians should use extended-release formulations, should keep track of pills and refills, and should obtain urine toxicology to determine if the patient is actually adherent with the treatment regimen or is engaging in substance misuse/abuse.

Psychosocial Interventions

Longitudinal Case, part 5: Tina has been taking her medication as prescribed and finds it helps her to focus on schoolwork and other important tasks. Despite significant improvements in her ADHD symptoms, she is still struggling with procrastination, time management, organizational challenges, and keeping up with her assignments. She is feeling overwhelmed and wants to know about other treatment options.

Evidence-based psychosocial interventions for young adults with ADHD include academic accommodations (for college or university students), possible workplace accommodations (addressed later in the chapter), coaching, and cognitive behavioral therapy (CBT) [23]. Academic accommodations include formal modifications of curriculum, teaching and testing approaches, and the incorporation of assistive technology and educational support. These are generally available to students with documented physical, sensory, or learning disabilities; ADHD; and psychiatric conditions (anxiety or mood disorders). The purpose of each accommodation is to compensate for specific aspects of the student's learning profile that puts them at a disadvantage in the usual academic setting. Examples include reduced course load, priority course registration, extended time on tests and long-term assignments, preferential seating, note taking, recordings of lectures, and test administration in a quiet room.

The amount of documentation that is required for academic modifications varies from school to school and often requires recent psychoeducational testing results (within the past 2 years). Informal modifications such as study groups, tutoring sessions, organizational skills instruction, and coaching sessions are more easily accessed than formal ones and usually do not require extensive documentation. The effectiveness of academic accommodations and assistive technologies for students with ADHD and LD has not been well studied. Nevertheless, given anecdotal reports of their helpfulness, and in view of existing policies and practices at institutions of higher learning, it is reasonable to recommend that students with learning challenges make use of them.

ADHD coaching has become a widely accepted, evidence-based intervention to improve executive functioning in individuals with ADHD [40]. It aims to help individuals develop skills, strategies, and behaviors to better cope with the impairments in executive functioning that are commonly associated with ADHD: planning, time management, goal setting, organization, and problem-solving [41].

Coaching is highly collaborative and aimed at providing practical guidance and accountability for tackling common obstacles to successful attainment of personal, academic, and other valued goals. Coaching sessions are provided in person or remotely via telephone or video conferencing and consist of helping the individual with ADHD identify their goals; set objectives and priorities; define key responsibilities; develop implementation plans; manage distractions; maintain motivation and focus; and work in a consistent fashion so as to complete prioritized tasks. Coaches monitor their clients' progress toward task completion and offer suggestions for overcoming barriers to success. Coaching is offered in either individual or group formats, and increasingly, colleges and universities are offering skills-based coaching in their student learning centers. Published studies of formal coaching programs based in institutions of higher learning have documented positive outcomes for students who attend sessions regularly and practice the skills and coping strategies provided. There are a growing number of studies of ADHD coaching for adults who are not enrolled in higher education. Preliminary results indicate generally positive outcomes and favorable perceptions of these services [42].

Cognitive behavioral therapy for adults with ADHD is an adaptation of CBT, which addresses the common problems faced by adults with ADHD. It differs from coaching insofar as it helps individuals understand how ADHD is affecting their lives (especially with respect to daily functioning), explores the impact of dysfunctional thinking and behavior, assists patients to develop more effective coping strategies, explores how events influence the completion of tasks and goals, and provides a framework for building resilience and adaptation. Several manualized treatments have been developed in both individual and group formats. Two recent meta-analytic reviews of CBT for adult ADHD report strong evidence for its effectiveness in reducing symptoms and improving functioning using a variety of outcome measures [43, 44]. Standard mean differences from 32 studies ranged from 0.51 to 1.00, indicating a medium to large effect size for the intervention, with variations seen depending upon whether the control group was active or passive.

Elements of CBT for adult ADHD [23, 45]	
Education	Psychoeducation, accepting the diagnosis, understanding the cognitive model (including how negative beliefs and distortions affect emotions and behaviors)
Planning	Managing time, developing organizational skills, setting priorities, modifying the environment so as to reduce distractions
Goal setting	Committing to change, minimize procrastination, adaptive thinking, manage stress, think before acting (i.e., improving impulse control), reduce risks, handle frustration, develop and sustain motivation in the face of obstacles, improve relationships
Healthy lifestyle	Managing diet, sleep, and exercise
Specific inventions	Cognitive modification, behavioral modification and coping skills, acceptance, mindfulness, persistence, and implementation strategies

In addition to CBT, other "possibly effective" psychosocial interventions for adults with ADHD include neurofeedback, cognitive remediation therapy, mindfulness meditation training, and computer-assisted cognitive training [46]. While more research is needed before these can be considered evidence-based, preliminary studies (mostly open-label) indicate that these approaches can be helpful as adjunctive treatments for this population.

Transition Preparation

Case: Pablo is an 18-year-old senior in high school who was diagnosed with ADHD at age 8 years. His parents wake him up every day and remind him about important school obligations, which they check on the school's online system and through communications with teachers. He is also not particularly attentive about keeping his room clean or putting away his clothes after they have been laundered by his mother. Next year, he is planning to go away to college. In view of his difficulty managing day-to-day responsibilities, his parents are worried about his readiness for school and are asking for advice.

Teenagers with ADHD and/or LD struggle more than their peers with disorganization, lack of self-management skills, substance use, and emotional problems as seniors in high school. Boys also report more disengagement, partying, and time spent on TV, video games, and computer games [47]. These difficulties along with other concerns about executive functioning should be addressed well in advance of the young person's senior year in college through a process referred to as *transition planning*. This includes *educational* transition planning (i.e., making sure realistic goals educational goals are set, suitable college choices are made, appropriate resources are available and in place prior to arrival at school) and *self-care* transition planning (i.e., managing daily routines; getting proper sleep, exercise, and diet; preparing for the demands of college life; and demonstrating appropriate knowledge and skills to manage specific mental health challenges such as medication and psychosocial treatment adherence). It is important that sufficient psychoeducation be provided to ensure that both the young adult and family members are aware of the potential pitfalls and problems that can arise on campus and to identify appropriate resources (academic supports, counseling, medical and psychiatric care).

It is also important to identify potential mindset barriers that might interfere with successful transition to college [48]. "Fear of not belonging" leads some students to pursue relationships in a reckless fashion and succumb to peer pressure.

Others avoid social situations out of concerns about being rejected which is especially true if they have been discriminated against, ostracized, or bullied in the past. "Fear of not making it" arises when students feel unprepared for the academic challenges of college and/or when they experience less-than-desired grades. If their expectations are too high (e.g., straight As in every course), it is easy for them to mistakenly believe that they are not suited for college. They may equate these setbacks as indicators that they will never succeed in the future. "Fear of being different" arises when students with ADHD, LD, or mental health issues experience stigma about their differences and feel ashamed of themselves. This may arise from a perception that others are intolerant of individuals with differences or from a self-rejecting mindset that inhibits feelings of self-compassion and self-acceptance. Overcoming these mindset barriers is an important developmental milestone for young adults with ADHD/LD to master.

Along with overcoming mindset barriers, successful transition to college requires that young people develop social-emotional readiness skills, including [49]:

1. *Conscientiousness* – the ability to "own" one's actions and to take responsibility for their behavior. Reliability, predictability, honesty, integrity, and trustworthiness are all vital aspects of conscientiousness.
2. *Self-Management* – the ability to take care of day-to-day activities on one's own. This means being able to wake up on time, prepare for the day, remember tasks and carry them out, develop routines, adjust one's schedule as needed, and fall asleep at a reasonable time each night.
3. *Interpersonal Skills* – the ability to form the basis for getting along with others such as working in teams, making and keeping friends, maintaining good communication with classmates, handling conflicts appropriately, and participating in the social events at school.
4. *Self-Control* (or "willpower") – the ability to set limits on oneself and to resist urges/desires when necessary. It results from the interaction of two sets of forces: those that trigger us to seek rewards and those that help us to hold back as needed.
5. *Grit* – the ability to cope with frustration, disappointment, and failure and to persist in the face of setbacks and obstacles to success. The ability to keep going in the face of delayed gratification or of unexpected hardship is highly predictive of success in later life.
6. *Risk Management* – This involves the ability to have fun and experiment with risky behaviors without taking foolish or dangerous chances. Individuals have to decide how much they will allow themselves to engage in activities like smoking, drinking, partying, and having sex and how to draw the line when it becomes necessary to avoid harm.
7. *Self-Acceptance* (or "self-compassion") – the ability to accept one's faults, tolerate one's mistakes, and deal with one's shortcomings without excessive amounts of guilt and shame. It is a cornerstone of mental health and has been found to be highly protective against anxiety disorders and depression in college students.
8. *Open Mindset/Help-Seeking* – This involves the ability to recognize when things aren't going well and to ask for help when problems appear to be impossible to solve. It involves a willingness to overcome "denial" that anything could be wrong and to accept the idea that "tincture of time" isn't always the best way to approach potential problems.

The ideal way to prepare for a successful transition to college is for patients, family members, and healthcare providers to structure a series of sessions aimed at identifying critical steps to enable the young adult to practice readiness skills and to formulate concrete plans for engaging helping professionals at school. Facilitating a discussion about the parameters of continued family involvement and help is critical since the loss of parental "scaffolding" may make it difficult for the young person to manage on their own. Finally, healthcare providers should draw up the transition plan and share it with the helping professionals with whom the patient will be working next (i.e., "warm hand-off"). Constructing an effective social safety net that provides the right amount of support and supervision to the college student with ADHD, LD, or other mental health concerns is now widely considered to be an evidence-based standard of care for vulnerable youth [47].

Workforce Issues

Case: Mark is a 22-year-old man with a history of ADHD and dyslexia brought in for an evaluation by his parents. They say he "flunked out of college" and has worked at a grocery store, bank, and fast-food restaurant since. He was fired by two jobs and quit the third. Methylphenidate helped with some symptoms but has not significantly altered his trajectory. They are thinking of "shipping him off to the army" and are worried, frustrated, and seeking advice.

Mark's story is not uncommon. Adults with ADHD struggle in the workforce. They are more likely to be unemployed [9] and less likely to have full-time jobs [2].

Mark was unable to succeed in the transition to college, likely due to the combination of increased demands on his executive functioning and decreased support from school and home compared to childhood. The accommodations he had received through his 504 plan to assist him in high school are not likely to be extended to the workplace. Workplace modifications are usually limited to those that do not create significant financial hardship for his employers [50].

The same factors that impacted Mark's transition to college have likely affected workforce performance. Children diagnosed with ADHD are more likely to be financially dependent on their parents as adults and attain a lower social class than their families [9]. Mark may have been overly dependent on parents and teachers for support with planning, organization, and follow-through. He is anticipated to require support to earn and budget money, pay bills, figure out taxes, and carry out a variety of other activities required for adult life.

Entering the job market is challenging with ADHD. Poor organization skills and difficulties with completing tasks will likely impair job performance. Adults with ADHD may struggle to find a good job "fit" despite being highly intelligent and motivated. Highly structured or sedentary jobs that require repetitive and detail-oriented work, like many office-based jobs, challenge the core symptoms of ADHD and may result in more errors and unmet expectations. With Mark's difficulty sustaining focus, especially on repetitive or detail-oriented tasks, it is easy to understand why entry-level jobs he attempted quickly became boring. Frustrated with the monotony and inflexibility of work, adults with ADHD may quit or act out impulsively. Adults with ADHD get fired and quit more often and have shorter employment [2].

Like Mark, adults with ADHD change jobs more often [51]. This may be related to the need to explore more careers in order to find the right fit. Novelty-seeking related to impulsivity and easy boredom, along with suboptimal job performance, is highly associated with getting fired or quitting more frequently. People with ADHD tend to gravitate toward flexible jobs that are stimulating and challenging and allow for independence [50].

While ADHD itself presents challenges to finding employment, treatment may also, ironically, limit job prospects. Some organizations ban those who have been diagnosed with ADHD regardless of the level of their impairment. Other organizations may employ people with ADHD, but only under the condition that they do not take medications to treat their condition.

The Armed Forces and certain law enforcement jobs are not an option for Mark. While amphetamine preparations were used to improve performance and reduce fatigue in armed forces in World War II, the use of these medications is now banned for military personnel, even when it is prescribed for ADHD and used as directed by a physician [52, 53]. The military requires no stimulant use for 2 years prior to recruitment [29]. Pilots (commercial and private) cannot have ADHD – they must be tested by an approved neuropsychologist after at least 90 days off stimulant medications to confirm the absence of ADHD [54]. Higher-level sports either ban or require therapeutic use exemptions for stimulants for ADHD [55].

This can be frustrating for adults with ADHD, as treatment can improve workplace outcomes.

Stimulant treatment positively impacts workplace productivity for adults with ADHD [56], though data is limited and general improvement in occupational functioning has not been demonstrated [50].

If stimulants are banned from a sector or industry, non-stimulant medications should be considered, and non-medication treatments should be maximized. CBT and coaching may be useful to adults with ADHD entering the workforce, or when navigating issues that arise from work. Job training programs and assistance in job searching and placement have been found to be beneficial for young adults with ADHD [57].

Legal Rights and Protections

Case continued: Pablo and his family have worked together to improve his self-management skills and have fashioned a realistic transition plan to facilitate his entry into college. At this point, their main concerns center on the availability of resources, services, and accommodations at his future school. They wonder if he is entitled by law to receive academic modifications in college like those he was granted in high school under his individualized education plan (IEP).

Children, adolescents, and young adults between the ages of 3 and 21 years who have a qualifying disability that adversely affects their education are covered by the Individuals with Disabilities Education Act (IDEA) of 2004 [58]. IDEA stipulates that schools are required to provide individualized specialized educational plans (IEPs), services, and accommodations in the least restrictive learning environment in order to guarantee that disabled individuals receive an adequate education. *Disability* is defined as a "physical or mental impairment that substantially limits one or more aspects of a person's life" [59]. Specific learning disabilities are among the qualifying criteria for IDEA, but ADHD is not specifically named and is not always protected. It is listed in the statute as an "other health impairment," a category which includes chronic health problems like asthma, diabetes, epilepsy, Tourette syndrome, and lead poisoning, among others. Young adults lose the legal protection of IDEA (including IEPs) when they either graduate from high school or when they turn 22 years old.

The Rehabilitation Act (RA) of 1973 and the Americans with Disabilities Act (ADA) of 1990 are two important Congressional statutes that were passed to protect individuals with disabilities. The Rehabilitation Act made discrimination against individuals with disabilities unlawful in three areas: (1) employment by the executive branch of the federal government, (2) employment by most federal contractors, and (3) activities that are funded by federal subsidies or grants.

Section 504 of the RA provides access to services to individuals with physical or mental impairment at any age but does not support or fund these services [60]. Schools that receive federal funding must provide accommodations such as increased support, extended testing time, behavioral plans, and mental health and health services. Compared to IEPs, 504 plans are less restrictive and allow students to participate in regular education; hence, they are expected to meet regular educational standards. Educational institutions that do not receive federal funds are not subject to the RA. Colleges that accept federal funding must continue to comply with Section 504, but eligibility criteria for disability and availability of accommodations vary in secondary and higher education, and most colleges do not provide the extent of assistance that students may have received under their IEPs. Pablo and his family need to be advised of this fact so they can approach his future school with realistic expectations.

Post-secondary institutions are regulated by the RA and ADA in three key domains: (1) testing (for admissions, evaluation of academic performance and graduation), (2) delivery of curriculum/course materials, and (3) non-academic aspects of campus life (residential settings, recreational facilities, dining areas, etc.).

Case law regarding the definitions and boundaries of the requirements for accommodations under RA/ADA is highly complex and beyond the scope of this chapter. In general, there is an expectation that "*discrimination* against individuals with disabilities is prohibited, and *qualified individuals* with disabilities are entitled to *reasonable accommodations* in meeting the *essential requirements* of the educational program" [59]. The italicized terms indicate where legal disputes have been centered. For instance, colleges are not obliged to provide an individualized course of study for a disabled individual. They are required to provide equal access to classroom and course materials. They are also mandated to select and administer tests in ways that enable the individual to demonstrate the disabled individual's aptitude or achievement level. While these issues are subject to interpretation, post-secondary institutions are *not* required to lower their curricular content, academic standards, or their requirements for graduation. Furthermore, individuals with disabilities are required to request accommodations and must provide reasonable documentation to support the requested modifications. Returning to Pablo's case, it is important that he and his parents fully understand the college's academic requirements, that he request only those accommodations that he can legitimately verify, and that he make available the necessary documentation to substantiate his request. This can entail providing prior testing results, evaluations, and IEPs or 504 plans, as well as supporting letters from qualified health professionals.

With respect to employment, the ADA stipulates that employers, state and local governments, employment agencies, and labor unions cannot discriminate against qualified individuals with disabilities regarding job applications, hiring, firing, career advancement, compensation, or training. Employers may not ask applicants about the existence, nature, or severity of a disability, and may only query their ability to perform specific job functions. Employers must allow reasonable accommodation like job restructuring, modifying work schedules, use of equipment or devices, adjusting examinations, and training.

Conclusion

ADHD and LD are often incorrectly viewed as disorders exclusively of childhood. Instead, ADHD and LD represent inherent differences in understanding and processing information, acquiring skills, and solving problems. These differences are neurologically "hard-wired," emerge in early childhood, and persist into adulthood, even when they may not cause noticeable impairments in early life. Moreover, these conditions are highly associated with multiple developmental challenges including delays in emotional and cognitive maturation, persistent executive functioning deficits, and serious, long-term health risks.

Most research supporting the diagnosis and treatment of ADHD and LD is derived from studies of pediatric populations. Children diagnosed with ADHD and LD receive assistance from parents and schools, including instructional and testing accommodations, that are backed by stronger legal protections than those afforded to adults.

While most children with ADHD and LD suffer from symptoms well into adolescence, far less is known about how to help young adults. If already diagnosed, they face declining structural and interpersonal support after finishing high school. If not yet evaluated, young adults will likely struggle to get diagnosed and treated due to an amalgamation of complex factors including stigma, misunderstandings about these diagnoses and their treatments, bias, cost, and provider shortages.

Unfortunately, the symptoms of ADHD and LD do not diminish at the same rate that social and education support and protections are removed as adolescents move into young adulthood. In fact, symptoms may even become worse and more debilitating as environmental demands rise and the individual's coping strategies cannot keep up. Entering adulthood with ADHD and LD poses a serious set of challenges to the individual's functionality and chances for success. ADHD also threatens financial, physical, and emotional health.

Treating adults with ADHD can be complicated, time-consuming, and risky. Young adults are likely to struggle with medication adherence and some may misuse their medications. Stimulants have received a lot of negative press related to the misuse that commonly occurs on college campuses. However, all medications are associated with risks, and the critical question is not whether risks exist, but if these are outweighed by potential benefits.

If the purpose of medical care is to enhance quality of life, improve functionality, and reduce mortality, ADHD should be treated throughout adulthood. There are significant and compelling risks associated with withholding treatment, including, most notably, increased rates of car accidents, nearly half of which are preventable with medication treatment with stimulants [18]. The risk of early mortality in adult ADHD should be carefully considered and compared with any potential risks of treatment.

The transition to college and to the workforce should be anticipated to be especially challenging for those with ADHD or LD. It should be planned carefully and realistically using all available resources to ensure the best outcomes. Psychosocial interventions and educational supports should be utilized to the greatest extent possible. The transition to adult medical providers and other healthcare professionals needs to be initiated during late adolescence. Holistic care plans should be developed that promote wellness and resilience so that individuals can successfully cope with the multiple challenges that living with ADHD and LD entails.

To summarize, ADHD and LD are common and treatable. They pose threats to the success and well-being of about one in ten children. These threats do not disappear in adulthood. The learning and executive functioning concerns that impacted grade school performance are likely to impair success in higher education, work, and relationships. Young adults should be prepared for these difficulties and supported socially, academically, medically, and psychologically as they face a multitude of new expectations and attempt to transition to greater independence.

The following organizations are resources for information, treatment, and advocacy for ADHD and LD:

(a) Attention Deficit Disorder Association – www.add.org
(b) Children and Adults with Attention-Deficit/Hyperactivity Disorder – www.chadd.org
(c) National Resource Center for ADHD – www.help4add.org
(d) Association on Higher Education and Disability – www.ahead.org
(e) Learning Disabilities Association of America – www.ldaamerica.org
(f) National Center for Learning Disabilities – https://www.ncld.org/
(g) ADD Resources – www.addresources.org

References

1. Faraone SV, Asherson P, Banaschewski T, Biederman J, Buitelaar JK, Ramos-Quiroga JA, et al. Attention-deficit/hyperactivity disorder. Nat Rev Dis Prim [Internet]. 2015;1(1):15020. Available from: https://doi.org/10.1038/nrdp.2015.20.
2. Hechtman L, Swanson JM, Sibley MH, Stehli A, Lakes KD, Owens EB, et al. Functional adult outcomes 16 years after childhood diagnosis of attention-deficit/hyperactivity disorder: MTA results. J Am Acad Child Adolesc Psychiatry. 2016;55(11):945–52.
3. Barkley RA, Fischer M. Hyperactive child syndrome and estimated life expectancy at young adult follow-up: the role of ADHD persistence and other potential predictors. J Atten Disord. 2019;23(9):907–23.
4. Xu G, Strathearn L, Liu B, Yang B, Bao W. Twenty-year trends in diagnosed attention-deficit/hyperactivity disorder among US children and adolescents, 1997–2016. JAMA Netw Open. 2018;1(4):e181471.
5. Altarac M, Saroha E. Lifetime prevalence of learning disability among US children. Pediatrics. 2007;1:S77–89.
6. Biederman J, Faraone SV, Spencer T, Wilens T, Mick E, Lapey KA. Gender differences in a sample of adults with attention deficit hyperactivity disorder. Psychiatry Res. 1994;53(1):13–29.
7. Weyandt LL, DuPaul GJ. College students with ADHD: current issues and future directions. College students with ADHD: current issues and future directions. New York: Springer; 2013.
8. Barkley RA, Fischer M, Smallish L, Fletcher K. The persistence of attention-deficit/hyperactivity disorder into young adulthood as a function of reporting source and definition of disorder. J Abnorm Psychol. 2002;111(2):279–89.
9. Biederman J, Monuteaux MC, Mick E, Spencer T, Wilens TE, Silva JM, et al. Young adult outcome of attention deficit hyperactivity disorder: a controlled 10-year follow-up study. Psychol Med. 2006;36(2):167–79.

10. Cascade E, Kalali AH, Weisler RH. Short-acting versus long-acting medications for the treatment of ADHD. Psychiatry (Edgmont). 2008;5(8):24–7.
11. Rommelse N, Antshel K, Smeets S, Greven C, Hoogeveen L, Faraone SV, et al. High intelligence and the risk of ADHD and other psychopathology. Br J Psychiatry. 2017;211(6):359–64.
12. Ashinoff BK, Abu-Akel A. Hyperfocus: the forgotten frontier of attention. Psychol res [internet]. 2019;(0123456789). Available from: https://doi.org/10.1007/s00426-019-01245-8.
13. Wilens TE, Isenberg BM, Kaminski TA, Lyons RM, Quintero J. Attention-deficit/hyperactivity disorder and transitional aged youth. Curr Psychiatry Rep. 2018;20(11):100.
14. Kessler RC, Adler L, Berkley R, Biederman J, Conners CK, Demler O, et al. The prevalence and correlates of adult ADHD in the United States: results from the National Comorbidity Survey Replication. Am J Psychiatry. 2006;163(4):716–23.
15. American Psychiatric Association. Diagnostic and statistical manual of mental disorders, 5th Edition. 2013. Arlington: American Psychiatric Association.
16. Taylor A, Deb S, Unwin G. Scales for the identification of adults with attention deficit hyperactivity disorder (ADHD): a systematic review. Res Dev Disabil. 2011;32:924.
17. von Hahn LE. Specific learning disabilities in children: evaluation. [Internet]. UPTODATE. Available from: uptodate.com.
18. Swanson JM. Debate: are stimulant medications for attention-deficit/hyperactivity disorder effective in the long term? J Am Acad Child Adolesc Psychiatry. 2019;58(10):936–8.
19. Catalá-López F, Hutton B, Núñez-Beltrán A, Page MJ, Ridao M, Saint-Gerons DM, et al. The pharmacological and non-pharmacological treatment of attention deficit hyperactivity disorder in children and adolescents: a systematic review with network meta-analyses of randomised trials. PLoS One. 2017;12:e0180355.
20. Chang Z, Quinn PD, Hur K, Gibbons RD, Sjölander A, Larsson H, et al. Association between medication use for attention-deficit/hyperactivity disorder and risk of motor vehicle crashes. JAMA Psychiat. 2017;74(6):597–603.
21. Lichtenstein P, Halldner L, Zetterqvist J, Sjölander A, Serlachius E, Fazel S, et al. Medication for attention deficit-hyperactivity disorder and criminality. N Engl J Med. 2012;367(21):2006–14.
22. McCabe SE, Veliz P, Wilens TE, Schulenberg JE. Adolescents' prescription stimulant use and adult functional outcomes: a national prospective study. J Am Acad Child Adolesc Psychiatry. 2017;56(3):226–33.
23. Ramsay JR, Rostain A. College students with ADHD. In: Attention-deficit hyperactivity disorder in adults and children. Cambridge: Cambridge University Press; 2015. p. 366–77.
24. Cortese S, Adamo N, Del Giovane C, Mohr-Jensen C, Hayes AJ, Carucci S, et al. Comparative efficacy and tolerability of medications for attention-deficit hyperactivity disorder in children, adolescents, and adults: a systematic review and network meta-analysis. Lancet Psychiatry. 2018;5(9):727–38.
25. Wilens T, Carellas N, Biederman J. ADHD and substance misuse. In: Oxford textbook of attention deficit hyperactivity disorder; Oxford University Press in Oxford, United Kingdom. 2016.
26. Cunill R, Castells X, Tobias A, Capellà D. Atomoxetine for attention deficit hyperactivity disorder in the adulthood: a meta-analysis and meta-regression. Pharmacoepidemiol Drug Saf. 2013;22(9):961–9.
27. Maneeton N, Maneeton B, Srisurapanont M, Martin SD. Bupropion for adults with attention-deficit hyperactivity disorder: meta-analysis of randomized, placebo-controlled trials. Psychiatry Clin Neurosci. 2011;65:611–7.
28. Wilens TE, Biederman J, Prince J, Spencer TJ, Faraone SV, Warburton R, et al. Six-week, double-blind, placebo-controlled study of desipramine for adult attention deficit hyperactivity disorder. Am J Psychiatry. 1996;153(9):1147–53.
29. Medical standards for appointment, enlistment, or induction into the military service. Office of the Under Secretary of Defense for Personnel and Readiness; 2018. p. 44. https://www.esd.whs.mil/Portals/54/Documents/DD/issuances/dodi/613003p.pdf.
30. Asherson P, Bushe C, Saylor K, Tanaka Y, Deberdt W, Upadhyaya H. Efficacy of atomoxetine in adults with attention deficit hyperactivity disorder: an integrated analysis of the complete database of multicenter placebo-controlled trials. J Psychopharmacol. 2014;28(9):837–46.
31. Sumner CR, Gathercole S, Greenbaum M, Rubin R, Williams D, Hollandbeck M, et al. Atomoxetine for the treatment of Attention-Deficit/Hyperactivity Disorder (ADHD) in children with ADHD and dyslexia. Child Adolesc Psychiatry Ment Health. 2009;3(40):1–9.
32. Rostain A. Medications affecting behavior and learning. In: Goldstein S, Naglieri J, editors. Learning and attention disorders in adolescence and adulthood – a comprehensive guide for practitioners. John Wiley & Sons Hoboken, NJ; 2011.
33. Adler LD, Nierenberg AA. Review of medication adherence in children and adults with ADHD. Postgrad Med. 2010;122(1):184–91.
34. Gajria K, Lu M, Sikirica V, Greven P, Zhong Y, Qin P, et al. Adherence, persistence, and medication discontinuation in patients with attention-deficit/hyperactivity disorder - a systematic literature review. Neuropsychiatr Dis Treat. 2014;10:1543–69.
35. Gray WN, Kavookjian J, Shapiro SK, Wagoner ST, Schaefer MR, Rawlinson AR, et al. Transition to college and adherence to prescribed attention deficit hyperactivity disorder medication. J Dev Behav Pediatr. 2018;39(1):1–9.
36. Rostain AL. "Time is not on my side": a college student with ADHD and a reading disability. In: Martel

AL, Derenne J, Leebens P, editors. Promoting safe and effective transitions to college for youth with mental health conditions. 2018th ed. New York: Springer; 2018. p. 95–102.
37. Manos M. Sustainable change: treatment adherence in ADHD. In: Adler L, Spencer T, Wilens T, editors. Attention deficit hyperactivity disorder in adults and children. New York: Cambridge University Press; 2015. p. 353–65.
38. Martins SS, Ghandour LA. Nonmedical use of prescription drugs in adolescents and young adults: not just a Western phenomenon. World Psychiatry [Internet]. 2017;16(1):102–4. Available from: https://www.ncbi.nlm.nih.gov/pubmed/28127929.
39. Faraone SV, Rostain AL, Montano CB, Mason O, Antshel KM, Newcorn JH. Systematic review: nonmedical use of prescription stimulants: risk factors, outcomes, and risk reduction strategies. J Am Acad Child Adolesc Psychiatry [Internet]. 2020;59(1):100–12. Available from: https://doi.org/10.1016/j.jaac.2019.06.012.
40. Prevatt F. Coaching for college students with ADHD. Curr Psychiatry Rep. 2016;18(12):110.
41. Goudreau SB, Knight M. Executive function coaching: assisting with transitioning from secondary to postsecondary education. J Atten Disord. 2018;22(4):379–87.
42. Ahmann E, Tuttle L. A descriptive review of ADHD coaching research: implications for college students. J Postsecond Educ Disabil. 2018;31(1):17–39.
43. Jensen CM, Amdisen BL, Jørgensen KJ, Arnfred SMH. Cognitive behavioural therapy for ADHD in adults: systematic review and meta-analyses. ADHD Atten Deficit Hyperact Disord. 2016;8(1):3–11.
44. Knouse LE, Teller J, Brooks MA. Meta-analysis of cognitive-behavioral treatments for adult ADHD. J Consult Clin Psychol. 2017;85(7):737–50.
45. Ramsay J. Rethinking adult ADHD – helping clients turn intentions into actions. Washington, DC: American Psychological Press; 2020.
46. Lofthouse N, Hurt E, Arnol J. Complementary and alternative treatments for pediatric and adult ADHD. In: Attention-deficit hyperactivity disorder in adults and children. Cambridge: Cambridge University Press; 2015. p. 307–17.
47. DuPaul GJ, Pinho TD, Pollack BL, Gormley MJ, Laracy SD. First-year college students with ADHD and/or LD: differences in engagement, positive core self-evaluation, school preparation, and college expectations. J Learn Disabil. 2017;50(3):238–51.
48. Hibbs B, Rostain A. The stressed years of their lives: helping your kid survive and thrive during their college years. New York: St. Martin's Press; 2019.
49. Martel A, Derenne J, Leebens P. Promoting safe and effective transitions to college for youth with mental health conditions. Promoting safe and effective transitions to college for youth with mental health conditions. New York: Springer; 2018.
50. Gordon CT, Fabiano GA. The transition of youth with ADHD into the workforce: review and future directions. Clin Child Fam Psychol Rev. 2019;22:316–47.
51. Kuriyan AB, Pelham WE, Molina BSG, Waschbusch DA, Gnagy EM, Sibley MH, et al. Young adult educational and vocational outcomes of children diagnosed with ADHD. J Abnorm Child Psychol. 2013;41(1):27–41.
52. Rasmussen N. Medical science and the military: the Allies' use of amphetamine during World War II. J Interdiscip Hist [Internet]. 2011;42(2):205–33. Available from: https://doi.org/10.1162/JINH_a_00212.
53. Defalque RJ, Wright AJ. Methamphetamine for Hitler's Germany: 1937 to 1945. Bull Anesth Hist [Internet]. 2011;29(2):21–32. Available from: http://www.sciencedirect.com/science/article/pii/S1522864911500162.
54. Airman information – ADHD/ADD evaluation [Internet]. Available from: https://www.faa.gov/about/office_org/headquarters_offices/avs/offices/aam/ame/guide/media/AI_ADHD_ADD.pdf.
55. Garner AA, Hansen AA, Baxley C, Ross MJ. The use of stimulant medication to treat attention-deficit/hyperactivity disorder in elite athletes: a performance and health perspective. Sports Med. 2018;48(3):507–12.
56. Wigal T, Brams M, Gasior M, Gao J, Squires L, Giblin J. Randomized, double-blind, placebo-controlled, crossover study of the efficacy and safety of lisdexamfetamine dimesylate in adults with attention-deficit/hyperactivity disorder: novel findings using a simulated adult workplace environment design. Behav Brain Funct. 2010;6:34.
57. Glynn K, Schaller J. Predictors of employment outcomes for transition-age state-federal vocational rehabilitation consumers with attention-deficit/hyperactivity disorder. J Vocat Rehabil. 2017;47(2):159–74.
58. Individuals With Disabilities Education Act of 2004, Pub. L. No. 108–446, 104 Stat. 327 [Internet]. United States; 2004. p. 2647–808. Available from: http://spannj.org/pti/IDEA-504Overview.pdf.
59. Latham P, Latham P. Learning and attention disorders in adolescence and adulthood – a comprehensive guide for practitioners. In: Goldstein S, Naglieri J, editors. . New York: John Wiley & Sons; 2011.
60. Smith TEC. Section 504, the ADA, and public schools. Remedial Spec Educ. 2001;22:335.

13 Disruptive, Impulse-Control, and Conduct Disorders: Prognosis, Assessment, and Treatment of Youth "Grown-Up"

Shelley Co, Margaret Wohlleber, and Cathryn A. Galanter

Key Points

- The disruptive, impulse-control, and conduct disorders (DICCDs) include oppositional defiant disorder, conduct disorder, and intermittent explosive disorder. These conditions typically have first onset in childhood but can also first emerge in adulthood.
- Integrating childhood and adolescent history with the transitional age youth's current life circumstances is crucial for accurate assessment and treatment of transitional age youth with DICCD symptoms. Certain childhood and adolescent psychosocial elements have implications in adulthood.
- A pediatric DICCD diagnosis increases the risk of having certain psychiatric disorders including depression, anxiety, antisocial personality and substance use disorders in adulthood.
- Most of the DICCD treatments with evidence for efficacy are psychotherapeutic rather than psychopharmacologic.
- There are no US FDA-approved medications for the treatment of children, adolescents, or transitional age youth with a DICCD. Medications can be helpful in treating co-occurring conditions.

Introduction

Disruptive, impulse-control, and conduct disorders (DICCDs) are a diverse set of conditions now categorized together in the *Diagnostic and Statistical Manual of Mental Disorders, 5th Edition* (DSM-5) [7]. These disorders are characterized by emotional and behavioral self-control that vary in their degree of violation of societal normative behaviors, interpersonal conflicts, and problems with authority [7]. Although these disorders often begin in childhood or adolescence, they can cause significant and substantial impairments to individuals and society-at-large as the developmental cycle progresses. An early-

S. Co · C. A. Galanter (✉)
State University of New York Downstate Health Sciences University/Kings County Hospital Center, Brooklyn, NY, USA
e-mail: shelley.co@downstate.edu; cathryn.galanter@downstate.edu

M. Wohlleber
Emory University School of Medicine, Atlanta, GA, USA
e-mail: mwohlle@emory.edu

V. Chan, J. Derenne (eds.), *Transition-Age Youth Mental Health Care*,
https://doi.org/10.1007/978-3-030-62113-1_13

intervention approach with skillful, thoughtful care is required and, ideally, mitigates the consequences of these devastating conditions. This chapter focuses on oppositional defiant disorder (ODD), conduct disorder (CD), and intermittent explosive disorder (IED) as they evolve in transitional age youth (TAY), briefly reviews antisocial personality disorder, and does not review other or unspecified related disorders, pyromania, or kleptomania.

Epidemiology of the Disruptive, Impulse-Control, and Conduct Disorders in Children and Adolescents

DICCDs are quite common in children and adolescents. In community samples, ODD prevalence has been shown to range from 0.6% to 11%, averaging 3.3% [27] (Table 13.1), and is more common in boys than girls [9, 37]. ODD has significant comorbidity with DSM-III-R CD, attention-deficit/hyperactivity disorder (ADHD), depression, and overanxious disorder [105].

Studies of CD demonstrate rates ranging from about 1% to 12% with median rate around 4% [38] (Table 13.1). CD is more common in boys [66] and is significantly comorbid with ODD, depression, and overanxious disorder [105]. The association between CD/ODD and ADHD is stronger for ODD than CD [37].

There is limited research on rates of IED in children and adolescents. Data from the National Comorbidity Survey Replication Adolescent Supplement (NCS-A) indicated rates ranging from 1.7% to 6.2% [72] (Table 13.1).

Table 13.1 Prevalence of disruptive, impulse-control, and conduct disorders

Diagnosis	Child/adolescent rates	Adult rates
Oppositional defiant disorder	0.6–11% with average at 3.3% [27]	1.2% [79]
Conduct disorder	1–12% with median rate around 4% [38]	1.4% [79]
Intermittent explosive disorder	1.7–6.2% in adolescents [72]	6.2% [31]

Specifically, of the 63.3% of 13–17 years old who reported lifetime anger attacks (destroying property, threatening violence, or engaging in violence), 7.8% met DSM-IV/World Health Organization Composite International Diagnostic Interview (CIDI) criteria for lifetime IED [72]. The prevalence of lifetime IED was the same in both genders [72]. Comorbidities are also common: 63.9% of NCS-A respondents with lifetime IED met criteria for at least one other mental illness; associations were strongest for agoraphobia, panic disorder, and social phobia. In this survey, however, those with a lifetime history of ADHD, ODD, or CD were excluded from the study [72].

Epidemiology of the Disruptive, Impulse-Control, and Conduct Disorders in Young Adulthood

The epidemiological data on ODD and CD in adulthood is limited, as these conditions were not included in most studies of adults. DICCDs typically have first onset in childhood but can also emerge in adulthood. DSM-5 criteria do not preclude the diagnosis of a DICCD in adulthood [7]. This is a particular distinction in the DSM-5, despite earlier versions of the DSM, which place ODD and CD in the section, "Disorders Usually First Diagnosed in Infancy, Childhood, or Adolescence" [5, 6]. Additionally, in previous versions of the DSM, the diagnosis of ODD was prohibited if a patient also mets criteria for CD. This is not true for DSM-5. All of these nosological changes have contributed to limitations in the estimated rates of the DICCD in adulthood.

The 12-month prevalence of ODD among those 18–29 years old in the National Comorbidity Survey Replication (NCS-R) was 1.2% [79] (Table 13.1). Overall lifetime prevalence for ODD in those 18 years or older in the NCS-R was 10.2% with rates higher in males at 11.2% compared to females at 9.2% [83]. Additionally, the median age-of-onset of ODD was 12 years of age [83].

The 12-month prevalence of CD among those 18–29 years old in the NCS-R was 1.4% [79] (Table 13.1). Lifetime prevalence of CD in those 18 years or older in the NCS-R was 9.5% with males at 12% and females at 7.1% with a median onset age of 11.6 years [82]. A different population-based study determined the prevalence of CD in adults 18 years and older to be 2.2% [20].

IED prevalence from a clinical sample of 18- to 24-year-old participants was 6.2% (Table 13.1), while lifetime prevalence for the same group was 9.2% [31]. Furthermore, a cross-national study among adults at least 18 years old found lifetime prevalence of IED ranging from 0.1% to 2.7% with 12 month and 30-day prevalence for IED at 0.4% and 0.3%, respectively [99]. The same study found the median age of onset for IED to be 17 years old [99]. The age at onset is earlier for males than for females, but overall, females are as likely as males to develop IED [31].

Where It Often Begins: Disruptive, Impulse-Control, and Conduct Disorders in Children

Case: DICCD in Childhood

Identifying Information: *Kevin was a 10-year-old boy who lived with his mother and 14-year-old half-sister and was in 4th grade in an integrated co-teaching class.*

Chief Complaint: *He presented for an intake at an intensive day treatment program referred by his outpatient therapist due to multiple aggressive outbursts at school and at home.*

History of Present Illness: *For the past 5 months, he had exhibited worsening irritability and tantrums involving screaming at peers and teachers for up to 30 minutes twice a week. Teachers stated that he was able to sit still and do his classwork until he did not get his way. He then became disruptive and argumentative. Kevin's mother also reported that he was disrespectful and did not listen to her. He was restless at home and required redirection to do his homework.*

Past Psychiatric and Psychosocial History: *Kevin started having attention problems and disruptive behavior 3 years ago. His symptoms were mild at first but escalated at age 8 years, after social services became involved due to his teacher's concern for neglect and excessive corporal punishment. Kevin was then removed from his mother's custody, placed with his maternal grandmother, and began outpatient mental health treatment. He was diagnosed with ADHD, began psychotherapy, and was prescribed amphetamine-dextroamphetamine mixed salts and clonidine. His mother participated in a social services' required parenting program. Kevin's mother was able to have supervised visits. These interventions resulted in improved behavior. Kevin returned to living with his mother about 6 months ago, and within a month of living with his mother, his explosive and aggressive behavior returned.*

Developmental History: *Kevin was born full term* via *Cesarean section. His mother smoked cigarettes while pregnant with him. He had no reported developmental delays.*

Educational History: *Kevin had been in an integrative co-teaching (ICT) class per his individualized education program (IEP) for the past year, since having to repeat 3rd grade.*

Family History: *Kevin's mother had a history of depression, and his father, who had been incarcerated for years, reportedly had behavioral problems as a child.*

Kevin's History and Its Implications

Conceptualizing the various diagnoses, relevant psychosocial factors, and treatment history for Kevin, or a child like him, is useful in determining how to best evaluate and treat his DICCD symptoms. Clarifying the differential diagnosis can be challenging and painstaking. In Kevin's case, there were multiple historians who had differing perspectives on his behavior. There were also many considerations in Kevin's differential diagnosis, which may have varying consequences for his development and longitudinal course. For example, an adjustment or mood disorder may be fairly transient, while diagnoses of ADHD, learning disorders, and post-traumatic stress disorders may have long-lasting consequences. Specifically, the diagnosis of ODD is associated with increased risk for future psychopathology [95, 113] and adverse outcomes in young adults such as interpersonal difficulties with peers, parents, and romantic partners [26].

Kevin's childhood history will be important to track as he ages into a TAY. Certain childhood elements have consequences even in adulthood. Childhood history may be overlooked however, due to factors like time or poor recall. Relevant childhood domains include psychosocial context, trauma, and developmental history. A case conceptualization examining Kevin's predisposing, precipitating, persisting, and protective factors helps to organize the clinician [47]. For example, Kevin's predisposing factors included his father having a history of childhood "behavioral problems" as well as incarceration and Kevin's exposure to tobacco in utero. Kevin's precipitating factors included being physically abused by his mother and not having a relationship with his biological father. Kevin also experienced many household disruptions. One persisting factor was the entrenched parenting interactions of his mother, while protective factors included his grandmother's involvement, medication adherence, and being engaged in treatment and school. The significance of these factors is not just confined to childhood. For instance, maternal smoking during pregnancy is tied to an elevated risk of antisocial behavior in adulthood [86]. Childhood maltreatment is associated with an increased risk of poor mental and physical health outcomes in adulthood [10], and being raised in a single-parent home is associated with violent behavior in adulthood [44]. The next section will discuss more psychosocial risk factors that are key in the history taking of TAY.

Significance of Childhood and Adolescent History in Early Adulthood

Acquiring data on childhood and adolescent diagnoses, psychosocial risk factors, and pharmacological and psychotherapeutic interventions is essential for evaluating and treating TAY. Both child and adult psychiatric providers have key roles. Child and adolescent clinicians should monitor patients for evolving diagnoses and risk factors and prepare patients and families for future challenges. Providers who work with adult patients should be aware of their patients' childhood and adolescent histories and the ways in which they impact current symptom presentations. Children with behavioral issues may meet criteria for a DICCD diagnosis, as well as other DSM-5 diagnoses in the future. For instance, both active and remitted ODD [83] as well as CD [82] have been associated with increased risks for future psychiatric disorders.

The evaluation of TAY involves gathering a complete past psychiatric history by integrating significant life events and outlining the evolution of childhood, adolescent, and adult symptoms on a timeline. Certain psychosocial elements such as childhood home environment, abuse history, peer support, and relationship with parents also have effects persisting in adulthood – these will be discussed in more detail in this section.

History of Aggression and Risk-Taking Behavior

Obtaining details on past aggressive and risk-taking behaviors is key in assessing all patients with DICCD symptoms. Aggressive behavior in adolescence has been associated with various outcomes in young adulthood including substance use, depression, criminal activity, and lack of educational attainment [16, 75]. There is also evidence that adolescent risk-taking is associated with violence in young adulthood [50].

When evaluating a TAY, gathering information about childhood aggressive and risk-taking behaviors aids in determining whether a childhood DICCD has been present. To distinguish among the DICCD diagnoses, the circumstances surrounding the childhood misbehavior should be clarified. Risk-taking behaviors such as lying, school truancy, running away, and staying out late may be diagnostic features of CD. The nature of aggressive attacks can be different among the various DICCDs. It can be helpful to understand the co-occurring conditions at the time. For example, are the behaviors only occurring during a mood episode? If so, they might not be indicative of a DICCD. It can also be helpful to understand the precipitants. Eliciting whether the childhood misbehavior is premeditated is useful for distinguishing among the DICCD. Those with CD with the specifier of limited prosocial emotions are more likely than those without the specifier to engage in planned aggression for self-gain. Misbehavior in IED is impulsive and involves an instant overreaction to a particular stressor. Finally, it is helpful to understand the nature and intensity of the aggressive or impulsive act. Aggression in ODD involves arguing with or talking back to authority figures and refusal to follow rules. Aggressive actions in CD are more intense and may involve assaulting people, animals, or property. The aggression in IED, on the other hand, can involve either verbal or physical attacks.

Risk Assessment

A safety evaluation including collateral informants is important due to the concern over impulsivity, self-violence, aggression toward others, and/or destruction of property in patients with a DICCD. This assessment involves outlining the patient's past acts of hostility, self-injurious behavior, suicide attempts, and placing these in the context of current symptoms and intent to engage in future aggressive actions. If a patient exhibits severe symptoms with serious threats to harm themselves or others, then an inpatient psychiatric hospitalization is necessary. Law enforcement may need to be involved if the patient presents a threat to harm specific individuals due to duty to warn or duty to protect obligations which vary by state [54].

Childhood and Adolescent Psychosocial Elements

Identifying childhood and adolescent psychosocial and environmental risk factors is valuable in evaluating a patient of any age and especially for TAY.

Home Environment Factors such as having a large family size (i.e., four or more siblings) in childhood and experiencing childhood separation from a parent for reasons other than death or hospitalization have been shown to predict antisocial behavior in young adults [43]. Another study found that children left home alone at a very young age (3 years old) were involved in more crimes in young adulthood compared to groups in which young children were cared for by mothers, siblings, or other relatives [120].

Parental Styles How parents deal with their child's behavior is another important consideration. Harsh physical punishment in childhood has been associated with adult antisocial behavior [92]. Parenting styles involving limited supervision and inconsistent rules in adolescence have been associated with violence in young adulthood [50].

Temperament The TAY's childhood disposition is another factor that can explain their behavior in childhood and, later, adulthood. There is evidence that young children with an undercontrolled temperament (i.e. irritable, impulsive, emotionally labile) have been found to be impulsive and unreliable and demonstrate antisocial traits as young adults [28]. Children with interpersonal callousness have also been found to have violent behavior in adulthood [87]. Moreover, power struggles may occur between parents and children with undercontrolled temperaments. One study showed that mothers with low perceived power as caregivers were reactive to children with difficult temperaments; they also reported greater use of harsh control practices like spanking [68]. This has consequences in adulthood as outlined in the above section on "Parental Styles."

Developmental and Educational History Developmental delays and educational history are important factors in evaluating TAY. For example, investigators have shown that language impairment at age 5 years was associated with increased risk of delinquent behavior in young adulthood [22]. Reading problems in childhood and adolescence have been tied to crime in early adulthood [106] and low academic performance in childhood and adolescence has been associated with violence in young adulthood [50].

Trauma History Witnessing domestic violence in childhood has been correlated with antisocial behavior in adulthood [40]. Experiencing or witnessing violence in early life has also been associated with an increase in lifetime risk of IED [99]. Furthermore, the more violence a patient experiences in childhood, the greater the association with antisocial behaviors in adulthood [1]. Neglect, emotional abuse, physical abuse, and sexual abuse have also been associated with an increased risk of adult antisocial behavior [41].

Peer Association Having a delinquent peer group in adolescence has been associated with an increased risk of antisocial behavior in young adulthood [106, 119]. Peers become less influential in the progression from adolescence to adulthood, and the association between having deviant peers in young adulthood and antisocial behavior is less than what is seen in adolescence [78].

Outcome Studies on the Disruptive, Impulse-Control, and Conduct Disorders

This next section focuses on what is known about the DICCD from prospective studies of children with DICCD and retrospective studies of adults examining their childhood histories of DICCD. Such studies can inform future practice with the goal of early intervention to improve functional and psychopathological outcomes in emerging adulthood.

Oppositional Defiant Disorder "Grown-Up": Prospective Studies

Children with ODD are at increased risk of developing CD in adolescence. They are also at risk of developing anxiety and major depressive disorders as adults. Evidence for these trajectories vary. Investigators have described a cumulative developmental pathway for antisocial personality disorder (ASPD) wherein children with ODD are at risk for developing CD during adolescence, and those with CD in adolescence are at risk for developing ASPD as adults [65]. Studies have shown that very few adolescents with ODD progress to ASPD without also having intermediate CD [62, 67]. More recently, investigators have examined the factors which may lead to these outcomes. For example, Rowe and colleagues suggested that ODD is a significant predictor of later CD in boys but not in girls, after controlling for comorbid and subthreshold CD and subthreshold CD symptomatology [94, 95]. ODD has also been found to be predictive of future anxiety and depressive disorders [25]. Data from the Great Smoky Mountain Study and other population-based and clinical samples demonstrated that childhood ODD predicted development of adult depression [19, 25, 35, 83] and that male adolescents with ODD were at increased risk of later developing anxiety disorders including later generalized anxiety disorder and panic disorder without agoraphobia [35]. Moreover, researchers have demonstrated that different symptom clusters of ODD were predictive of adult psychopathology. For example, irritability symptoms of ODD have been associated with later development of mood disorders [114] and neuroticism, i.e., negative disposition to emotional distress as measured on the NEO Personality Inventory (neuroticism, extraversion, openness) [24], while defiance has been most associated with adult disruptive behavior and criminality [3]. Beyond psychopathology, ODD confers unique risk for specific types of functional problems in adulthood, including poor interpersonal outcomes such as reduced quality and number of positive peer relationships, romantic relationships, relationships with parents, and whether or not anyone is willing to provide a recommendation for a job application [26].

Conduct Disorder "Grown-Up": Prospective Studies

Childhood and adolescent CD have been shown to predict ASPD. This pathway was incorporated into the diagnostic frameworks of ASPD in both DSM-IV and DSM-5, which require the presence of CD in childhood. Yet, this developmental association persists when investigators used modified ASPD criteria which did not require evidence of CD before age 15 [35]. CD in youth also predicts substance use disorders in adults [39]. Some studies linked pediatric CD and depressive disorders in adulthood, both in children with and without childhood mood disorders [110], while in other samples, these findings lost their significance when controlling for childhood mood disorders [36]. Additionally, gender and trajectory may moderate outcomes. CD that is limited to childhood is associated with mood disorders, whereas CD that persists from childhood into adulthood is associated with externalizing problems later in life [100]. CD that begins in adolescence and continues into adulthood is also associated with externalizing problems (i.e., aggression and rule-breaking behavior) [14, 77, 84, 100].

Juvenile Justice Offender "Grown-Up"

Several studies have examined outcomes of children who have a history of delinquency including the well-known Pittsburgh Youth Study (PYS), a longitudinal study of inner-city boys. Findings from the PYS showed that participants who began committing delinquent or criminal offenses (e.g., theft, violence, drug dealing) at an early age continued these behaviors up to age 30 years, and their acts escalated in frequency as they aged [53]. These results demonstrate the need to design intervention programs to reduce recidivism.

Beyond difficulties with recidivism, criminological theories suggest that juvenile justice offenders suffer from an inordinate amount of poor health outcomes compared to nonoffenders. These include injury, cardiovascular disease, psychological disorders, and neurological disorders [43, 76, 89, 103]. Given the high negative impact of offending, other researchers have sought to identify early risk factors in an attempt to understand and ultimately prevent serious and persistent delinquent behavior. They found that aggressive or disruptive behavior, alcohol/drug abuse, poor relationships with peers or family, emotional problems, risky sexual behavior, poor academic achievement or low IQ, unstable job record, high rates of crime in one's community or neighborhood, health problems, and having a positive attitude toward delinquency have been shown to be associated with poor outcomes [8, 11, 55].

Follow-Back Studies on Oppositional Defiant Disorder and Conduct Disorder

Follow-back studies show that a majority of children with CD had prior ODD, and most adults with ASPD had prior CD. This is in contrast to the follow-forward studies that have shown that most ODD children do not develop CD and most CD children do not develop ASPD. Studies have shown that childhood and adolescent ODD and CD precede a heterogenous array of adult psychiatric disorders. Adult ASPD, mania, schizophreniform disorder, and eating disorders were associated with childhood ODD and/or CD [60]. In addition, childhood and adolescent rule-breaking is associated with adult disruptive behaviors [51]. These findings led to an important conclusion regarding DICCDs in childhood: they represent a vital prevention opportunity for reducing burden associated with many major adult psychiatric disorders. Yet, given the complexity of diagnosis and management, DICCDs are often left free to take their unfavorable course.

Intermittent Explosive Disorder "Grown-Up"

Of the epidemiologic studies that have examined IED, few have focused on the adult outcomes of childhood or adolescent IED. Both the National Comorbidity Survey Replication Adolescent Supplement (NCS-A) and the National Comorbidity Study-Replication (NCS-R) included IED, both for the past 12 months and for lifetime occurrence. In the NCS-A, investigators found that IED had an early age of onset (mean age 12 years) and was highly persistent as 80.1% of lifetime cases met current (past 12 months) criteria for IED [72]. McLaughlin and colleagues excluded from their analyses participants with bipolar disorder, ADHD, ODD, and CD given the reports of overlap with IED. Investigators analyzing adult data from the NCS-R found that IED usually began in childhood or adolescence (per retrospective reports), was persistent over the life course (averages of 6.2–11.8 years with attacks), was associated with substantial role impairment, and was highly comorbid with other DSM-IV mood, anxiety, and substance use disorders [59]. They also demonstrated that 44.9% of adults with IED have a history of child or adolescent ADHD, OD, or CD. Unpublished data from NCS-R using within-person analyses demonstrated that IED frequently precedes many of the other DSM-IV disorders with which it is comorbid, especially major depressive, generalized anxiety, panic, and substance use disorders. The vast majority of respondents reported that their IED began at an earlier age indicating the importance of intervening early with IED in hopes of preventing future adverse outcomes [59].

Growing Up: Disruptive, Impulse-Control, and Conduct Symptoms in Transitional Age Youth

Differential diagnoses for patients who present with DICCD symptoms are numerous. In addition to ODD, CD, and IED, one should consider medical conditions and neurodevelopmental, mood, and personality disorders (Table 13.2). These considerations will be discussed in more depth in the next section.

Table 13.2 Differential diagnoses of disruptive, impulse-control, and conduct disorders

Medical conditions
Delirium
Substance intoxication
Substance withdrawal
Neurodevelopmental disorders
Attention-deficit/hyperactivity disorder
Autism spectrum disorder
Intellectual disability
Learning disability
Mood disorders
Bipolar disorder
Depressive disorders
Personality disorders
Antisocial personality disorder
Borderline personality disorder

Case: DICCD in TAY

Identifying Information: Angelique was a 22-year-old, single, unemployed female of Puerto Rican descent who lived with her mother.

Chief Complaint: "I want to hang myself."

History of Present Illness: One week prior to admission to the psychiatric inpatient service, Angelique attacked her girlfriend, gave her two black eyes, and destroyed her girlfriend's car after seeing her girlfriend text an ex-girlfriend. In the ensuing week, she became remorseful and acutely suicidal, so her mother brought her to the hospital. On admission, Angelique admit-

ted to having poor sleep and feeling guilty and dysphoric since attacking her girlfriend. She punched walls when feeling angry and had done so several times over the past 2 months since being released from prison. Since then, Angelique had stopped taking her medications: sertraline 200 mg daily and quetiapine 200 mg daily and 400 mg at bedtime.

Past Psychiatric History: Angelique had multiple past diagnoses and psychiatric hospitalizations. She had been told she had major depressive, anxiety, bipolar, and borderline personality disorders. At 14 years old, she started cutting her arm superficially without intent to kill herself after a breakup with her boyfriend. The following year, she was hospitalized for cutting school, fighting, and using marijuana; she was prescribed unknown medications which she states helped her mood. She was hospitalized again at age 16 when, after an argument with her mother, she smashed her hand through a car window, resulting in nerve damage in her arm. Both Angelique and her mother denied Angelique ever having symptoms consistent with mania or psychosis. Both also reported that her depressive episodes generally consisted of poor sleep, appetite, and concentration as well as low energy and anhedonia with intermittent suicidal ideation.

Substance Use History: She tried marijuana for the first time at 14 years old, but had been clean for the past year. She stated the most she ever used marijuana was about twice a week on weekends around when she was 18 years old.

Legal History: Angelique was incarcerated twice, once after a robbery at age 18 years old and then again a year ago after she physically attacked her roommate in an argument over rent payments.

Developmental and Educational History: Angelique had mild delays in speech and reading. She was in regular education with multiple behavioral problems in elementary school and suspensions throughout middle school and high school. She dropped out early in her senior year of high school. She received her GED while in prison.

Social History: Angelique had no children and identified as bisexual. Angelique's mother was financially supporting her. Angelique's mother raised Angelique and her father was not involved in her childhood.

Family History: Angelique's biological father had a reported diagnosis of bipolar disorder. No other family members had identified mental illness or substance use disorders.

Angelique's Differential Diagnoses

Angelique's history and presentation demonstrate the complexities involved in working with TAY. Based on information at presentation, Angelique met criteria for IED and major depressive disorder (MDD). Over a 1-year period, she had attacked her girlfriend and former roommate and destroyed her girlfriend's car. She also punched walls when angry and engaged in verbal arguments. In her teen years, she punched a car window. These outbursts were grossly out of proportion to the triggering incidents. While these incidents at times co-occurred with depressive episodes, they could not be fully be explained by a mood disorder. Nevertheless, Angelique had episodes of MDD as demonstrated by recurring, discrete episodes of neurovegetative symptoms with intermittent suicidal ideation. She had no history of a manic or hypomanic episode to date.

Other diagnoses to be considered included ODD, CD, substance use disorder, and personality disorder. Angelique often lost her temper and was easily angered or annoyed, but had not engaged in frequent oppositional behaviors. She was not purposefully annoying others, argumentative, actively defying rules, nor blaming others for her behavior. Thus, she did not meet criteria for ODD. Similarly, for CD, she only had two out of the three required symptoms (e.g., physical aggression toward people and property). Whether Angelique had suffered from these disorders as a child is also important to consider, yet more childhood data would be necessary to determine that definitively.

Substance use was another factor that may have been playing a role in her presentation. Based on her history, she did not appear to have been dependent on marijuana. Her use of substances should be periodically assessed due to the strong correlation between intermittent explosive disorder and substance use issues [33].

In addition, it is helpful to consider whether Angelique had a personality disorder or traits, such as borderline or antisocial. She demonstrated impulse-control issues, intense anger episodes, and aggressiveness. Evidence for borderline personality disorder included Angelique having mood instability along with unstable interpersonal relationships. For a diagnosis of ASPD, Angelique must have demonstrated evidence of CD before the age of 15 years. The history gathered during her hospital stay did not substantiate this.

Comorbidities with Disruptive, Impulse-Control, and Conduct Disorders in Adults

Adult comorbidity rates of DICCD are limited as many studies report lifetime rates of DICCD. Data from the National Comorbidity Survey Replication (NCS-R) revealed that 92.4% of adult participants with lifetime ODD met criteria for at least one other lifetime disorder; data from the NCS-R demonstrated that 45.8% had a lifetime mood disorder, 62.3% had a lifetime anxiety disorder, and 47.2% had a lifetime substance use disorder [83].

Data from the NCS-R demonstrated that participants with a lifetime diagnosis of CD were at increased risk for all disorders, especially impulse-control disorders and substance use disorders, with the exception of agoraphobia [82]. CD was also found to occur before comorbid mood disorders and substance use disorders, but not impulse-control disorders and specific and social phobias [82]. Moreover, patients may not have CD symptoms as their primary condition. A cross-sectional study involving adult substance users found that 39% met criteria for conduct disorder; 43% of those with substance use issues and conduct disorder also had ADHD [98].

In an epidemiological sample, investigators have found that for adults with lifetime IED, 81.7% had at least one other lifetime disorder; comorbidity was highest for alcohol abuse at 36.5% and depression at 35.2% [99]. In a clinical research sample, investigators have found the most frequent comorbid condition in adults with current IED was depressive disorder at 21.1% followed by phobic anxiety disorder at 12.4%, non-phobic anxiety disorder at 11.9%, PTSD at 11.1%, and bulimia/binge eating disorder at 2.9% [30].

Connecting the Past and Present: The Transitional Age Youth's Childhood and Adolescent History and Current Psychosocial Situation

Integrating childhood and adolescent history with the TAY's current life circumstances is crucial for accurate assessment and treatment. As discussed earlier in the chapter, certain childhood and adolescent psychosocial factors have effects in young adulthood.

Key components to consider when assessing a TAY's level of functioning and degree of impairment include current home environment, parental/family engagement, peer network, financial situation, and current involvement in higher education or employment. The TAY's living situation may be different from what they experienced in childhood. Family members may have entered or left the household. The young adult may be living by themselves or caring for their own children, and they may have varying levels of support from their parents, families, peers, and romantic partners. Finances may significantly impact symptom evolution and treatment planning. The young adult may be unemployed and reliant on government assistance, financially supported by family, or successfully working a job. Others may be completing high school or engaged in post-secondary education.

Importance of Collateral Information

Determining whether a TAY has a current or past DICCD may be difficult if the evaluating clinician relies only on self-report. TAY may minimize their past and present symptoms, especially in situations where there is the potential for secondary gain if certain symptoms are modified, exaggerated, or omitted. Others may genuinely be unaware of their childhood behaviors and/or diagnoses.

Obtaining collateral information from the TAY's family (with the patient's permission) can be helpful for assessment and for engaging family in treatment planning. Parents, or other significant adults, can act as safety nets when the young adult is experiencing a crisis [115]. Young adults with frequent parental involvement experience greater life satisfaction [46]. Acquiring past records from inpatient and/or outpatient mental health treatment may be especially useful to confirm or fill in any missing gaps from the patient's history. This is key because in some cases, the TAY's parents or guardians become less involved in the patient's life. This is especially true if the youth is progressing toward income attainment and intimate partnership [115].

Treatment of the Disruptive, Impulse-Control, and Conduct Disorders

Treatment in Children and Adolescents

Familiarity with evidence-based DICCD treatments in children and adolescents is necessary when working with TAY, especially when these are part of the youth's past history. Most of the DICCD treatments with evidence for efficacy are psychotherapeutic. There are no US Food and Drug Administration (FDA)-approved medications for the treatment of children and adolescents with DICCD. If medications are used, they are largely adjunctive to psychotherapeutic interventions. They can also be used to treat comorbid conditions when they occur.

DICCD Treatment in Childhood

In the first case example, Kevin was referred to an intensive day treatment (IDT) program because his behavior was becoming unmanageable at home and at school. Kevin's treatment at the IDT program included being restarted on stimulants, which had led to improved ADHD symptoms and oppositional behavior in the past. His mother also became engaged in a parent training program to help her more effectively set limits at home. Additionally, Kevin started individual psychotherapy to better understand whether he had a mood disorder that was contributing to his irritability and disruptive behavior.

Psychotherapy has a major role in DICCD treatment. There is more literature in support of psychotherapeutic interventions in treating pediatric ODD and CD, but less so for IED. The psychotherapeutic treatment of IED in children and adolescents is limited as many studies focus on adult treatment (this is addressed more in the section "DICCD Treatment in TAY").

Evidence supports parent management training (PMT) in treating children with ODD symptoms. PMT focuses on training parents in child behavior management techniques. These include delivering focused attention, positive reinforcements and praise, labeling behaviors, giving appropriate directions/commands, and levying timely consequences such as "time-outs" [21, 73, 116]. Additionally, some PMTs provide instruction on token economies to shape behaviors, family agreements/contracts, and how to conduct structured family meetings [21, 73, 116]. PMTs

Table 13.3 Empirically supported psychotherapies for oppositional defiant disorder

Program type	Age of child	Session participants
Helping the Noncompliant Child [73]	3–8 years	Parent and child
Parent-Child Interaction Therapy (PCIT) [21]	2–7 years	Parent and child
Incredible Years [116, 117]	2–12 years	Parent and child
Triple P – Positive Parenting Program [96]	Birth – 16 years	Parent
Parent Management Training – Oregon Model [88]	3–12 years	Parent

require active role play on the part of the therapist and regular practice on the part of parents and caregivers. PMT treatments with evidence for treating ODD symptoms include Helping the Noncompliant Child [118], Parent-Child Interaction Therapy [12, 81], the Incredible Years [42, 93], Triple P – Positive Parenting Program [17], and Parent Management Training – Oregon Model [85, 104] (Table 13.3).

Conduct disorder, which is often considered more refractory to interventions, may require additional therapies. Evidence-based interventions for CD, presented by order of treatment intensity, include problem-solving skills training (PSST) [57, 58], functional family therapy (FFT) [2, 102], multisystemic therapy (MST) [18, 48, 97], and multidimensional treatment foster care (MTFC) [64, 107] (Table 13.4).

Problem-solving skills training (PSST) incorporates cognitive-behavioral therapy techniques to teach children how to deal with interpersonal conflicts [56]. PSST delivers interventions using a "5 Problem Solving Step" format and offers this practice in a game-playing, token economy structure [56]. PSST attempts to generalize the problem-solving solutions into actual, hypothetical, then outside-treatment behaviors [56].

FFT is a short-term intervention that involves improving intrafamilial communication toward higher respect, empathy, and understanding and engaging the systems in which the family is embedded (e.g., school, neighborhood, justice system) [101]. The FFT model intends to engage the family in motivational change, by guiding families to eventually reflect on the functional aspects of maladaptive behaviors and communications and to recharacterize behaviors into relational transactions [101]. Many FFT programs offer interventions intensely for 3–6 months' durations [101].

Table 13.4 Empirically supported psychotherapies for conduct disorder

Problem-solving skills training (PSST) [56]	Utilizes cognitive-behavioral therapy techniques to teach youth how to deal with interpersonal conflicts Delivers interventions using a "5 Problem Solving Step" format
Functional family therapy (FFT) [101]	Focuses on improving intrafamilial communication Encourages families to reflect on the functional aspects of the youth's maladaptive behaviors Interventions can last for 3–6 months
Multisystemic therapy (MST) [49]	Addresses how the youth's various systems (e.g., peers, school, family, community) influence the youth's behavior Involves week-to-week assessment and evaluation of problem behaviors Average duration is 6 months with 24 hour-a-day/7-day-per-week team support
Multidimensional treatment foster care (MTFC) [29]	Delinquent foster youth who have been removed from their homes are placed in a community-based, specially trained, foster family so that the youth's misbehavior can be modified with the help of a treatment team MFTC families work intensively on a weekly basis with a high degree (i.e., 24/7) of therapeutic support

Multisystemic therapy (MST) focuses on how the child's various systems (e.g., peers, school, family, community) influence the child's behavior [49]. MST incorporates but does not specifically instruct on individual therapy modalities, such as cognitive behavior therapy and motivational interviewing [49]. Characterized by "fit circles," MST case formulation requires week-to-week assessment and evaluation of problem behaviors and their multisystemic solutions [49]. MST is often offered for an average of 6 months' duration with 24 hour-a-day/7-day-per-week team support [49].

MTFC is a multisystemic treatment specific to delinquent foster youth who have been removed from their homes [29]. MTFC requires that only one or two youth are placed in a community-based, specially trained, foster family so that the youth's misbehavior can be modified with the help of a treatment team [29]. As an alternative to higher levels of care, MFTC families work intensively on a weekly basis with a high degree (i.e., 24/7) of therapeutic support [29].

Pharmacological approaches for ODD, CD, and IED involve treating comorbid conditions and targeting symptoms (e.g., hyperactivity, impulsivity, and aggression) to improve DICCD behavior (Table 13.5). Long-acting methylphenidate has been shown to be effective in the treatment of oppositional-defiant and aggressive behavior in children and adolescents with ADHD [108]. Methylphenidate has also been found to decrease antisocial behaviors in children with CD with or without comorbid ADHD [61]. One RCT demonstrated that children with ADHD and ODD treated with guanfacine extended release had improvements in oppositional behavior as well as ADHD symptoms [34]. Another RCT of children with ADHD and comorbid ODD demonstrated that atomoxetine led to improvement of ADHD and ODD symptoms although the impovement in ODD symptoms was not maintained at the 8-week endpoint [13]. Risperidone has also been shown to decrease disruptive behavior and aggression in youth with a DSM-IV disruptive behavior disorders diagnosis and subaverage IQ [4, 23, 109] and to decrease aggression in youth with average IQ and CD [45].

Table 13.5 Evidence-based psychopharmacological treatment for children and adolescents with DICCDs

Methylphenidate
Decreases oppositional-defiant and aggressive behavior in children and adolescents with ADHD [108]
Decreases antisocial behaviors in children with CD with or without comorbid ADHD [61]
Guanfacine
Improves oppositional behavior in children with ODD and ADHD [34]
Atomoxetine
Short-term improvement of ODD symptoms in children with comorbid ADHD and ODD [13]
Risperidone
Decreases disruptive behavior and aggression in youth with a DSM-IV disruptive behavior disorders diagnosis and subaverage IQ [4, 23, 109]
Decreases aggression in youth with average IQ and CD [45]

Treatment in Transitional Age Youth

Evidence on psychotherapeutic and pharmacological interventions in ODD, CD, and IED in TAY is limited. There are no treatment studies for ODD and CD in TAY and no FDA-approved medications to treat ODD, CD, and IED in children or adults. There are a small number of studies examining related symptoms such as anger, violence, and aggression. Because of the limited evidence, treatment approaches for DICCD in TAY often focus on treating any comorbid conditions with evidence-based treatments.

The few studies which examine IED medication treatment in adults demonstrate the potential of medications to target IED symptoms. Fluoxetine has been shown to reduce impulsive aggression in adult patients with IED [32]. Divalproex has been found to decrease impulsive aggression in adult patients with IED and cluster B personality disorders [52, 112]. Investigators have demonstrated that oxcarbazepine, phenytoin, and carbamazepine reduced impulsive aggression in adult patients with IED [69, 112]. Levetiracetam, on the other hand, has not been effective in IED patients with impulsive aggression [70].

The best psychotherapeutic evidence on IED supports group and individual cognitive-behavioral therapy to improve anger control and decrease aggression, anger, and hostile thinking [71].

DICCD Treatment in Transitional Age Youth

Angelique met criteria for comorbid MDD and IED. Her most recent medication regimen before being hospitalized involved sertraline and quetiapine. Gathering further history from Angelique, her past providers, and her mother about her response and adverse effects to her most recent and prior medications was important in determining her treatment. This guided the decision on whether the sertraline and quetiapine should be restarted. The inpatient psychiatric team also considered other medications like the mood stabilizers, which have data, albeit limited, for efficacy in treating IED in adults. In addition, it was important for Angelique to engage in individual and group psychotherapy. Angelique's mother was also encouraged to attend family sessions on the unit. The treatment team also connected Angelique to an agency for assistance in searching for a job upon discharge.

Treatment: Antisocial Personality Disorder

Given the pathway from CD to ASPD, we briefly address the treatment of ASPD. There is no consistent evidence regarding the pharmacological and psychotherapeutic treatment of ASPD. One study found that divalproex decreased impulsive aggression and irritability in subjects with cluster B disorders [52]. Other studies have focused on ASPD symptoms (e.g., aggression and impulsivity) rather than an actual ASPD diagnosis. Phenytoin and carbamazepine have been found to decrease impulsive aggression [15, 111, 112]. In addition, many studies have examined ASPD's comorbidities and their treatments. For instance, one study has demonstrated that alcohol-dependent subjects with ASPD (DSM III-R) on nortriptyline compared to placebo had more improvement in scores on the Severity of Alcohol Dependence Questionnaire (SADQ), number of drinking days, and abstinence at 6-month follow-up [90]. Another study demonstrated that naltrexone and disulfiram were effective in decreasing drinking for alcohol-dependent participants with comorbid ASPD [91]. Another study of cocaine- and opioid-dependent patients on methadone maintenance revealed that those with ASPD had a worse prognosis than those without [63]. They also exhibited a poorer response to pharmacotherapy trials with desipramine and amantadine [63].

There is also limited evidence examining the psychotherapy treatments for ASPD. Contingency management and CBT have been found to improve outcomes related to substance use in those with ASPD [74, 80]. Because there are no interventions targeting ASPD specifically, its management involves treating co-occurring conditions – this is the fundamental principle in managing ODD, CD, and IED in adults as well.

Conclusion

A DICCD diagnosis at any age has implications for quality of life and functioning across several domains. Some children may continue to have a DICCD when they become adults. Other patients may experience the first onset of a DICCD in adulthood. Obtaining childhood data from collateral sources is important in evaluating TAY. Childhood diagnoses as well as certain psychosocial and environmental elements (e.g., childhood home environment, parental management, childhood temperament, educational and trauma history, childhood peer association, engagement of family and other support networks in treatment) have implications, even in adulthood. There is a dearth of studies on ODD, CD, and IED in adults, especially in the TAY population. More research on these disorders in TAY and adults is needed to maximize the clinical utility of these diagnoses and improve outcomes.

References

1. Afifi TO, Fortier J, Sareen J, Taillieu T. Associations of harsh physical punishment and child maltreatment in childhood with antisocial behaviors in adulthood. JAMA Netw Open. 2019;2(1):e187374.
2. Alexander JF, Parsons BV. Short-term behavioral intervention with delinquent families: impact on family process and recidivism. J Abnorm Psychol. 1973;81(3):219–25.
3. Althoff RR, Kuny-Slock AV, Verhulst FC, Hudziak JJ, van der Ende J. Classes of oppositional-defiant behavior: concurrent and predictive validity. J Child Psychol Psychiatry. 2014;55(10):1162–71.
4. Aman M, De Smedt G, Derivan A, et al. Double-blind, placebo-controlled study of risperidone for the treatment of disruptive behaviors in children with subaverage intelligence. Am J Psychiatry. 2002;159(8):1337–46.
5. American Psychiatric Association. Diagnostic and statistical manual of mental disorders, Third Edition-Revised. Washington, DC: American Psychiatric Association; 1987.
6. American Psychiatric Association. Diagnostic and statistical manual of mental disorders, Fourth Edition Text Revision. Washington, DC: American Psychiatric Association; 2000.
7. American Psychiatric Association. Diagnostic and statistical manual of mental disorders. Fifth ed. Arlington: American Psychiatric Association; 2013.
8. Andrews D, Bonta J. The pathology of criminal conduct. 5th ed. New Providence: Matthew Bender & Company, Inc., LexisNexis Group; 2010.
9. Angold A, Erkanli A, Farmer EM, et al. Psychiatric disorder, impairment, and service use in rural African American and white youth. Arch Gen Psychiatry. 2002;59(10):893–901.
10. Archer G, Pereira SP, Power C. Child maltreatment as a predictor of adult physical functioning in a prospective British birth cohort. BMJ Open. 2017;7(10):e017900.
11. Assink M, van der Put CE, Hoeve M, et al. Risk factors for persistent delinquent behavior among juveniles: a meta-analytic review. Clin Psychol Rev. 2015;42:47–61.
12. Bagner DM, Eyberg SM. Parent-Child Interaction Therapy for disruptive behavior in children with mental retardation: a randomized controlled trial. J Clin Child Adolesc Psychol. 2007;36(3):418–29.
13. Bangs ME, Hazell P, Danckaerts M, et al. Atomoxetine for the treatment of attention-deficit/hyperactivity disorder and oppositional defiant disorder. Pediatrics. 2008;121(2):314–20.
14. Barker ED, Maughan B. Differentiating early-onset persistent versus childhood-limited conduct problem youth. Am J Psychiatry. 2009;166(8):900–8.
15. Barratt ES, Stanford MS, Felthous AR, Kent TA. The effects of phenytoin on impulsive and premeditated aggression: a controlled study. J Clin Psychopharmacol. 1997;17(5):341–9.
16. Bongers IL, Koot HM, Van der Ende J, Verhulst FC. Predicting young adult social functioning from developmental trajectories of externalizing behavior. Psychol Med. 2008;38:988–99.
17. Bor W, Sanders MR, Markie-Dadds C. The effects of the Triple P-Positive Parenting Program on preschool children with co-occurring disruptive behavior and attentional/hyperactive difficulties. J Abnorm Child Psychol. 2002;30(6):571–87.
18. Borduin CM, Mann BJ, Cone LT, Henggeler SW, Fucci BR, Blaske DM, Williams RA. Multisystemic treatment of serious juvenile offenders: long-term prevention of criminality and violence. J Consult Clin Psychol. 1995;63(4):569–78.
19. Boylan K, Vaillancourt T, Boyle M, Szatmari P. Comorbidity of internalizing disorders in children with oppositional defiant disorder. Eur Child Adolesc Psychiatry. 2007;16(8):484–94.
20. Breslau J, Saito N, Tancredi DJ, Nock M, Gilman SE. Classes of conduct disorder symptoms and their life course correlates in a US national sample. Psychol Med. 2012;42(5):1081–9.
21. Brinkmeyer M, Eyberg SM. Parent-child interaction therapy for oppositional children. In: Kazdin AE, Weisz JR, editors. Evidence-based psychotherapies for children and adolescents. New York: Guilford; 2003. p. 204–23.
22. Brownlie EB, Beitchman JH, Escobar M, Young A, Atkinson L, Johnson C, Wilson B, Douglas L. Early language impairment and young adult delinquent and aggressive behavior. J Abnorm Child Psychol. 2004;32(4):453–67.
23. Buitelaar JK, van der Gaag RJ, Cohen-Kettenis P, Melman CT. A randomized controlled trial of risperidone in the treatment of aggression in hospitalized adolescents with subaverage cognitive abilities. J Clin Psychiatry. 2001;62(4):239–48.
24. Burke JD. An affective dimension within oppositional defiant disorder symptoms among boys: personality and psychopathology outcomes into early adulthood. J Child Psychol Psychiatry. 2012;53(11):1176–83.
25. Burke JD, Loeber R, Lahey BB, Rathouz PJ. Developmental transitions among affective and behavioral disorders in adolescent boys. J Child Psychol Psychiatry. 2005;46(11):1200–10.
26. Burke JD, Rowe R, Boylan K. Functional outcomes of child and adolescent oppositional defiant disorder symptoms in young adult men. J Child Psychol Psychiatry. 2014;55(3):264–72.
27. Canino G, Polanczyk G, Bauermeister JJ, et al. Does the prevalence of CD and ODD vary across cultures? Soc Psychiatry Psychiatr Epidemiol. 2010;45(7):695–704.
28. Caspi A. The child is father of the man: personality continuities from childhood to adulthood. J Pers Soc Psychol. 2000;78(1):158–72.

29. Chamberlain P. The Oregon multidimensional treatment foster care model: features, outcomes, and progress in dissemination. Cogn Behav Pract. 2003;10(4):303–12.
30. Coccaro EF. Psychiatric comorbidity in intermittent explosive disorder. J Psychiatr Res. 2019;118:38–43.
31. Coccaro EF, Posternak MA, Zimmerman M. Prevalence and features of intermittent explosive disorder in a clinical setting. J Clin Psychiatry. 2005;66(10):1221–7.
32. Coccaro EF, Lee RJ, Kavoussi RJ. A double-blind, randomized, placebo-controlled trial of fluoxetine in patients with intermittent explosive disorder. J Clin Psychiatry. 2009;70(5):653–62.
33. Coccaro EF, Fanning JR, Lee R. Intermittent explosive disorder and substance use disorder: analysis of the National Comorbidity Survey Replication sample. J Clin Psychiatry. 2017;78(6):697–702.
34. Connor DF, Findling RL, Kollins S, et al. Effects of guanfacine extended release on oppositional symptoms in children aged 6–12 years with attention-deficit hyperactivity disorder and oppositional symptoms: a randomized, double-blind, placebo-controlled trial. CNS Drugs. 2010;24(9):755–68.
35. Copeland WE, Shanahan L, Costello EJ, et al. Childhood and adolescent psychiatric disorders as predictors of young adult disorders. Arch Gen Psychiatry. 2009;66(7):764–72.
36. Copeland WE, Shanahan L, Erkanli A, et al. Indirect comorbidity in childhood and adolescence. Front Psych. 2013;4:144.
37. Costello EJ, Mustillo S, Erkanli A, Keeler G, Angold A. Prevalence and development of psychiatric disorders in childhood and adolescence. Arch Gen Psychiatry. 2003;60(8):837–44.
38. Costello EJ, Egger H, Angold A. 10-year research update review: the epidemiology of child and adolescent psychiatric disorders: I. methods and public health burden. J Am Acad Child Adolesc Psychiatry. 2005;44(10):972–86.
39. Costello EJ, Copeland W, Angold A. Trends in psychopathology across the adolescent years: what changes when children become adolescents, and when adolescents become adults? J Child Psychol Psychiatry. 2011;52(10):1015–25.
40. Dargis M, Koenigs M. Witnessing domestic violence during childhood is associated with psychopathic traits in adult male criminal offenders. Law Hum Behav. 2017;41(2):173–9.
41. Degli Esposti M, Pinto Pereira SM, Humphreys DK, Sale RD, Bowes L. Child maltreatment and the risk of antisocial behaviour: a population-based cohort study spanning 50 years. Child Abuse Negl. 2020;99:104281.
42. Drugli MB, Larsson B, Fossum S, Mörch W. Five- to six-year outcome and its prediction for children with ODD/CD treated with parent training. J Child Psychol Psychiatry. 2010;51(5):559–66.
43. Farrington DP. Childhood origins of teenage antisocial behaviour and adult social dysfunction. J R Soc Med. 1993;86(1):13–7.
44. Fergusson DM, Boden JM, Horwood LJ. Exposure to single parenthood in childhood and later mental health, educational, economic, and criminal behavior outcomes. Arch Gen Psychiatry. 2007;64(9):1089–95.
45. Findling RL, McNamara NK, Branicky LA, et al. A double-blind pilot study of risperidone in the treatment of conduct disorder. Am Acad Child Adolesc Psychiatry. 2000;39(4):509–16.
46. Fingerman KL, Cheng YP, Wesselmann ED, et al. Helicopter parents and landing pad kids: intense parental support of grown children. J Marriage Fam. 2012;74(4):880–96.
47. Henderson SW, Martin A. Case formulation and integration of information in child and adolescent mental health. In: Rey JM, editor. IACAPAP e-textbook of child and adolescent mental health. Geneva: International Association for Child and Adolescent Psychiatry and Allied Professions; 2014.
48. Henggeler SW, Melton GB, Smith LA. Family preservation using Multisystemic Therapy: an effective alternative to incarcerating serious juvenile offenders. J Consult Clin Psychol. 1992;60:953–61.
49. Henggeler SW, Schoenwald SK, Borduin CM, Rowland MD, Cunningham PB. Multisystemic therapy for antisocial behavior in children and adolescents second edition. Guilford: New York; 2009.
50. Herrenkohl TI, Maguin E, Hill KG, et al. Developmental risk factors for youth violence. J Adolesc Health. 2000;26(3):176–86.
51. Hofstra MB, van der Ende J, Verhulst FC. Child and adolescent problems predict DSM-IV disorders in adulthood: a 14-year follow-up of a Dutch epidemiological sample. J Am Acad Child Adolesc Pyschiatry. 2002;41(2):182–9.
52. Hollander E, Tracy KA, Swann AC, Coccaro EF, McElroy SL, Wozniak P, Sommerville KW, Nemeroff CB. Divalproex in the treatment of impulsive aggression: efficacy in cluster B personality disorders. Neuropsychopharmacology. 2003;28(6):1186–97.
53. Jennings WG, Loeber R, Pardini DA, Piquero AR. Offending from childhood to young adulthood: recent results from the Pittsburgh Youth Study. New York: Springer; 2016.
54. Johnson R, Persad G, Sisti D. The Tarasoff rule: the implications of interstate variation and gaps in professional training. J Am Acad Psychiatry Law. 2014;42(4):469–77.
55. Jolliffe D, Farrington DP, Piquero AR, Loeber R, Hill KG. Systematic review of early risk factors for life-course-persistent, adolescence-limited, and late-onset offenders in prospective longitudinal studies. Aggress Violent Behav. 2017;33:15–23.
56. Kazdin A. Problem-solving skills training and parent management training for oppositional defiant disorder and conduct disorder. In: Weisz JR, Kazdin AE, editors. Evidence-based psychotherapies for children and adolescents. 2nd ed. New York: Guilford; 2010. p. 211–26.
57. Kazdin A, Esveldt-Dawson K, French N, Unis A. Problem-solving skills training and relationship

therapy in the treatment of antisocial child behavior. J Consult Clin Psychol. 1987;55(1):76–85.
58. Kazdin AE, Siegel TC, Bass D. Cognitive problem-solving skills training and parent management training in the treatment of antisocial behavior in children. J Consult Clin Psychol. 1992;60(5):733–47.
59. Kessler RC, Coccaro EF, Fava M, Jaeger S, Jin R, Walters E. The prevalence and correlates of DSM-IV intermittent explosive disorder in the national comorbidity replication. Arch Gen Psychiatry. 2006;63(6):669–78.
60. Kim-Cohen J, Caspi A, Moffitt TE, Harrington H, Milne BJ, Poulton R. Prior juvenile diagnoses in adults with mental disorder: developmental follow-back of a prospective-longitudinal cohort. Arch Gen Psychiatry. 2003;60(7):709–17.
61. Klein RG, Abikoff H, Klass E, Ganeles D, Seese LM, Pollack S. Clinical efficacy of methylphenidate in conduct disorder with and without attention deficit hyperactivity disorder. Arch Gen Psychiatry. 1997;54(12):1073–80.
62. Lahey BB, Loeber R, Burke JD, Applegate B. Predicting future antisocial personality disorder in males from a clinical assessment in childhood. J Consult Clin Psychol. 2005;73:389–99.
63. Leal J, Ziedonis D, Kosten T. Antisocial personality disorder as a prognostic factor for pharmacotherapy of cocaine dependence. Drug Alcohol Depend. 1994;35(1):31–5.
64. Leve LD, Chamberlain P, Reid JB. Intervention outcomes for girls referred from juvenile justice: effects on delinquency. J Consult Clin Psychol. 2005;73:1181–5.
65. Loeber R, Burke JD. Developmental pathways in juvenile externalizing and internalizing problems. J Res Adolesc. 2011;21(1):34–46.
66. Loeber R, Burke JD, Lahey BB, et al. Oppositional defiant and conduct disorder: a review of the past 10 years, part I. J Am Acad Child Adolesc Psychiatry. 2000;39(12):1468–84.
67. Loeber R, Burke JD, Lahey BB. What are the adolescent antecedents to antisocial personality disorder? Crim Behav Ment Health. 2002;12:24–36.
68. Martorell GA, Bugental DB. Maternal variations in stress reactivity: implications for harsh parenting practices with very young children. J Fam Psychol. 2006;20(4):641–7.
69. Mattes JA. Oxcarbazepine in patients with impulsive aggression: a double-blind, placebo-controlled trial. J Clin Psychopharmacol. 2005;25(6):575–9.
70. Mattes JA. Levetiracetam in patients with impulsive aggression: a double-blind, placebo-controlled trial. J Clin Psychiatry. 2008;69(2):310–5.
71. McCloskey MS, Noblett KL, Deffenbacher JL, et al. Cognitive-behavioral therapy for intermittent explosive disorder: a pilot randomized clinical trial. J Consult Clin Psychol. 2008;76(5):876–86.
72. McLaughlin KA, Green JG, Hwang I, et al. Intermittent explosive disorder in the National Comorbidity Survey Replication Adolescent Supplement. Arch Gen Psychiatry. 2012;69(11):1131–9.
73. McMahon RJ, Forehand RL. Helping the noncompliant child: family based treatment for oppositional behavior. 2nd ed. New York: Guilford; 2003.
74. Messina N, Farabee D, Rawson R. Treatment responsivity of cocaine-dependent patients with antisocial personality disorder to cognitive-behavioral and contingency management interventions. J Consult Clin Psychol. 2003;71(2):320–30.
75. Miller S, Malone PS, Dodge KA. Developmental trajectories of boys' and girls' delinquency: sex differences and links to later adolescent outcomes. J Abnorm Child Psychol. 2010;38:1021–32.
76. Moffitt TE. Life-course-persistent versus adolescence-limited antisocial behavior. In: Cicchetti D, Cohen DJ, editors. Developmental psychopathology: risk, disorder, and adaptation. New York: Wiley; 2006. p. 570–98.
77. Moffitt TE, Arseneault L, Jaffee SR, Kim-Cohen J, Koenen KC, Odgers CL, et al. Research review: DSM-V conduct disorder: research needs for an evidence base. J Child Psychol Psychiatry. 2008;49:3–33.
78. Monahan KC, Steinberg L, Cauffman E. Affiliation with antisocial peers, susceptibility to peer influence, and antisocial behavior during the transition to adulthood. Dev Psychol. 2009;45(6):1520–30.
79. National Comorbidity Survey: 12-month prevalence of DSM-IV/WMH-CIDI disorders by sex and cohort. Harvard Medical School, 2005. https://www.hcp.med.harvard.edu/ncs/ftpdir/NCS-R_12-month_Prevalence_Estimates.pdf. Accessed 28 Feb 2020.
80. Neufeld KJ, Kidorf MS, Kolodner K, King VL, Clark M, Brooner RK. A behavioral treatment for opioid-dependent patients with antisocial personality. J Subst Abus Treat. 2008;34(1):101–11.
81. Nixon RD, Sweeney L, Erickson DB, Touyz SW. Parent-child interaction therapy: a comparison of standard and abbreviated treatments for oppositional defiant preschoolers. J Consult Clin Psychol. 2003;71:251–60.
82. Nock MK, Kazdin AE, Hiripi E, et al. Prevalence, subtypes, and correlates of DSM-IV conduct disorder in the National Comorbidity Survey Replication. Psychol Med. 2006;36(5):699–710.
83. Nock MK, Kazdin AE, Hiripi E, Kessler RC. Lifetime prevalence, correlates, and persistence of oppositional defiant disorder: results from the national comorbidity survey replication. J Child Psychol Psychiatry. 2007;48(7):703–13.
84. Odgers CL, Caspi A, Broadbent JM, Dickson N, Hancox RJ, Harrington HL, Poulton R, Seras MR, Thomson WM, Moffitt TE. Prediction of differential adult health burden by conduct problem subtypes in males. Arch Gen Psychiatry. 2007;64:476–84.
85. Ogden T, Hagen KA. Treatment effectiveness of Parent Management Training in Norway: a randomized controlled trial of children with conduct problems. J Consult Clin Psychol. 2008;76(4):607–21.
86. Paradis AD, Shenassa ED, Papandonatos GD, Rogers ML, Buka SL. Maternal smoking during pregnancy and offspring antisocial behaviour:

findings from a longitudinal investigation of discordant siblings. J Epidemiol Community Health. 2017;71(9):889–96.
87. Pardini DA, Byrd AL, Hawes SH, Docherty M. Unique dispositional precursors to early-onset conduct problems and criminal offending in adulthood. J Am Acad Child Adolesc Psychiatry. 2018;57(8):583–92.
88. Patterson GR, Reid JB, Jones RR, et al. A social learning approach to family intervention, volume 1: families with aggressive children. Eugene: Castalia Publishing Co; 1975.
89. Piquero AR, Daigle LE, Gibson C, Piquero NL, Tibbetts SG. Research note: are life-course-persistent offenders at risk for adverse health outcomes? J Res Crime Delinq. 2007;44(2):185–207.
90. Powell BJ, Campbell JL, Landon JF, Liskow BI, Thomas HM, Nickel EJ, et al. A double-blind, placebo-controlled study of nortriptyline and bromocriptine in male alcoholics subtyped by comorbid psychiatric disorders. Alcohol Clin Exp Res. 1995;19(2):462–8.
91. Ralevski E, Ball S, Nich C, Limoncelli D, Petrakis I. The impact of personality disorders on alcohol use outcomes in a pharmacotherapy trial for alcohol dependence and comorbid Axis I disorders. Am J Addict. 2007;16(6):443–9.
92. Rebellon CJ, Straus M. Corporal punishment and adult antisocial behavior: a comparison of dyadic concordance types and an evaluation of mediating mechanisms in Asia, Europe, and North America. Int J Behav Dev. 2017;41(4):503–13.
93. Reid MJ, Webster-Stratton C, Hammond N. Follow-up of children who received the incredible years intervention for oppositional-defiant disorder: maintenance and prediction of two-year outcome. Behav Ther. 2003;34:471–91.
94. Rowe R, Maughan B, Pickles A, Costello EJ, Angold A. The relationship between DSM-IV oppositional defiant disorder and conduct disorder: findings from the Great Smoky Mountains study. J Child Psychol Psychiatry. 2002;43(3):365–73.
95. Rowe R, Costello EJ, Angold A, et al. Developmental pathways in oppositional defiant disorder and conduct disorder. J Abnorm Psychol. 2010;119(4):726–73.
96. Sanders MR. The Triple P-Positive parenting program: towards an empirically validated multilevel parenting and family support strategy for the prevention of behavior and emotional problems in children. Clin Child Fam Psychol Rev. 1999;2(2):71–90.
97. Sawyer AM, Borduin CM. Effects of multisystemic therapy through midlife: a 21.9-year follow-up to a randomized clinical trial with serious and violent juvenile offenders. J Consult Clin Psychol. 2011;79(5):643–52.
98. Schubiner H, Tzelepis A, Milberger S, Lockhart N, Kruger M, Kelley BJ, Schoener EP. Prevalence of attention-deficit/hyperactivity disorder and conduct disorder among substance abusers. J Clin Psychiatry. 2000;61(4):244–51.
99. Scott KM, Lim CC, Hwang I, et al. The cross-national epidemiology of DSM-IV intermittent explosive disorder. Psychol Med. 2016;46(15):3161–72.
100. Sentse M, Kretschmer T, de Haan A, Prinzie P. Conduct problem trajectories between age 4 and 17 and their association with behavioral adjustment in emerging adulthood. J Youth Adolesc. 2017;46(8):1633–42.
101. Sexton TL. Functional family therapy in clinical practice: an evidence-based treatment model for working with troubled adolescents. New York: Routledge; 2010.
102. Sexton T, Turner CW. The effectiveness of functional family therapy for youth with behavioral problems in a community practice setting. J Fam Psychol. 2010;24(3):339–48.
103. Shepherd J, Farrington D, Potts J. Impact of antisocial lifestyle on health. J Public Health. 2005;27(3):312–3.
104. Sigmarsdóttir M, Thorlacius Ö, Guðmundsdóttir EV, DeGarmo DS. Treatment effectiveness of PMTO for children's behavior problems in Iceland: child outcomes in a nationwide randomized controlled trial. Fam Process. 2015;54(3):498–517.
105. Simonoff E, Pickles A, Meyer JM, Silberg JL, Maes HH, Loeber R, Rutter M, Hewitt JK, Eaves LJ. The Virginia twin study of adolescent behavioral development. Arch Gen Psychiatry. 1997;54(9):801–8.
106. Simonoff E, Elander J, Holmshaw J, Pickles A, Murray R, Rutter M. Predictors of antisocial personality: continuities from childhood to adult life. Br J Psychiatry. 2004;184:118–27.
107. Sinclair I, Parry E, Biehal N, Fresen J, Kay C, Scott S, Green J. Multi-dimensional treatment foster care in England: differential effects by level of initial antisocial behaviour. Eur Child Adolesc Psychiatry. 2016;25(8):843–52.
108. Sinzig J, Dopfner M, Lehmkuhl G. Long-acting methylphenidate has an effect on aggressive behavior in children with attention-deficit/hyperactivity disorder. J Child Adolesc Psychopharmacol. 2007;17(4):421–32.
109. Snyder R, Turgay A, Aman M, et al. Effects of risperidone on conduct and disruptive behavior disorders in children with subaverage IQs. Am Acad Child Adolesc Psychiatry. 2002;41(9):1026–36.
110. Sourander A, Jensen P, Davies M, et al. Who is at greatest risk of adverse long-term outcomes? The Finnish from a Boy to a Man Study. J Am Acad Child Adolesc Psychiatry. 2007;46(9):1148–61.
111. Stanford MS, Houston RJ, Mathias CW, Greve KW, Villemarette-Pittman NR, Adams D. A double-blind placebo-controlled crossover study of phenytoin in individuals with impulsive aggression. Psychiatry Res. 2001;103(2–3):193–203.
112. Stanford MS, Helfritz LE, Conklin SM, et al. A comparison of anticonvulsants in the treatment of impulsive aggression. Exp Clin Psychopharmacol. 2005;13(1):72–7.

113. Stringaris A, Goodman R. Longitudinal outcome of youth oppositionality: irritable, headstrong, and hurtful behaviors have distinctive predictions. J Am Acad Child Adolesc Psychiatry. 2009;48(4):404–12.
114. Stringaris A, Cohen P, Pine D, Leibenluft E. Adult outcomes of youth irritability. A 20-year prospective community-based study. Am J Psychiatry. 2009;166:1048–54.
115. Swartz TT, Kim M, Uno M, et al. Safety nets and scaffolds: parental support in the transition to adulthood. J Marriage Fam. 2011;73(2):414–29.
116. Webster-Stratton C. The incredible years: a training series for the prevention and treatment of conduct problems in young children. In: Hibbs ED, Jensen PS, editors. Psychosocial treatments for child and adolescent disorders. Washington, DC: American Psychological Association; 2005. p. 507–55.
117. Webster-Stratton C, Reid MJ. The incredible years parents, teachers, and children training series: a multifaceted treatment approach for young children with conduct problems. In: Kazdin AE, Weisz JR, editors. Evidenced-based psychotherapies for children and adolescents. First ed. New York: The Guilford Press; 2003. p. 224–40.
118. Wells KC, Egan J. Social learning and systems family therapy for childhood oppositional disorder: comparative treatment outcome. Compr Psychiatry. 1988;29:138–46.
119. Wojciechowski TW. The development of deviant peer association across the life course and its relevance for predicting offending in early adulthood. J Dev Life-Course Criminol. 2018;4(1):73–91.
120. Wong KK, Raine A, Venables P. The effect of being left home alone at age 3 years on schizotypy and antisocial behavior at ages 17 and 23 years. J Psychiatr Res. 2018;105:103–12.

14 First-Episode & Early Psychosis in Transition-Age Youth

Pari Faraji, Charles Camp, Zhanna Elberg,
and Craigan Usher

Key Points

- The onset and course of schizophrenia in youth varies widely, though many individuals will have premorbid cognitive disruptions and experience an insidious functional decline prior to the appearance of psychotic symptoms.
- The onset of psychosis during youth is highly disruptive to normal neurobiological and psychosocial development, often resulting in long-term ramifications to lifetime functioning, a dilemma that coordinate specialty care (CSC) programs aim to address.
- Youth with psychosis are at significantly elevated risk for suicide, and it is imperative that all patients receive a thorough lethality assessment.
- Once psychosis is identified, antipsychotics should be started to help shorten the duration of untreated psychosis (DUP) and reduce the salience one ascribes to perceptual disturbances.
- Attempt to use a shared decision-making model, keeping in mind that a more authoritative approach may be important for some individuals and families and in certain cultural contexts.
- Aim for remission of symptoms while keeping in mind functional outcomes/patient goals.
- Where available, early intervention (EI) or coordinated specialty care (CSC) team intervention for individuals with first-episode psychosis (FEP) has proven superior to treatment as usual; referral to such programs is optimal.
- The most well-studied, effective psychotherapeutic approach to psychosis is cognitive behavioral therapy for psychosis (CBTp), which is focused on rapport building/alliance and examining one's relationship to symptoms, as opposed to trying to convince/dissuade individuals from delusional thoughts or that perceptual disturbances are not real.

P. Faraji (✉) · C. Usher
Oregon Health & Science University,
Portland, OR, USA
e-mail: faraji@ohsu.edu; ushercr@ohsu.edu

C. Camp · Z. Elberg
Jacobs School of Medicine and Biomedical Sciences,
University at Buffalo, Buffalo, NY, USA
e-mail: ctcamp@buffalo.edu; zelberg@buffalo.edu

V. Chan, J. Derenne (eds.), *Transition-Age Youth Mental Health Care*,
https://doi.org/10.1007/978-3-030-62113-1_14

Introduction

Schizophrenia is a neurodevelopmental disorder that typically presents in late adolescence through the mid-30s and is characterized by a decline in psychosocial functioning, perceptual disturbances, and fundamental deviations from shared reality. First-episode psychosis (FEP) refers to the first time a patient demonstrates frank psychotic symptoms, when most individuals receive diagnosis and treatment. Childhood-onset schizophrenia refers to the onset of illness prior to the age of 13 years. Early onset Schizophrenia (EOS) refers to onset of illness before age 18 years, and adult-onset schizophrenia refers to illness that begins after 18 years. Although EOS is less common, it is considered to be on the same spectrum as adult-onset schizophrenia, given its clinical presentation and course of illness.

Some but not all young people who develop psychosis demonstrate a period of mild psychotic symptoms prior to their FEP. Historically, this period was referred to as a "prodrome." However, this term should be used with caution as it may lead to the erroneous conclusion (1) that all people with attenuated symptoms develop the "syndrome" of psychosis and schizophrenia and (2) that someone without a prodrome cannot have psychosis. Attenuated psychosis syndrome (APS), included as a focus of research in the Diagnostic and Statistical Manual of Mental Disorders, Fifth Edition (DSM-5), involves mild symptoms wherein the individual experiences little distress and largely maintains insight [1, 2]. Attenuated symptoms are joined by two risk factors—having a family history of psychosis and transient bouts of psychosis—that place one at clinical high risk for psychosis (CHR-p) [3]. While details on CHR-p and APS are included later in this chapter, particularly around the subject diagnostic tools useful in early psychosis work, the main focus of this chapter is FEP.

The onset of psychosis often occurs in the late teens and early adulthood. For many transitional age youth (TAY), disruptions to thinking and perceiving in and of themselves can be devastating. Meanwhile, the diagnostic terms psychosis and schizophrenia are often associated with stigma and grim prognostic assumptions. In her award-winning book *The Collected Schizophrenias*, essayist Esmé Weijun Wang captures this well:

> Schizophrenia and its ilk are not seen by society as conditions that coexist with the potential for being high-functioning and are therefore terrifying. No one wants to be crazy, least of all truly crazy—as in psychotic. Schizophrenics are seen as some of the most dysfunctional members of society: we are homeless, we are inscrutable, and we are murderers [4].

Thus, for mental health practitioners working with transitional age youth (TAY) impacted by psychosis, combatting stigma and extending hope are essential. This is accomplished by adopting a collaborative and recovery-oriented stance, the philosophical anchors of coordinated specialty care (CSC) for first-episode psychosis teams. CSCs have emerged as the "gold standard" for treating TAY with psychosis. These teams vary in staffing and the treatments they offer, but nearly all provide family and support systems, psychoeducation, psychotherapy, supported education and employment, psychosocial support, and medication management.

These practices promote the idea that psychotic interruptions can be just that, interruptions that often necessitate a slowing down or "hitting the pause button" on plans and dreams, *and* provide encouragement that symptoms should not be considered the end of aspirations or development. These practices also promote a sense of identity separate from one's diagnosis. They bolster nonpharmacologic support around an individual so that they can engage in academic, professional, and social activities. Finally, CSC teams offer tools that help individuals, friends, and families accept some symptoms and difficulties (for example, auditory verbal hallucinations or executive function problems) without being overwhelmed by them, recognizing that people do well when they are not completely giving into symptoms nor fighting against them.

In hopes of helping practitioners—those participating in CSC programs and those providing treatment where CSC is not available—support youth who are impacted by psychosis and the support network around them, this chapter explores the phenomenology, differential diagnosis, assessment, and treatment of first-episode psychosis in TAY.

Epidemiology, Pathogenesis, and Risk Factors

The median lifetime prevalence of schizophrenia is 4.0 per 1000 persons [5, 6]. A systematic review completed by McGrathe et al. [6] reports that schizophrenia is more prevalent in migrants versus native-born residents. It is also more prevalent in developed countries versus less-developed countries and higher latitudes versus middle and low latitudes. Prevalence estimates can vary slightly depending on diagnostic criteria [7], race, and ethnicity [8].

The precise etiology and pathophysiology of schizophrenia is unknown; however, a neurodevelopmental model is widely accepted. This model suggests that the illness, a state of altered neural circuitry, develops through a complex interplay of disrupted development. This involves susceptibility genes, environmental factors and stressors such as *in utero* exposure to increased stress hormones or maternal famine, or later-life insults, including bullying, trauma, abuse, neglect, or refugee status, which ultimately lead to an imbalance of excitatory and inhibitory pathways resulting in psychotic symptoms [9, 10].

The risk factors for schizophrenia are divided into two categories: genetic and environmental. Genetic risk factors include de novo point mutations [11, 12], the risk of which may be increased by advanced paternal age, risk gene inheritance, and parental schizophrenia [13–15]. Some environmental risk factors include adverse childhood events and trauma [15], personal or family history of migration, and urban place of birth or residence [6, 16, 17]. Some maternal prenatal factors associated with greater risk include infection, use of analgesics, iron deficiency, stress or exposure to severe trauma, and maternal cannabis use [8, 18–20].

There is a high prevalence of substance use among individuals with FEP [21–24]. The causal relationship between substance use and schizophrenia has not been established, but substance use is considered a potential risk factor for the development of psychosis, at least in vulnerable individuals [25, 26]. Several studies showed correlation between substance use and earlier onset of psychosis [22, 23, 27]. Cannabis is the most reported substance among individuals with first-episode psychosis, followed by alcohol [21, 28, 29].

A correlation between cannabis use and the development of psychosis has been consistently reported. A 10-year prospective cohort study on over 3000 individuals between ages 14 and 24 years without a history of psychosis showed that cannabis use is a risk factor for the development of psychotic symptoms [30]. Meanwhile, a systematic metaanalysis showed that cannabis use is associated with earlier onset of symptoms [31]. However, it is possible that drug use is simply part of a wider risk cluster of teen-life behaviors/difficulties (e.g., school truancy, early sexual activity, decreased support) associated with mental illness wherein a straight line of causation cannot be drawn between cannabis and psychosis [32]. Other substance use can be implicated in the development of psychosis and will be discussed in the Differential Diagnosis section.

Diagnosis and Clinical Manifestations

The diagnosis of schizophrenia in children and adolescents is made using the same criteria as in adults: the presence of two or more of its core symptoms—hallucinations, delusions, disorganized speech, disorganized or catatonic behavior, and negative symptoms—for at least one month (unless adequately treated), with overall signs of illness lasting for at least 6 months. In order to meet the criteria for the diagnosis of schizophrenia, at least one of the following must be present: hallucinations, delusions, or disorganized speech [1]. These symptoms constitute psychosis, which is broadly understood as a break from reality characterized by perceptual disturbances, disordered and delusional thought processes, and aberrant behaviors. Psychosis, a more general term, has a wide range of etiologies, which includes schizophrenia spectrum disorders, as well as mood disorders, substance use, and various medical conditions [33]. Florid psychosis may be easy to detect. However, psychosis also begins in an insidious manner, and the heterogeneity of its presentation can make the diagnosis challenging. This is particularly true in the adolescent population, where youth are often reluctant to disclose internal experiences that they perceive to be outside the norm. Though the tendency may be to search directly for core features of psychosis, such as hallucinations and delusions, transitional age youth often present with nonspecific symptoms such as irritability, anxiety, poor concentration, worsening school performance, and social problems [33, 34].

The skilled clinician must then gently examine for the presence of psychosis that may underlie these social and behavioral changes. This is accomplished through careful and, ideally, separate interviews of the patient and family, a review of school records, and by completing a thorough psychiatric and medical history. Close attention to developmental history (birth history, temperament, presence of harassing or menacing imaginary friends that result in being awake at night, milestone delays, congenital diseases, or malformations), chronic or recurrent illness, chronic medications, cognitive functioning, substance use history, and trauma history is warranted [34]. Collateral data gathered from parents or other family members are often critical to developing a timeline of symptomatology and further define core symptoms (i.e., behavioral changes, disturbances in activities of daily living, social isolation, unusual thought content). School records are helpful in assessing the characteristic decline in academic performance and social functioning, and teachers and staff may be useful additional sources of information. Timely identification of symptoms is critical as reducing the duration of untreated psychosis (DUP) has been shown to improve outcomes [35].

While conducting an assessment, it is crucial to remember that reports of psychotic symptoms are somewhat common in children and adolescents and do not necessarily represent psychotic (schizophrenia spectrum) illness. Approximately 17% of children of ages 9–12 years and 7.5% of adolescents of ages 13–18 years describe psychotic-like experiences, compared to 5.8% of adults and 4.5% of the elderly, suggesting a course that is commonly self-limited [36]. Reports of psychotic symptoms that are situationally specific (e.g., hearing voices only when anxious), overly detailed, and/or lack associated thought or behavioral disorganization are atypical of genuine psychosis [33]. Psychotic-like symptoms in this population may instead represent developmental delays, manifestations of anxiety, trauma, dissociative symptoms, vivid imaginations, attention-seeking behavior, or simply misunderstanding of the question asked [37]. This does not mean that any reports of hallucinations or other perceptual disturbance are likely "nothing" or simply a transient phase. There is evidence to suggest that hallucinations in adolescence are more indicative of psychopathology in general, and children and teens who report psychotic experiences are at higher risk for anxiety, depression, behavioral problems, substance abuse, and self-injurious behavior [33, 36]. Youth who report only hallucinations usually display preserved social interactions, situationally specific triggers, fewer premorbid abnormalities, lower rates of associated distress, less-pervasive and functionally impairing symptoms, preserved social interactions, and lower rates of delusions, language abnormalities, and odd behavior [38, 39].

In assessing adolescents for psychosis, it is important to utilize predominately open-ended questions that can be more likely to elicit an accurate and detailed picture of a patient's thought form and content. Normalization can be a powerful tool to facilitate the discussion of uncomfortable thought content, and it is prudent to avoid medical jargon [34]. For patients who are guarded, it may be helpful to directly address their apprehensions by asking about thoughts and fears related to sharing information or inquiring if they are being instructed to remain silent by a voice or other agent (e.g., "I wonder if there is something happening inside your mind which makes answering my questions difficult. That can often happen.")

Hallucinations

Hallucinations, defined as erroneous perceptions in the absence of identifiable stimuli, are perhaps the most common feature of adolescent psychosis and early-onset schizophrenia (EOS), occurring in approximately 70–85% of cases [40, 41]. Single-voice auditory hallucinations are the most frequently reported and typically involve comments and commands. Multiple conversing voices are less common and more often seen in adults [34]. Children and adolescents are more likely to ascribe stereotypic names or physical characteristics to their hallucinations (e.g., "the monster," "the shadow man"). They are also more likely to experience multimodal hallucinations in which the auditory phenomenon includes a related visual or tactile component [34]. Rather than asking about hallucinations directly during an assessment (e.g., "Do you hear voices?"), consider starting with a subtler inquiry (e.g., "Have you ever heard things that others don't seem to notice or hear?"), which may be less threatening and more effective at eliciting information. Again, normalization is a powerful tool, especially for teens. For example, one might pose a question to a teen in this way: "Sometimes people can have experiences in which their mind plays tricks on them, causing them to see and hear things others do not. Has that ever happened to you?"

Most youth who report hallucinations do not meet the criteria for schizophrenia, nor have a psychotic illness [42]. A detailed and systematic exploration of these experiences is necessary to refine the clinician's understanding and determine the likelihood of an authentic psychotic process. Key features in this evaluation process include a full description of the phenomenon, its frequency, when it occurs, and under what context (e.g., in times of emotional distress, in specific locations, around certain people). Asking the patient about whether and how these experiences differ from their imagination or other ordinary thoughts and experiences can be helpful. Hallucinations of the psychotic/schizophrenia variety are typically vivid (grabbing and holding the person's attention), reaction provoking, and not especially detailed and cannot be willed away or easily ignored [34]. It is also prudent to assess whether the hallucinations are distressing to the patient.

Only about half of adolescents who report auditory hallucinations express being distressed by them, and evidence suggests that distress is more strongly associated with eventual conversion to psychosis [38]. Carefully screening for the presence of suicidal ideation is crucial as hallucinations have been shown to be a powerful independent risk factor for suicidal behavior in children and adolescents, which increases both short- and long-term risks [36].

New tools have recently been developed to aid clinicians in systematically and comprehensively assessing hallucinations in youth. The SOCRATES Assessment of Perceptual Abnormalities and Unusual Thought Content offers a structured interview guideline for the assessment of auditory hallucinations; this is free and available online [43]. The Auditory Vocal Hallucination Rating Scale Questionnaire (AVHRS-Q) is a brief (6-minute) self-report tool that can also be used to assess auditory hallucinations in adolescents [36]. For an "outside the box" approach, there is Multisensory Hallucinations Scale for Children (MHASC), a free mobile app with game-based visuals and an engaging interface that explores five sensory domains (auditory, visual, somatosensory, gustatory, and olfactory) and may help destigmatize symptom reporting [36]. It is likely best reserved for younger patients or those who have a developmental profile in the age range 8–12 years.

Delusions

Delusions, or false beliefs not amenable to change despite conflicting evidence, are also common in EOS, occurring with a frequency of 54–77% [41]. Delusions in teens and TAY tend to be less complex than in adults [1, 34, 39, 44]. Whereas adults commonly possess delusions that are specific and elaborately systematized, delusions in adolescents—particularly those under the age of 16 years—typically involve vague suspicions [34, 45]. This may be a consequence of their earlier stage of cognitive development, limited ability to articulate or rationalize aberrant perceptual experiences, or having had less time to internally process and solidify a narrative around the delusional content [44].

A broad array of delusional presentations exist, and these can be characterized as persecutory (often cited as the most common), referential, grandiose, somatic, erotomanic, mixed, unspecified, and with bizarre content [1, 34, 44, 46].

There is evidence to suggest that anxiety and negative schema may contribute to the development of persecutory delusions, and youth with psychotic symptoms may have higher rates of anxiety relative to their adult counterparts, perhaps resulting from their unique developmental life stressors [44]. Common examples of persecutory delusions include the sense that one is being harassed by peers or being monitored by cameras or tapped phones, again all examples of simpler delusions relative to the complex persecutory delusional systems often seen in adults [45]. These delusions may manifest as a pathological response to the social pressures of being in middle school, high school, or college/grad school settings or in new job environments. Referential delusions commonly involve receiving direct messages from the Internet, television, or other media sources [45]. Grandiose delusions include a sense of access to special knowledge or belief in the ability to make things happen through thought alone, while somatic delusions include erroneous belief in pregnancy (pseudocyesis) or the presence of a foreign object in the body [34]. Collateral information may be instrumental in identifying and characterizing delusional content in guarded adolescents reluctant to engage in clinical assessment.

Thought, Speech, and Behavioral Disorganization

Disorganization of thought, speech, and behavior is observable in 52–65% of EOS cases, although it may be challenging to differentiate these symptoms from premorbid or comorbid language and cognitive difficulties [34, 41]. TAY who develop schizophrenia commonly exhibit premorbid abnormalities in verbal reasoning, speech and language, working memory, attention, processing speed, and executive function [42]. These abnormalities may often precede the classical prodromal stage [42], an early phase of schizophrenia, which will be further described in the Clinical Course section. Frequently observed phenomena include poverty of thought and speech, tangentiality or derailment, perseveration, incoherence, loose associations, poor attention, and odd, purposeless, or repetitive behaviors [42, 47]. Together, hallucinations, delusions, and thought/speech/behavior disorganization are often called positive symptoms of schizophrenia due to their visibility, in contrast to negative symptoms, which represent absence deficits.

Negative Symptoms

Negative symptoms are a prominent feature of EOS, causing clinically relevant deficits in at least half of cases at the time of presentation. This is significantly higher than the estimated 15% negative symptom presentation of adult first-onset cases [41]. Negative symptoms in youth may accumulate undetected for years before the onset of positive symptoms [45]. Common features include progressive social withdrawal, avolition, decreased emotional expression, apathy, anhedonia, diminished self-care, inattention, blunted affect, and alogia [45, 48]. Avolition, apathy, anhedonia, and social withdrawal have been particularly associated with longer DUP, perhaps because they may be less likely to raise alarm than more overt symptoms like affective blunting or poor hygiene [35]. Of the negative symptoms, poor social functioning and diminished verbal fluency are particularly predictive of transition to frank psychosis in clinically high-risk (CHR) patients [49, 50].

Differential Diagnosis

Clarifying the various possible causes of psychosis in youth can be immensely challenging. When psychosis symptoms are reported, a provider's first thought may be to consider a diagnosis within the schizophrenia spectrum and other psychotic disorder category. However, adolescents with psychosis are just as likely to have a primary affective disorder as they are a primary thought disorder [34]. Myriad additional possibilities exist, including anxiety disorders, trauma-related disorders, developmental disorders, substance abuse, medical conditions, and nonpsychotic perceptual abnormalities [34, 39, 48]. Since reports of psychotic symptoms in youth are more common than in adults, clinicians who immediately equate the presence of hallucinations with psychotic illness should expect a significant false positive rate [36, 39]. Careful consideration of the numerous etiological possibilities should follow any psychotic symptom report, as well as a healthy dose of patience. Time is often the most critical diagnostic tool in youth with psychosis as an illness in the prodromal stage can take months or years to fully reveal itself [33].

Mood Disorders

Of the psychiatric illnesses, mood disorders and schizophrenia are the most common causes of psychosis [33]. Not only do they significantly overlap in symptomatology; these disorders also share similar peak ages of onset during young adulthood. Bipolar I disorder, in particular, has a peak onset between 15 and 24 years of age and is commonly confused with schizophrenia [51, 52]. Differentiating these illnesses can be especially challenging in youth, who often present with ill-defined symptoms. In assessing an adolescent with psychotic symptoms, it is important to first ask oneself whether affective symptoms appear to be present and, if so, whether there seems to be a temporal relationship between the two [39]. Psychotic symptoms fueled by affective illness should be entirely contained within mood episodes, whereas psychosis occurring independently of mood symptoms is more suggestive of schizophrenia.

Other clinical distinctions may be useful as well. Psychosis underlying mania will typically involve florid delusions and abundant thought content in contrast to the impoverishment characteristic of schizophrenia [33]. The onset of mania is also more likely to be abrupt than gradual, although a chronically developing course is possible [39]. When symptoms seem to cycle or fluctuate over time, this may be more consistent with affective illness [34]. Sleep disruptions are seen in both mania and schizophrenia. They may be differentiated by the underlying cause: abundant energy in the former and fear, anxiety, or disturbing perceptual experiences in the latter. Additionally, youth who develop schizophrenia usually have more long-standing premorbid abnormalities in cognition, language, and social functioning than do those who develop bipolar disorder [34, 39].

Unipolar depression is also common in early psychosis [53]. Clinicians must diligently avoid dismissing the "moody adolescent" without a careful assessment for associated negative and positive symptoms. Major depressive disorder with psychotic features presents its own diagnostic challenges and may be difficult to distinguish from schizophrenia. Delusions and hallucinations are common to both illnesses, though formal thought disorder is more specific to schizophrenia [34] and may be a helpful differentiator. Many negative symptoms of schizophrenia overlap with neurovegetative features of depression, such as inattention, fatigue, avolition, and insomnia. Alogia and blunted affect are more common in schizophrenia. Recognition of true negative symptoms is particularly meaningful diagnostically as they are more specific than positive symptoms and thus are more predictive of the presence of schizophrenia [39]. The youth's ability to describe their symptoms can also provide valuable insight; an individual with depression may be more likely to provide richer descriptions of their internal experience (e.g., prominent expression of sadness and self-criticism), whereas an individual with schizophrenia may be more likely to have difficulty conveying their internal experience (e.g., report feeling "blah" or use other vague descriptors) [34]. A depressed individual may also demonstrate a higher degree of insight into neurovegetative symptoms or social dysfunction relative to an individual with schizophrenia, who may appear undisturbed by mounting negative symptoms.

Longitudinal assessment is often the most important diagnostic tool, allowing the clinician to monitor for fluctuations in psychotic symptoms and their possible relationship with affective shifts. A careful distinction may also need to be made in longitudinal assessment to clarify any schizoaffective disorder diagnosis, which requires the continuation of psychosis symptoms for at least two weeks' duration after unipolar or bipolar syndromes have resolved.

Trauma and PTSD

Studies have repeatedly demonstrated a correlation between trauma and psychotic symptoms [38, 40, 42, 48]. Traumatized youth are three to four times more likely to report psychotic symptoms, and there appears to be a dose-response relationship, with three childhood traumas being predictive of developing hallucinations [38, 40, 48]. Traumatic experiences that have been shown to increase risk include sexual, physical, and emotional abuse; bullying; and neglect [40]. Sadly, the dose-response relationship appears to be bidirectional in nature: not only does trauma increase the risk for psychosis, but psychotic symptoms also increase the risk that an individual will experience trauma [36, 40].

Although not every child who experiences trauma will go on to develop psychotic symptoms, children with a high number of adverse childhood experiences (ACEs) represent a more vulnerable population with unique diagnostic considerations [36]. The presence of trauma in the history of an adolescent neither rules in nor rules out a diagnosis of schizophrenia but instead should alert the clinician to carefully differentiate trauma-associated pathology and posttraumatic stress disorder (PTSD) from primary psychotic illness [42]. Youth who have suffered trauma can experience intrusive thoughts, dissociative symptoms, mood and behavioral dysregulation, hypervigilance, and cognitive disturbances, which may mimic positive psychotic symptoms of schizophrenia [37, 39]. Furthermore, studies indicate that a large majority of adolescents who report auditory hallucinations also screen positive for a traumatic event directly around the time of symptom onset [40]. Assessment should investigate the temporal and contextual association between trauma and psychotic symptoms. Individuals suffering from PTSD-associated psychotic symptoms are more likely to have detailed hallucinations that relate to trauma content and occur transiently in times of stress [34]. If dissociative symptoms are present, functioning between episodes should be relatively preserved [34]. Situationally specific psychosis (i.e., during times of stress, around certain individuals, or in certain locations) in the absence of formal thought disorder, or behavioral disorganization is uncharacteristic of schizophrenia [33].

Anxiety Disorders and Obsessive-Compulsive Disorder

Anxiety is commonly comorbid with schizophrenia and appears to be particularly prevalent in youth who struggle with psychosis in the midst of significant developmental, school, and social pressures [45]. Youth who develop schizophrenia often present with nonspecific symptoms, of which anxiety is frequently prominent [34]. Furthermore, approximately 12% of youth at clinical high risk for psychosis meet the criteria for general anxiety disorder (GAD) or social phobia [48]. The clinician should thus be sure to gently explore for the presence of perceptual disturbances or abnormal thinking which may be hidden below the surface of a teen presenting with anxiety.

Obsessive-compulsive disorder (OCD) is often easily confused with schizophrenia [34]. It is well understood that OCD has a particularly high association with schizophrenia and is comorbid in approximately 25% of adolescent cases [54, 55]. Obsessive-compulsive symptoms most often manifest in the prodromal period leading up to FEP and have been linked with higher insidiousness of onset, increased negative symptoms, and male gender [54]. Overlapping symptoms between OCD and schizophrenia include odd and intrusive thoughts, unusual and repetitive behaviors, perseveration, inattention, and dysphoria [39]. One helpful distinguishing factor for OCD symptoms may be ego-dystonicity, in which the patient demonstrates intrusive thoughts and odd behaviors though maintains insight into their illogical nature. This insight may be lacking in a typical patient with schizophrenia. However, younger individuals and adolescents who are less metacognitively skilled may also lack insight and experience their intrusive thoughts as foreign or hallucinatory, contributing to diagnostic complexity [39]. Patients with schizophrenia can often be distinguished by having more severe premorbid abnormalities; a wider array of psychotic symptoms, including thought disorder and multimodal hallucinations; higher difficulty in articulating fears and obsessions; and more bizarre compulsions that are usually less anxiety relieving to the individual [34].

Neurodevelopmental Disorders

Studies conducted under DSM-IV nomenclature show that pervasive developmental disorders are frequently comorbid with EOS, co-occurring in approximately 12.5% of cases [48]. Many features of thought, speech, and behavioral disorganization significantly overlap with symptoms of autism spectrum disorder (ASD) and other developmental disabilities, which must be considered as differential diagnoses. Individuals with ASD will display pervasive abnormalities throughout development, whereas youth who develop schizophrenia undergo clearer deterioration in social and cognitive function [42]. The presence of hallucinations or delusions alongside thought and speech disorganization as a change from baseline functioning suggests the development of psychotic illness. ASD and attention-deficit/hyperactivity disorder (ADHD) co-occur the most commonly and have a complex pathophysiological relationship with psychosis and schizophrenia [33, 34, 56]. All three disorders seemingly result from disruptions in early brain development, likely share genetic determinants, and result in premorbid cognitive pathology that typifies adolescent schizophrenia [33, 34, 56]. Studies have shown that youth with ADHD are at particularly high risk of developing psychotic illness as they age, with inattention being the most consistent shared developmental symptom [56]. Other overlapping features include impulsivity, poor frustration tolerance, poor social functioning, and deficits in executive functioning and emotional processing [56]. Furthermore, youth with ADHD have significantly increased rates of substance abuse, which is hypothesized to contribute to the development of psychotic disorders [56]. ASD also shares a number of commonalities with schizophrenia, including perseverative thinking, odd beliefs, rigid behaviors, language deficits, and cognitive and social impairments [33, 48]. The most important distinguishing factor between these illnesses and schizophrenia is the presence of psychotic symptoms. Once hallucinations or delusions manifest for at least one month in an adolescent with features of ASD and/or ADHD, the diagnosis of a schizophrenia-spectrum illness would take precedence [33, 48]. It is also helpful to consider the illness course as youth who develop schizophrenia should demonstrate a stark decline inconsistent with baseline functional abnormalities [42].

Personality Disorders

Certain personality disorders may share overlapping features with EOS, with schizoid, schizotypal, and borderline personalities being the most commonly cited [39, 57, 58]. Shared features with Cluster A personality disorders include solitariness, magical thinking, eccentric behavior, and perceptual abnormalities. Impulsivity and behavioral disturbance, along with transient psychotic phenomena, are consistent with borderline pathology [39]. Although personality disorders should be considered as part of a complete differential, caution should be taken in ascribing personality disorders to youth who are still consolidating their identity and exploring new ways of navigating intrapsychic and interpersonal relationships.

Substance Use Risk Factors

Adolescence can be a period that marks a steep increase in illicit drug use. Many substances can induce psychotic symptoms [48]. The rate of substance abuse in adolescents with a schizophrenia spectrum disorder may near 70% at the upper estimated range [41]. Common culprits include cannabis, synthetic cannabinoids (e.g., "K2" or "spice"), cocaine, methamphetamine, 3,4-methyl enedioxymethamphetamine (MDMA or "ecstacy"), synthetic cathinones (bath salts), phencyclidine (PCP), lysergic acid diethylamide (LSD), dextromethorphan, peyote, opiates, psilocybin (shrooms), inhalants, and ketamine [34, 59]. Regulated medications that have been implicated in psychotic symptoms include steroids, antihistamines, isoniazid, serotonergic agents, psychostimulants, certain anesthetic agents, dopamine agonists, antihistamines, and certain antibiotics such as quinolones [34, 59].

When substance abuse precedes the development of psychotic symptoms, it can be extraordinarily difficult to differentiate between drug effects and a concomitantly developing primary psychotic illness [42]. There are several questions for a provider to consider in this workup: Was illicit drug use something the patient engaged in as part of a pattern of risk-taking behavior due to the early cognitive and impulse-control disruptions associated with psychosis? Was the patient attempting to treat their psychosis or escape symptoms by using drugs? Was there an underlying vulnerability or vulnerabilities (genes and environment) that substance use unmasked [42]? Is this a time-limited psychosis that will resolve once the patient no longer uses and is drug-free for a period of time?

Thorough history taking and a sustained period of abstinence often help answer these questions. However, the period needed to resolve substance-induced psychoses varies depending on the individual and the agents used [48]. Certain substances such as cannabis can persist in the system for many weeks, and many others, like methamphetamine, are known to cause psychotic symptoms well after discontinuation. Substance-associated psychosis symptoms in the absence of premorbid or progressive cognitive and social abnormalities associated with early-onset schizophrenia are more suggestive of substance-induced psychosis.

Medical Conditions

In the case of new-onset, unexplained psychosis in an adolescent, it is important for the clinician to keep medical conditions known to cause psychosis on the diagnostic radar. Broadly, medical disorders known to cause psychosis include neurologic, endocrine, metabolic, autoimmune, infectious, and genetic processes [34]. Most of these medical conditions are relatively rare, and indiscriminate screening should be avoided in favor of thoughtful evaluation dictated by the clinical presentation, physical symptoms, and history [33].

Key neurologic disorders to consider in youth include epilepsy, migraines, and neoplasms [34]. The prevalence of psychosis is 10–15% in patients with epilepsy and may be the first presenting symptom in youth [59]. It can occur during, after, and between seizures [34]. Foci in the temporal lobe are the most commonly implicated in psychotic symptoms, though they can also occur in association with all forms of seizures, ranging from partial to generalized [34, 59]. Migraine headaches may also be preceded or accompanied by perceptual disturbances, including hallucinations, though the symptoms should be limited to the time frame of the headache or its herald symptoms. Brain tumors are rare but can also cause psychosis, particularly when they affect the limbic system. Astrocytoma, ependymoma, and medulloblastoma tumors in the pituitary, visual cortex, and frontal and temporal lobes are commonly implicated in TAY psychosis and are capable of producing both hallucinations and delusions [34, 59]. Traumatic brain injury (TBI) should also be considered.

Endocrinopathies associated with psychosis include overactivity and underactivity of both the thyroid and parathyroid glands [59]. Hyper- and hypoglycemia have also been implicated, as well as electrolyte abnormalities in magnesium, phosphate, sodium, and calcium [59]. Elevated levels of heavy metals such as lead or copper have been associated, the latter of which may be seen in

Wilson's disease, which causes psychosis in nearly half of children who present clinically for treatment [59]. Other common genetic disorders associated with psychosis include fragile X, Turner syndrome, Marfan syndrome, velocardiofacial (VCFS)/DiGeorge syndromes (22q11 deletion syndromes), Friedrich's ataxia, Huntington's disease, tuberous sclerosis, acute intermittent porphyria, and Down's syndrome [34].

Several other rheumatological and inflammatory conditions can cause psychosis. Lupus has been shown to present with neuropsychiatric symptoms in 35% of cases in youth, with psychosis as well as cognitive, mood, anxiety, and attentional symptoms [59]. Childhood-onset multiple sclerosis and poststreptococcal syndromes are other autoimmune causes [59]. Paraneoplastic syndromes as a result of germline, ovarian, breast, and small cell lung cancers may lead to psychosis secondary to encephalitis [34]. Anti-N-methyl-D-aspartate (NMDA) receptor encephalitis, in particular, commonly presents with psychosis and is seen in young women with ovarian teratomas [59]. Infectious causes include HIV/AIDS, viral encephalitis, brain abscesses, Lyme disease, and parasitic infections of the central nervous system (CNS) [59].

Assessment and Workup

Labs and Tests

Although it is relatively rare to find general medical causes for psychosis symptoms in TAY, a comprehensive evaluation which may include laboratory tests and radiologic imaging is warranted in all patients to ensure that treatable conditions are not missed [34]. A preliminary workup should always include a complete blood count (CBC), a comprehensive metabolic panel (CMP), magnesium (Mg) levels, thyroid-stimulating hormone (TSH), thyroxine (free T4), and urine toxicology screens [34]. Detailed neurological examination should be universally performed, with subsequent brain MRI with contrast completed should any deficits be noted [34].

At present, there is inadequate evidence to suggest that brain imaging should be ordered in all new-onset cases, though it may be prudent in patients with a history of TBI or treatment-resistant symptoms [34]. An electroencephalogram (EEG) should only be requested if there is suspicion for seizures, including markedly episodic symptoms, automatisms, or postepisode confusion, with a 24- to 48-hour tracing or sleep-deprivation study preferred to increase the probability of detecting epileptic activity [34]. In some cases, video EEG (video telemetry) may be warranted. A genetics consultation may be considered if a disorder is suspected based on a characteristic dysmorphology or positive family history of schizophrenia spectrum disorders [34]. Other optional studies that may be obtained based on clinical suspicion include an erythrocyte sedimentation rate (ESR), antinuclear antibody (ANA) test, rapid plasma reagin (RPR) for syphilis, human immunodeficiency virus (HIV) testing, heavy metals, and copper/ceruloplasmin, and specialist consultation should be obtained if metabolic, storage, or infectious diseases are suspected [34, 59]. Anti-NMDA receptor encephalitis can be ruled out by testing cerebrospinal fluid (CSF) or blood for antibodies. Finally, coordination and exchange of data with the patient's primary care provider, if one exists, is beneficial.

Assessment Tools

A number of rating scales and surveys are available to aid in identifying and assessing psychotic symptoms in adolescents. These may be broadly divided into screeners (Table 14.1) and comprehensive assessment measures (Table 14.2). Screening tools are brief self-report measures geared toward quickly detecting at-risk individuals in need of further assessment, whereas comprehensive assessment measures are semi-structured clinical interviews aimed at thorough assessment and diagnosis. Many of the comprehensive assessment measures require training to administer properly, whereas screening tools do not.

Table 14.1 Screening tools utilized to assess psychosis risk and schizophrenia spectrum disorders

Name	Description	Training required
Prodromal Questionnaire—Brief Version (**PB-Q**)	21-item self-report questionnaire Assesses symptoms in the past month PQ-16 is a 16-item version [36, 60]	None
Early Psychosis Screener for Internet (**EPSI**)	64-item self-report survey Validated to detect risk of conversation to psychosis in 16 months EPS-26 is a 26-item paper version EPS-9 is a 9-item online version [61, 62]	None
Prevention Through Risk Identification, Management, and Education—Revised (**PRIME-R**)	12-item self-report questionnaire Developed from the SIPS comprehensive assessment tool [63]	None
Youth Psychosis At-Risk Questionnaire—Brief (**Y-PARQ-B**)	28-item self-report questionnaire Developed from the CAARMS comprehensive assessment tool [64]	None

Course and Outcome

The course of early-onset schizophrenia varies widely in its onset, progression, and chronic versus time-limited nature [42]. It can be particularly challenging to anticipate disease progression. However, certain characteristic patterns are discernible, and the early phase of illness, particularly the five years following an index episode of psychosis, often forecast long-term disease course [48].

Table 14.2 Comprehensive assessment measures utilized to assess psychosis and schizophrenia spectrum disorders

Name	Description	Training required
Structured Interview for Prodromal Syndromes (**SIPS**)	Structured interview used to diagnose prodromal psychosis syndromes [36, 65] Includes SOPS (Scale of Prodromal Symptoms)—a 19-item scale that measures the severity of prodromal symptoms and changes over time [63]	Extensive
Comprehensive Assessment of At-Risk Mental States (**CAARMS**)	Structured interview to assess for psychopathology indicating imminent development of first-episode psychosis Determines if UHR criteria are met [66]	Moderate
Kiddie Schedule for Affective Disorders and Schizophrenia (**K-SADS**)	Semi-structured interview that is generally briefer than SIPS Assesses for a broad range of psychopathology in addition to psychosis [67]	Some
Brief Psychiatric Rating Scale (**BPRS; BPRS-C** for children)	Clinician-rated 18–24-item 7-point Likert scale Measures psychiatric symptoms, including several symptoms specific to psychosis [68]	Some
Positive and Negative Syndrome Scale (**PANSS**)	Interviewer-rated 30-item 7-point Likert scale Measures positive, negative, and general psychopathology symptom severity of schizophrenia [69]	Moderate, interview must demonstrate standardized level of reliability

Clinical Course

The majority of youth affected by psychosis will first experience a period of progressive functional decline, often referred to as the "prodromal period" [42]. This may last from months to years and is commonly characterized by social withdrawal, decreased self-care, academic or occupational decline, dysphoria, and idiosyncratic preoccupations [42]. Typically, the first discernible prodromal symptoms are either negative symptoms or nonspecific depression, anxiety, social isolation, or functional decline [70]. Prodromal symptoms are frequently identified retrospectively once positive symptoms emerge, which may present in the form of an attenuated psychotic syndrome (APS). APS entails mild psychotic-like experiences of lower intensity, frequency, and duration than would be required for the diagnosis of a psychotic disorder [70]. Relative to full-threshold psychosis, attenuated symptoms of psychosis may occur on a weekly to monthly basis, last for only a few minutes, and be associated with lower levels of distress with greater preservation of insight. Should these symptoms become functionally impairing, or cause clinically significant distress yet remain a subthreshold for schizophrenia diagnosis, they would constitute the Attenuated Psychosis Syndrome specifier for the Other Specified Schizophrenia Spectrum or Other Psychotic Disorder diagnosis [1]. Looking back at the course of those who develop FEP, it appears that unusual, predelusional thought content, budding perceptual abnormalities, and subtle thought disorganization may become apparent [70].

Up to one-third of those at clinical high risk for psychosis (CHR-p)—a distinction anchored in having a positive family history of schizophrenia spectrum or schizoid disorders, one having attenuated psychotic symptoms or very brief, intermittent psychotic bouts—will convert to full-threshold psychosis [42, 48, 49, 70]. Conversion most often occurs within 2 years of disease onset, though it may take as long as 10–15 years in some cases [48]. A minority of patients will not have detectable prodrome and may present with an acute development of psychotic symptoms. Negative emotional content and heightened distress related to APS have been found to be predictive of conversion [48]. The majority of CHR-p clinical population go on to be diagnosed with nonpsychosis spectrum primary illnesses. [48]

The acute phase of schizophrenia spectrum conditions features prominent and persistent positive symptoms coupled with a drastic functional deterioration, necessitating treatment [42]. Hospitalization is commonly necessary depending on the degree of symptom burden or safety concerns. The duration of this phase depends on a number of factors, including the timeliness of intervention and treatment responsiveness, which are closely associated. A prolonged DUP has been shown to be correlated with treatment resistance, leading to a protracted acute phase and poorer outcomes [71].

Successful treatment can bring about remission of an acute psychotic episode and entry into the recovery phase, generally a period of several months with significant ongoing functional impairment [42]. Positive symptoms, the most responsive to antipsychotic treatment, become less prominent and may fully remit, while negative symptoms become more prominent and often frustrating to youth, families, friends, and other supports [42]. The emergence of postpsychosis depressive symptoms commonly occurs as insight returns. At this time, the young person must come to terms with the illness and its implications. These symptoms may take the form of a mild grief, an adjustment disorder, or a full major depressive episode requiring pharmacotherapy. This can be a particularly difficult time as youth attempt to negotiate reentry into school and are confronted with peers for whom life seems to have moved on, while the TAY was absent and/or continues to struggle.

The course following the first psychotic episode is heterogeneous, ranging from full symptom recovery to chronic positive and/or negative symptoms of greatly varying severity [72]. The majority of patients will experience at least a residual phase in which negative symptoms and mild positive symptoms persist rather than achieve full remission, and the prognosis is guarded [42]. The rate of relapse to the acute phase is highly variable and is dependent on many factors, including the degree of treatment responsiveness, treatment adherence, medication persistence, comorbid substance use, and family support. Abstinence from drugs, particularly cannabis, is helpful in preventing relapse.

Impact and Outcomes

The prognosis of earlier onset schizophrenia is not abundantly clear, but many studies show a trend toward poorer outcomes than seen in the adult-onset population [73]. This is likely attributable to the interruption of crucial neurobiological maturation and psychosocial development processes integral to childhood, adolescence, and emerging adulthood [73]. Key developmental areas impacted include identity formation, solidifying peer relations, enhancing empathy and mentalizing, affect regulation, impulse control, learning about intimacy, sexuality, abstract thought, moral reasoning, honing creativity, celebrating academic achievement, and occupational productivity [48].

Interrupting both the neurobiological underpinnings of these activities and the psychological development associated with these developmental events can have life-long ramifications, significantly impacting an adolescent's ability to individuate and transition into an independent and productive adult. School interruption by means of cognitive blunting, isolation from peers, and disease-related absence is particularly disruptive. This can impair one's ability to gain foundational academic and social knowledge, along with a sense of agency associated with navigating these. Supporting this notion is the fact that younger ages of onset, and thus greater degrees of developmental interruption, have been correlated with worse long-term outcomes [73].

Occupational participation is significantly impacted as well, with approximately 30% of individuals applying for disability benefits within a year of accessing early intervention services and 60% within 5 years [74]. Thus, optimal psychiatric care must aim not simply to reduce or ameliorate symptoms but instead to address the psychosocial implications of psychosis and its interruptions to scholastic, social, and employment goals. It is important to help young people to see psychosis as an interruption opposed to a termination of the process of achievement and connection to others.

In addition to its disruptive effects on development, school, and work, EOS also profoundly impacts the family. Adolescents and adults with schizophrenia rank family as one of their leading sources of stress [75]. Given the stress-sensitive nature of the illness, this can significantly influence course and outcome. Families may react to mental illness in a myriad of ways. Some may grow more supportive, while others may try to exert more control. Anger, confusion, skepticism, exasperation, empathy, fear, and despair are common. Families and supports may rally around their loved one, distance themselves for fear of how the young person will react, hover over them, or push to an extent that sparks conflict. Psychosis more often provokes irritability, criticism, and interruptions from caregivers, while affective symptoms tend to elicit empathy, constructive talk, and gentle physical contact [74]. Adolescents with psychosis are at uniquely elevated risk for family conflict, which has been shown to directly correlate with positive symptom burden, thought disorganization, and negative long-term outcomes [74]. Despite this, it is crucial to avoid blaming families but rather actively enlist them in treatment. This can be done in a variety of ways, including support groups, multifamily workshops, family therapy, and psychoeducation [76, 77]. Cultivating a network of supportive family, friends, and other important figures is key in helping affected youth navigate their illness and work toward physical, emotional, and social recovery.

Alongside younger age of onset, longer DUP, and high family conflict, other negative prognostic factors include lower premorbid functioning and insidious onset without a precipitating stressor. High negative symptom burden, positive family history of schizophrenia spectrum disorders, absence of mood symptoms, lower degree of recovery after initial hospitalization, frequent hospitalizations, and co-occurring substance use also predict poorer outcomes [39, 41, 48, 52, 70,

78]. Substance use is of particular concern as it is a modifiable factor that is highly prevalent in youth with psychosis and has been independently associated with longer duration of psychotic episodes, increased hospitalization rates, and poorer lifetime functioning [70]. There is evidence suggesting that youth at risk or actively experiencing psychosis are uniquely sensitive to the psychoactive effects of substances [70]. Furthermore, substances exacerbate developmental disruption by interfering with brain maturation, education, and social and emotional learning and are thus a key target for intervention [70].

Unfortunately, youth with psychosis and those at CHR-p are at high risk for suicide [79, 80]. About 50–75% of affected individuals report current or past suicidal ideation, 20% report a past attempt, and 8–10% die by suicide [79–81]. Suicide risk in adolescents has been consistently found to be greater than their adult counterparts, particularly during and directly following a first psychotic episode, which accounts for approximately half of all psychosis-related attempts [81, 82]. Risk factors for suicide include longer DUP, high negative symptom burden, substance abuse, recent hospital discharge, suicidal gestures or past attempts, command hallucinations, living alone, impaired functioning, higher IQ, and depressive symptoms [81]. All adolescents presenting with psychotic symptoms must be comprehensively evaluated for suicide, including frequency and intensity of ideation, intent, plan, access to means, past attempts, and self-harming behavior. Related to this, a suicide prevention plan/safety plan should follow through history taking, with clinicians helping the individual identify early warning signs of heightened suicide risk. They should also review tools that the TAY can use to remain alive and language they would like to use around suicide and help identify who the patient trusts to reach out to in times of crisis.

Despite the substantial risk of chronically disabling disease in early-onset schizophrenia, fortunately not all individuals will experience a poor outcome. In fact, the advent of coordinated specialty care (CSC) programs such as NAVIGATE has appeared to significantly improve 2-year outcomes with regard to quality of life, symptom burden, treatment retention, and participation in work and school [83]. Remission rates 2 years following the first psychotic episode may be as high as 61% following admission to an early psychosis program, with over half of adolescents engaging in work or school within that time frame [78]. However, these outcomes continue to be significantly influenced by DUP, and thus early identification and treatment remain crucial [83].

Treatment

Most mental health clinicians providing psychiatric care for individuals with psychosis are familiar with widely available and accepted clinical practice guidelines. Examples include those guidelines published by the American Psychiatric Association (APA) [84] or treatment recommendations put forth by the National Institute for Health and Care Excellence (NICE) [85]. In this section, we focus on evidence-based pharmacological and psychosocial interventions (EBPs) for individuals with FEP. There is a growing body of evidence on the positive impact of early and effective treatment of psychosis on prognosis and course of illness [86–90]. Specialized treatment programs, or coordinated specialty care (CSC), to treat first-episode psychosis have been developed and implemented in many parts of the world, with available model of manualized practices, and have been shown to have better treatment outcomes compared to standard treatment [91–94].

Coordinated specialty care (CSC) refers to multicomponent, team-based, recovery-oriented, and person-centered care that utilizes shared decision-making to provide support, education, and treatment to youth with first-episode psychosis and their families. CSC teams require specialized training (on core values and components of CSC) and ongoing support for its team members. CSC focuses on outreach and early engagement, with the goal of decreasing the length of untreated psychosis. The treatment approach of the team is optimally trauma informed, based on shared decision-making and collaboration with youth by focusing on recovery and defining personal goals. CSC team members meet regularly for collaboration and coordination of care.

Although there is a variability among CSC teams in terms of team composition and therapeutic modalities offered, CSC typically involves personalized pharmacological management and intensive case management. Therapy interventions are focused on problem-solving and are anchored in psychoeducation and cognitive behavioral therapy for psychosis (CBTp) principles, which are offered in individual, family/support network, and group settings. TAY are also offered specialized support to meet their educational and vocational goals. Peer support specialists are available in some CSC programs, and although their role is not well defined as others, they usually support youth by drawing upon their lived experience of coping with mental challenges, negotiating school and work difficulties, and navigating the mental healthcare system [76]. Families and support systems are highly encouraged to participate in psychoeducation and structured problem-solving skills for support. Table 14.3 summarizes components of CSC.

Although CSC programs were well established internationally, the rise of CSC in the United States started in 2008 with the Recovery After an Initial Schizophrenia Episode (RAISE) initiative. This was a research initiative funded by the National Institute of Mental Health (NIMH) to test the effectiveness and feasibility of CSC programs in the United States, which has a differ-

Table 14.3 Program components of coordinated specialty care (CSC) [76]

Team leadership	Team leaders are familiar with all aspects of coordinated specialty care and provide ongoing consultation to team members about the principles of early psychosis intervention. They may coordinate program services such as screening potential clients, leading weekly team meetings, overseeing treatment planning and case review, and developing outreach and referral strategies. They are the public face of the program and sometimes, also deliver direct intervention services.
Psychotherapist/ primary clinician	Psychotherapy for FEP is based upon cognitive and behavioral treatment principles and emphasizes resilience training, helps process trauma, reduces feelings of stigma, focuses on illness and wellness management, and works to improve general coping skills. Treatment consists of core and supplemental modules and is tailored to each client's needs. Clients and psychotherapists work one-on-one or in groups, meeting weekly or biweekly, with the duration and frequency of sessions personalized for each individual. This primary clinician often serves as the main coordinator for a client's care
Supported employment and education (SEE)	Supported employment and education specialists support each individual's return to work or school, as well as attainment of expected vocational and educational milestones. The SEE specialist strives to integrate vocational and mental health services; is the CSC team liaison with outside educators and employers, and frequently works with the individual in the community to enhance school or job performance.
Family education and support	Family education and support specialists educate family members about psychosis and its treatment and strengthen their capacity to aid in the consumer's recovery by reducing family stress through improved communication and problem-solving skills. They ensure that family members are included in all aspects of a consumer's care (consistent with the consumer preferences). Family support can be offered on an individual basis or through multifamily groups.
Case management	Case managers assist clients with problems-solving to ensure that their immediate practical needs are met. Case managers have frequent in-person contact with clients and their families to address issues related to housing, transportation, income, criminal justice involvement, and medical care.
Peer support	Peer specialists works with program participants and family members to support and advocate for the participant within the context of the team.
Prescriber services, pharmacotherapy, and coordination with primary care	Along with interventions and supports consistent with team goals, providers monitor patients' symptoms and side effects (especially cardiometabolic risk) and address attitudes toward medication treatment at each patient visit. Prescribers maintain close contact with primary care providers to assure optimal medical treatment for risk factors related to cardiovascular disease and diabetes, as well as the range of possible health and side effects that may occur.

ent payor system than other parts of the world, leading to challenges in delivering integrated, multicomponent models of care. RAISE consisted of two main projects, the RAISE-Early Treatment Program (RAISE-ETP) and the RAISE Connection Program Implementation and Evaluation Study (RAISE-IES), both aimed at developing, testing, and implementing interventions to improve long-term outcomes and the prognosis of schizophrenia through early intervention.

The RAISE-ETP study evaluated the effectiveness of the team-based NAVIGATE approach in a cluster randomized controlled trial compared with the usual community treatment [83]. NAVIGATE is based on three conceptual frameworks:

- The recovery model, which is a person-centered approach emphasizing hope that one can work to regain function and strive to achieve *a priori* or new goals
- The stress-vulnerability model, which encourages individuals and families to work to reduce the stresses that can trigger and exacerbate mental health conditions
- The rehabilitation model, which supports the fact that one can work to regain functioning and develop new skills [95]

As described in Table 14.4, NAVIGATE is made up of various team components.

The RAISE-IES study assessed the feasibility and implementation of a CSC program in "real world" circumstances [96]. This study gave rise to OnTrackNY, a CSC program similar to NAVIGATE.

The RAISE-ETP study and the RAISE-IES study demonstrate that CSC programs are cost-effective and can be successfully implemented in community settings [96–98]. RAISE participants stayed in treatment longer and had more improvement in overall symptom severity, depression, and quality of life. The duration of untreated psychosis (DUP) was shown to moderate the outcome, meaning participants with shorter DUP (less than 74 weeks) benefited more from CSC than participants with longer DUP. CSC also helped improve work and school participation and decreased rate of hospitalization and length of hospitalization stay.

CSC programs have been expanding in recent years, with NAVIGATE and OnTrackNY as examples; the Specialized Treatment Early in Psychosis (STEP) program and the Early Assessment and Support Alliance (EASA) are other examples of US CSC programs. Table 14.4 compares the components of three CSC programs, of which the authors have first-hand knowledge.

While not every area in the country has a CSC team, many do, and these can be found by looking online at tools like the Substance Abuse and Mental Health Services Administration

Table 14.4 Composition of three coordinate specialty care (CSC) teams

OnTrackNY[a]	NAVIGATE	Early Assessment and Support Alliance (EASA)[a, b]
Team leader Case manager Supported employment and education specialist Psychotherapist/primary clinician Pharmacotherapist Family education specialist Peer specialist	Team leader/family educator Pharmacotherapist Supported employment and education specialist Individual resiliency trainer (primary clinician) Case manager Peer specialist	Team leader Nurse Occupational therapist Peer support specialist Pharmacotherapist (licensed medical provider (LMP)) Service coordinator Supported employment and education specialist Supported housing specialist

[a]In smaller teams, roles may be combined and still meet program fidelity standards.

[b] In EASA, many team members may serve as multifamily group (MFG) facilitator, and insofar as possible, the team operates via a transdisciplinary model, with members offering services that may traditionally be covered by a different specialist if they are a better fit for the client or for the team at the time.

(SAMHSA) website's Early Serious Mental Illness Treatment Locator (https://www.samhsa.gov/esmi-treatment-locator). For those clinics and settings where CSC is not available, we recommend modeling the treatment, as best as possible, after high-quality CSC programs. These emphasize frequent contact, family/support network involvement that helps optimize one's living environment and promote positive social contact, individual skill-enhancing treatment, psychiatric medication treatment, and academic/employment support. It is important to keep in mind that CSC requires specialized training, which is becoming more widely available. In this chapter, we emphasize two treatment modalities that medical professionals are likely to offer transition-age youth with psychosis: pharmacotherapy and psychotherapy.

Transitional age youth with first-episode psychosis experience a wide range of emotional, psychological, interpersonal, and social stressors. The common goals of psychological interventions for FEP are to:

- Engage the individual and their support network in treatment.
- Help them understand and process the experience of psychosis.
- Bolster the person's strengths and resources and develop new coping skills to help manage symptoms and stressors.
- Identify personal goals and strengths and keep hope alive that psychotic symptoms are an imposition but that the diagnosis of psychosis is not tantamount to one needing to abandon their dreams. Romantic partnership, employment, and academic achievement are still possible and achievable.

Optimizing support for individuals with FEP can take many evidence-based forms, including individual and multifamily supportive psychotherapy groups. Psychoeducation, as well as individualized support for employment, scholastic, and interpersonal goals, are delivered by a range of professionals [99, 100]. For the sake of brevity, it is important to note that family involvement has repeatedly been shown to improve outcomes for individuals with FEP. Where the individual is comfortable with their family (or those that they consider to be part of their family) being involved, we urge making them part of the treatment.

Pharmacological Treatment: Adopting a Collaborative Stance

Studies and clinical experience show that individuals with schizophrenia or first-episode psychosis are interested in being active participants, as opposed to passive recipients of psychiatric care. They are eager to make decisions and are able to do so [101, 102] (Fig. 14.1).

Practitioners can work to understand the subjective concerns of an individual. One young person characterized this as taking an "ME before MEDS" approach to visits with their psychiatrist. It is important to be very clear about symptom targets and the potential benefits and risks of the treatments they are proposing. It is also essential to be methodical about reviewing medication efficacy while avoiding undue burden secondary to side effects. Table 14.5 offers five tips that help set the stage for collaborating with transition-age youth surrounding medication treatment.

Pharmacotherapy

Antipsychotic medications, which sometimes have been called "major tranquilizers," have their primary action in dopamine receptor blockade. There has been a movement toward neuroscience-based nomenclature to possibly lessen the stigma around psychotropic drugs and to increase their name association with underlying neuroscience (https://www.cinp.org/nomenclature, https://www.ecnp.eu/research-innovation/nomenclature). However, these medications may not only have action in dopamine antagonism as some medications have both dopamine agonist and antagonist actions, while others may also have serotonin and other neurotransmitter consequences. Regardless, this category of medications are the first-line pharmacological agents for

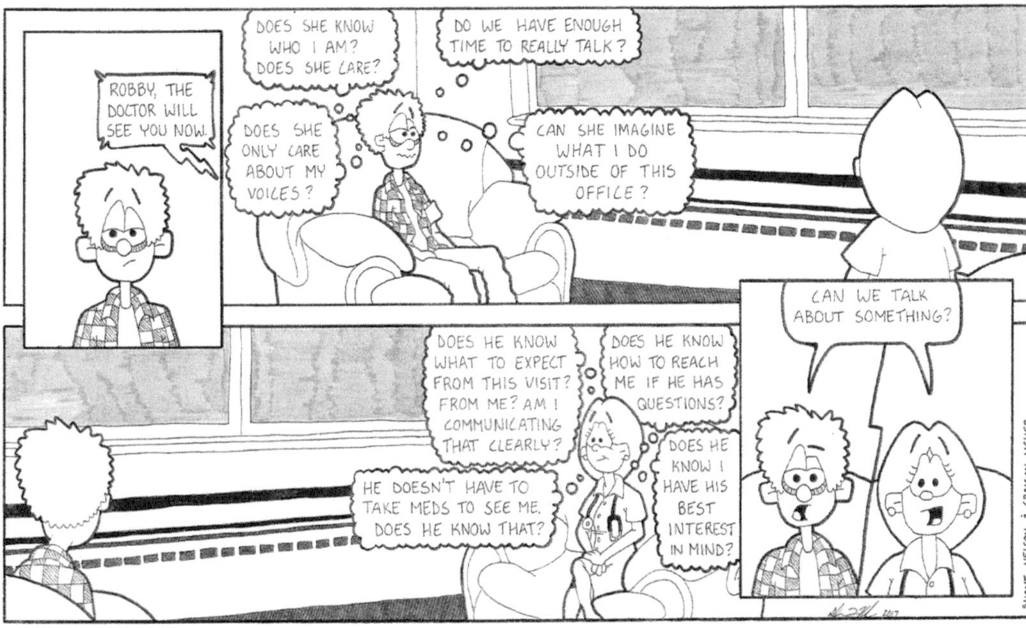
ROBBY, THE DOCTOR WILL SEE YOU NOW.
DOES SHE KNOW WHO I AM? DOES SHE CARE?
DO WE HAVE ENOUGH TIME TO REALLY TALK?
DOES SHE ONLY CARE ABOUT MY VOICES?
CAN SHE IMAGINE WHAT I DO OUTSIDE OF THIS OFFICE?
CAN WE TALK ABOUT SOMETHING?
DOES HE KNOW WHAT TO EXPECT FROM THIS VISIT? FROM ME? AM I COMMUNICATING THAT CLEARLY?
DOES HE KNOW HOW TO REACH ME IF HE HAS QUESTIONS?
HE DOESN'T HAVE TO TAKE MEDS TO SEE ME. DOES HE KNOW THAT?
DOES HE KNOW I HAVE HIS BEST INTEREST IN MIND?
SHANE NELSON & CRAIGAN USHER

Fig. 14.1 Things providers and participants need to talk about. (Art by Shane Nelson and dialog by Craigan Usher included in Conrad SK, Farris MS, Nicoli D, Ly R, Hobson K, Morenz R, Schmick E, Myers J, Smart K, Shenoy A, Usher C. Early Assessment & Support Alliance Center for Excellence (EASA C4E) medication guide. EASA Community website. December 8, 2017. Available at: http://www.easacommunity.org/PDF/easa-med-guide.pdf)

Table 14.5 Moving from a "med check" to a meaningful meeting

Learn what is important to the participant.	Repeat back what you learned for clarity. For example, "It sounds like what is most important to you is not feeling so tired. Is that right?" Make explicit when what is most important to the individual sounds or appears different from what their family members, their friends, or others feel is most important: "From what I'm hearing, it sounds like your parents are concerned about seeing you angry and frustrated. Would you say that's right?" Or "Do you agree with your parents' point of view? Is this something that you think is important to work on?"
Explicitly invite participants in decision-making.	Here is an example: "Today I would like to talk with you about medications. I would like to share with you what I know, learn what you know about medications, and then make a decision together."
Present options and provide information on benefits and risks.	Participants need to know about the full array of management strategies—writing this down can be helpful. For example, why would they want to take quetiapine instead of lurasidone? What are the benefits? What side effects might be more common with one versus the other?
Facilitate deliberation and decision-making.	Let participants know they have time to think things over and ask what else they might need to know to feel confident about their decision(s).
Develop a shared blueprint.	Executive function challenges are something nearly all of us face, but TAY with psychosis may be particularly vulnerable to these. It can be greatly helpful to write down HOW TO: Access medications (What pharmacy? How will they pay for this?) Take medications (Where will the bottle/pack sit?) Transition (titrate, taper) medications Assess if medications are working (rating scales or simple questions you will pose in the future) Consider typing this up, writing it down and making copies, or sketching this on a dry-erase board and having the participant take a picture of it with their phone.

Adapted from National Learning Consortium's Shared Decision-Making Fact Sheet. https://www.healthit.gov/sites/default/files/nlc_shared_decision_making_fact_sheet.pdf Published December 2013. Accessed on September 28, 2015 the treatment of adolescents and young adults with schizophrenia spectrum disorders, and these terms will be used interchangeably throughout this chapter. Dopamine antagonist agents are often grouped into two categories: first-generation antipsychotics (FGAs) and second-generation antipsychotics (SGAs), which differ based on when they were developed and their pharmacological properties/mechanism of action.

Although existing guidelines for psychopharmacological treatment of schizophrenia are widely used [103–105], there is a growing evidence base for pharmacological treatment specific to first-episode/early psychosis necessitating a more targeted approach [106]. Several studies looking at response rates in FEP patients show that they tend to have a high response rate [107] with minimal differences in response rates between antipsychotic medications [108–110], implying that a patient with FEP is just as likely to respond to haloperidol as they are to aripiprazole or even clozapine. More than half of FEP patients will experience complete remission of positive symptoms with their first antipsychotic trial; thus, the goal of treatment is resolution of symptoms. Although more limited, similar results are seen in studies of adolescents with early psychosis [111, 112]. Individuals with FEP also tend to need lower doses of antipsychotics than multiepisode patients [113, 114]. Additionally, those with FEP tend to take longer than multiepisode patients to respond to antipsychotic trials. Their symptoms may take up to 16 weeks to respond while not appearing to respond to early antipsychotic switching [115, 116]. This has significant implications for the existing system of care, where hospitalizations tend to be brief and medications are quickly titrated and often switched due to "poor response." Individuals with FEP are therefore at risk of ending up on high doses of antipsychotics and are thought to "fail" antipsychotic trials when in fact a more measured and watchful approach may yield a better outcome. Monotherapy is preferred, especially due to increased risk of side effects with multiple medications. FEP patients are also more sensitive to antipsychotic side effects despite low dosing strategies [108, 117, 118].

Antipsychotic medications differ with regard to the side effects they commonly produce. Therefore, the choice for the initial pharmacological agent is often driven by the side-effect profile and not concerns about efficacy since FEP patients tend to respond similarly to different dopamine blocking agents [108]. This is understandable as nearly all young adults and their families/support are eager to make sure that both the symptoms *and* side effects of treatments are short-lived. Young people with FEP are very sensitive to weight gain, and it is important to be mindful of each medication's propensity to cause it. The greatest weight gain has been associated with olanzapine and quetiapine, with aripiprazole—though still contributing to weight gain—having the most favorable profile [108, 119–123]. An additional study involving adults found that switching from olanzapine, quetiapine, or risperidone to aripiprazole can be associated with decreased low-density lipoproteins, serum triglycerides, and weight and modest reduction in the ten-year risk of coronary heart disease [124, 125]. Nonadherence to medication regimen is common and should be expected in TAY, who often have difficulty accepting that they have an illness, especially once they start feeling better. Adherence strategies include ongoing assessment of treatment adherence, communication regarding the need for maintenance and risk of relapse, engagement of the entire family in psychoeducation, and encouragement to maintain adherence.

Long-Acting Injectable Antipsychotic Medication (LAIs)

For many reasons, long-acting injectable (LAI) antipsychotic medications play an important role in the treatment of psychosis in transition-age youth [105, 126]. TAY with housing instability or those who live outdoors and wish to remain on antipsychotic treatment may find that LAIs are useful because they do not have to carry medications. College students may also prefer that their friends or roommates not know that they take medications, so they may be more comfortable to come in for an injectable agent at regular appointments. Furthermore, long-acting injectable medications may also reduce conflicts between individuals and their families, often parents, whose encouragement to take medications (e.g., "Did you take your meds?") may feel burdensome. As one patient intoned: "I found it easier to make the choice once a month opposed to having to hear about meds and make that choice every day."

Importantly, LAIs have been shown to be quite effective in terms of improving adherence and outcomes [127]. For example, Tiihonen and colleagues compared the use of LAI versus oral antipsychotics in 2588 individuals with schizophrenia who were hospitalized for the first time, which showed threefold decrease in the risk of rehospitalization in those on LAIs versus oral medications [126]. Two different 2-year studies compared LAI use with paliperidone palmitate vs oral medication, and aripiprazole monohydrate compared to usual care, with time to relapse significantly longer for patients on LAIs [128, 129]. However, it should be noted that even with LAI treatment, some individuals experience breakthrough symptoms. Thus, individuals should be warned that additional treatment, sometimes temporarily combining LAI with the same antipsychotic in oral form to achieve a higher dose or with an additional agent may be necessary [130].

Despite the excitement about LAIs, they are not for everyone. First, some settings may feel that they lack the resources to make certain that individuals can obtain their prescriptions and have a sufficiently safe place to receive their injections. For others, problems like needle phobia, insufficient trial periods of oral medications, and a history of neuroleptic malignant syndrome/catatonia spectrum disorders can make LAIs difficult to use. Finally, financial and insurance barriers or a wish for a fine-tuned taper or titration of medications may preclude the use of LAIs.

CSC programs for FEP utilize evidence-based practices in their approach to psychopharmacological management. The RAISE study demonstrated that patients enrolled in NAVIGATE and the Connection Program were more likely to be prescribed an antipsychotic conforming to FEP treatment principles, such as using lower doses and implementing longer medication trials, while being mindful of side-effect profiles and using shared decision-making in choosing medications [83, 131–133]. NAVIGATE supports using measurement-based care to obtain information about patient problems that then allows the selection of evidence-based options that are presented in shared decision-making processes [133]. In NAVIGATE, patients have their vital signs taken at each visit and complete a self-report of symptoms, side effects, adherence, substance use, and preferences about changing or keeping their current medications. Prescribing clinicians then assess symptoms and side effects guided by patient self-report, and decisions are made after providers and patients review evidence-based treatment possibilities. Patients are seen at least monthly but possibly more often if they are more symptomatic.

The NAVIGATE antipsychotic treatment algorithm is grouped into stages based on available data in FEP and the medication side effects. Table 14.6 summarizes NAVIGATE stage 1 antipsychotic recommendations.

NAVIGATE stage 2 medications include chlorpromazine, haloperidol, and olanzapine. Meanwhile, in this protocol, clozapine is reserved as a stage 3 agent for patients who have persistent positive symptoms after two antipsychotic medication trials. Incidentally, OnTrackNY employs a similar treatment approach as NAVIGATE but includes loxapine and perphenazine in its treatment algorithm for first-line medication agents, given their decreased risk to cause metabolic side effects and EPS [132] .

When prescribing for adolescents with FEP, special consideration should be given to agents that are approved by the US Food and Drug Administration (FDA), such as aripiprazole, lurasidone, olanzapine, paliperidone, quetiapine, olanzapine, quetiapine, and risperidone, while recognizing that ziprasidone and asenapine do not have FDA approval in adolescents. It should be noted that studies have shown that ziprasidone [134] and asenapine [135] were not superior to placebo for treating schizophrenia in adolescents and may not be appropriate agents to use in the treatment algorithm for schizophrenia spectrum disorders in patients under 18 years of age.

Table 14.6 Navigate stage 1 antipsychotic recommendations

Medication	Advantages	Disadvantages
Aripiprazole	Favorable metabolic profile, may have better efficacy for depression and negative symptoms, has long-acting formulations	Higher risk of akathisia
Quetiapine	Sedative effects may be useful in acute treatment	Higher risk for metabolic side effects; sedative effects may not be desirable long term
Risperidone (paliperidone if >2 week LAI)	Has the most data from first-episode studies, has fewer metabolic effects than quetiapine but more than aripiprazole, has long-acting formulations that can last up to 3 months between injections	Causes hyperprolactinemia, no direct paliperidone first-episode studies
Ziprasidone	Favorable metabolic profile	BID dosing and need to take with food can be a barrier to patient adherence

From Robinson, D, Quick Guide to Navigate Psychopharmacological Treatment. 2019

TAY with FEP may struggle with depressive symptoms during the acute course of illness, but these symptoms usually resolve with antipsychotic monotherapy as psychosis remits. If depressive symptoms are severe, or if other interventions to address the symptoms are ineffective, providers may consider initiating antidepressants. Prescribers may need to keep in mind that no guidelines for initiating antidepressants in FEP are available. In the RAISE-ETP study, continuous use of antipsychotic medications during the two years of study was recommended. Patients and families often wonder about the length of treatment and when discontinuation of antipsychotics should take place. There are limited data to guide discontinuation, and studies show that discontinuation during the first few years of illness increases risk of relapse [136–138]. There are some data, although limited, that suggest that some people do not relapse after medication discontinuation [139]. However, until there is a way to identify those individuals who can safely discontinue medication, the best strategy may be to continue prescribing maintenance dopamine antagonist agents at the lowest effective dose.

Minimizing Side Effects

It is very important to establish the comprehensive treatment goals at the outset of treatment outlined in Table 14.6 and to relate and assess pharmacotherapy's role in helping or hindering those goals. This means assessing symptoms and reviewing side effects. While many health systems have electronic medical records with automatic alerts prompting clinicians to check for side effects, many clinics do not enjoy this luxury. Practitioners who prescribe antipsychotic medications for youth need to check necessary vital signs (height, weight, body mass index (BMI)) at every visit. They also must complete fasting labs, including blood glucose and a lipid profile at regular interviews: pretreatment, at the 3-month mark, at the 6-month mark, and at 1-year posttreatment initiation. Where indicated, we also recommend obtaining electrocardiograms prior to treatment and after the treatment is initiated. This includes situations in which ziprasidone is prescribed and where patients have an underlying heart condition that would place them at increased risk for complications with prolonged repolarization. Clinicians should systematically screen for extrapyramidal symptoms (EPS), including acute dystonia, akathisia, parkinsonism, and tardive dyskinesia (TD). The management of EPS will be discussed further in the chapter.

As previously stated, patients treated with antipsychotic medications, especially SGAs, are at an increased risk for weight gain, and multiple strategies have been suggested for the management of SGA-induced weight gain and metabolic derangement. While a discussion of this is worthy of its own book chapter, we can simply write that there is evidence that multimodal treatment, including education around nutrition and helping young people think about ways that they can keep their bodies moving, is key [140–143]. Terms like "exercise" or "diet" or making broad "boiler plate" recommendations are not helpful. These recommendations often have the quality of making the practitioner feel better and the patient worse and result in few, if any, changes. Instead, it is important to take a genuine interest in an individual's lifestyle, drilling down on the specifics of how one moves their body or does not. Providers should explore with patients the opportunities they have to be active in safe situations. Similarly, writing a nutrition journal with a patient and taking a non-shaming stance as one inquires about nutrition choices and food security is crucial. There is evidence for the use of metformin in mitigating antipsychotic-related weight gain [144, 145] and dyslipidemia [146] in adults and weight gain in adolescents [147]. Table 14.7 presents some general guidelines on commonly used SGAs.

Table 14.7 Second-generation antipsychotic medications (SGAs)

Generic Name	Brand Name	Long acting formulation	FDA approved for adolescents	Sedation	Weight gain	Notes
Aripiprazole	Abilify Abilify Maintena	Yes 4 weeks	Yes (13–17 y/o)	+	+	Can be activating
Asenapine	Saphris	No	No	+++	+++	Tablet "melts" in the mouth May not eat or drink for 10 minutes after taking
Brexpiprazole	Rexulti	No	No	?	+++?	Serotonin and dopamine receptor modulator
Iloperidone	Fanapt	No	No	+++	+++	
Lurasidone	Latuda	No	Yes (13–17 y/o)	+++	Short term: +++ Long term: +	Must be taken with food (min 350 calories)
Olanzapine	Zyprexa	No	Yes (13–17 y/o)	++++	++++	
Paliperidone	Invega Invega Sustena Invega Trinza	Yes 4 weeks 3 months	Yes (13–17 y/o)	+++	+++	Active metabolite of risperidone
Quetiapine	Seroquel	No	Yes (13–17 y/o)	++++	+++	Sedation dose dependent Check thyrotropin and free T4 at baseline and follow-up Eye exam at baseline and at 6 months
Risperidone	Risperdal Risperdal Consta	Yes 2 weeks	Yes (13–17 y/o)	+++	+++	High risk for elevated prolactin (obtain level if symptomatic)
Ziprasidone	Geodon	No	No	++	+	Must be taken with food (min 350 calories) Obtain ECG at baseline, during titration, and at maximum dose
Clozapine	Clozaril	No	No	++++	++++	Proven to reduce suicides in schizophrenia Drooling can be an issue Obtain ECG at baseline Associated with orthostatic hypotension, tachycardia, myocarditis, and cardiomyopathy

Adapted and revised, from Conrad SK, Farris MS, Nicoli D, Ly R, Hobson K, Morenz R, Schmick E, Myers J, Smart K, Shenoy A, Usher C. Early Assessment & Support Alliance Center for Excellence (EASA C4E) medication guide. EASA Community website. December 8, 2017. Available at: http://www.easacommunity.org/PDF/easa-med-guide.pdf

Table 14.8 First-generation antipsychotics (FGAs)

Drug name	Brand Name (all ®)	Long-acting injectable	FDA approval for adolescents	Sedation	Weight gain	Notes
Chlorpromazine	Thorazine	No	No	++++	+++	Excellent for short-term use, but risk of TD can limit long-term use
Fluphenazine	Prolixin Prolixin Decanoate	Yes 2 weeks	No	++	++	Less sedation and orthostatic hypotension but more EPS risk
Haloperidol	Haldol Haldol Decanoate	Yes 4 weeks	Yes (3–17 y/o)	++	++	Can be used for tic disorders
Loxapine	Loxitane	No	No	+++	+	
Perphenazine	Trilafon	No	Yes (12–17 y/o)	+++	+++	
Thioridazine	Mellaril	No	Yes	+++	+++	Very limited availability Associated with prolonged QTc
Thiothixene	Navane	No	Yes (12–17 y/o)	++	+	
Trifluoperazine	Stelazine	No	Yes (6–12 y/o)	+++	+	

Adapted and revised from Conrad SK, Farris MS, Nicoli D, Ly R, Hobson K, Morenz R, Schmick E, Myers J, Smart K, Shenoy A, Usher C. Early Assessment & Support Alliance Center for Excellence (EASA C4E) medication guide. EASA Community website. December 8, 2017. Available at: http://www.easacommunity.org/PDF/easa-med-guide.pdf

While SGAs are more prone to be associated with cardiometabolic side effects, first-generation antipsychotic medications have been more commonly associated with EPS compared to SGAs in the treatment of first-episode psychosis [148]. Table 14.8 organizes prescribing information on commonly used FGAs.

All patients who are started on antipsychotic agents should be evaluated for extrapyramidal symptoms weekly, until the medication dose has not been increased for at least 2 weeks. After dose stabilization, the frequency for EPS evaluation should depend on the side-effect profile of each antipsychotic medication and the patient's vulnerability. For monitoring, clinicians can use the Abnormal Involuntary Movement Scale (AIMS) [149], the Neurological Rating Scale [150], or the Barnes Akathisia Scale [151], and can rely on direct observation and obtain a detailed history about extrapyramidal symptoms.

Acute dystonia is a sustained involuntary muscle spasm or abnormal posture (particularly in the head and neck) that typically occurs shortly after starting treatment with an antipsychotic agent. It can occur shortly after increasing the dosage of medication, as well as anytime during the course of treatment. It may be more common in young patients and with higher medication dosages and typically ends with discontinuation of the offending agent. Dystonia can be treated with an anticholinergic medication such as diphenhydramine or benztropine [152].

Akathisia is the most common movement disorder side effect. It usually occurs hours to days after starting the dopamine-blocking agents but can happen at any time. Akathisia usually presents with increased psychomotor activity, restlessness, and inability to sit still. It may also present as a subjective intense feeling of restlessness. Akathisia can be managed by cautiously lowering the dose or switching to another agent. There is also evidence for the use of beta blockers, benzodiazepines, and benztropine [153, 154].

Parkinsonism (i.e., any condition that causes movement problems similar to those seen in Parkinson's disease) can present with tremor, muscle rigidity, bradykinesia, or difficulty with walking. These symptoms generally occur two weeks to one month after starting an antipsychotic or increasing the dose but can happen at any time during treatment and usually stops with discontinuation of the offending agent. Treatment of parkinsonism includes lowering the dose of the antipsychotic, switching to an SGA or one less often associated with EPS, or using other medications to specifically treat these side effects [155, 156]. Medications commonly used to treat parkinsonism include benztropine, trihexyphenidyl, and amantadine [157, 158].

Tardive dyskinesia is an involuntary repetitive movement that typically occurs a few months after receiving antipsychotic treatment and will persist at least after a month after discontinuation of the offending agent [1]. These movements usually involve the tongue, lower face, and jaw but can also involve the torso or the respiratory muscles. Risk factors include older age, longer duration of treatment [159], and developing EPS at early stages of treatment with antipsychotic medications [160]. Despite these risk factors and common presentation, TD can be seen in TAY. The treatment of tardive dyskinesia is complex, and therefore the emphasis is on early detection and frequent monitoring. Treatment strategies may include reducing the dose or switching from first-generation antipsychotic agents to second generation, in particular clozapine or quetiapine [161]. Valbenazine is an FDA-approved [162] agent for the treatment of tardive dyskinesia in adults and showed efficacy in short-term treatment [163, 164]. There is limited evidence for the use of benzodiazepines [165], tetrabenazine, or botulinum toxin injections [166], but these choices should be considered if clinically appropriate.

No discussion of antipsychotic treatment is complete without mentioning clozapine. Clozapine has shown superior efficacy, compared to the other antipsychotics, for both adults and adolescents [121, 138, 166]. However, due to the risk of agranulocytosis and the need for frequent blood draws and monitoring, lowering of the seizure threshold, myocarditis, and weight gain associated with clozapine treatment, this is not the first-line treatment for first-episode psychosis and is usually reserved for treatment-resistant patients.

Psychotherapeutic Interventions

Optimizing support for individuals with FEP can take many evidence-based forms, including individual and multifamily supportive psychotherapy groups. Psychoeducation, as well as individualized support for employment, scholastic, and interpersonal goals [99], is delivered by a range of professionals. Briefly, it is important to note that family involvement has repeatedly been shown to improve outcomes for individuals with FEP [100]. When TAY are comfortable with their family (or those that they consider to be part of their family) being involved, it is ideal that they are part of the treatment.

The multi-family group (MFG) with psychoeducation model was developed by McFarland and colleagues in Portland, Maine. Many programs including Oregon's CSC teams, the Early Assessment and Support Alliance (EASA) utilize this model as a therapeutic intervention [167]. In these groups, multiple families (which includes anyone the client identifies as "family" or members of their support network) and clients (who have the choice to participate or opt out) join with two trained facilitators for problem-solving-focused sessions. The typical format of MFGs involves some time for socializing, then going around the room and reviewing the week's events and reviewing how families utilized "Family Guidelines" to either de-escalate tensions or anticipate and manage problems. These guidelines are posted in the meeting space and contain practical maxims like "keep it cool" or encouragement to "suspend expectations, temporarily." In the review, usually families or individuals bring up problems to be solved, and then the group, together, decides which of these to address that week. The group then spends at least 45 minutes defining the problem, generating possible solutions/management strategies, and weighing the pros and cons of each of these approaches. The family/individual then chooses which of these strategies they would like to employ over the next 2 weeks, and they determine who is responsible for implementing the various aspects of their preferred solution. The family/individual then returns to the next MFG for a report on how things went and if the strategy was useful. Thus, the entire multifamily group contributes to and learns from the process. The MFG format may be adapted for work with individual families and for clinicians/families working outside of CSCs.

While many individual psychotherapeutic approaches have been studied for addressing FEP, the most well-studied psychotherapeutic approach and the anchoring treatment from which many other modified approaches are derived is cognitive behavioral therapy (CBT) [88]. CBT for psychosis (abbreviated CBTp) has been shown to effectively reduce positive and negative symptoms [168] with effect sizes reported between 0.40 and 0.65 [169, 170]. CBTp has also been shown to impact overall functioning, mood, and social anxiety, and it can be modified for individual, family, and group treatment [171, 172].

As informed by Brabban and colleagues, the fundamental principles of CBTp include the following: (1) collaborating on a formulation that helps inform how and where psychotic symptoms arise and are maintained, (2) normalizing the psychotic experience as an extension/hyperactive extension of human experiences, and (3) accepting psychotic symptoms as information/sensory input that one is receiving that one does not necessarily need to act upon. For example, one can resist acting in accordance with a command auditory hallucination or, in opposition to a symptom, attempting to get rid of it [173]. In this way, CBTp may be a powerful adjunct to pharmacotherapy as one may experience medications as a means of turning the volume down on signals/symptoms that one may be receiving, allowing them to accept their presence without needing to take drastic symptom-syntonic or -dystonic action.

As with all forms of psychotherapy, developing a strong therapeutic rapport and working alliance is key. This is particularly essential in CBTp, where due to one's psychosis and the jarring, traumatic nature of urgent treatment (including emergency department visits and hospitalizations), trusting others may be very difficult. Again, since this may be due to paranoia, a potential history of trauma, and/or an individual's traumatic experiences of coercive emergency treatment prior to engaging in outpatient work, taking a slow history and growing to understand the individual's subjective experience are key. Practitioners utilizing CBTp are encouraged to proceed very slowly, making certain that there is a strong working alliance before moving to the next phase of treatment.

In the second phase of treatment, the CBTp therapist sits with their chair alongside or at a 45-degree angle to the patient and looks out of the window wondering how the individual experiences the world and how they put together their understanding. At this point, CBTp therapists adopt a very neutral stance, potentially sharing some of what they see happening in the world but not challenging the patient's view. In the third phase of CBTp, therapists work with individuals to link how the experiences or events in a person's life are interpreted and how this interpretation links to thoughts, feelings, and actions. At this phase, the therapist may encourage the individual to examine how certain actions and behaviors may be adaptive or maladaptive.

In the fourth phase of CBTp, the formulation is put into action, introducing new coping skills that address some of the concerns outlined. For example, each time a college student with FEP went to class, he found himself panicking because he felt everyone was reading his thoughts. This led him to leave class early, or avoid class completely. This young man then found his grades dropping. In therapy, he shared that he still believed that, even when he was not present for the class, others could read his thoughts. In response, this student worked with his therapist to outline the pros and cons of attending class and on some adaptive coping strategies. The student reasoned that because he suspected that no matter what he did he would sense that people were reading his thoughts, it was better that he attend class because that way he took notes and got credit for attending. Further, the student worked to arrive early and get a seat in the back so he could monitor others and not have people sitting behind him. To do so, he had to set reminders on his smartphone to get to class on time.

While CBTp as articulated in traditional manuals and literature certainly contains some of the classic evaluation of evidence for and against a cognitive distortion or delusion, contemporary CBTp very much focuses on the extent to which one's relationship to a given symptom is working for them [174]. CBTp is an attempt not to correct (or coerce) beliefs but to help individuals function more adaptively and flexibly.

Suicide Risk, Thinking About Support, and Relapse Response

While the precise rate of suicide in schizophrenia spectrum disorders has been disputed, the literature is clear that the riskiest period for suicide attempts is in the year following a first episode, and all-cause mortality in individuals 16–30 years old is as high [175] as 24 times that of same-age peers [176]. Vigilance around suicide is extremely important. Tools such as the Columbia Suicide Severity Rating Scale may be useful in systematically assessing suicide risk [177]. In addition to standard assessments of suicide, within the emerging adult early psychosis population, we recommend inquiring about a history of suicide attempts and rehearsing suicide or suicidal gestures. Further, clinicians should assess one's sense of being a burden to others, an individual's sense of belonging or not belonging, access or lack thereof to supportive people, and future-orientation versus hopelessness. A family history of suicide and connection to friends and peers or identification with famous figures (artists, musicians, actors, athletes) who died by suicide should also be assessed. One of the most common problems identified in chart reviews of suicide risk assessment in FEP is the failure to document how, based on the information gathered in such assessments, the clinician(s); supports for the client/patient, including friends/family; and the individual will alter their approach. Developing a comprehensive plan to address risk factors and lethal-means reduction as part of early treatment planning is key.

The term "relapse" with regard to FEP is fraught as in the lay use of the term there is the implication that relapse is something one chooses. Further, while studies generally demonstrate a response to treatment, this can sometimes fall short of something one might, themselves, consider remission. For example, in a study by Phahladira and colleagues that followed 98 individuals with FEP over two years, 70% of the individuals achieved symptom remission, yet less than half that number [29] met the criteria for a complete, functional recovery [178]. It may be offensive to many individuals, who subjectively do not feel their symptoms are sufficiently addressed or their functioning adequately restored or who may not experience their symptoms as problematic, to hear language of remission and recovery. Thus, care should be taken when talking to individuals and families about the relapse of symptoms following stabilization of a first episode of psychosis. Using phrases like "the return of symptoms" or "a period of worsening" can be helpful. Still, in medical vernacular, relapses are common in FEP, and preparing for them is an important part of empowering young people. The core components of a relapse prevention and contingency plan include identifying events or situations that triggered or signaled previous episodes and a list of early warning signs that one is at risk for the exacerbation of underlying symptoms. It is also important to determine what the patient thinks might be helpful should such a thing occur, who the individual believes would be helpful, and who they can reach out to (and how) in an emergency.

Conclusion

Transition-age youth with first-episode psychosis experience a wide range of emotional, psychological, interpersonal, and social stressors. The common goals of interventions for FEP are to (1) engage the individual and their support network in treatment, (2) help them understand and process the experience of psychosis, (3) facilitate drawing on the person's strengths and resources and developing new coping skills to help manage symptoms and stressors, and (4) identify personal goals and strengths and keep hope alive that psychotic symptoms are an imposition but that the diagnosis of psychosis is not tantamount to one needing to abandon their dreams. Romantic partnership, employment, and academic achievement are still possible. CSC programs have been designed to achieve these goals by (1) providing support and psychoeducation to individuals and their support network, (2) reducing the impact of symptoms by pharmacotherapy, (3) decreasing symptoms burden and impact on social aspects of life by psychotherapy and family interventions, (4) providing vocational services to support education and employment, and (5) providing case management and peer support to help with problem-solving and advocacy.

References

1. American Psychiatric Association. Diagnostic and Statistical Manual of Mental Disorders, Fifth Edition (DSM-5), American Psychiatric Association, Arlington, VA 2013.
2. de Pablo GS, Catalan A, Fusar-Poli P. Clinical validity of DSM-5 attenuated psychosis syndrome: advances in diagnosis, prognosis, and treatment. JAMA Psychiatry. 2020;77(3):311–20.
3. Fusar-Poli P. The Clinical High-Risk State for Psychosis (CHR-P), Version II. Schizophr Bull. 2017;43(1):44–47.
4. Wang EW. The collected schizophrenias: essays. Minneapolis: Graywolf Press; 2019.
5. Saha S, Chant D, Welham J, McGrath J. A systematic review of the prevalence of schizophrenia. PLoS Med. 2005;2(5):e141.
6. McGrath J, Saha S, Chant D, Welham J. Schizophrenia: a concise overview of incidence, prevalence, and mortality. Epidemiol Rev. 2008;30:67–76.
7. Perälä J, Suvisaari J, Saarni SI, Kuoppasalmi K, Isometsä E, Pirkola S, et al. Lifetime prevalence of psychotic and bipolar I disorders in a general population. Arch Gen Psychiatry. 2007;64(1):19–28.
8. Kahn RS, Sommer IE, Murray RM, Meyer-Lindenberg A, Weinberger DR, Cannon TD, et al. Schizophrenia. Nat Rev Dis Primers. 2015;1:15067.
9. Rapoport J, Giedd J, Gogtay N. Neurodevelopmental model of schizophrenia: update 2012. Mol Psychiatry. 2012;17(12):1228–38.
10. Lieberman JA, Small SA, Girgis RR. Early detection and preventive intervention in schizophrenia: from fantasy to reality. Am J Psychiatry. 2019;176(10):794–810.
11. Gejman PV, Sanders AR, Duan J. The role of genetics in the etiology of schizophrenia. Psychiatric Clinics. 2010;33(1):35–66.
12. Cross-Disorder Group of the Psychiatric Genomics Consortium. Identification of risk loci with shared effects on five major psychiatric disorders: a genome-wide analysis. Lancet. 2013;381(9875):1371–9.
13. Lichtenstein P, Yip BH, Björk C, Pawitan Y, Cannon TD, Sullivan PF, et al. Common genetic determinants of schizophrenia and bipolar disorder in Swedish families: a population-based study. Lancet. 2009;373(9659):234–9.
14. Arendt M, Mortensen PB, Rosenberg R, Pedersen CB, Waltoft BL. Familial predisposition for psychiatric disorder: comparison of subjects treated for cannabis-induced psychosis and schizophrenia. Arch Gen Psychiatry. 2008;65(11):1269–74.
15. Procopio M. Paternal age and schizophrenia: one swallow does not make a summer. BMJ. 2005;330(7483):147–8; author reply 8
16. Dealberto MJ. Ethnic origin and increased risk for schizophrenia in immigrants to countries of recent and longstanding immigration. Acta Psychiatr Scand. 2010;121(5):325–39.
17. Hollander AC, Dal H, Lewis G, Magnusson C, Kirkbride JB, Dalman C. Refugee migration and risk of schizophrenia and other non-affective psychoses: cohort study of 1.3 million people in Sweden. BMJ. 2016;352:i1030.
18. Sørensen HJ, Mortensen EL, Reinisch JM, Mednick SA. Association between prenatal exposure to analgesics and risk of schizophrenia. Br J Psychiatry. 2004;185:366–71.
19. Insel BJ, Schaefer CA, McKeague IW, Susser ES, Brown AS. Maternal iron deficiency and the risk of schizophrenia in offspring. Arch Gen Psychiatry. 2008;65(10):1136–44.
20. Khashan AS, Abel KM, McNamee R, Pedersen MG, Webb RT, Baker PN, et al. Higher risk of offspring schizophrenia following antenatal maternal exposure to severe adverse life events. Arch Gen Psychiatry. 2008;65(2):146–52.
21. Sevy S, Robinson DG, Holloway S, Alvir JM, Woerner MG, Bilder R, et al. Correlates of substance misuse in patients with first-episode schizophrenia and schizoaffective disorder. Acta Psychiatr Scand. 2001;104(5):367–74.
22. Bühler B, Hambrecht M, Löffler W, an der Heiden W, Häfner H. Precipitation and determination of the onset and course of schizophrenia by substance abuse–a retrospective and prospective study of 232 population-based first illness episodes. Schizophr Res. 2002;54(3):243–51.
23. Mauri M, Volonteri LS, De Gaspari IF, Colasanti A, Brambilla MA, Cerruti L, et al. Substance abuse in first-episode schizophrenic patients: a retrospective study. Clin Pract Epidemiol Ment Health. 2006;2(1):1–8.
24. Cantwell R, Brewin J, Glazebrook C, Dalkin T, Fox R, Medley I, et al. Prevalence of substance misuse in first-episode psychosis. Br J Psychiatry. 1999;174:150–3.
25. Mueser KT, Yarnold PR, Levinson DF, Singh H, Bellack AS, Kee K, et al. Prevalence of substance abuse in schizophrenia: demographic and clinical correlates. Schizophr Bull. 1990;16(1):31–56.
26. Mueser KT, Yarnold P, Bellack AS. Diagnostic and demographic correlates of substance abuse in schizophrenia and major affective disorder. Acta Psychiatr Scand. 1992;85(1):48–55.

27. Allebeck P, Adamsson C, Engström A. Cannabis and schizophrenia: a longitudinal study of cases treated in Stockholm County. Acta Psychiatr Scand. 1993;88(1):21–4.
28. Rabinowitz J, Bromet E, Lavelle J, Carlson G, Kovasznay B, Schwartz JJ. Prevalence and severity of substance use disorders and onset of psychosis in first-admission psychotic patients. Psychol Med. 1998;28(6):1411–9.
29. Hambrecht M, Häfner H. Substance abuse and the onset of schizophrenia. Biol Psychiatry. 1996;40(11):1155–63.
30. Kuepper R, van Os J, Lieb R, Wittchen HU, Höfler M, Henquet C. Continued cannabis use and risk of incidence and persistence of psychotic symptoms: 10 year follow-up cohort study. BMJ. 2011;342:d738.
31. Large M, Sharma S, Compton MT, Slade T, Nielssen O. Cannabis use and earlier onset of psychosis: a systematic meta-analysis. Arch Gen Psychiatry. 2011;68(6):555–61.
32. Gage SH, Hickman M, Zammit S. Association between cannabis and psychosis: epidemiologic evidence. Biol Psychiatry. 2016;79(7):549–56.
33. McClellan J. Psychosis in children and adolescents. J Am Acad Child Adolesc Psychiatry. 2018;57(5):308–12.
34. Sikich L. Diagnosis and evaluation of hallucinations and other psychotic symptoms in children and adolescents. Child Adolesc Psychiatr Clin N Am. 2013;22(4):655–73.
35. Birnbaum ML, Wan CR, Broussard B, Compton MT. Associations between duration of untreated psychosis and domains of positive and negative symptoms. Early Interv Psychiatry. 2017;11(5):375–82.
36. Maijer K, Hayward M, Fernyhough C, Calkins ME, Debbané M, Jardri R, et al. Hallucinations in children and adolescents: an updated review and practical recommendations for clinicians. Schizophr Bull. 2019;45(45 Suppl 1):S5–s23.
37. McClellan J. Clinically relevant phenomenology: the nature of psychosis. J Am Acad Child Adolesc Psychiatry. 2011;50(7):642–4.
38. Loberg EM, Gjestad R, Posserud MB, Kompus K, Lundervold AJ. Psychosocial characteristics differentiate non-distressing and distressing voices in 10,346 adolescents. Eur Child Adolesc Psychiatry. 2019;28:1353.
39. Masi G, Mucci M, Pari C. Children with schizophrenia: clinical picture and pharmacological treatment. CNS Drugs. 2006;20(10):841–66.
40. Jardri R, Bartels-Velthuis AA, Debbane M, Jenner JA, Kelleher I, Dauvilliers Y, et al. From phenomenology to neurophysiological understanding of hallucinations in children and adolescents. Schizophrenia bulletin. 2014;40(Suppl 4):S221–32.
41. Stentebjerg-Olesen M, Pagsberg AK, Fink-Jensen A, Correll CU, Jeppesen P. Clinical characteristics and predictors of outcome of schizophrenia-spectrum psychosis in children and adolescents: a systematic review. J Child Adolesc Psychopharmacol. 2016;26(5):410–27.
42. McClellan J, Stock S, American Academy of C, Adolescent Psychiatry Committee on Quality I. Practice parameter for the assessment and treatment of children and adolescents with schizophrenia. J Am Acad Child Adolesc Psychiatry. 2013;52(9):976–90.
43. Kelleher I, Cannon M. SOCRATES Assessment of Perceptual Abnormalities and Unusual Thought Content. Royal College of Surgeons in Ireland, 2014. Available from: https://repository.rcsi.com/articles/preprint/SOCRATES_Assessment_of_Perceptual_Abnormalities_and_Unusual_Thought_Content/10795397.
44. Russell AT. The clinical presentation of childhood-onset schizophrenia. Schizophrenia bulletin. 1994;20(4):631–46.
45. Hafner H, Maurer K, Loffler W, Riecher-Rossler A. The influence of age and sex on the onset and early course of schizophrenia. Br J Psychiatry. 1993;162:80–6.
46. Rajapakse T, Garcia-Rosales A, Weerawardene S, Cotton S, Fraser R. Themes of delusions and hallucinations in first-episode psychosis. Early Interv Psychiatry. 2011;5(3):254–8.
47. Ayer A, Yalincetin B, Aydinli E, Sevilmis S, Ulas H, Binbay T, et al. Formal thought disorder in first-episode psychosis. Compr Psychiatry. 2016;70:209–15.
48. Chan V. Schizophrenia and psychosis: diagnosis, current research trends, and model treatment approaches with implications for transitional age youth. Child Adolesc Psychiatr Clin N Am. 2017;26(2):341–66.
49. Addington J, Liu L, Perkins DO, Carrion RE, Keefe RS, Woods SW. The role of cognition and social functioning as predictors in the transition to psychosis for youth with attenuated psychotic symptoms. Schizophr Bull. 2017;43(1):57–63.
50. Devoe DJ, Farris MS, Townes P, Addington J. Interventions and social functioning in youth at risk of psychosis: a systematic review and meta-analysis. Early Interv Psychiatry. 2019;13(2):169–80.
51. Rowland TA, Marwaha S. Epidemiology and risk factors for bipolar disorder. Ther Adv Psychopharmacol. 2018;8(9):251–69.
52. Werry JS, McClellan JM, Chard L. Childhood and adolescent schizophrenic, bipolar, and schizoaffective disorders: a clinical and outcome study. J Am Acad Child Adolesc Psychiatry. 1991;30(3):457–65.
53. Fulford D, Niendam TA, Floyd EG, Carter CS, Mathalon DH, Vinogradov S, et al. Symptom dimensions and functional impairment in early psychosis: more to the story than just negative symptoms. Schizophr Res. 2013;147(1):125–31.
54. Baytunca B, Kalyoncu T, Ozel I, Erermis S, Kayahan B, Ongur D. Early onset schizophrenia associated with obsessive-compulsive disorder: clinical

features and correlates. Clin Neuropharmacol. 2017;40(6):243–5.
55. Poyurovsky M, Faragian S, Shabeta A, Kosov A. Comparison of clinical characteristics, comorbidity and pharmacotherapy in adolescent schizophrenia patients with and without obsessive-compulsive disorder. Psychiatry Res. 2008;159(1-2):133–9.
56. Levy E, Traicu A, Iyer S, Malla A, Joober R. Psychotic disorders comorbid with attention-deficit hyperactivity disorder: an important knowledge gap. Can J Psychiatry. 2015;60(3 Suppl 2):S48–52.
57. Sevilla-Llewellyn-Jones J, Camino G, Russo DA, Painter M, Montejo AL, Ochoa S, et al. Clinically significant personality traits in individuals at high risk of developing psychosis. Psychiatry Res. 2018;261:498–503.
58. Bedwell JS, Donnelly RS. Schizotypal personality disorder or prodromal symptoms of schizophrenia? Schizophr Res. 2005;80(2-3):263–9.
59. Algon S, Yi J, Calkins ME, Kohler C, Borgmann-Winter KE. Evaluation and treatment of children and adolescents with psychotic symptoms. Curr Psychiatry Rep. 2012;14(2):101–10.
60. Loewy RL, Pearson R, Vinogradov S, Bearden CE, Cannon TD. Psychosis risk screening with the Prodromal Questionnaire–brief version (PQ-B). Schizophr Res. 2011;129(1):42–6.
61. Brodey BB, Addington J, First MB, Perkins DO, Woods SW, Walker EF, et al. The Early Psychosis Screener (EPS): item development and qualitative validation. Schizophr Res. 2018;197:504–8.
62. Brodey BB, Girgis RR, Favorov OV, Bearden CE, Woods SW, Addington J, et al. The Early Psychosis Screener for Internet (EPSI)-SR: predicting 12 month psychotic conversion using machine learning. Schizophr Res. 2019;208:390–6.
63. Miller TJ, Cicchetti D, Markovich PJ, Woods S. The SIPS Screen: a brief self-report screen to detect the schizophrenia prodrome. Schizophr Res. 2004;70(1):78.
64. Fonseca-Pedrero E, Ortuño-Sierra J, Chocarro E, Inchausti F, Debbané M, Bobes J. Psychosis risk screening: Validation of the youth psychosis at-risk questionnaire – brief in a community-derived sample of adolescents. Int J Methods Psychiatr Res. 2017;26(4):e1543.
65. Miller TJ, McGlashan TH, Rosen JL, Cadenhead K, Cannon T, Ventura J, et al. Prodromal assessment with the structured interview for prodromal syndromes and the scale of prodromal symptoms: predictive validity, interrater reliability, and training to reliability. Schizophr Bull. 2003;29(4):703–15.
66. Yung AR, Yuen HP, McGorry PD, Phillips LJ, Kelly D, Dell'Olio M, et al. Mapping the onset of psychosis: the Comprehensive Assessment of At-Risk Mental States. Aust N Z J Psychiatry. 2005;39(11-12):964–71.
67. Tsuji T, Phalen P, Rakhshan Rouhakhtar P, Millman Z, Bussell K, Thompson E, et al. Using the K-SADS psychosis screen to identify people with early psychosis or psychosis risk syndromes. Clin Child Psychol Psychiatry. 2019;24(4):809–20.
68. Overall JE, Gorham DR. The brief psychiatric rating scale. Psychiatry Res. 1962;10(3):799–812.
69. Kay SR, Fiszbein A, Opler LA. The positive and negative syndrome scale (PANSS) for schizophrenia. Schizophr Bull. 1987;13(2):261–76.
70. Larson MK, Walker EF, Compton MT. Early signs, diagnosis and therapeutics of the prodromal phase of schizophrenia and related psychotic disorders. Expert Rev Neurother. 2010;10(8):1347–59.
71. Demjaha A, Lappin JM, Stahl D, Patel MX, MacCabe JH, Howes OD, et al. Antipsychotic treatment resistance in first-episode psychosis: prevalence, subtypes and predictors. Psychol Med. 2017;47(11):1981–9.
72. Parellada M, Castro-Fornieles J, Gonzalez-Pinto A, Pina-Camacho L, Moreno D, Rapado-Castro M, et al. Predictors of functional and clinical outcome in early-onset first-episode psychosis: the child and adolescent first episode of psychosis (CAFEPS) study. J Clin Psychiatry. 2015;76(11):e1441–8.
73. Clemmensen L, Vernal DL, Steinhausen HC. A systematic review of the long-term outcome of early onset schizophrenia. BMC Psychiatry. 2012;12:150.
74. Boychuk C, Lysaght R, Stuart H. Career decision-making processes of young adults with first-episode psychosis. Qual Health Res. 2018;28(6):1016–31.
75. Salinger JM, O'Brien MP, Miklowitz DJ, Marvin SE, Cannon TD. Family communication with teens at clinical high-risk for psychosis or bipolar disorder. J Fam Psychol. 2018;32(4):507–16.
76. Heinssen RK, Goldstein AB, Azrin ST. Evidence-based treatments for first episode psychosis: components of coordinated specialty care.: National Institute of Mental Health; 2014 [Retrieved July 12, 2020]. Available from: https://www.nimh.nih.gov/health/topics/schizophrenia/raise/evidence-based-treatments-for-first-episode-psychosis-components-of-coordinated-specialty-care.shtml.
77. Drapalski AL, Piscitelli S, Lee RJ, Medoff D, Dixon LB. Family involvement in the clinical care of clients with first-episode psychosis in the RAISE connection program. Psychiatr Serv. 2018;69(3):358–61.
78. Pencer A, Addington J, Addington D. Outcome of a first episode of psychosis in adolescence: a 2-year follow-up. Psychiatry Res. 2005;133(1):35–43.
79. Gill KE, Quintero JM, Poe SL, Moreira AD, Brucato G, Corcoran CM, et al. Assessing suicidal ideation in individuals at clinical high risk for psychosis. Schizophr Res. 2015;165(2-3):152–6.
80. D'Angelo EJ, Lincoln SH, Morelli N, Graber K, Tembulkar S, Gonzalez-Heydrich J. Suicidal behaviors and their relationship with psychotic-like symptoms in children and adolescents at clinical high risk for psychosis. Compr Psychiatry. 2017;78:31–7.

81. Falcone T, Timmons-Mitchell J. Psychosis and suicidality in adolescents. Psychiatr Times. 2013;30(12):20.
82. Taylor PJ, Hutton P, Wood L. Are people at risk of psychosis also at risk of suicide and self-harm? A systematic review and meta-analysis. Psychol Med. 2015;45(5):911–26.
83. Kane JM, Robinson DG, Schooler NR, Mueser KT, Penn DL, Rosenheck RA, et al. Comprehensive versus usual community care for first-episode psychosis: 2-year outcomes from the NIMH RAISE early treatment program. Am J Psychiatry. 2016;173(4):362–72.
84. APA Practice Guideline for the Treatment of Patients with Schizophrenia.: American Psychiatric Association; 2019. Available from: https://www.psychiatry.org/psychiatrists/practice/clinical-practice-guidelines.
85. Psychosis and schizophrenia in adults: treatment and management. London: National Institute for Health and Clinical Excellence; 2014. Available from: https://www.nice.org.uk/guidance/cg178/evidence/full-guideline-490503565.
86. Perkins DO, Gu H, Boteva K, Lieberman JA. Relationship between duration of untreated psychosis and outcome in first-episode schizophrenia: a critical review and meta-analysis. Am J Psychiatry. 2005;162(10):1785–804.
87. Loebel AD, Lieberman JA, Alvir JM, Mayerhoff DI, Geisler SH, Szymanski SR. Duration of psychosis and outcome in first-episode schizophrenia. Am J Psychiatry. 1992;149(9):1183–8.
88. Bird V, Premkumar P, Kendall T, Whittington C, Mitchell J, Kuipers E. Early intervention services, cognitive-behavioural therapy and family intervention in early psychosis: systematic review. Br J Psychiatry. 2010;197(5):350–6.
89. Alvarez-Jiménez M, Parker AG, Hetrick SE, McGorry PD, Gleeson JF. Preventing the second episode: a systematic review and meta-analysis of psychosocial and pharmacological trials in first-episode psychosis. Schizophr Bull. 2011;37(3):619–30.
90. Sigrúnarson V, Gråwe RW, Morken G. Integrated treatment vs. treatment-as-usual for recent onset schizophrenia; 12 year follow-up on a randomized controlled trial. BMC Psychiatry. 2013;13:200.
91. Cullberg J, Levander S, Holmqvist R, Mattsson M, Wieselgren IM. One-year outcome in first episode psychosis patients in the Swedish Parachute project. Acta Psychiatr Scand. 2002;106(4):276–85.
92. Craig TK, Garety P, Power P, Rahaman N, Colbert S, Fornells-Ambrojo M, et al. The Lambeth Early Onset (LEO) Team: randomised controlled trial of the effectiveness of specialised care for early psychosis. BMJ. 2004;329(7474):1067.
93. Petersen L, Jeppesen P, Thorup A, Abel MB, Øhlenschlaeger J, Christensen T, et al. A randomised multicentre trial of integrated versus standard treatment for patients with a first episode of psychotic illness. BMJ. 2005;331(7517):602.
94. Srihari VH, Tek C, Kucukgoncu S, Phutane VH, Breitborde NJ, Pollard J, et al. First-episode services for psychotic disorders in the U.S. Public Sector: a pragmatic randomized controlled trial. Psychiatr Serv. 2015;66(7):705–12.
95. Mueser KT, Penn DL, Addington J, Brunette MF, Gingerich S, Glynn SM, et al. The NAVIGATE program for first-episode psychosis: rationale, overview, and description of psychosocial components. Psychiatr Serv. 2015;66(7):680–90.
96. Dixon LB, Goldman HH, Bennett ME, Wang Y, McNamara KA, Mendon SJ, et al. Implementing coordinated specialty care for early psychosis: the RAISE connection program. Psychiatr Serv. 2015;66(7):691–8.
97. Rosenheck R, Leslie D, Sint K, Lin H, Robinson DG, Schooler NR, et al. Cost-effectiveness of comprehensive, integrated care for first episode psychosis in the NIMH RAISE early treatment program. Schizophr Bull. 2016;42(4):896–906.
98. Nossel I, Wall MM, Scodes J, Marino LA, Zilkha S, Bello I, et al. Results of a coordinated specialty care program for early psychosis and predictors of outcomes. Psychiatr Serv. 2018;69(8):863–70.
99. Meyer PS, Gottlieb JD, Penn D, Mueser K, Gingerich S. Individual resiliency training: an early intervention approach to enhance well-being in people with first-episode psychosis. Psychiatr Ann. 2015;45(11):554–60.
100. McFarlane WR. Family interventions for schizophrenia and the psychoses: a review. Fam Process. 2016;55(3):460–82.
101. Hamann J, Cohen R, Leucht S, Busch R, Kissling W. Do patients with schizophrenia wish to be involved in decisions about their medical treatment? Am J Psychiatry. 2005;162(12):2382–4.
102. Barry MJ, Edgman-Levitan S. Shared decision making--pinnacle of patient-centered care. N Engl J Med. 2012;366(9):780–1.
103. Barnes TR, Drake R, Paton C, Cooper SJ, Deakin B, Ferrier IN, et al. Evidence-based guidelines for the pharmacological treatment of schizophrenia: updated recommendations from the British Association for Psychopharmacology. J Psychopharmacol. 2020;34(1):3–78.
104. Buchanan RW, Kreyenbuhl J, Kelly DL, Noel JM, Boggs DL, Fischer BA, et al. The 2009 schizophrenia PORT psychopharmacological treatment recommendations and summary statements. Schizophr Bull. 2010;36(1):71–93.
105. Hasan A, Falkai P, Wobrock T, Lieberman J, Glenthoj B, Gattaz WF, et al. World Federation of Societies of Biological Psychiatry (WFSBP) Guidelines for Biological Treatment of Schizophrenia, part 1: update 2012 on the acute treatment of schizophrenia and the management of treatment resistance. World J Biol Psychiatry. 2012;13(5):318–78.
106. Robinson DG, Woerner MG, Delman HM, Kane JM. Pharmacological treatments for first-episode schizophrenia. Schizophr Bull. 2005;31(3):705–22.

107. Sheitman BB, Lee H, Strous R, Lieberman JA. The evaluation and treatment of first-episode psychosis. Schizophr Bull. 1997;23(4):653–61.
108. McEvoy JP, Lieberman JA, Perkins DO, Hamer RM, Gu H, Lazarus A, et al. Efficacy and tolerability of olanzapine, quetiapine, and risperidone in the treatment of early psychosis: a randomized, double-blind 52-week comparison. Am J Psychiatry. 2007;164(7):1050–60.
109. Lieberman JA, Phillips M, Gu H, Stroup S, Zhang P, Kong L, et al. Atypical and conventional antipsychotic drugs in treatment-naive first-episode schizophrenia: a 52-week randomized trial of clozapine vs chlorpromazine. Neuropsychopharmacology. 2003;28(5):995–1003.
110. Robinson DG, Gallego JA, John M, Petrides G, Hassoun Y, Zhang JP, et al. A Randomized comparison of aripiprazole and risperidone for the acute treatment of first-episode schizophrenia and related disorders: 3-month outcomes. Schizophr Bull. 2015;41(6):1227–36.
111. Pagsberg AK, Jeppesen P, Klauber DG, Jensen KG, Rudå D, Stentebjerg-Olesen M, et al. Quetiapine extended release versus aripiprazole in children and adolescents with first-episode psychosis: the multicentre, double-blind, randomised tolerability and efficacy of antipsychotics (TEA) trial. Lancet Psychiatry. 2017;4(8):605–18.
112. Sikich L, Frazier JA, McClellan J, Findling RL, Vitiello B, Ritz L, et al. Double-blind comparison of first- and second-generation antipsychotics in early-onset schizophrenia and schizo-affective disorder: findings from the treatment of early-onset schizophrenia spectrum disorders (TEOSS) study. Am J Psychiatry. 2008;165(11):1420–31.
113. Schooler N, Rabinowitz J, Davidson M, Emsley R, Harvey PD, Kopala L, et al. Risperidone and haloperidol in first-episode psychosis: a long-term randomized trial. Am J Psychiatry. 2005;162(5):947–53.
114. Emsley RA. Risperidone in the treatment of first-episode psychotic patients: a double-blind multicenter study. Risperidone Working Group. Schizophr Bull. 1999;25(4):721–9.
115. Robinson DG, Woerner MG, Napolitano B, Patel RC, Sevy SM, Gunduz-Bruce H, et al. Randomized comparison of olanzapine versus risperidone for the treatment of first-episode schizophrenia: 4-month outcomes. Am J Psychiatry. 2006;163(12):2096–102.
116. Kahn RS, Winter van Rossum I, Leucht S, McGuire P, Lewis SW, Leboyer M, et al. Amisulpride and olanzapine followed by open-label treatment with clozapine in first-episode schizophrenia and schizophreniform disorder (OPTiMiSE): a three-phase switching study. Lancet Psychiatry. 2018;5(10):797–807.
117. Chatterjee A, Chakos M, Koreen A, Geisler S, Sheitman B, Woerner M, et al. Prevalence and clinical correlates of extrapyramidal signs and spontaneous dyskinesia in never-medicated schizophrenic patients. Am J Psychiatry. 1995;152(12):1724–9.
118. Chakos MH, Alvir JM, Woerner MG, Koreen A, Geisler S, Mayerhoff D, et al. Incidence and correlates of tardive dyskinesia in first episode of schizophrenia. Arch Gen Psychiatry. 1996;53(4):313–9.
119. Robinson DG, Gallego JA, John M, Petrides G, Hassoun Y, Zhang J-P, et al. A randomized comparison of aripiprazole and risperidone for the acute treatment of first-episode schizophrenia and related disorders: 3-month outcomes. Schizophr Bull. 2015;41(6):1227–36.
120. Jensen KG, Correll CU, Rudå D, Klauber DG, Decara MS, Fagerlund B, et al. Cardiometabolic adverse effects and its predictors in children and adolescents with first-episode psychosis during treatment with quetiapine-extended release versus aripiprazole: 12-week results from the tolerance and effect of antipsychotics in children and adolescents with psychosis (TEA) trial. J Am Acad Child Adolesc Psychiatry. 2019;58(11):1062–78.
121. Leucht S, Cipriani A, Spineli L, Mavridis D, Orey D, Richter F, et al. Comparative efficacy and tolerability of 15 antipsychotic drugs in schizophrenia: a multiple-treatments meta-analysis. Lancet. 2013;382(9896):951–62.
122. De Hert M, Yu W, Detraux J, Sweers K, van Winkel R, Correll CU. Body weight and metabolic adverse effects of asenapine, iloperidone, lurasidone and paliperidone in the treatment of schizophrenia and bipolar disorder: a systematic review and exploratory meta-analysis. CNS Drugs. 2012;26(9):733–59.
123. Casey DE, Haupt DW, Newcomer JW, Henderson DC, Sernyak MJ, Davidson M, et al. Antipsychotic-induced weight gain and metabolic abnormalities: implications for increased mortality in patients with schizophrenia. J Clin Psychiatry. 2004;65(Suppl 7):4–18; quiz 9–20
124. Stroup TS, McEvoy JP, Ring KD, Hamer RH, LaVange LM, Swartz MS, et al. A randomized trial examining the effectiveness of switching from olanzapine, quetiapine, or risperidone to aripiprazole to reduce metabolic risk: comparison of antipsychotics for metabolic problems (CAMP). Am J Psychiatry. 2011;168(9):947–56.
125. Stroup TS, Byerly MJ, Nasrallah HA, Ray N, Khan AY, Lamberti JS, et al. Effects of switching from olanzapine, quetiapine, and risperidone to aripiprazole on 10-year coronary heart disease risk and metabolic syndrome status: results from a randomized controlled trial. Schizophr Res. 2013;146(1-3):190–5.
126. Tiihonen J, Haukka J, Taylor M, Haddad PM, Patel MX, Korhonen P. A nationwide cohort study of oral and depot antipsychotics after first hospitalization for schizophrenia. Am J Psychiatry. 2011;168(6):603–9.
127. Subotnik KL, Casaus LR, Ventura J, Luo JS, Hellemann GS, Gretchen-Doorly D, et al. Long-acting injectable risperidone for relapse prevention and control of breakthrough symptoms after a recent first episode of schizophrenia. A randomized clinical trial. JAMA Psychiatry. 2015;72(8):822–9.

128. Schreiner A, Aadamsoo K, Altamura AC, Franco M, Gorwood P, Neznanov NG, et al. Paliperidone palmitate versus oral antipsychotics in recently diagnosed schizophrenia. Schizophr Res. 2015;169(1-3):393–9.
129. Kane JM, Schooler NR, Marcy P, Achtyes ED, Correll CU, Robinson DG. Patients with early-phase schizophrenia will accept treatment with sustained-release medication (long-acting injectable antipsychotics): results from the recruitment phase of the PRELAPSE Trial. J Clin Psychiatry. 2019;80(3):18m12546.
130. Emsley R, Asmal L, Rubio JM, Correll CU, Kane JM. Predictors of psychosis breakthrough during 24 months of long-acting antipsychotic maintenance treatment in first episode schizophrenia. Schizophr Res. 2019. https://doi.org/10.1016/j.schres.2019.11.025.
131. Kreyenbuhl JA, Medoff DR, McEvoy JP, Smith TE, Hackman AL, Nossel IR, et al. The RAISE Connection Program: psychopharmacological treatment of people with a first episode of schizophrenia. Psychiatr Serv. 2016;67(12):1300–6.
132. Buchanan RW, Kreyenbuhl K, Henry C, Stroup S, Nossel I. OnTrackNY medical manual. 2016. Available from: https://www.ontrackny.org/portals/1/Files/Resources/Medical%20Manual%20FINAL%202016.pdf.
133. NAVIGATE Psychopharmacological Treatment Manual. 2014. Available from: http://www.navigateconsultants.org/wp-content/uploads/2017/05/Prescribers-Manual.pdf.
134. Findling RL, Cavuş I, Pappadopulos E, Vanderburg DG, Schwartz JH, Gundapaneni BK, et al. Ziprasidone in adolescents with schizophrenia: results from a placebo-controlled efficacy and long-term open-extension study. J Child Adolesc Psychopharmacol. 2013;23(8):531–44.
135. Findling RL, Landbloom RP, Mackle M, Pallozzi W, Braat S, Hundt C, et al. Safety and efficacy from an 8 week double-blind trial and a 26 week open-label extension of asenapine in adolescents with schizophrenia. J Child Adolesc Psychopharmacol. 2015;25(5):384–96.
136. Wunderink L, Nienhuis FJ, Sytema S, Slooff CJ, Knegtering R, Wiersma D. Guided discontinuation versus maintenance treatment in remitted first-episode psychosis: relapse rates and functional outcome. J Clin Psychiatry. 2007;68(5):654–61.
137. Chen EY, Hui CL, Lam MM, Chiu CP, Law CW, Chung DW, et al. Maintenance treatment with quetiapine versus discontinuation after one year of treatment in patients with remitted first episode psychosis: randomised controlled trial. BMJ. 2010;341:c4024.
138. Robinson D, Woerner MG, Alvir JMJ, Bilder R, Goldman R, Geisler S, et al. Predictors of relapse following response from a first episode of schizophrenia or schizoaffective disorder. Arch Gen Psychiatry. 1999;56(3):241–7.
139. Wunderink L, Nieboer RM, Wiersma D, Sytema S, Nienhuis FJ. Recovery in remitted first-episode psychosis at 7 years of follow-up of an early dose reduction/discontinuation or maintenance treatment strategy: long-term follow-up of a 2-year randomized clinical trial. JAMA Psychiatry. 2013;70(9):913–20.
140. Yarborough BJ, Stumbo SP, Yarborough MT, Young TJ, Green CA. Improving lifestyle interventions for people with serious mental illnesses: qualitative results from the STRIDE study. Psychiatr Rehabil J. 2016;39(1):33–41.
141. Usher C, Thompson A, Griebeler M, Senders A, Seibel C, Ly R, et al. Meals, Mindfulness, & Moving Forward: a feasibility study to a multi-modal lifestyle approach in early psychosis. Early Interv Psychiatry. 2019;13(1):147–50.
142. Thompson A, Senders A, Seibel C, Usher C, Borgatti A, Bodden K, et al. Qualitative analysis of the Meals, Mindfulness, & Moving Forward (M(3)) lifestyle programme: cultivating a 'safe space' to start on a 'new path' for youth with early episode psychosis. Early Interv Psychiatry. 2020;
143. Gates J, Killackey E, Phillips L, Álvarez-Jiménez M. Mental health starts with physical health: current status and future directions of non-pharmacological interventions to improve physical health in first-episode psychosis. Lancet Psychiatry. 2015;2(8):726–42.
144. de Silva VA, Suraweera C, Ratnatunga SS, Dayabandara M, Wanniarachchi N, Hanwella R. Metformin in prevention and treatment of antipsychotic induced weight gain: a systematic review and meta-analysis. BMC Psychiatry. 2016;16(1):341.
145. Maayan L, Vakhrusheva J, Correll CU. Effectiveness of medications used to attenuate antipsychotic-related weight gain and metabolic abnormalities: a systematic review and meta-analysis. Neuropsychopharmacology. 2010;35(7):1520–30.
146. Wu R, Zhang F, Gao K, Ou J, Shao P, Jin H, et al. Metformin treatment of antipsychotic-induced dyslipidemia: an analysis of two randomized, placebo-controlled trials. Mol Psychiatry. 2016;21(11):1537.
147. Ellul P, Delorme R, Cortese S. Metformin for weight gain associated with second-generation antipsychotics in children and adolescents: a systematic review and meta-analysis. CNS Drugs. 2018;32(12):1103–12.
148. Zhang JP, Gallego JA, Robinson DG, Malhotra AK, Kane JM, Correll CU. Efficacy and safety of individual second-generation vs. first-generation antipsychotics in first-episode psychosis: a systematic review and meta-analysis. Int J Neuropsychopharmacol. 2013;16(6):1205–18.
149. Lane RD, Glazer WM, Hansen TE, Berman WH, Kramer SI. Assessment of tardive dyskinesia using the abnormal involuntary movement scale. J Nerv Ment Dis. 1985;173(6):353–7.

150. Simpson GM, Angus JW. A rating scale for extrapyramidal side effects. Acta Psychiatr Scand Suppl. 1970;212:11–9.
151. Barnes TR. A rating scale for drug-induced akathisia. Br J Psychiatry. 1989;154:672–6.
152. Miyamoto S, Miyake N, Jarskog L, Fleischhacker W, Lieberman JJ. Pharmacological treatment of schizophrenia: a critical review of the pharmacology and clinical effects of current and future therapeutic agents. Mol Psychiatry. 2012;17(12):1206–27.
153. Kane JM, Fleischhacker WW, Hansen L, Perlis R, Pikalov A 3rd, Assunção-Talbott S. Akathisia: an updated review focusing on second-generation antipsychotics. J Clin Psychiatry. 2009;70(5):627–43.
154. Adler LA, Peselow E, Rosenthal M, Angrist B. A controlled comparison of the effects of propranolol, benztropine, and placebo on akathisia: an interim analysis. Psychopharmacol Bull. 1993;29(2):283–6.
155. Di Fabio R, De Filippis S, Cafariello C, Penna L, Marianetti M, Serrao M, et al. Low doses of rotigotine in patients with antipsychotic-induced parkinsonism. Clin Neuropharmacol. 2013;36(5):162–5.
156. Lohr JB, Liu L, Caligiuri MP, Kash TP, May TA, Murphy JD, et al. Modafinil improves antipsychotic-induced parkinsonism but not excessive daytime sleepiness, psychiatric symptoms or cognition in schizophrenia and schizoaffective disorder: a randomized, double-blind, placebo-controlled study. Schizophr Res. 2013;150(1):289–96.
157. Ebadi M, Srinivasan S. Pathogenesis, prevention, and treatment of neuroleptic-induced movement disorders. Pharmacol Rev. 1995;47(4):575–604.
158. DiMascio A, Bernardo DL, Greenblatt DJ, Marder JE. A controlled trial of amantadine in drug-induced extrapyramidal disorders. Arch Gen Psychiatry. 1976;33(5):599–602.
159. Tarsy D. Tardive Dyskinesia. Curr Treat Options Neurol. 2000;2(3):205–14.
160. Novick D, Haro JM, Bertsch J, Haddad PM. Incidence of extrapyramidal symptoms and tardive dyskinesia in schizophrenia: thirty-six-month results from the European schizophrenia outpatient health outcomes study. J Clin Psychopharmacol. 2010;30(5):531–40.
161. Tarsy D, Baldessarini RJ, Tarazi FI. Effects of newer antipsychotics on extrapyramidal function. CNS Drugs. 2002;16(1):23–45.
162. McEvoy JP. FDA-Approved Medications to Treat Tardive Dyskinesia. J Clin Psychiatry. 2019;81(1):NU18041BR3C.
163. Hauser RA, Factor SA, Marder SR, Knesevich MA, Ramirez PM, Jimenez R, et al. KINECT 3: a phase 3 randomized, double-blind, placebo-controlled trial of valbenazine for tardive dyskinesia. Am J Psychiatry. 2017;174(5):476–84.
164. Sarva H, Henchcliffe C. Valbenazine as the first and only approved treatment for adults with tardive dyskinesia. Expert Rev Clin Pharmacol. 2018;11(3):209–17.
165. Thaker GK, Nguyen JA, Strauss ME, Jacobson R, Kaup BA, Tamminga CA. Clonazepam treatment of tardive dyskinesia: a practical GABAmimetic strategy. Am J Psychiatry. 1990;147(4):445–51.
166. Bhidayasiri R, Fahn S, Weiner WJ, Gronseth GS, Sullivan KL, Zesiewicz TA. Evidence-based guideline: treatment of tardive syndromes: report of the Guideline Development Subcommittee of the American Academy of Neurology. Neurology. 2013;81(5):463–9.
167. McFarlane WR, Lukens E, Link B, Dushay R, Deakins SA, Newmark M, et al. Multiple-family groups and psychoeducation in the treatment of schizophrenia. Arch Gen Psychiatry. 1995;52(8):679–87.
168. Zimmermann G, Favrod J, Trieu VH, Pomini V. The effect of cognitive behavioral treatment on the positive symptoms of schizophrenia spectrum disorders: a meta-analysis. Schizophr Res. 2005;77(1):1–9.
169. Wykes T, Steel C, Everitt B, Tarrier N. Cognitive behavior therapy for schizophrenia: effect sizes, clinical models, and methodological rigor. Schizophr Bull. 2008;34(3):523–37.
170. Gould RA, Mueser KT, Bolton E, Mays V, Goff D. Cognitive therapy for psychosis in schizophrenia: an effect size analysis. Schizophr Res. 2001;48(2-3):335–42.
171. Lecomte T, Leclerc C, Corbière M, Wykes T, Wallace CJ, Spidel A. Group cognitive behavior therapy or social skills training for individuals with a recent onset of psychosis? Results of a randomized controlled trial. J Nerv Ment Dis. 2008;196(12):866–75.
172. Saksa JR, Cohen SJ, Srihari VH, Woods SW. Cognitive behavior therapy for early psychosis: a comprehensive review of individual vs. group treatment studies. Int J Group Psychother. 2009;59(3):357–83.
173. Brabban A, Byrne R, Longden E, Morrison AP. The importance of human relationships, ethics and recovery-orientated values in the delivery of CBT for people with psychosis. Psychosis. 2017;9(2):157–66.
174. Kingdon DG. Cognitive-behavioral therapy of schizophrenia. New York: Guilford Press; 1994.
175. Dutta R, Murray RM, Hotopf M, Allardyce J, Jones PB, Boydell J. Reassessing the long-term risk of suicide after a first episode of psychosis. Arch Gen Psychiatry. 2010;67(12):1230–7.
176. Schoenbaum M, Sutherland JM, Chappel A, Azrin S, Goldstein AB, Rupp A, et al. Twelve-month health care use and mortality in commercially insured young people with incident psychosis in the United States. Schizophr Bull. 2017;43(6):1262–72.
177. Posner K, Brown GK, Stanley B, Brent DA, Yershova KV, Oquendo MA, et al. The Columbia-Suicide Severity Rating Scale: initial validity and internal consistency findings from three multisite studies with adolescents and adults. Am J Psychiatry. 2011;168(12):1266–77.
178. Phahladira L, Luckhoff HK, Asmal L, Kilian S, Scheffler F, Plessis SD, et al. Early recovery in the first 24 months of treatment in first-episode schizophrenia-spectrum disorders. NPJ Schizophr. 2020;6(1):2.

15 Dilemmas in Disability

Jana Dreyzehner, Karen Goldberg,
Stephanie Sims, and Celine Turco

Key Points

- The number and magnitude of changes for transitional age youth (TAY) with disabilities require more planning for a successful transition and frequently exceed those for typical TAY.
- Effective transition plans center around the youth's strengths, needs, and preferences inclusive of "self-determination" and the "dignity of risk."
- Planning for a successful transition should start well before the transition date and include representatives from all systems of care.
- Multiple life domains must be examined, including legal capacity needs, housing, accessing funds and benefits, and transitioning health care from pediatrics to adult care.
- Medicaid is the primary funding source of community-based long-term health care and living supportive services through its home- and community-based services (HCBS) waivers that are defined by each state.
- Youth with continuing education or employment goals are more likely to find themselves in situations providing the three key elements for happiness – meaningful activity, relationships, and goals.

Introduction

Transition to adulthood is an exciting milestone that presents unique challenges for persons with disabilities. There are various types of disabilities including those that affect a person's thinking, learning, communication, vision, hearing, movement, social relationships, and mental health. Typically developing transitional age youth (TAY) experience enhanced levels of responsibilities when they turn 18 years old and often continue to receive some level of support from their primary caretakers well into adulthood. For children with disabilities, the transition into adulthood includes additional challenges, may be more abrupt, and is too often synonymous with drastic and sudden change in support. It is not unusual for youth with disabilities aging out of

J. Dreyzehner (✉) · K. Goldberg · C. Turco
Life Connect Health, LLC, Nashville, TN, USA
e-mail: DrD@LifeConnectHealth.com

S. Sims
Department of Psychiatry, University of Florida College of Medicine-Jacksonville and UF Health-Jacksonville, Jacksonville, FL, USA

V. Chan, J. Derenne (eds.), *Transition-Age Youth Mental Health Care*,
https://doi.org/10.1007/978-3-030-62113-1_15

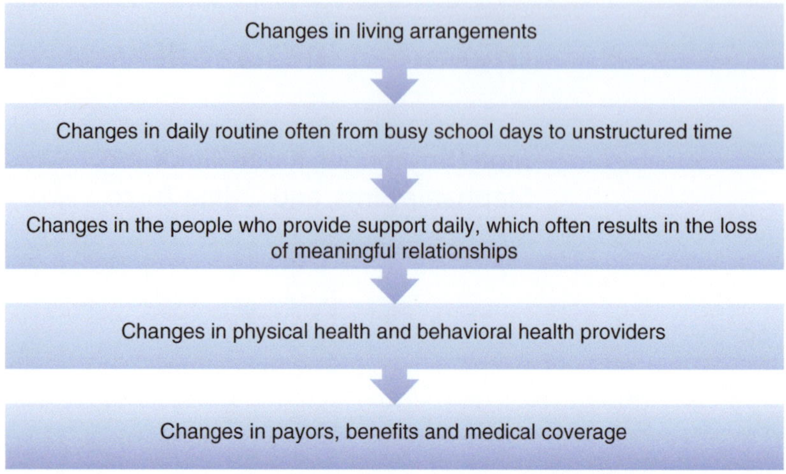

Fig. 15.1 Changes to supports for TAY with disabilities

the school system to experience changes that can cause significant disruptions (Fig. 15.1).

A comprehensive transition plan can be a highly effective process to eliminate some of the highlighted challenges and support the youth with developing *their* vision for *their* future. In this chapter, as we examine the elements of successful transition planning for youth with various disabilities, it is appropriate to begin with the guiding principle of self-determination.

Key Principles of Transition Planning: Self-Determination, Timeliness, and Cross-System Planning

Self-Determination

Self-Determination: "free choice of one's own acts or states without external compulsion" [1].

The American Association on Intellectual and Developmental Disabilities (AAIDD) and The Arc, the largest national advocacy organization for intellectual and developmental disabilities (I/DD), have jointly authored a position paper that details the right of individuals to self-determination including the right "to opportunities, respectful support, and the authority to exert control in their lives, to direct their services, and to act on their own behalf…the individual must be able to advocate for themselves with the assurance that their desires, interests, and preferences will be respected and honored" [2].

Commonalities in the many definitions of self-determination include an individual taking control and responsibility for one's life, setting goals, taking the initiative to reach these goals, and making choices motivated primarily by internal desires, rather than being motivated by external pressures or rewards. Self-determinism realizes that one has a real choice to control one's destiny, but it does not mean being entirely independent or self-sufficient. Similarly, the concept of autonomy does not mean being entirely independent from others [3, 4]. This is particularly important for youth with disabilities who frequently lack opportunities to learn self-determination skills. Adults or teams of adults tend to make well-intentioned decisions for youth with disabilities to protect them from unwanted consequences. While this may protect individuals, it conveys an erroneous assumption that the individual who has disabilities is incapable of independent decision-making. Additionally, it denies the individual the personal freedom to experience an essential self-esteem milestone, the "dignity of risk." This is the concept that self-determination and risk-taking allow an individual to both make a choice and experience the consequences of their choice [5, 6]. There are many resources on developing self-determination skills in youth with disabilities. The National Center on Secondary Education and Transition (NCSET) has a publication that includes the table titled, "Promoting Self-Determination in Youth with Disabilities: Tips for Families and Professionals" [7] which succinctly lists valuable teaching or coaching strategies in the following domains:

- Promote Choice Making
- Encourage Exploration of Possibilities
- Promote Reasonable Risk Taking
- Encourage Problem Solving
- Promote Self Advocacy
- Facilitate Development of Self-Esteem
- Develop Goal Setting and Planning
- Help Youth Understand Their Disabilities

An Individualized Education Plan (IEP) can be utilized to memorialize goals and objectives related to building self-determination skills and to reflect effective strategies to implement across environments by all systems of care. Early implementation of these strategies affords TAY opportunities to practice these skills prior to transitioning from high school [4].

A key to success in the transition process is to guarantee the youth's central role in the transition plan development. The end product ideally accurately reflects the youth's preferences and contains realistic, appropriate life-stage choices. Transition planning often necessarily focuses on the youth's vulnerabilities and strategies to minimize risks for the future. However, it is critical that the plan provides equal focus on the youth's preferences and dreams for the future. The team's role is to carefully assess the youth's abilities and needs and formulate choices that relate directly to his or her ambitions. This can be a difficult process, as many youth have not yet had life experiences that promote self-determination. It is common for youth nearing adulthood to struggle with articulating a vision for their future, but it is the supporting team's responsibility and privilege to help them formulate it. There are a number of ways to do so, such as interviewing TAY to establish preferences in the type of living environment they hope for, exposing them to job sampling and career fairs which can be facilitated through a meaningful IEP, and obtaining feedback from primary caretakers. There are formal resources such as the Happiness Assessment [8] which help individuals articulate their future goals. In some situations, youth may present dreams and goals that the supporting team may think are unrealistic. Teams must proceed cautiously when providing feedback, as they do not want youth to feel hopeless about the possibility of achieving their dreams. Rather, the team has an opportunity to help the youth identify and prioritize essential elements of their dreams and determine how to incorporate them in the transition plan. For example, a youth may state his vocational goal is to become a National Basketball Association (NBA) professional basketball player. Instead of judging NBA eligibility as unreachable, adults can help the youth explore what is really important to him about that goal. For example, a supporter may ask if being part of a team is important, and if so, look at jobs that involve teams of workers. If the youth remains focused on being on an NBA team, then supporters may assist in breaking down the steps needed to achieve this dream. For example, an individual may be able to see that playing recreationally on a local team (e.g., offered by the Special Olympics) to improve basketball skills is a step leading toward his ultimate goal. If he struggles with punctuality and use of public transportation, the supporters may be able to use this to provide new motivation to work on specific life skills in order to make it to the team practice. Helping a youth set realistic stepwise expectations and goals for his or her future that are based on preferences and dreams is the most effective way to meaningfully engage the youth in his or her own transition process.

Timeliness

Planning for a successful transition begins as early as possible (i.e., a minimum of 2 years prior to the youth's 18th birthday) and is an ongoing process throughout adolescence. IEP meetings are great opportunities to further define educational and vocational goals for the future, identify skill-building opportunities that relate directly to those goals, and continue to offer opportunities for exploration. Vocational and educational domains are critical areas of focus in preparing for adulthood, but defining a life plan needs to be inclusive of additional domains (i.e., social relationships, meaningful activities in the community, health and wellness, housing). Existing resources such the "transition toolkit" developed by the Parent Information Center (https://picnh.org/wp-content/uploads/2018/06/Transition-Toolkit-2018v2.pdf) or the toolkit created by the National Technical Assistance Center on Transition (https://transitionta.org/) can help organize the transition planning milestones in an actionable format across environments. Helping TAY define their preferences across domains and assessing their needs and abilities in each area is a lengthy process that best occurs concurrently with the development of vocational and educational goals. The more time the youth is afforded to explore options and receive feedback and education, the more likely they are to feel empowered to make decisions and be hopeful about their future.

Cross-System Planning

As a transition date (18th birthday) approaches and a plan becomes actionable, it is extremely helpful when individuals who will support the youth once they have crossed into adulthood participate in the planning. It is not unusual for a youth and their team to initially feel confident about the plan defined. However, problems with information-sharing results in elements of the plan not being implemented. The best safeguard to prevent such a situation is including future support representatives in the planning stages rather than simply providing a "warm hand-off" between the current and future supporters. Representatives from the following future systems should be considered: residential providers, behavioral health services providers, employment training and support providers, and case management services. This allows the youth to build rapport with the individuals who will champion the plan in the future and further builds the youth's trust and engagement in the process. Additionally, those who have expertise in resources and opportunities in adult services can greatly enrich the discussion. Participation in transition planning also helps the adult system support team obtain rich knowledge about the youth's abilities, needs, and preferences.

Elements of a Successful Transition Plan

In addition to defining goals for the future, there are a number of critical elements to consider in a comprehensive transition plan to ensure appropriate supports are in place and to avoid unnecessary challenges such as lapses in services, loss of important supports, and missed opportunities for benefits during the course of transition to adulthood.

Legal Capacity Needs

One of the instant and inherent changes of turning 18 years old is becoming one's own guardian by default. During the transition planning process, it is important to examine an individual's abilities to manage affairs with the help and support of their existing and future teams. In some cases, there may be concerns that a youth lacks the competency to make major life decisions even with support. Consequently, he or she may be at risk for substantial harm and may need to become a ward who is afforded special protections. When that is the case, the team may want to explore options for guardianship, a lengthy legal process ideally initiated early, at least 1 year prior to the youth's 18th birthday. In some states, distinctions are made between guardianships and conservatorships, but both are legal mechanisms for legal authority to be awarded to others. The team can attempt to first identify natural supportive individuals who could petition the court for guardianship or conservatorship. If none exist or are willing, the team must explore options for a state-appointed guardian or paid guardian, depending on the programs available in the state of residence.

There are different types of guardianships and conservatorships. Full guardianship is applicable to all life decisions, while others are limited to a certain domain, such as medical, psychiatric, or financial decisions. Guardianship can be temporary or permanent depending on the situation. As part of the legal filing process, a medical professional will conduct an assessment and make recommendations as to which type of guardianship is necessary, and the court will make the final determination.

It is important to recognize that seeking guardianship or conservatorship for a person is a serious matter, as it strips the person's autonomy to make choices. A 2019 joint position statement from AAIDD and The Arc states that "guardianship has been over-used by those who were unaware of less intrusive alternatives or who simply wanted to have their views prevail over the wishes of the individual" [9]. When considering guardianship or conservatorship, supporting teams must not confuse the youth's *competency* (or lack of) to make decisions with the perceived *quality* of the decisions made. People have the right to make decisions that others may view as "bad." Physicians are well aware that many people who are very competent (i.e., capable) often make choices contrary to their best long-term interest. For example, many people have heard their doctors' recommendations to stop smoking, lose weight, or exercise regularly but do not take the advice and choose to eat donuts, smoke cigarettes, and skip the gym membership in favor of a movie channel subscription. Persons with disabilities have the same right to make choices as long as they are competent, meaning they have the ability to understand the consequences of their choice.

Living Arrangements and Access to Funds

Planning for housing and having sufficient funding for adulthood can be a lengthy and complex process. Understanding the basics of the options available and how those options may be financed is critical and can save time and frustration on everyone's part. There are resources helpful in deciphering the "alphabet soup" of acronyms encountered on this topic such as the Center for Parent Information and Resources website list, "Disability and Special Education Acronyms," available at https://www.parentcenterhub.org/acronyms/. It is important for supporting teams to both understand all of the options that are available to the youth and also define what supports are needed for the youth to be safe and integrated in their community.

Understanding the Waiver

Medicaid is the primary funding source of community-based health-care long-term services, primarily through its *home- and community-based services (HCBS) waivers (Section 1915 [c] or [i] waivers)* [10]. While state and federal Medicaid together provide over 75 percent of the funding for services for people with I/DD nationwide, many states have lengthy waiting lists, and many eligible individuals are unable to access the needed supports [11]. Eligibility for these Medicaid programs is determined on a state by state basis but generally requires that the young adult has received a diagnosis of intellectual and/or developmental disabilities before age 21 years and their income and assets must not exceed the threshold set by Medicaid (updated annually). Individuals with assets exceeding the threshold may be required to spend down their assets (sometimes referred to as Medicaid Buy-In programs) prior to qualifying for HCBS waiver.

The Section 1915(c) Waiver

Section 1915(c) of the Social Security Act authorizes the Medicaid HCBS waiver program which, in turn, authorizes states to request the option of providing home- and community-based alternatives to institutional care. This effectively waives certain requirements in Medicaid law so that states may offer intensive community-based services comparable to an institutional level of care for those individuals who choose to receive services in their home or community making it possible for persons with disabilities to live and work among family and friends rather than in an institutional setting [10].

HCBS waivers can provide general assistance for individuals with mental illness, intellectual disabilities, and/or physical disabilities of any age. Both medical and nonmedical services can be provided depending on the Medicaid program though persons eligible for Medicare benefits (usually 2 years after being granted disability) often have medical services covered by Medicare as a primary insurance and Medicaid as their secondary payor. Nonmedical services, such as respite care, skills support and development, transportation, case management, home health aide, day programs, funding for special diets, and in-home modifications for accessibility, often can be covered by Medicaid in addition to traditional speech, hearing, occupational, or physical therapies.

The 1915(i) SPA (State Plan Amendment) The 1915(i) SPA was created in the Deficit Reduction Act of 2005 (DRA, P.L. 109-171) and was updated by the Patient Protection and Affordable Care Act (ACA, P.L. 111-148, as amended) to allow states to provide HCBS services under their Medicaid state plans without obtaining a waiver from Centers for Medicare and Medicaid Services (CMS). Unlike Section 1915(c) waivers, the 1915(i) SPA allows states to set the qualifying level for HCBS at either an institutional level of care or lower.

Like the Section 1915(c) waiver, the 1915(i) SPA allows states to design service packages targeted to people with specific needs, including special services for those who have developmental disabilities, physical disabilities, mental illness, or substance use disorders. States may offer benefits to a specific age group without regard to comparability of services for those who do not receive the 1915(i) services, although they must abide by the statewideness rule, dictating that state Medicaid programs cannot exclude enrollees or providers because of where they live or work in the state [10].

Understanding Some Additional Terms

Long-Term Services and Supports (LTSS) Refers to medical and/or personal care and support services needed by individuals who require assistance with activities of daily living (ADLs such as eating, toileting, and self-care activities) and with instrumental activities of daily living (IADLs such as housework, shopping, preparing meals, managing money) and are determined by the payor to be necessary for the long term using a level of care assessment (e.g., community living supports and supported employment services).

Managed Long-Term Services and Supports (MLTSS) Refers to the LTSS being managed/administered by a managed care organization (MCO) rather than services paid directly by the state Medicaid agency without being managed. Movement nationally has been toward MLTSS to help with cost containment as this has historically been one of the most "expensive" populations for total cost of care. In an effort to reduce costs and to add value to the cross-system support team around an individual receiving LTSS services, many MCOs have programs that actively include an MCO staff person who is clinically trained in nursing, social work, or therapy/behavioral health. For example, Tennessee is the first state in the nation to require all Medicaid recipients be enrolled in a TennCare MCO. TennCare MCOs 1915(c) waiver program is called Employment and Community First Choices and has a defined role for the MCO clinical staff person as the "Support Coordinator" who partners with the providers and the individual. While this may seem to blur the line between provision of payment and provision of service, the specific role identifies eligible individuals and administers the level of care assessments necessary to determine needed services. The Support Coordinator then assists the individual in accessing the needed services while staying within their benefit budget.

Level of Care (LOC) The service delivery setting that meets the requirements deemed necessary for the individual's needs. Levels of care range from outpatient service settings and intensive outpatient programs (IOPs) to residential treatment settings (RTCs), supported housing (SH), and intermediate care facilities (ICFs). The highest LOC is inpatient or acute hospitalization.

Settings Final Rule This refers to the requirements for home- and community-based settings as defined in Section 1915(c) of the Social Security Act. A summary of the key provisions of the HCBS Settings Final Rule provided by CMS explains that the provisions in this final rule establish a more outcome-oriented definition of home- and community-based settings defined by the quality of the individual's experience rather than based solely on a setting's location, geography, or physical characteristics. The settings requirements are meant to maximize the opportunities for waiver participants to have access to the benefits of community living, including receiving services in a home or community setting [12]. The Center for Medicaid and CHIP services (CMCS) offers a Home and Community Based Settings Requirements Compliance Toolkit which is a summary of the regulatory requirements. The primary requirements are presented in Table 15.1 [13].

Table 15.1 Regulatory requirements for home- and community-based settings

For 1915(c) home- and community-based waivers and for 1915(i) State Plan home- and community-based services, home- and community-based settings must have all of the following qualities defined at §441.301(c) [4] and §441.710, respectively, and such other qualities as the Secretary determines to be appropriate, based on the needs of the individual as indicated in their person-centered service plan:
The setting is integrated in and supports full access of individuals receiving Medicaid HCBS to the greater community, including opportunities to seek employment and work in competitive integrated settings, engage in community life, control personal resources, and receive services in the community, to the same degree of access as individuals not receiving Medicaid HCBS.
The setting is selected by the individual from among setting options including non-disability-specific settings and an option for a private unit in a residential setting. The setting options are identified and documented in the person-centered service plan and are based on the individual's needs, preferences, and, for residential settings, resources available for room and board.
Ensures an individual's rights of privacy, dignity and respect, and freedom from coercion and restraint.
Optimizes, but does not regiment, individual initiative, autonomy, and independence in making life choices, including, but not limited to, daily activities, physical environment, and with whom to interact.
Facilitates individual choice regarding services and supports and who provides them.

Navigating the Waiver Process

It is important to understand the process to help TAY qualify for adult services and funding well in advance of the transition, ideally at least 2 years prior to the youth's 18th birthday. Each state defines the services that are available within their funding option, establishes an eligibility process, and ultimately administers the waiver in accordance with federal guidelines. Transition planning is therefore dependent on the state where the youth resides and begins with a review of the youth's state waiver to understand the eligibility criteria, enrollment process, and availability of services.

Once the enrollment process begins, the youth and team can expect to undergo a level of care assessment. States utilize specific assessment tools to determine the level of needs and support services the youth will require upon transition. This is very important as it determines eligibility for services, and in most states, such assessment is also used as a rate-setting tool that determines the annual funding available to the youth for services. This assessment is an opportunity to summarize and share all the findings of the needs evaluation that should be taking place throughout the transition planning process. It should be noted that each state has the flexibility to select which level of care assessment tool is utilized, and that information can be found in the state-specific HCBS 1915(c) document.

Planning for Living Arrangements

It is important to understand that although funding for services is available through the states' Medicaid waivers, the youth will be expected to contribute to their housing cost because "room and board" is specifically excluded from the 1915 [c] waiver coverage [14]. Similarly, Medicaid waivers do not provide funding for personal needs expenses. Social Security benefits can be used to cover room and board and personal expenses. It is important that support teams help the youth with applying for Social Security benefits prior to their 18th birthday. Previous Social Security policies allowed the individual to apply 30 days prior to their birthday, but the application processing time has been so lengthy that the 30-day timeline often left youth with no benefit for several months after transition. The policy has since changed to allow youth to apply 90 days prior to their 18th birthday to reduce the occurrence of gaps in benefits. In conjunction with securing eligibility for services, the support team needs to help the youth articulate their preferences in regard to their living environment. Some of the topics to discuss include:

- *Geography*: establishing housing is important. For example, the youth may want to remain within a certain area where family and friends live to maintain in-person contact. Or, the youth may still be enrolled in high school, and a change of school due to moving locations may cause additional stress. When evaluating different locations, a team consideration is the availability of other ancillary services and accessibility to recreational and vocational activities.
- *Physical plant*: in addition to accommodations that may be required for medical needs, a youth may have preferences or needs regarding the physical plant. For example, a youth may be ambulatory, but may prefer a ground floor bedroom, or may want to live in a home where it is possible to have a private bedroom and/or bathroom.
- *Living with others*: most housing options are inclusive of living with one or two housemates. Choice in housemates is an individual's right under the requirements of the HCBS Settings Final Rule. It is important to understand from the youth what characteristics are critical in a housemate and plan for meet and greets with potential housemates so each individual is in agreement.

It is equally important to work with the youth on setting realistic expectations, as they may not find living arrangements that meet all of their preferences and fall within their benefit budget. Unfortunately, the adult services infrastructure has historically struggled to keep pace with consumer needs. Therefore, working on the youth's preparedness to compromise on some preferences may help prevent disappointment and negative feelings about the options offered.

Once the youth is presented with options from adult services providers, it is time for the youth to evaluate the options. This may include tours of potential housing options, meeting potential housemates and support staff, and exploring the nearby community. Being able to envision what their living environment could look like will empower them to make an informed decision and feel confident that they were afforded choice, and their plan incorporates their individual preferences and goals.

Health-Care Transition

Many facets of transitioning youth's health-care management drastically change with the transition to adulthood. Too often, TAY with Medicaid coverage aging out of pediatric health-care experience lapse in health insurance coverage. Although most continue to be eligible for Medicaid coverage, a redetermination process needs to be completed when transitioning into adulthood in order to secure health insurance coverage. Therefore supporting teams must understand and facilitate the process of enrollment as well as recognize the differences in coverage, as some services such as occupational therapy and speech therapy are not included in general adult Medicaid coverage.

The transition from pediatric to adult care presents significant risk to youth with complex health-care needs if not managed properly. Got Transition®, the federally funded national resource center on health-care transition (HCT) has developed guidance for practitioners from both systems to help support successful transition in its "Six Core Elements of Health Care Transition™" [15]. The guidance recommends initiating the transition timeline at age 12 years and culminates at ages 23–26 years when the young adult is integrated into adult care. Unfortunately, as noted in a PolicyLab issued by the Children's Hospital of Philadelphia, "although this guidance is readily available, we know that it is not consistently implemented in pediatric and adult medical settings across the country. Many young adults with special health care needs face potentially life-threatening barriers to getting the care they need, such as lapses in insurance coverage, not seeing appropriate providers, and losing access to necessary medications and medical equipment, among many other issues" [16]. This highlights the importance of the supporting teams taking a central role in championing the health-care transition and minimizing potential lapses in critical services.

There are a number of strategies the team can employ to support a successful health-care transition:

- *Identifying providers*: It is important for the supporting team to state the "identification of adult providers" as an actionable item in the transition plan. It can be very challenging to find qualified providers who accept Medicaid payments and also have the experience needed to work with persons with disabilities. It has been reported that individuals with intellectual disability must contact on average 50 physicians before they can find one who has expertise with persons with disabilities [17]. Due to the paucity of experienced providers, travel and transportation to visits may be more challenging as an adult so exploring telehealth options may offer additional possibilities.
- *Facilitating exchange of critical health information*: Once new providers have been identified, the next step is identifying a champion from the support team who is charged with gathering critical medical records so they are accessible to the new providers. A summary of care and assessment of needs should be obtained from the pediatrics medical providers and shared with the new providers.
- *Preparing the youth to manage their own health care as independently as possible*: Once the youth has become an adult, unless guardianship has been established, he or she will function as his or her own medical decision-maker. The team can identify steps to prepare the youth for this new responsibility. Activities toward preparedness could include education on the youth's chronic conditions and practice identifying and communicating symptoms, medication side effects, and other relevant information. They may need to practice preparing the logistics of a medical appointment. The individual may need scaffolding with making and attending appointments until they demonstrate competency in independent management of health-care needs. The I/DD toolkit [18] created by the Vanderbilt Kennedy Center provides various resources, including checklists and training to support individuals with I/DD to access improved health care.

Accessing Meaningful Activities and Relationships

"The key to happiness is having something to do, someone to love, and something to look forward to" [19]. This is a quote attributed to many over the years that seems to pass the popular intuition test. In addition, it had been described by psychiatrist Viktor Frankl and, in modern times, has been supported by research in the literature on positive psychology. Martin Seligman, the psychologist who has coined the term positive psychology in the late 1990s, has studied happiness or well-being and in his book *Flourish* outlines the five elements of well-being: pleasure, engagement, relationships, achievement, and meaning. Seligman's research shows a relationship between meaning and happiness. People who have a strong sense of meaning or purpose in their lives have the highest level of happiness [20]. Applying this to the quote above, we may translate "something to do" as "engaging in meaningful and pleasurable activities"; "someone to love" as "having meaningful and pleasurable relationships"; and "something to look forward to" as "having meaningful goals that lead to a sense of achievement once accomplished."

Karyn Harvey, building from Seligman's findings, has applied these principles of happiness and well-being to individuals with I/DD in her work on *Trauma Informed Behavioral Interventions* for persons with intellectual and developmental disabilities. Harvey has created a "Happiness Assessment" recognizing the importance of supporting individuals in their pursuit of happiness rather than solely trying to control their behavior with outside rewards. The Happiness Assessment is an interview tool used to support individuals in identifying their sources of pleasure, engagement, relationships, achievement, and meaning [8]. In each of the five sections, there are 3–8 statements prompting the individual to list relevant answers. For example, "These are the things I like to do when I want to totally relax" or "I am happiest when I am doing this (an activity)." As described earlier, this information is the first step in self-determination. The individual must be able to identify personal preferences and sources of happiness in order to use them to determine interests and guide life choices.

Transitional age youth generally have had the experience of a day structured around school, where they hopefully have been presented opportunities to learn and socialize with others. Because these opportunities have generally been carefully crafted and scheduled in the students' day, individuals likely have not had experience with finding these opportunities on their own. The activities in which the transitioning youth will engage in their new communities are critical. Unstructured time and boredom can result in loss of acquired skills, feelings of isolation and depression, and, ultimately, a loss of hope for a fulfilling life.

TAY with continuing education or employment goals are more likely to find themselves in situations providing the three key elements for happiness – meaningful activity, relationships, and goals. For youth who do not express interest in either continuing education or employment, their need to engage in meaningful activities and relationships remains just as important. The challenge for the supporting team becomes how to encourage TAY to consider additional options for active participation in the community and provide access to social interactions. Use of the Happiness Assessment [8] as an evolving conversation that takes place over one or more sessions with a trusted adult support may help illuminate options for meaningful engagement in activity that the youth may not otherwise be able to independently produce or verbalize. These could include creative volunteering opportunities (e.g., animal shelters, local food pantries, libraries) or engaging in structured recreational and community activities (e.g., participating in Special Olympics or joining a local church group).

In addition to identifying meaningful activities for the transitional age youth, conversations facilitated through the Happiness Assessment are opportunities to strengthen a positive relationship with a trusted adult and also support the youth's development of a positive identity and self-image. Individuals with I/DD often are unhappy and frustrated when the focus is on the negatives and what he or she is *not* (e.g. *not* the person who gets married, drives, or plays on a professional sports team). The Happiness Assessment conversation allows for focus on the positives (e.g., preferences and strengths) which support positive identity development [21].

Some transitional age youth continue to experience significant behavioral health challenges that may prevent meaningful involvement in community activities in which they would like to be able to participate. Very often, these TAY lack the skills to manage their emotions, which often results in maladaptive behavioral expression of feelings commonly labeled "challenging behaviors." Applied behavioral analysis (ABA) has long been considered the gold standard for treatment of challenging behaviors in children with I/DD. ABA, simply put, is determining the function of a behavior (e.g., access to attention or tangibles or sensory stimulation; escape/avoidance) and then changing the environment (offering positive reinforcements) in order to change the specific behavior. While ABA can be very effective in a highly structured and controlled training environment (e.g., special school), it can be difficult to generalize effectively in a less-controlled community setting. In addition, a frequent critique is that ABA fosters dependence on external control and reward for specific behaviors rather than fostering internal growth and development of skills contributing to healthy and effective emotion regulation. Because replacement behaviors in ABA plans do not tend to integrate instruction of comprehensive skills to build internal emotion regulation capacity, pairing of ABA behavior strategies and emotion regulation skills training can be valuable for TAY.

For TAY with I/DD who are experiencing challenging behaviors, incorporating social and emotional skills training as early as possible in the transition plan may be helpful with increasing the individual's potential for successful interactions in the community. One evidence-informed adaptation of dialectical behavior therapy (DBT) skills training for the I/DD population is described by Julie Brown, MSW, PhD. In her "Emotion Regulation Skills System for Cognitively Challenged Clients: A DBT®-Informed Approach," she provides a path for individuals to learn to manage and cope with strong emotions internally themselves rather than having to be managed by others externally (using medications, restraints or restrictions, hospitalizations or incarcerations) [22]. Individuals using the Skills System® learn tangible self-regulation skills. The Skills System® is a set of nine skills and three system tools that guides the person through a process of becoming aware of their current situation, intentionally directing their attention, and activating behaviors that are in service of personal goals.

The first three skills in the Skills System® are a core progression that forms the foundation for skills use. The first skill, named Clear Picture, leads the person in being aware of, or having a "clear picture" of the current moment (mindfulness) that includes naming and rating their current feeling using the Feelings Rating Scale (0- to 5-level scale). This scale is used later in the progression by individuals to choose which skills they can use effectively at their feeling level and how many skills are needed to manage the current situation. Getting a Clear Picture also includes noticing current thoughts and urges. When using the second skill, called On-Track Thinking, individuals appraise whether their current urges will be helpful ("on-track") in reaching their goal, or would be antithetical ("off-track") to their goal. If the urge is "off-track," the individual turns around off-track thoughts, uses cheerleading, and makes a Skills Plan. The third skill, called On-Track Action, assists the individual to execute goal-directed behaviors.

Skills 1, 2, and 3 are the foundation of an individual's Skills Plan. Skills 4–9 offer the individual a repertoire of adaptive responses that are added to this foundation depending on their level of emotion and the needs of the situation. For example, Skill 4, labeled Safety Plan, offers scaffolding to manage risky situations. Skill 5 describes New-Me Activities: activities that help focus, self-soothe, distract, or have fun. Skills 1–5 (Clear Picture, On-Track Thinking, On-Track Action, Safety Plan, and New-Me Activities) are designed to help individuals downregulate and maintain safety, if they are at higher levels of emotion. The remaining skills, 6–9, can only be used effectively when a person is calm enough to be thinking clearly. These "Calm-Only" skills provide structured strategies for problem-solving, expressing oneself, getting something that one wants from another person, and having on-track relationships with oneself and others [22].

Special Considerations for Blind and Visually Impaired TAY

According to the Centers for Disease Control and Prevention's Vision and Eye Health Surveillance System (VEHSS), 1.7% of children less than 18 years of age in the United States have a vision problem that cannot be corrected with eyeglasses or contact lens [23]. Visual acuity is historically measured by the clarity or sharpness of vision of an average person reading a standardized chart at 20 feet distance (i.e., "20/20" vision). Variances to visual acuity compare to this standard (e.g., an individual with 20/40 vision reads at 20 feet what the majority of people can read at 40 feet distance). The World Health Organization [24] defined blindness as a visual field of less than ten degrees or visual acuity less than 0.05, with optimal correction in the stronger eye. Low vision

(LV) was defined as a visual field of less than 20 degrees or visual acuity less than 0.3 but equal to or greater than 0.05, with optimal correction in the stronger eye [24]. The term "visually impaired" (VI) includes both LV and blindness. In the United States, the definition of "legally blind" is visual acuity of 0.1 (20/200) or less in the better eye with the best possible correction, or visual field of 20 degrees or less [25].

Visual impairment in children and adolescents is heterogeneous in etiology, and causes of vision loss in children can include genetic factors, alterations in embryonic development, central nervous system damage, perinatal complications, trauma, progressive disorders, and infectious diseases of the eye. In higher-income countries, cortical visual impairment (CVI) and optic nerve anomalies (i.e., optic nerve hypoplasia and optic nerve atrophy) are the most common causes of pediatric visual impairment, while retinopathy of prematurity (ROP), cataracts, glaucoma, and non-accidental injury are the most common avoidable causes of pediatric VI. The causes of childhood VI in lower-income countries have historically involved congenital anomalies, infectious diseases of the eye (e.g., measles), and nutritional deficiencies (e.g., vitamin A deficiency), but this pattern is shifting over time to resemble the causes seen in higher-income countries [26]. Some youth with visual impairment have additional disabilities including learning disabilities, deafness/hard of hearing, medical diagnoses, and/or physical limitations which must also be taken into consideration when planning for transition. Students who are deaf or hard of hearing in addition to visual impairment have very unique needs, and this population of students will be covered later in this chapter.

According to the National Center for Education Statistics (2017), 1% of high school completers and 1% of undergraduates reported having a vision disability [27]. As with all transitional age youth, youth with blindness and low vision have variability in their transition preferences and requirements. The interests and aspirations of TAY with visual impairment should provide direction for transition planning. As is the case for sighted youth, individual goals for TAY with VI may include postsecondary education, vocational training, supported employment, adult services, independent living services, and/or community participation.

According to the US Department of Education's *Digest of Education Statistics* (2017), 53.1% of transitional age youth with disabilities were competitively employed, while only 34.1% of youth with visual impairments were competitively employed [28]. Several barriers to successful transitioning have been identified for youth with VI including transportation limitations, limited access to assistive technology (AT), lack of access to coordinated transition services while in high school, and negative employer attitudes about hiring individuals with VI [29]. A 2015 study on vocational rehabilitation (VR) services and outcomes for transitional age youth with VI documented the importance of individualizing VR services to promote long-term career success for TAY with VI [30]. Each transition plan requires a coordinated effort among team members including the youth, their families, teachers, guidance counselors, and rehabilitation professionals. The youth's team should discuss issues related to orientation and mobility needs such as using public transportation, getting around as a non-driver or driver with low vision, and the options of using a white cane or a guide dog. (Of note, the majority of dog guide programs require handlers to be a minimum of 16 years of age to be partnered with a dog guide.) The team should also discuss the youth's skills related to money management, time management, organizational skills, compensatory skills, and daily living skills.

Successful transitioning for youth with VI requires recognition that becoming independent is not equivalent to doing everything oneself. Independent adults also know how to seek and obtain necessary supports. Some of the rehabilitation professionals who work with and provide support to individuals with VI include:

- *Teachers of Students with Visual Impairments (TVI)*: Professionals with training in how VI affects development and learning
- *Certified Orientation and Mobility Specialists (COMS)*: Professionals who teach individuals with VI to travel safely and independently in

their environments (including use of canes and/or guide dogs when necessary)

- *Low Vision Specialists/Certified Low Vision Therapists (CLVT)*: Professionals (often optometrists or ophthalmologists) who are trained in low vision and assist individuals with maximizing functioning of useful vision, such as use of optical devices.
- *Certified Vision Rehabilitation Therapists (CVRT)*: Professionals who instruct persons with vision impairments in the use of compensatory skills and assistive technology
- *Certified Assistive Technology Instructional Specialists for People with Visual Impairments (CATIS)*: Professionals who help determine which assistive technology (AT) will best meet a person's needs, such as electronic video magnifiers or computers with screen-reading software
- *Vocational Rehabilitation Counselors*: Professionals who assist youth with employment by providing guidance and counseling, vocational assessment, job placement, and/or other services

High school students with VI are expected to receive instruction in the Expanded Core Curriculum (ECC) which includes education in nine areas: *assistive technology (AT), career education, compensatory skills, independent living skills, orientation and mobility (O&M), recreation and leisure, self-determination, sensory efficiency, and social interaction skills*. The ECC includes individualized instruction, as needed, in reading and writing with Braille, using optical devices, and visual and sensory efficiency. As students with VI progress through high school, one standard goal is to become increasingly independent in advocating for their own visual needs in all settings and to know their rights and responsibilities. Students are encouraged to set goals for their future while understanding their own unique assets, challenges, and needs for accommodations. For students with VI, the high school educational team ideally will continuously review the student's Individualized Education Plan (IEP) and develop an Individual Plan for Employment (IPE) in line with the student's vocational strengths, capabilities, and interests. The education team must help the student understand their disability and how to self-advocate for accommodations in higher education and employment settings.

An important aspect of transitioning to college or the workforce for youth with VI is proficiency in the use of assistive technology (AT). According to the Assistive Technology Act of 1998, assistive or adaptive technology refers to "...products, devices, or equipment…that are used to maintain, increase or improve the functional capabilities of individuals with disabilities." AT enables people with disabilities to accomplish daily living tasks by assisting in communication, education, work, or recreation activities, thus enhancing independence and quality of life. For individuals with VI, AT refers to any adaptive device or software program that helps to overcome the barriers presented by vision loss. Examples of AT for individuals with VI include screen readers, screen magnification devices, video magnifiers (closed-circuit television system or CCTV system), adaptive keyboards, and Braille displays. It is common for individuals with VI to use a combination of AT to perform tasks effectively and efficiently.

Transitioning to College

For some students, transition planning will include transitioning to a college or university program. Vision loss can increase the challenges a student has in college, so students must master skills from the ECC prior to attending a secondary institution. College students with VI must self-advocate in order to have a successful on-campus experience. The US Department of Education's Office for Civil Rights (OCR) notes that it is very important for transitioning youth to have accurate knowledge about their civil rights under legislation including Section 504 of the Rehabilitation Act of 1973, the Individuals with Disabilities Education Act (IDEA) of 1990, and the Americans with Disabilities Act Amendments Act (ADAAA) of 1990 [31]. Colleges and universities are not permitted to make any "preadmission inquiry" about a student's disability status. Colleges and universities may inquire about an applicant's ability to meet essential program requirements provided that such inquiries are not designed to reveal disability status. If an applicant meets the essential requirements for admission, an institution may not deny that applicant admission simply because of a disability.

In order to be successful, college-bound students with VI must be taught specific skills including how to request appropriate accommodations for common college entrance exams (i.e., SAT, ACT) which may include use of Braille, large print, extended testing time, frequent breaks, and/or fewer items on each page. Students must learn how to apply for scholarships or loans. There are multiple scholarships made available specifically to VI students. College-bound students must be able to order educational materials in accessible formats (such as large print, Braille version, or audio version). The student must establish a relationship with the college's Office for Students with Disabilities and coordinate services with a vocational rehabilitation (VR) agency. Students with VI must develop a plan for how to travel/navigate independently on campus and how to self-advocate with professors. Students must be proficient in their use of necessary assistive technology and know how to hire and work with a "live reader." Even with all the available technology, there are times when enlisting a human reader is the best option. Electronic devices can break down or may not handle needed material such as handwritten documents or complicated charts, diagrams, or mathematical and scientific formulae.

Many colleges and universities are implementing Universal Design for Learning (UDL) which is a framework for inclusive education and is key for integrating blind and visually impaired students into the college classroom. UDL addresses and modifies course curricula that exclude any student, particularly those with a disability that affects their ability to learn in a class setting. For students with VI, this includes making auditory software, large-font presentations, and/or Braille materials available. Other components of UDL include making note-takers, readers, and scribes available in classes; ensuring that classrooms and on-campus facilities are accessible; and allowing students to take exams and give presentations using alternative formats.

Transitioning to the Workforce

Transitional age youth with VI entering the workforce must also learn specific skills in workplace readiness. On-the-job training opportunities, internships, and job shadowing experiences can teach students with VI basic employability skills and help students determine what type of career they may wish to pursue.

The Workforce Innovation and Opportunity ACT (WIOA) of 2014 requires states to reserve funds to provide pre-employment transition services to youth with VI [32]. Vocational rehabilitation (VR) agencies are responsible for making five required activities available to students with VI:

- Job exploration counseling
- Work-based learning experiences
- Counseling on opportunities for enrollment in comprehensive transition or postsecondary educational programs at institutions of higher education
- Workplace readiness training to develop social skills and independent living skills
- Instruction in self-advocacy

Vocational rehabilitation services provided to VI youth entering the workforce can include disability-related augmentative skills training such as orientation and mobility, training in the use of low vision devices, and training in Braille in addition to job search assistance, job placement assistance, on-the-job supports, transportation services, and reader services.

TAY seeking employment must know their legal rights as a person with a visual impairment under the Americans with Disabilities Act Amendments Act (ADAAA) [33]. Individuals must know how to communicate their accommodation needs to their employer. Employers are not legally required to provide all requested accommodations. Employers are not legally allowed to ask if the job seeker is visually impaired; however, if one has an obvious visual impairment, then the employer can ask about potential need for accommodations. Employers can ask about one's ability to perform essential functions of the potential job. The potential employee does not legally have to disclose their visual impairment prior to getting a job unless an accommodation is needed. Employers must provide reasonable accommodations to employees with disabilities unless the accommodation would pose an undue hardship such as a significant difficulty or expense to the employer. Examples of reasonable accommodations for employees with VI include use of a larger monitor or optical magnifier and better lighting at one's work station. Personal items (such as eyeglasses or cane) that are used both on and off the job are the responsibility of the employee. Potential employees can develop a disclosure statement to share during interviews describing how they access printed information and electronic information, how they produce written communication, and how they use visual devices. AT Giesen et al. [29] showed that risk factors for lower success rates for competitive employment for youth with VI include female gender, African American race, greater severity of visual impairment, and having additional disabilities (both cognitive and non-cognitive). This study also showed that factors promoting successful employment include early work experience, services related to job placement, and college attendance [29]. Cimera et al. [30] revealed that increased intensity of VR services, on-the-job supports, job placement services, job development services, receipt of qualified reader services, and receipt of assistive technology were associated with successful employment outcomes for transitional age youth with VI [30].

Overall, successful transition from youth to adulthood for students with blindness or low vision depends on creating a realistic, thorough transition plan. Whether a youth with VI wishes to pursue postsecondary education or enter the workforce, an individualized transition plan can increase the likelihood of a positive outcome.

Special Considerations for Deaf, Hard of Hearing, and Deaf-Blind TAY

This section will focus on the unique challenges impacting individuals who are deaf, hard of hearing, or deaf-blind as they navigate the transition to young adulthood via starting college or entering the workforce. According to the American Community Survey for 2018, there are over 11.5 million deaf or hard of hearing individuals in the United States; and of these, approximately 300,000 are between the ages of 5 and 17 years of age, and over 600,000 are between the ages of 18 and 34 years [32]. There is a critical need to prepare these young people for independent living and postsecondary life.

Deafness can be defined as any degree of hearing loss that affects the audiological and medical condition of hearing [33]. Medically, the terminology of hearing impairment has been associated with someone who has any degree of hearing loss. Culturally, however, the definition of deafness excludes the use of the term hearing impairment but focuses more on the self-identification and culturalization of the individual as a member of the Deaf community. Individuals with full or profound hearing loss prefer the term Deaf, with a capital D, to refer to their cultural identity, their sense of shared experiences, shared language, shared history, and a shared sense of identity. The use of the term deaf, with the small d, is representative of the medical and audiological condition of deafness, without the identification of cultural identification as seen with Deaf. Hard of hearing individuals are those with any degree of hearing loss outside of severe to profound deafness. They may retain some hearing, aided or unaided. They may or may not consider themselves part of the Deaf community. Deaf-blindness is a unique classification for individuals with any degree of hearing loss in conjunction with any degree of visual impairment. In terms of cultural identity, these individuals often self-identify with the Deaf community, and communication often consists of some form of tactile sign language (interpreter signing within the hand of the individual) [34].

There are three basic types of hearing loss [35]:

- *Conductive Hearing Loss*: Happens when sound cannot get through the outer and middle ear; sound transmission is blocked. This may be due to fluid in the middle ear (such as from colds or allergies), ear infection, damage to the eardrum itself (such as a hole or tear), or due to blockage in the ear canal (ear wax or benign tumor). Conductive hearing loss makes it harder to hear soft sounds and may muffle louder sounds. Depending on the underlying reason, this type of hearing loss may not be permanent.
- *Sensorineural Hearing Loss*: Happens when there is damage to the inner ear or the nerve from the ear to the brain. This type of hearing loss is permanent, ranging in severity from mild to profound.
- *Mixed Hearing Loss*: This is a combination of the other two types of hearing loss. While the sensorineural part of the hearing loss tends to be permanent, the conductive part may be correctable.

Every state and territory in the United States has instituted the Early Hearing Detection and Intervention (EHDI) program in which all newborns are screened for hearing loss. The goal is early identification and early intervention for those in need of services [36]. Newborns who do not pass the screening undergo a diagnostic evaluation by 3 months of age and then are enrolled in early intervention programs by 6 months. Throughout childhood and adolescence, children are enrolled in programs and provided with assistive technologies to aid in their communication throughout their schooling. Nonetheless, many of these individuals still experience challenges with communication and may have variable levels of proficiency for the English language, written as well as spoken.

Hearing assistive technology systems (HATS) are devices to aid in hearing and oral communication for individuals who are hard of hearing. Individuals who are profoundly deaf may or may not benefit from assistive technologies, and many tend to prefer sign language as primary mode of communication [37]. For individuals with hearing loss who would benefit from hearing assistive technology systems, there are several that can be helpful:

- *FM Systems*: Frequency modulation systems; works like a tiny radio with its own frequency. Consists of two parts: the microphone that the speaker wears and the receiver that the individual with hearing loss wears (worn separately or as part of the hearing aid).
- *Infrared Systems*: Uses light waves to send sound waves across a room. Infrared systems change sounds to light waves and sends them to a receiver worn by the individual with hearing loss (worn separately or as part of the hearing aid). The receiver turns the light waves back into sound.
- *Induction Loop Systems*: These systems work with hearing aids. A loop wire is placed throughout the room (either under the carpet or through the ceiling). The wire is connected to a microphone for the speaker. An electrical current moves through the wire creating an electromagnetic field in the room. Most hearing aids have a setting on them to pick up the signal so the individual can hear the speaker.
- *One to one Communicators*: Similar system as FM but more direct for communication with just one person. A microphone is used by an individual, and the sound goes directly to the person with hearing loss for more direct communication.
- *Coupling Accessories*: These are augmentation accessories for hearing aids or cochlear implants that can connect directly to media devices to enhance hearing on the phone, through a computer/tablet or use with a television.

There are assistive visual technology programs which convey information visually for deaf and hard of hearing individuals. These types of programs are often used in conjunction with hearing assistive technologies for optimal access to information. Examples of assistive visual technology include [38]:

- *Visual Alerting Systems*: These devices help alert individuals to sound using visual support. These include specially designed alarm clocks, smoke detectors, doorbells, timers, baby monitors, and phone alerting equipment. These devices may also use vibration to enhance alerting.
- *Captioning*: This is a crucial means to aid deaf/hard of hearing individuals access to media such as television or movies. Most televisions enable closed captioning options (logo of CC in a box). Many movie theaters offer both closed captioning (only the individual who requests the captioning can see it through a special device used in the theater) or open captioning (where the captions appear on the screen and everyone can see them).
- *Real-Time Transcription*: These are transcription services that provide instant translation of spoken word into written English. One commonly used system is the communication access real-time translation (CART) which transcribes oral English into text, word for word. The CART provider may be on-site or remote. There are some available technologies which provide automatic translation of spoken language to text, although this is more prone to errors and may complicate communication, particularly if the speaker has an accent or if the system is not used to the speaker's unique patterns.

Research has shown that deaf and hard of hearing youth tend to lag behind their hearing peers in readiness for college and postsecondary young adult life, often scoring lower on college entrance examinations such as the SAT and the ACT [39]. Much of this is likely due to the differences in proficiency in English language skills. However, it has been noted that deaf and hard of hearing students tend to perform better on the ACT than the SAT because the ACT asks questions on what students learn in high school [40]. The National Deaf Center on Postsecondary Outcomes published findings in their publication "Deaf People and Educational Attainment: 2017." This publication notes that as of 2015, 83% of deaf adults graduated high school compared to 89% of their hearing counterparts, leaving a gap of 6%. The largest gap was noted in completion of bachelor's degree in which 18% of deaf and hard of hearing students graduated college compared to 33% of their hearing counterparts, a gap of 15%. Statistics such as these emphasize the need for effective transition planning and preparation for deaf and hard of hearing students [41].

Transition programs help students and parents plan for life after high school and help students develop the skills necessary for independent living. Deaf and hard of hearing students need additional preparation to aid them in the transition process. Given the unique challenges as a result of their hearing loss, deaf and hard of hearing students need to be prepared to navigate communication barriers and learn how to self-advocate to ensure appropriate accommodations in postsecondary education settings as well as in the job force. The National Deaf Center in their published document Transition Planning Tip Sheet notes that effective transition planning is one that (a) is student focused, (b) is student involved, (c) is family involved, (d) utilizes transition assessments as needed for additional information, (e) regularly checks with student about barriers encountered and accommodations needed, and (f) includes annual reviews with updates and revisions as indicated [42].

With these goals in mind, transition planning starts at an early age for deaf/hard of hearing students. In 2006, the Transitional Skills Guidelines was developed at the Laurent Clerc National Deaf Education Center K-12 Program at Gallaudet University. The Transition Skills Guidelines provide a hierarchy of specific skills to prepare the young deaf/hard of hearing student over the course of their K-12 education for a successful transition to adulthood. The transition skill sets are arranged in five distinct standards [43, 44] (Table 15.2).

Table 15.2 Transition Skills Guidelines, Laurent Clerc National Deaf Education Center K-12 Program at Gallaudet University

Standard 1: Student demonstrates the skills necessary to advocate for him/herself
Self-awareness
Rights and responsibilities
Advocacy/empowerment
Interpreting
Standard 2: Student demonstrates knowledge of educational and career exploration, preparation, and planning
Career exploration and planning
Career materials exploration
Educational planning
Learning/study skills
Life-role planning
Standard 3: Student develops positive and practical work habits, skills, and attitudes within a work environment
Pragmatics/social courtesies
Conflict resolution
Teamwork
Work attitudes
Work habits
Time management
Resource management
Workplace communication
Feedback
Performance and self-assessment
Self-management
Technology and equipment
Standard 4: Student demonstrates the knowledge of one's community, one's role in the community, and available resources
Emergency and environmental safety
Personal safety
Money/banking
Purchasing/negotiating
Nutrition
Clothing
Hygiene
Standard 5: Student demonstrates the knowledge of one's community, one's role in the community, and available resources
Travel
Community roles and responsibilities
Leisure
Community resources
Community services

Transitioning to College and Postsecondary Education

In a position statement on Communication Access Services for Students who are Deaf or Hard of Hearing at Colleges and Universities, the National Association of the Deaf posited that "American colleges and universities and vocational rehabilitation agencies are responsible for providing communication services for students who are deaf or hard of hearing. By doing so, this allows for equal access to academic and postsecondary educational programs as required by the Americans with Disabilities Act Amendments Act and by the Rehabilitation Act. Services included under this provision include sign language and oral interpreters, computer assisted real time transcription services (CART), captioning service, note-taking services, assistive listening systems and related communication accommodations (determined by the needs of the student)" [45].

The Individuals with Disabilities Education Act (IDEA) was originally enacted in 1975 to ensure that children with disabilities are afforded a free and appropriate public education, just like other children. There have been revisions over the years including the Individuals with Disabilities Education Improvement Act of 2004, with additional specifications and objectives for children with disabilities ages 3–22 years [46].

Per IDEA and Americans with Disabilities Act Amendments Act (ADAAA), all public colleges and universities must ensure deaf and hard of hearing students have equal access to the full educational experience and that accommodations are provided for each student in attendance. Typically, the college or postsecondary education setting will have a formal office for student support services. In earlier education settings, accommodations are made through an Individualized Education Plan (IEP). However, once the young person goes to college, they will need to have the ability to self-advocate and request the accommodations that they need to be successful in college [47]. Typical basic accommodations for academic success at the college level for the deaf/hard of hearing student may include any or all of the following:

- Certified American Sign Language Interpreting Services
- Hearing assistive technology systems
- Assistive visual technology
- Note-taking services (so the student can focus on the lecture)
- Examination accommodations (extended time, signed examinations)
- Student life accommodations (such as visual fire alarms in classroom buildings and dormitories)

Basic accommodations are put into place so that the deaf/hard of hearing student can access auditory information in the classroom. However, the basic level of accommodation does not provide the students with full access to the learning environment which often extends to outside the classroom and is not always associated with positive outcomes. In this regard, the National Deaf Center on Postsecondary Outcomes gathered literature and research to develop a model of accommodations to meet the needs of deaf/hard of hearing students. They identified six key components of access to ensure a fuller, richer experience for the deaf/hard of hearing student (using the acronym ACCESS) [48]:

- **Attitudes**: Campus climate that welcomes and integrates deaf/hard of hearing students in all aspects of campus life
- **Campus Technology**: Flexible technologies that are readily available in all campus settings – from classrooms to locker rooms – for deaf students to fully access and experience the college environment
- **Communications**: Efficient and effective communication and information delivery that allows deaf students to maximize formal and informal learning opportunities
- **Environment**: Accessible physical and online spaces that accommodate and adapt to a wide variety of deaf student experiences
- **Services**: Comprehensive accommodations for deaf students that are readily available, reliably provided, individually customized, and monitored for quality and success
- **Social Engagement**: The complete immersion in a campus experience that seamlessly includes deaf students in all events and opportunities to socialize, network, and connect

Transitioning to the Workforce

There is a notable gap in employment data between deaf and hearing people in the United States. In the report "Deaf People and Employment: 2016" published by the National Deaf Center on Postsecondary Outcomes, they note that in 2014, only 48% of deaf people were employed, compared to 72% of hearing people. Deaf and hard of hearing youth who transition directly to the workforce will also need transition skills to prepare them for the labor market [49]. As is true for students transitioning to college, those going directly into the workforce need a comprehensive transition program. The Transition Skills Guidelines, noted earlier in this section, is utilized whether the student ultimately chooses college or straight to work. The Pre-Employment Transition Services (Pre-ETS) Guide is a program to aid students in preparation for work and career pathways. It is a program utilized in conjunction with vocational rehabilitation (VR) to aid students in their transition from high school to vocational training, college, and the workforce mandated by the Workforce Innovation and Opportunity Act (WIOA). WIOA requires 15% of every state VR agency's federal budget be allocated to provide specific education and training to prepare students with disabilities for postsecondary pathways. The National Deaf Center on Postsecondary Outcomes has further adapted the Pre-Employment Transition Services Guide to address the unique needs of deaf and hard of hearing students [50].

The Pre-ETS categories of consideration are:

- *Job exploration counseling*: Includes discussion on student's interests, abilities, and capabilities in relation to careers and activities to increase career awareness and labor market

- *Work-based learning experiences*: Provides immersive learning opportunities for students to understand the working world and develop knowledge and skills for future careers
- *Counseling on postsecondary opportunities*: Includes discussions on student's career pathway; involves planning for postsecondary training and education depending on the interests and capabilities of the student and their aspirations
- *Workplace readiness training*: Involves the development of social and independent living skills required for any career
- *Instruction in self-advocacy*: Includes strategies to empower deaf students to assert, pursue, and take responsibility for their needs and goals necessary for life after high school

Since its launch in 2017, the National Deaf Center for Postsecondary Outcomes (housed at the University of Texas at Austin) has maintained its mission to "close the substantial gaps in education and employment that exist for deaf people in the United States and its territories" [51]. They are a technical assistance and dissemination center federally funded by the Department of Education's Office of Special Education Programs (OSEP) and Rehabilitation Services Administration to provide evidence-based strategies at the local, state, and national levels. Their website offers practical guidelines based on literature review and evidence-based strategies for students, families, and educators to maximize the potential for student success in their postsecondary lives. Role models are critical to anyone interested in a particular career path, and this is particularly true for deaf and hard of hearing students. In response, the National Deaf Center highlights success stories in their series #DeafAtWork (also showcased on the National Association of the Deaf's website) as well as #DeafSuccess [52].

Deaf and hard of hearing youth need to be educated about their legal rights in the workforce. These are governed by federal and state laws. The laws are outlined on the National Association of the Deaf's website page on Employment Laws and Regulations. For federal employees, the rights are covered under Section 501 of the Rehabilitation Act of 1973 which requires the federal government to practice affirmative action to hire and promote employees with a disability. The regulations of this law also require equal access to training and promotion opportunities and to make reasonable accommodations for employees with disabilities. For employees of private companies or state/local government, the rights are protected by Title I of the Americans with Disabilities Act Amendments Act (ADAAA), which prohibits discrimination against persons with disabilities and to make reasonable accommodations available [53].

"Reasonable accommodations" refers to modifications or adjustments to a job or work environment such that the individual with disability will have access to an equal employment opportunity. Per ADAAA, reasonable accommodations ensure:

- An equal opportunity in the application and interview process
- An employee to perform essential functions of the job
- An employee to enjoy equal benefits and privileges of employment

Reasonable accommodations for deaf and hard of hearing individuals may include:

- Video phones, captioned telephones, amplified phones
- Instant messaging and email services
- Assistive listening systems and devices
- Visual alerts for audible alarms and messages
- Modifications to reduce ambient noise levels
- Captioned audiovisual information
- Service animals in the workplace
- Policies and procedures for qualified interpreters or CART services as needed

Transition Issues for Students Who Are Deaf-Blind

The discussion on special considerations for transitional age youth who are deaf would be remiss if there were no additional discussion of the considerations for youth who are deaf-blind. Deaf-blindness means any combination of hearing loss with visual impairments. It is the combination of these sensory-related losses that could cause such severe communication and other developmental and educational needs that they cannot be accommodated in special education programs solely for children with deafness or children with blindness [54].

Transition issues present unique challenges for students who have deaf-blindness as there is so much variability based on the severity of either the hearing loss or vision loss. The prevailing misperception is that individuals who are deaf-blind have full and total loss of both senses, but the reality is that deaf-blindness encompasses any degree of hearing loss with any degree of visual impairment. Even a mild or moderate loss of one of these senses can cause significant challenges when combined with some degree of loss of the other sense. The potential to achieve and succeed for deaf-blind individuals often depends on how much the deaf-blind individual uses their residual vision and/or hearing as well as appropriate accommodations and individual interventions. Helen Keller is probably the most recognized US citizen with deaf-blindness. She made the astute observation that "Because I cannot see or hear, the thoughtless suppose life must be a blank for me" [55]. Nothing could be further from the truth given her legacy and successes in all areas of her life.

One of the most important areas to consider when working with a student who is deaf-blind is the ability to access information in their environment and communicate with others. This impacts all areas of an individual's life including learning, relationships, recreation, and vocation. Transition planning is as critical for individuals who are deaf-blind as it is for those with deafness or blindness. It is important to take the unique challenges that someone with both vision loss and hearing loss face as they make transition to young adulthood. The same types of transitional guidelines previously discussed for other students with sensory loss are useful with students with deaf-blindness, incorporating the needs of both sensory losses.

In 2008, the Perkins School for the Blind worked with experts in deaf-blindness to develop the guide called *Deafblindness: Educational Service Guidelines* [56]. These guidelines provided a framework to provide programming for students who are deaf-blind including transitional planning. In 2016, the National Center on Deaf-Blindness (NCDB) Transition Work Group revised their transition planning guide to reflect current practices, requirements, trends in education, transition planning, and vocational rehabilitation [57]. Transition planning helps students with deaf-blindness prepare for their future lives, should they opt for college, vocational training, employment, as well as aid in their community and personal lives in adulthood. As with all transition planning, it is critical to start early. While the IDEA mandates transition planning by the age of 16 years, the process for transition planning for deaf blindness is best if started even earlier. Transition planning is an individualized process that includes the student, the family, and the educational system with collaboration with vocational rehabilitation and adult developmental disability agencies. The NCDB converted their transition planning guide into a format that can be easily used by students, families, and professionals. The guide was renamed the READY Tool (Readiness Evaluation of Transition to Adulthood for Deaf-Blind Youth) [58].

The READY Tool is organized by four age groups: prior to age 14 years; ages 14–17 years; ages 18–21 years; and ages 22–26 years. With each age range, the tool is further divided into three areas which are rated on the status or progress ("started," "progressing," or "completed"):

- **Transition Assessment**: Includes recommendations regarding assessment processes and practices to help the team gather information needed for transition and adult-life planning
- **Transition-Related Education Programming**: Describes best practices for educational programming to prepare students and young adults for all aspects of adult life (e.g., independence, adult living, employment, community engagement)
- **Team Collaboration and Adjustments**: Outlines practices to ensure the team has the right members and processes at each stage of transition planning and instruction

Successful transition from childhood to young adulthood involves early, intensive, and individualized transition planning for students who are deaf, hard of hearing, and deaf-blind. Comprehensive resources are available for students, parents, and educators to promote a successful transition to postsecondary endeavors. Given the special and unique needs facing deaf, hard of hearing, and deaf-blind students, the collaborative approach with adult vocational rehabilitation services and disability services are integral components to the transition.

Conclusion

Youth with disabilities will experience multiple changes over the course of their transition to adulthood which require navigating complex systems to access and secure supports and services specific to the needs of the individual. A comprehensive well-coordinated transition plan is helpful in alleviating challenges and preventing loss of critical supports and benefits. An effective plan uses the guiding principles of self-determination, timeliness, and cross-system collaboration and addresses anticipated challenges across life domains including housing, meaningful activities, relationships, professional services, legal capacity needs, and benefits. There are multiple types of disabilities that can affect a person's thinking, learning, communication, vision, hearing, movement, social relationships, and mental health. Special considerations for youth with low vision, blindness, or deafness have been examined, as well as additional psychosocial therapy for youth with emotion regulation skills deficits. Assessing the individual's abilities and preferences in each life domain helps create a transition plan reflective of the individual's abilities and needs while being aligned with the person's hopes for their future.

References

1. Merriam-Webster. (n.d.). Self-determination. In Merriam-Webster.com dictionary. Retrieved July 2020 from https://www.merriam-webster.com/dictionary/self-determination.
2. Joint position statement of AAIDD and The Arc. Self-determination. 2018. Retrieved July 2020 from: https://www.aaidd.org/news-policy/policy/position-statements/self-determination.
3. Ryan RM, Deci EL. Self-determination theory: basic psychological needs in motivation, development, and wellness. New York: Guilford Publishing; 2017.
4. PACER Center, Inc. National Parent Center on Transition and Employment. Self determination. 2019. Retrieved from: https://www.pacer.org/transition/learning-center/independent-community-living/self-determination.asp.
5. Perske R. The dignity of risk and the mentally retarded. Ment Retard. 1972;10(1):24–7.
6. Wolpert J. The dignity of risk. Trans Inst Br Geogr. 1980;5(4):391–401.
7. Bremer CD, Kachgal M, Schoeller K. The National Center on Secondary Education and Transition (NCSET). Self-determination: supporting successful transition. Table: "promoting self-determination in youth with disabilities: tips for families and professionals". 2003. Retrieved July 2020 from http://ncset.org/publications/viewdesc.asp?id=962.
8. Harvey K. Positive identity development: an alternative treatment approach for individuals with mild and moderate intellectual disabilities The NADD Press, 2009 addendum for happiness assessment download. Retrieved July 2020 from: http://pid.thenadd.org/.
9. Joint Position Statement of AAIDD and The Arc- Guardianship. 2019. Retrieved July 2020 from https://www.aaidd.org/news-policy/policy/position-statements/guardianship.
10. Centers for Medicare and Medicaid Services. Home and community-based services. Retrieved July 2020 from: https://www.medicaid.gov/medicaid/home-community-based-services/home-community-based-services-authorities/home-community-based-services-1915c/index.html. http://www.ssa.gov/OP_Home/ssact/title19/1915.htm and https://www.macpac.gov/subtopic/behavioral-health-services-covered-under-hcbs-waivers-and-spas/.
11. Position statement of The Arc – Medicaid. Retrieved July 2020 from: https://thearc.org/policy-advocacy/medicaid/.
12. Regulatory requirements for home and community-based settings. Retrieved July 2020 at: https://www.medicaid.gov/sites/default/files/2019-12/requirements-for-home-and-community-settings.pdf.
13. Home and community based settings toolkit. Retrieved July 2020 at: https://www.medicaid.gov/medicaid/home-community-based-services/guidance/home-community-based-settings-requirements-compliance-toolkit/index.html.
14. Compilation of the Social Security Laws. Provisions respecting inapplicability and waiver of certain requirements of this title. Retrieved July 2020 from: https://www.ssa.gov/OP_Home/ssact/title19/1915.htm.
15. Got Transition. Six core elements of health care transition. Retrieved July 2020 from: https://www.gottransition.org/six-core-elements/).

16. Caren Steinway, Jennifer Gable, Sophia Jan | policylab.chop.edu (Spring 2017).
17. Corbin S, Holder M, Engstrom K. Changing attitudes, changing the world: the health and health care of people with intellectual disabilities. Washington, DC: Special Olympics International; 2005.
18. Vanderbilt Kennedy Center. The IDD Toolkit. Retrieved July 2020 from: https://iddtoolkit.vkcsites.org/.
19. The quote is by the American clergyman George Washington Burnap (1802–1859), published in Burnap's *The Sphere and Duties of Woman: A Course of Lectures (1848)*, Lecture IV.
20. Seligman M. Flourish. New York: Free Press; 2015.
21. Harvey K. Positive identity development: an alternative treatment approach for individuals with mild and moderate intellectual disabilities: The NADD Press; 2009.
22. Brown J, editor. The emotion regulation skills system for cognitively challenged clients: a DBT informed approach. New York: Guilford Press; 2015.
23. Vision & Eye Health Surveillance System (VEHSS), Centers for Disease Control and Prevention, Vision Health Initiative, [online] [accessed Nov 11, 2019]. URL: https://www.cdc.gov/visionhealth/vehss/project/index.html.
24. World Health Organization. International classification of diseases for mortality and morbidity statistics (11th Revision). 2018. Retrieved from https://icd.who.int/browse11/l-m/en.
25. Social Security Act of 1935, Pub. L. No. 74-271, Stat. 620 (1935).
26. Solebo AL, Teho L, Rahi J. Epidemiology of blindness in children. Arch Dis Child. 2017;102(10):853–7. https://doi.org/10.1136/archdischild-2016-310532.
27. U. S. Department of Education. National Center for Education Statistics. Characteristics and outcomes of undergraduates with disabilities. NCES 2018-432. December 2017. Retrieved from https://nces.ed.gov/pubs2018/2018432.pdf.
28. U.S. Department of Education, National Center for Education Statistics. Digest of education statistics: Among special education students out of high school up to 8 years, percentage attending and completing postsecondary education, living independently, and working competitively, by type of disability: 2007 and 2009. 2017. Retrieved from https://nces.ed.gov.
29. Giesen J, Cavenaugh B. Transition-age youths with visual impairments in vocational rehabilitation: a new look at competitive outcomes and services. J Visual Impair Blind. 2012;106(8):475–87.
30. Cimera R, Rumrill P, Chan F, Kaya C, Bezyak J. Vocational rehabilitation services and outcomes for transition-age youth with visual impairments and blindness. J Vocation Rehabilit. 2015;43(2):103–11.
31. U.S. Department of Education, Office for Civil Rights. Transition of students with disabilities to postsecondary education: a guide for high school educators. Washington, D.C. 2011. Retrieved from http://www.ed.gov.
32. U.S. Census Bureau, American Community Survey. Disability characteristics. 2018. Retrieved from https://data.census.gov/cedsci/table?q=S18&d=ACS%201-Year%20Estimates%20Subject%20Tables&tid=ACSST1Y2018.S1810.
33. National Association of the Deaf. Community and culture: frequently asked questions. 2020. Retrieved from https://www.nad.org/resources/american-sign-language/community-and-culture-frequently-asked-questions/.
34. Miles B. Overview of deaf-blindness. 2008. Retrieved from https://www.nationaldb.org/info-center/deaf-blindness-overview/.
35. American Speech-Language-Hearing Association. Types of hearing loss. 2020. Retrieved from https://www.asha.org/public/hearing/Types-of-Hearing-Loss/.
36. American Speech-Language-Hearing Association. Early hearing detection and intervention (EHDI). 2020. https://www.asha.org/Advocacy/federal/Early-Hearing-Detection-and-Intervention/.
37. American Speech-Language-Hearing Association. Hearing assistive technology. 2020. Retrieved from https://www.asha.org/public/hearing/Hearing-Assistive-Technology/.
38. Laurent Clerc National Deaf Education Center. Assistive technologies for individuals who are deaf or hard of hearing. 2014. Retrieved from https://www3.gallaudet.edu/clerc-center/info-to-go/assistive-technology/assistive-technologies.html.
39. Qi S, Mitchell R. Large-scale academic achievement testing of deaf and hard-of-hearing students: past, present, and future. J Deaf Studies Deaf Educ. 2012;17(1):1–18.
40. Raising Deaf Kids. Getting ready for college. 2020. Retrieved from http://www.raisingdeafkids.org/learning/transition/college/preparing.php.
41. Garberoglio C, Cawthon S, Sales A. National Deaf Center on Postsecondary Outcomes: deaf people and educational attainment in the United States. 2017. Retrieved from https://www.nationaldeafcenter.org/sites/default/files/DeafPeopleandEducational_Attainment_white_paper.pdf.
42. National Deaf Center on Postsecondary Outcomes. Transition planning. 2020. Retrieved from https://www.nationaldeafcenter.org/resource/transition-planning.
43. Anderson K. Transition planning for adulthood. 2012, updated 2016. Retrieved from https://successforkidswithhearingloss.com/for-professionals/transition-planning-for-adulthood.
44. Laurent Clerc National Deaf Education Center. Transition skills guidelines. 2006. Retrieved from https://www.chs.ca/sites/default/files/uploads/transition_skills_guidelines_2006.pdf.
45. National Association of the Deaf. Position statement on communication access services for students who are deaf or hard of hearing at colleges and universities. 2002. Retrieved from https://www.nad.org/about-us/position-statements/position-statement-on-colleges-and-universities/.

46. Individuals with Disabilities Education Act. About IDEA. 1975. Retrieved from https://sites.ed.gov/idea/.
47. National Association of the Deaf. Americans with Disabilities Act. 2020. Retrieved from https://www.nad.org/resources/civil-rights-laws/americans-with-disabilities-act/.
48. Palmer J, Cawthon S, Garberoglio C, Ivanko T. ACCESS is more than accommodations: 2018–2019 deaf college student national accessibility report. National Deaf Center on Postsecondary Outcomes. 2019. Retrieved from https://www.nationaldeafcenter.org/sites/default/files/POD_Report_WEB.pdf.
49. Garberoglio C, Cawthon S, Bond M. Deaf people and employment in the United States. National Deaf Center on Postsecondary Outcomes. 2016. Retrieved from https://www.nationaldeafcenter.org/sites/default/files/Deaf%20Employment%20Report_final.pdf.
50. National Deaf Center on Postsecondary Outcomes. Pre-employment transition services guide. 2020. Retrieved from https://www.nationaldeafcenter.org/topics/pre-ets.
51. National Deaf Center on Postsecondary Outcomes. Our mission. 2020. Retrieved from https://www.nationaldeafcenter.org/mission.
52. National Deaf Center on Postsecondary Outcomes. #DeafSuccess. 2020. Retrieved from https://www.nationaldeafcenter.org/deafsuccess.
53. National Association of the Deaf. Employment laws and regulations. 2020. Retrieved from https://www.nad.org/nerc/laws-and-regs/.
54. Individuals with Disabilities Education Act. Statutes and regulations. 2017. Retrieved from https://sites.ed.gov/idea/statuteregulations/.
55. Center for Disabilities, Sanford School of Medicine, University of South Dakota. Transition guide for students who are deaf-blind. 2008. Retrieved from http://www.transitionplanningasia.org/sites/tpa.perkins-dev1.org/files/uploaded-files/transitionguide.pdf.
56. Perkins School for the Blind. Deafblindness: educational service guidelines. 2008. Retrieved from https://www.nationaldb.org/media/doc/DESG_Final.pdf.
57. National Center of Deafblindness. Transition planning. 2020. Retrieved from https://www.nationaldb.org/info-center/educational-services/transition-planning/.
58. National Center of Deafblindness. READY tool: readiness evaluation of transition to adulthood for deaf-blind youth. 2017. Retrieved from https://www.nationaldb.org/products/ready-tool/.

16 Emerging Personality Structures in Transitional-Age Youth

Erin Ursillo, Kristen Sundin,
and Gerrit I. van Schalkwyk

Key Points

- Transitional age youth may have vulnerabilities in their personality structure which impact their ability to function and engage in mental health treatment.
- Given the developmental nature of this period, these vulnerabilities may change and evolve over time and with the influence of treatment.
- It is therefore necessary to conceptualize patients across multiple dimensions, and not to rely purely on a categorical diagnosis of a personality disorder.
- A strengths-based approach to formulating and treating transitional age youth with personality vulnerabilities assumes patients can achieve functional recovery while the work of understanding the determinants of their personality is ongoing.

E. Ursillo · K. Sundin
Adolescent and Young Adult Services, Butler Hospital, Providence, RI, USA
e-mail: eursillo@butler.org; ksundin@butler.org

G. I. van Schalkwyk (✉)
University of Utah Department of Pediatrics, Salt Lake City, UT, USA
e-mail: gerrit.vanschalkwyk@hsc.utah.edu

Introduction

During transition from adolescence to adulthood, the abrupt change in environment from school to college or the workplace poses new challenges. Biological vulnerabilities may begin to manifest with psychiatric symptoms. Transitional age youth (or young adults, as we will refer to them in the text of this chapter) will approach these challenges with diverse core beliefs, values, and coping mechanisms – these and other dimensions define their emerging personality structure. The personality structure of a young adult is of importance when they are in treatment for mental health concerns, as the structure can drive behaviors that may interfere with, complicate, or enhance treatment.

Personality should be understood in developmental terms, and yet there is limited longitudinal data informing our understanding of how vulnerable personality styles may shift over time. In one systematic review [9], a core finding from the 18 included studies was the persistence of symptomatic and functional difficulties for individuals diagnosed with borderline personality disorder prior to age 19 into middle adulthood. A particularly informative longitudinal, twin study identified both the general decline in borderline personality traits from adolescence into adulthood, the potential variability of symptoms over the lifespan, and the increasing importance of genetic factors in influencing symptom presenta-

V. Chan, J. Derenne (eds.), *Transition-Age Youth Mental Health Care*,
https://doi.org/10.1007/978-3-030-62113-1_16

tion in adulthood relative to adolescence [4]. One way to make sense of existing data is to conclude that there is a significant relationship between adolescent and adult symptoms of borderline personality traits but that the potential for variability – and, indeed, improvement – exists.

Transitional age youth who continue to struggle with personality vulnerabilities are an important focus of clinical attention. It is important that the reality of their challenges be acknowledged and not minimized, but a strengths-based approach remains indicated, as there is hope for significant improvement over time. In this chapter, we begin with a conceptual overview wherein we (1) situate personality within the broader biopsychosocial formulation, (2) contrast the framework of "emerging personality structure" from the categorical term "personality disorder," and (3) substantiate the case for a strengths-based approach with a focus on specific unhelpful behaviors rather than an attempt to understand the origins of personality vulnerabilities.

We then discuss how specific clinical services can be designed to best support the care of young adults, given how we make sense of their emerging personality structures in treatment. This will include descriptions of how patients are cohorted according to age and developmental context and the importance of levels of care that provide necessary clinical support without negatively reinforcing unhelpful behaviors.

Finally, we use a case example of an individual with a poorly integrated sense of self, and diverse, primitive coping mechanisms. We describe the clinical approach both in terms of individual and group engagement and, most importantly, how the overall continuum and context of care helped the patient access strengths, avoid crisis, and show clinical improvement.

The goals of this chapter are to describe a specific theoretical approach to personality structure in young adults, to outline how we have designed clinical services to be responsive to this approach, and to bring the material to light through a case example. We hope that this will leave readers with a usable description that feels both conceptually robust and clinically resonant.

Personality Structure in a Biopsychosocial Context

Personality disorders are conceptualized in diverse ways. In the *Diagnostic and Statistical Manual of Mental Disorders* (DSM-IV), personality disorders were operationalized as categorical disorders, with specific signs, symptoms, and a threshold symptom burden required in order to make the diagnosis [1]. When revised for the DSM-5, consideration was given to adopting a more dimensional approach to personality disorders that would allow for situating patients on certain personality spectrums. However, this approach was ultimately not adopted, and a categorical approach remains prominent [2]. A contrasting, psychoanalytic-informed approach described by McWilliams [7] situates patients both in terms of the level of organization of their personality (e.g., neurotic, borderline, or psychotic) and its quality (e.g., obsessional, histrionic, and others). In this schema, level of organization is determined by the extent to which there are an integrated sense of self, a capacity for reality testing, and the maturity of defense mechanisms. As such, patients may, for example, be viewed as primarily narcissistic or obsessional, but at a borderline level of organization, allowing for more nuance in characterizing the overall personality style.

In addition to the approach taken in organizing the patient's personality, it is also important to consider how their personality fits into a broader formulation of their overall presentation. Within the biopsychosocial approach, personality disorders are frequently situated within the psychological dimension of the formulation (whereas constructs like a depressive episode may more commonly be understood as part of the biological formulation). However, emerging findings in neuroscience emphasize the importance of brain-based factors in driving some of the features which characterize personality vulnerabilities including concepts like emotion regulation, belief formation, and sensory factors [6, 8]. The distinction between what is characterized as "biological" vs "psychological" is largely informed by tradition or the degree of neuroscientific understanding that may be applied to a specific area, and although clinically useful at times, the arbitrary nature of this distinction must be appreciated.

Given this nuance, it is important to consider whether a strict, categorical approach to personality diagnosis is suitable for the clinical task at hand. In young adults, there are additional reasons to believe that a more sophisticated lens is necessary. Firstly, the brains and identities of young adults continue to be in a state of development, and it is possible that certain vulnerabilities may lose clinical significance later in life. Secondly, the young adult period is frequently characterized by exposure to fast-changing and complex environments which may amplify specific emotional and behavioral patterns; in adult life, a more predictable and selected environment might mitigate these vulnerabilities (e.g., obsessional tendencies may be impairing in college but of minor significance in certain career paths). Thirdly, there exists the availability of robust treatment approaches to support the development of resilience, emotion regulation, affect awareness, and other psychological strengths within young adults, and a conceptual approach to personality disorders should be able to capture the potential for improvement in the underlying vulnerabilities over time.

The approach taken to emerging personality structure within our young adult programs is rooted within the biopsychosocial formulation but involves a more in-depth consideration of how biological, psychological, and social factors may act to influence individual examples of thoughts, feelings, and behaviors. For example, rather than attributing self-injury as a symptom of borderline personality disorder, we would seek to define the ways in which this symptom is driven. We would consider biological vulnerabilities (such as abnormal impulse control, negative attention bias, sensory integration deficits, and others), psychological weaknesses (e.g., a tendency to rely on dramatic behaviors to gain the attention of others), and social factors (e.g., the presence of accommodation, in the form of a family member who quickly provides care for a self-inflicted injury). Through this approach, we are able to empathize with the patient by validazting that some aspects of their experience are outside of their control (such as the degree of anger, sadness, or anxiety they feel in response to a specific trigger) and that we will seek to provide them with evidence-based tools to address these challenges (e.g., medication). We also frankly state that the patient's choices affect the underlying problem and that their style of interacting with the world and meeting their own emotional needs is maladaptive. Evidence-based psychotherapeutic interventions are offered to address these vulnerabilities, and the importance of agency, choice, and engagement are strongly emphasized.

Although patients are given freedom to reflect on the early determinants of their personality structure, this is de-emphasized in their initial treatment. Rather, the focus is on helping patients live a life in accordance with their own values. Addressing core vulnerabilities in personality structure and functional recovery can proceed while the ongoing work of understanding earlier experiences occurs in parallel. In the next section, we describe how clinical services may be structured in order to safely support this approach to both conceptualizing and supporting the emerging personality structure of young adults.

Strengths-Based Programs for Youth with Emerging Personality Vulnerabilities

Although empirically based treatments exist for working with individuals with personality disorders, these approaches do not fully define how to best organize clinical services to maximize safety and engagement. In this section we describe a strengths- and resilience-based approach to the task and review how this approach may facilitate the feasible and safe delivery of care to young adults with personality vulnerabilities. This approach is currently implemented within the adolescent and young adult service line at Butler Hospital. For context, the full list of programs in our adolescent and young adult service line can be found in Table 16.1. The approach will be

Table 16.1 Organization of services at Butler Hospital, where approach is applied

Adolescent and young adult service line		
Levels of care	Programs for ages 13–17	Programs for ages 18–26
Inpatient	Adolescent Inpatient Unit	General Adult Inpatient
Partial hospital (PHP)	Adolescent Partial Hospital	Young Adult Partial Hospital
Intensive outpatient (IOP)		College IOP for college students True Self IOP for LGTBQ+ individuals Pathfinders IOP for those with college/workplace delay Connect IOP for individuals with social difficulties
Outpatient	Transitional Outpatient Clinic for post-inpatient/PHP visits	Transitional Outpatient Clinic for post-inpatient/PHP visits Ongoing outpatient psychiatric treatment Aftercare groups

described in more general chapters for the remainder of the chapter.

The first consideration that warrants discussion is why should young adult services exist at all? In many systems, individuals aged 18–26 years old will access treatment with adults of all ages. However, there are critical advantages to providing a separate treatment environment for young adults. Notably, young adults have a more consistent set of themes to their social experiences, including differentiation from parents, college attendance, early engagement in the workforce, and the pursuit of increasingly serious romantic relationships. The college experience, in particular, is characterized by a unique set of stressors which may influence the development of mood symptoms [5]. To the extent that PHP and IOP treatment models rely on group therapy, it is more likely that peer identification and the therapeutic benefits of shared experience and camaraderie will be achieved within this narrower age cohort.

A young adult program facilitates the strength-based approach which characterizes the overall treatment philosophy described in this chapter. Individuals with emerging personality vulnerabilities are exposed to age-matched peers who work toward success in their social, personal, academic, and vocational lives. This influence offers models for more adaptive styles of engagement with the world and, indeed, in treatment. In our experience, patients in young adult-specific programs are, on average, significantly more motivated and hopeful for a goal of good functional recovery since many are newer to treatment. This provides a more promising environment for fostering motivation for change in those with vulnerable styles, in contrast to cohorts who have chronic mental health issues and long-term functional impairment who may foster less adaptive perspectives on treatment and recovery which can negatively impact a group-based program.

A second important feature is the availability of both full-day and after-school programs. This offers a practical range of schedules, delivering care without negatively reinforcing patterns of avoidance, addressing provider enmeshment (e.g., a patient who appears to rely on crisis situations to connect with a preferred provider may benefit from being cared for in a setting where that provider is not involved in their care), escalating level of care without readmission, and titrating containment (e.g., by asking patients to initially take responsibility for their safety for an evening, then for a weekend, and then for the days when the program is not active). For example, if an individual appears to be accessing a PHP in order to avoid an emotionally taxing work environment, we may empathically suggest that they instead access IOP in order to work through this challenge without engaging in avoidance. On the other hand, individuals who request frequent check-ins for unsafe thoughts in IOP may be better cared for in a PHP until they are more contained.

Programs that allow for more intense clinical contact have substantial advantages at certain times for individuals with emerging personality disorders. These settings may allow the team to more quickly gather the rich clinical data necessary for the crafting of a detailed biopsychosocial formulation. This formulation may guide treatment within the PHP/IOP setting and also when individuals step down to outpatient care. Further, these treatment environments, which provide daily clinical support and safety planning, may allow for individuals to remain in the home environment despite ongoing high-risk behaviors [3]. PHP and IOP may provide the necessary scaffolding to help patients with emerging personality disorders maintain safety and some degree of functioning during crisis.

Inpatient settings may achieve many of the same goals as PHP and IOP but may fail to meet the patient's clinical needs and preferences. A frequent narrative, expressed particularly by college students in our community, is that they withhold reporting feelings of hopelessness and suicidality to prevent being hospitalized. PHP and IOP greatly extend the ability of providers to tolerate such high-risk thoughts, as one need only be reassured that patients will commit to safety for the hours between program days, rather than days to weeks. Inpatient settings may also serve to negatively reinforce avoidant behaviors, in so far as admission temporarily removes all obligations toward schools, friends, and family and even for one's own ability to stay safe. Although inpatient admission may be critical for some, there are considerable advantages to having an alternative. In the next section, we will describe a case of an individual with significant features of an emerging personality disorder, and how both the clinical approach and structure of services were important in facilitating her care.

A Case Example

Sarah was a 24-year-old, single, white, straight female who presented to our partial program as a referral from an outside psychiatric facility for continued treatment of depression after an overdose attempt on aspirin.

Socio-cultural History

Sarah, the patient, was born in South Carolina to married parents and has a younger sister. They moved together to Brattleboro, Vermont, when she was 4 years old. The patient reports her parents were divorced when she was 12 years old. Her father moved out and eventually remarried. She now has a step-sibling and a step-mother. She reports that she and her younger sister lived with her mother for the remainder of their childhood. As a child she experienced physical abuse at the hands of a family friend – no legal charges were pressed after this was discovered. The patient attended regular elementary, middle, and high school. She required support in high school related to difficulties with self-injury. She did acceptably academically aside from missing a high number of days in high school for mental health treatment. She completed some college but has not been able to continue in classes due to mood. She has never successfully held a job. She reported that she has few friends, no significant history of romantic relationships, and a significantly strained relationship with her parents and sister. She has no specific religious or spiritual beliefs.

Past Psychiatric History

Sarah identified feeling depressed and anxious as early as middle school. She received her first therapy when her parents divorced at age 12 years. She entered treatment again when her family found out that she had been physically abused. She was in and out of treatment programs and individual therapy during high school due to the mood symptoms and self-injury and received services in school to address this concern. She had two suicide attempts after high school which she greatly minimizes and was treated on an inpatient unit on both of these occasions. She did not find any level of care she had experienced helpful to date. She reported that most of the treatment she had received actually made her feel worse.

Events Leading to Hospitalization

Prior to this psychiatric event, the patient was on medical leave for college related to ongoing mental health difficulties and was living with her mother. She shared that her main goals at this time were to complete school, get a job, and become independent of her family. She felt the current living arrangement was triggering for her both because of her relationship with her mother and because of how disconnected she felt in her home community, having previously attended college at a school in a neighboring state. The patient felt that her decline in mood would be best managed by again attending an out of state school – she then chose to move across the country alone to Oregon and try to make a life for herself there. While in the new environment in Oregon, she attempted to re-focus on her goals to complete college and find a job. Unfortunately, she did not get accepted into any of the schools she applied to, nor was she successful in holding down a job.

As a result of mood decline and lack of success in Oregon, the patient then had to move back home with her mother. At home, she became quickly overwhelmed as it reminded her of how far she was from her goals. These feelings were further complicated by the knowledge that her sister was succeeding independently at college. She endorsed increased sleep, over-eating, low energy, amotivation, anhedonia, and feelings of hopelessness and worthlessness. As her symptoms worsened, she reported feeling quite stuck with no sense of purpose. It was at this time that she attempted overdose on ibuprofen and was psychiatrically hospitalized and sent to our program for further treatment.

Mental Status

The patient engaged with good eye contact and was neatly dressed and groomed. She was articulate with a normal rate, volume, and rhythm of speech. She had a restricted, negative affect, and her mood was depressed and irritable. Her thought form was linear, and her thought content was characterized by negative self-worth and hopelessness. She showed no perceptual disturbances or cognitive difficulties and sustained attention well. She had limited insight into many aspects of how her own choices intersected with her current situation, and her judgment appeared poor as it related to her choices in how she navigated interpersonal challenges.

Biology

The patient endorsed feelings of worthlessness, hopelessness, anhedonia, low mood, suicidal thoughts, increased sleep, and increased appetite. She showed a tendency to filter information around her through a negative lens which complicated her ability to experience positive emotions. She met criteria for a major depressive episode and did report a history of depression.

Psychology

Interpersonally, the patient was dismissive of the philosophy of the program and at times devalued treatment, group leaders, physicians, peers in groups, and her individual therapist. She expressed irritation with her parents for "forcing" her into treatment and not providing her what she felt was necessary for her to succeed in Oregon (financial means). She expressed distorted beliefs of what parents and treatment providers should be able to do for her as well as a significant misunderstanding of what her role should be in therapy (i.e., that therapy would "fix" her with little effort on her part; this belief appeared to underlie why no treatment had been successful thus far). She appeared to have little awareness into how her personality structure might interfere with her ability to succeed in school, in work, or in relationships. She appeared to have strong defenses that made her seem off-putting and difficult to build rapport with. She appeared to have poor distress tolerance creating difficulties in all spheres of her life.

Treatment Engagement

Sarah had a difficult time engaging in both individual and group sessions. She tended to focus on the ineffectiveness of the program and how groups would not be helpful for her. She frequently challenged group leaders and made no efforts to mingle with her peers. She used individual sessions to criticize the therapist rather than considering her role in her own wellness.

Treatment Course

Sarah completed 4 days of treatment in the partial hospital setting, where the average length of stay is 5–7 days. Due to her mental status, lack of treatment engagement, and personality structure, the treatment team encouraged her to focus on her role in treatment, rather than focusing on her perceived limitations of the program. We highlighted and emphasized the concept of radical acceptance: no treatment is perfect, but no treatment will be successful until she fully engages and accepts the help. She was dismissive of these recommendations and of all attempts to shift treatment discussions in that direction. She was offered treatment with a low dose of quetiapine in addition to the SSRI she was taking prior to admission to target her irritability, poor mood, and anxiety, but the patient was unwilling to participate in other aspects of treatment to the extent necessary that these interventions could be implemented and monitored safely.

Formulation

Sarah allowed us to conduct a family meeting on the last day of treatment in our program where we presented the following formulation:

Biologically, Sarah has symptoms and views consistent with depression. She has episodes of low mood, anhedonia, poor sleeping and eating patterns, feelings of worthlessness, hopelessness, and suicidal thoughts. She has difficulties with her ability to experience positive emotions and tends to negatively filter information. Psychologically, she has significant difficulty with distress tolerance, struggles to use effective coping mechanisms, and tends to undermine and end situations rather than experience vulnerability and anxiety. These vulnerabilities had an impact on the patient's ability to engage in the program much like all of her past treatment experiences. Socially, the patient had not experienced consistent and significant consequences for her avoidance, which had led to accommodation of symptoms both by the patient and her caretakers. This also contributed to a low threshold for tolerating distressing, challenging, or unwanted feelings, making it nearly impossible for the patient to achieve her main goals in life.

Recommendations

Going forward, it was strongly recommended that her parents clearly communicate expectations to avoid any accommodation of symptoms and drive the patient toward adaptive coping and recovery. It was recommended that the family create a new plan for supporting the patient's return to independence. This plan was advised to include a healthy balance of financial support (to foster some independence while she got back on her feet) and engagement in mental health treatment, something they had not been successful in clearly defining prior to this treatment.

Outcome

Although the patient was not pleased with her partial hospital experience, both the patient and parents were able to say that they had never before been presented with a clear formulation of the patient's difficulties. The parents were able to agree upon a clear set of expectations and guidelines for the patient after discharge that seemed feasible and realistic. The family reported a greater understanding of what each needed to do to promote wellness.

The Case in Context

This case, despite its complexity and challenges, illustrates how the approach to personality structure described in this chapter helped to conceptualize a difficult patient, communicate a formulation to the family, make some progress in treatment, and identify barriers to ongoing recovery. Further, it highlights some of the considerations relevant to the structure of young adult services.

At the outset, the patient described concern about being in a psychiatric hospital, and a PHP offered an alternative which was somewhat more acceptable. Despite the presence of both dynamic and static risk factors for suicide, the PHP allowed us to both provide the patient with treatment in a setting that met her needs and maintain good oversight of her safety. Secondly, the patient's thoughts and feelings were in line with themes that are particularly relevant to the young adult experience – college attendance, stress related to social media, and negotiating emerging independence with parents. It is likely that engagement would have been even more difficult to achieve if the patient had not been cohorted with peers who could hold some perspective on these issues.

Our therapeutic approach was first informed by our formulation, with a focus on immediate opportunities to improve the patient's functioning. An awareness of the patient's emerging personality vulnerabilities facilitated clear treatment team communications around the importance of her choices and engagement on her overall recovery. We were able to support the family in identifying sources and examples of accommodation. We minimized opportunities where the patient would be able to regress, or unproductively restate her disempowered narrative where nothing was helpful and there were no solutions. Although the patient marginally made use of the tools she was being offered, we were able to reach a shared understanding of what would need to change if she were to recover.

Conclusion

Supporting young adults with significant vulnerabilities in their personality structure is a significant clinical challenge, but may be best facilitated by a structured and nuanced approach to formulation, combined with optimally designed clinical services. In this chapter, we described an approach taken at one hospital and illustrate the ways in which formulation and thoughtful organization of clinical services may support teams working with challenging cases. Although it is rare that we are able to completely describe every vulnerability in a young adult's personality, we consider it a success if we are able to help develop a shared understanding of what these vulnerabilities are, where they intersect with the brain and environment, what we can do to help, and what critical choices the individual will need to make to promote sustained recovery.

References

1. American Psychiatric Association. DSM-IV. Washington, DC; 1994.
2. American Psychiatric Association. DSM-5; 2013.
3. Bateman A, Fonagy P. Effectiveness of partial hospitalization in the treatment of borderline personality disorder: a randomized controlled trial. Am J Psychiatry. 1999;156(10):1563–9. https://doi.org/10.1176/ajp.156.10.1563.
4. Bornovalova, Marina A., et al. "Stability, change, and heritability of borderline personality disorder traits from adolescence to adulthood: A longitudinal twin study." Development and psychopathology. 2009;21(4):1335.
5. Byrd DR, McKinney KJ. Individual, interpersonal, and institutional level factors associated with the mental health of college students. J Am Coll Heal. 2012;60(3):185–93. https://doi.org/10.1080/07448481.2011.584334.
6. Fineberg SK, Steinfeld M, Brewer JA, Corlett PR. A computational account of borderline personality disorder: impaired predictive learning about self and others through bodily simulation. Front Psych. 2014;5:AUG), 1–7. https://doi.org/10.3389/fpsyt.2014.00111.
7. McWilliams N. Psychoanalytic diagnosis: understanding personality structure in the clinical process. New York, NY: Guilfrod Press; 2020.
8. Vega D, Soto À, Amengual JL, Ribas J, Torrubia R, Rodríguez-Fornells A, Marco-Pallarés J. Negative reward expectations in Borderline Personality Disorder patients: neurophysiological evidence. Biol Psychol. 2013;94(2):388–96. https://doi.org/10.1016/j.biopsycho.2013.08.002.
9. Winsper, Catherine, et al. "Clinical and psychosocial outcomes of borderline personality disorder in childhood and adolescence: a systematic review." Psychological medicine. 2015;45(11):2237–51.

Part III

Special Populations

17 What's Next After High School: Exploring Options Through Identification of Individual Strengths and Needs

Edwin Williamson, Walter E. Wilson Jr, Kayla Pope, and Catherine Fuchs

Key Points

- A subset of transitional age youth (TAY) with mental illness do not attend a 4-year college.
- Child and adolescent psychiatrists need to be familiar with the demographics of this group of TAY and understand the unique challenges they face in managing their psychiatric conditions.
- Research on effective support for adolescent development may be helpful in identifying opportunities to support the transition to adulthood.
- A unique subset of TAY with mental illness includes those in the juvenile justice system.

E. Williamson (✉) · W. E. Wilson Jr · C. Fuchs
Vanderbilt University Medical Center, Department of Psychiatry & Behavioral Sciences and Pediatrics, Nashville, TN, USA
e-mail: Edwin.williamson@vumc.org; Catherine.fuchs@vumc.org

K. Pope
Winnebago Mental Health Institute, Oshkosh, WI, USA

Introduction

Child and adolescent psychiatrists (CAPs) play a significant role in guiding teens through the transition to young adulthood. The transition team should revolve around the young person as the central figure and include parents or guardians, clinicians, and support services. Youth have many paths to a successful transition to adulthood, including unique educational tracks, entering the workforce, or joining the military or through the juvenile justice system. Educational pursuits often include options such as trade school or community college. It is also possible that a young person will struggle to get a job or succeed in an independent living situation outside the home.

TAY refers to older adolescents (15–16 years) to young adults (24–26 years) [1]. Quantification of this stage is complicated by the nuances of culture, brain development, and the intersection of environment and genetics. Clinicians, parents, teachers, and administrators must consider the impact of mental illness onset and progression on development. Dr. Maryann Davis, Ph.D., Professor of Psychiatry at the University of Massachusetts, defines developmental transition as "the natural process of maturation and increased competence and the social changes that are associated with this natural process." Davis explores the impact of mental illness on psychological development while considering the addi-

V. Chan, J. Derenne (eds.), *Transition-Age Youth Mental Health Care*,
https://doi.org/10.1007/978-3-030-62113-1_17

tional challenges facing TAY due to institutional transitions which may lead to loss of services [1].

Access to institutional resources varies with ethnicity, socioeconomic status, adverse life events including victimization, and the impact of mental illness on developmental milestones. Cognitive development may be inconsistent due to the high comorbidity between behavioral disorders and learning disorders. Individuals with mental illness may have compromised problem-solving skills; this may be exacerbated by the presence of complicated family systems. Disadvantaged youth with mental illness may have additional risk factors as they transition to adulthood due to the potential absence of necessary skills for independent living [1].

Studies in neuroscience recognize the ongoing maturation of the brain at least to the age of 25 years, introducing opportunity for the continued development of executive function skills, reasoning, and impulse control [2]. Epigenetics emphasizes the consideration of the dynamics between the environment and individual development [2]. This highlights the value of thoughtfully considering the stepwise trajectories available to TAY with mental illness as they determine their social, educational, and vocational paths [3].

Successful transition requires a juxtaposition of developmental pathways with individual goals. This process varies with individual life circumstances. Too often, normal is defined as achieving developmental milestones "on time." An alternative construct is to recognize that individual vulnerabilities and strengths lead to variability in when youth achieve developmental milestones [4]. The CAP should review the domains of development including emotional and cognitive growth, motor skills, social skills, and language acquisition including language processing and receptive and expressive language. CAPs can work with youth to identify the infrastructure and supports necessary to achieve goals, as well as assist with planning and accountability.

It is important to consider the perceptions and preferences of TAY as they shift their care from child to adult mental health services. A literature review by Embrett et al. identified that, as youth make the transition to adult services, they often perceive the adult services as less supportive or less helpful. This introduces increased risk that the patient may not follow through on the adult mental health referrals. A review of the US healthcare system identified that between ages of 16–17 years and 18–19 years, use of mental health services declined by 45%; service use then increased after age 20 years but never attains the level experienced at age 16 years. Similarly, the study identified that in the UK, 61% of youth receiving child services stopped participating in mental healthcare at 18 years, and 24% stopped participating in mental healthcare after age 16 years [5].

Embrett et al. reported several barriers to transition including lack of communication and collaboration between the child and adult services, silos in funding of child vs. adult services creating financial barriers, lack of education about the purpose of transition, and the cultural differences between family-focused child services and individually focused adult services. Of note, in the USA, 47 states have a disparity between the criteria for mental health services in children and adolescents and the criteria for adult mental health services based upon how mental illness is defined, with adult services reported as more limited in scope than child and adolescent services. It is notable that there is limited research on the benefits of transition programs for TAY with mental illness. The review identified characteristics of successful transition programs. Critical factors include a "lifespan approach" which addresses skill gaps in maneuvering relationships and accessing education programs or vocational services. Peer support is also helpful, as are bridge programs and transfer meetings that include case management and wraparound services to promote the transition. The CAP working with TAY should be familiar with common challenges in transition of services and should be able to help facilitate successful moves from child to adult mental health services. While clinicians and support staff are focusing on the transition of services, parents are often simultaneously thinking about goals for their child. Parents must be able to encourage appropriate separation and individuation while also providing a realistic safety net for their children. This may challenge the parents to recalibrate their hopes, dreams, and expectations. Systemic or institutional factors create barriers, potentially disrupting the TAY's ability to utilize their strengths. The CAP can serve as a guide who encourages youth to optimize strengths while also encouraging patients and families to recognize barriers [1].

We present a number of potential postsecondary pathways for at-risk TAY, challenging the perception that matriculating at 4-year college is the definition of success. We recognize that there is variability among the TAY who select different pathways. This discussion is focused on TAY with a history of mental illness prior to graduation from high school.

Vignettes

Note that all cases are a compilation of several clinical scenarios and do not represent a specific patient.

"E" is a 17-year-old girl who first presented to her psychiatrist at age 14 years with aggression, mood liability, and poor insight and judgment. Her family history was significant for bipolar disorder (bp), and she was diagnosed with bipolar disorder (BP 1). Her course included multiple medication trials and psychiatric hospitalizations, which impacted her academic progression and social experience at school. She was ultimately stabilized on an atypical antipsychotic and a mood stabilizer. She had an intact family consisting of married parents and two brothers. Her father was an accountant, and her mother was a stay-at-home-mother. While the family always expected that "E" would attend a 4-year college, the illness prevented her from being academically, socially, and emotionally prepared. As her mental status improved, she was able to identify that she felt as though she had missed out on "normal teenage activities" and used her lack of knowledge of popular movies and music as evidence. "E" chose to attend a community college for the first 2 years to prepare for transition to a 4-year college. The CAP working with her focused on stabilizing her illness in the context of her unique strengths while facilitating her transition to a general adult psychiatrist. She ultimately decided to enter the workforce after community college.

"J" is a 19-year-old young man who presented to the adult clinic as a first-year student in community college. He had a history of adolescent-onset major depressive disorder (MDD) which negatively impacted his motivation in school. His parents had a strong cultural bias against engaging in treatment for mental illness. "J" was resistant to accepting the need for support, both institutional and individual. During his first year of community college, an advisor noted him to be increasingly withdrawn and encouraged "J" to attend a mental health assessment. He initially refused, so his advisor accompanied him to the appointment in an attempt to facilitate trust in the system. At the appointment, "J" reported relapsing symptoms of MDD complicating his social, academic, and emotional development. He did not want his parents informed of his struggles due to cultural stigma and concern about cost of care potentially impacting his family. Over several months, he was ultimately able to develop a trusting relationship with his psychiatrist, who addressed his ambivalence by focusing on the conflict between his desire for treatment and his family's cultural beliefs. He completed community college and successfully transitioned to the workforce.

"M" is a 21-year-old young man who originally encountered the mental health system when he was hospitalized for suicidal ideation at the age of 16 years. Over the next several months, he was diagnosed with autism spectrum disorder (ASD) and attention-deficit/hyperactivity disorder (ADHD). He had never enjoyed school and had switched from his zoned public school to an alternative school due to emotional and academic struggles. After his hospitalization, his parents withdrew him from the alternative school, with worries that he was "in the wrong crowd" and that suicidality was "being normalized." He was referred for psychological testing; results were consistent with ASD and ADHD. He had significant mood and cognitive side effects from even small, introductory doses of mixed amphetamine salts, lisdexamfetamine and methylphenidate. He tolerated atomoxetine 18 mg but was not able to tolerate an upward titration and discontinued the medication at various intervals because he did not like how it made him feel. He enrolled in a home school program, where he struggled with organization and structure. He completed high school a year later than initially anticipated. After graduating from high school, he attended community college and failed his first semester. He worked with his CAP to have another trial of atomoxetine while applying for a job. As part of his transition care plan, the CAP guided him toward the identification of adult psychiatric services.

Demographics and Resources: Matching Who We Are and What We Need

For the large number of young adults in America who do not attend a 4-year college, community colleges and trade schools offer educational opportunities, while the military and entry-level jobs can provide employment. Despite these many options, some still struggle to find success in education or employment. The child and adolescent psychiatrist can play a crucial role in assisting the subset of TAY dealing with mental illness by supporting both the patient and their family in further personal, emotional, and social development to help them successfully navigate this developmental stage. There are some key differences in the demographics of TAY who do not attend university compared to those who matriculate at a 4-year college. Knowing the demographics of this group can help mental health clinicians understand TAY needs and potential options.

Socioeconomic Factors

Socioeconomic status is correlated with post-high school status. TAY who do not attend a 4-year college have on average a lower socioeconomic status than those who do. In public institutions, 55% of students at four colleges have parents who earn over $65,000 per year, while that is true of only 42% of students at 2-year colleges [6]. In recent years, several states have created initiatives to reduce or eliminate costs for higher education with scholarships like the Tennessee Promise program, which provides community college and technical education with no tuition cost for high school graduates, regardless of income. Other programs include the California College Promise program, the Maryland Community College Promise program, and programs in six other states, with more states considering legislation to lower or eliminate tuition [7]. Psychiatrists can assist families by addressing economic barriers and being aware of programs and opportunities outside of 4-year colleges.

Entering the Workforce

Since 1990, the percentage of TAY directly entering the workforce has decreased. For the 20–24 year age group, the percentage enrolled in school has steadily climbed, from 29% in 1990 to 38% in 2014 [8]. While the trend is increasing, most TAY are not enrolled in school. Unemployment in this group has decreased in the last 10 years, from close to 20% in the 16–24 year age group in 2010 to close to 10% in 2014, but of all age groups, this group still has the highest unemployment rate [9]. At the same time, the earning gap between those with and without college degrees has doubled in the last four decades [10]. Managing expectations and assessing developmental skills can help psychiatrists, patients, and families navigate these years.

Educational Attainment

TAY who are not enrolled in a 4-year college have diverse pathways toward educational attainment. Some have graduated from high school and attended and, subsequently, left a 4-year college. Some have not finished high school or have obtained a GED. Others are choosing to enter the workforce directly from high school. For those who hope to continue in school, factors that affect persistence and graduation rates include socioeconomic status and academic preparedness [11, 12]. Mental illness is also a large factor and is estimated to account for roughly half of school failures [13]. Knowing the multiple, often nonlinear paths that young adults take as they traverse this transitional age toward adulthood can help psychiatrists prepare patients and their families for the future.

Community College

Most research on college mental health has been focused on 4-year college populations, but there is an increasing body of research on the large community college population. In one comparison between the two populations, researchers found that while community college students were less likely than traditional college students to report diagnoses of anxiety and depression, they were more likely to report diagnoses of severe mental illness like bipolar disorder, schizophrenia, and substance abuse. Despite a higher frequency of severe mental health reports, community colleges provide less psychoeducation to their students. Some mental health protective factors, like living in a residence hall (which can be protective against suicide), are less common at community colleges as well [14]. Knowing about the higher rates of severe mental health disorders and potential resource limitations at community colleges can help psychiatrists work with students to plan for mental health needs in these academic settings.

Military

Since 1990, the military population has decreased, from over 2 million members to 1.29 million in 2016 [15]. Of the 1 million enlisted service members, about half, or 550,000, are age 25 years and younger. While the overall numbers have decreased, the military remains a stable job for many TAY. The US Department of Defense defines certain mental illnesses as disqualifying for military service. The list of mental health conditions that are identified as disqualifying can be found in the *Medical Standards for Appointment, Enlistment, or Induction in the Armed Forces* [16]. According to the Army Times 2018, eligibility for military service requires a waiver if a recruit has a history of mood disorders, substance use disorders, or self-injurious behavior. During the 13 months from October 1, 2016, to October 31, 2017, the military authorized slightly more than 1000 waivers in these categories. Documentation of treatment, remission, and current condition can be submitted for review by a military psychiatrist. Factors including date of diagnosis, current ability to handle stressful situations, and score on the Armed Forces Qualification Examination (https://afqttest.com/) affect whether a waiver will be approved [17]. The criteria for a waiver have generated discussion within the military leadership. A review of mental healthcare in the military in multiple countries identified that, once in the military, access to care is variable with multiple factors contributing to barriers and facilitators to care. Barriers include individual concerns regarding the impact of mental healthcare upon one's career, the logistics of access to care in various settings, stigma, and attitudes toward care. Factors contributing to help-seeking include support system, greater impairment in level of functioning, and beliefs about mental illness [18]. The effectiveness of interventions is difficult to study given the broad range of job and career opportunities in the military. This review suggests that screening and referral is important but contingent upon available resources. Psychoeducation is indicated in part to reduce barriers to care, peer support is useful, and availability of evidence-based interventions is important. The CAP should be familiar with the complexities of mental healthcare in the military when working with an individual transitioning into the military during the TAY years.

Substance Use in TAY

The Monitoring the Future Survey compares college (including 2-year college) to noncollege

TAY from 1975 to 2017. There has been an overall increase in the annual prevalence of marijuana use in both groups in the last decade. The lowest rates were in 2006 for college students at 30% and in 2007 for noncollege students at 32%, with an increase to 39% for college students and 41% for noncollege students in 2016, the highest in three decades. Rates of nonmedical amphetamine use were slightly higher among college students. This is likely due to attempts to improve academic performance. Opiate misuse declined during this period for the noncollege group from 9.6% to 3.2%. The overall trends for all substances have been mostly stable or slightly increasing in the last two decades, down from the higher rates seen in the 1980s. While the rates are lower than in the 1980s, the annual prevalence of any illicit drug use in TAY is over 40%. In 2018, the Monitoring the Future survey explored vaping nicotine in young adults and found that annual prevalence in college age youth was 26% (30-day prevalence, 16%) compared to noncollege age youth at 21% (30-day prevalence, 13%) [19]. Experts encourage screening for substance use in the TAY population [20].

In the military, alcohol use disorders are the primary form of substance use. Binge drinking was identified in one of every three service members in 2014 compared to one in four in the general population. Rates vary by gender with men demonstrating greater binge alcohol use than women. Close to 11% of veterans seeking care within the VA system have a substance use disorder. This population's risks include the stress of deployment, transition back to civilian life, and potential combat exposure [21]. Knowing the risks of exposure and use within this age group can help psychiatrists work with patients and families to minimize disruptions to military service due to substance abuse and to incorporate substance use-specific treatment into the overall plan.

Healthcare Access

The ability to access healthcare can change according to age. The age group with the largest portion of people without health insurance is those from ages 18 to 29 years, which encompasses the TAY population. While this group saw a dramatic decrease in the rates of uninsured after the passage of the Affordable Care Act (from 32% in 2010 to 16.9% in 2015), one in six TAY do not have health insurance [22]. Young adults as a group tend to use mental health outpatient services less than older adults but use inpatient services more frequently. Variation in insurance coverage is one factor in this pattern [23].

For those with Medicaid, depending on the specific state laws, eligibility can change at age 18 or 21 years, making it harder to obtain Medicaid in adulthood. Some patients in state custody may no longer be eligible for Medicaid as adults. The income threshold for Medicaid eligibility may be stricter at age 19 than at age 17 years. For those with private health insurance, most plans allow children to stay on their parents' health plans up to the age of 26 years. Identifying how patients will pay for ongoing outpatient care, acute episodes requiring hospitalization and medications can help patients and families plan for a more stable transition period.

TAY Involved with Juvenile Justice

The resource matching, academic access, occupational opportunity, and general adult transitions are even more complicated for TAY who have been involved with the juvenile justice system. A significant number of TAY are involved in the juvenile justice system, although the number differs from state to state due to variability in the upper age of jurisdiction of juvenile courts (15–17 years old) and the age that youth are transferred from juvenile to adult systems (18–24 years old) [24]. Transitional age youth who are justice-involved have several characteristics that make them especially vulnerable to poor developmental outcomes, contributing to a more perilous transition to adulthood. These include higher rates of mental health and substance abuse problems. They are also more likely to come from disadvantaged backgrounds, with less family support, and are more likely to have experienced trauma [25].

Mental health problems in transitional age youth who are justice- involved are significantly higher than a community-based sample. Disruptive behavior disorders are the most prevalent mental health problem, but anxiety disorders, mood disorders, and substance abuse are also significant issues. Studies looking at nonresidential justice- involved youth find 45% of males and 50% of females have met diagnostic criteria for a mental health disorder [26].

Among youth placed in a residential facility, 65–70% meet criteria for a mental health issue. Comorbidity rates are also very high. It has been estimated that 79% of justice-involved youth have met criteria for two or more mental health issues and 60% have met criteria for a substance abuse problem [27].

There are several unique barriers to accessing care for TAY in the juvenile justice system. Many are also involved in the child welfare system which can lead to diffusion of agency responsibility and problems with communication and coordination of care. Further, many juvenile justice systems have resource and insurance limitations that impact access to mental health and substance abuse treatment. One study has found that only 15% of system-involved transitional age youth with mental health problems received services to address their mental health needs [28].

Upon reentry from an out-of-home placement, TAY face additional challenges. Detention or transitions in placement may adversely affect the educational process, leading to delays in completing high school or disruption in vocational training in preparation for entering the workforce. In addition, system involvement may preclude experience in the workforce. One study has found that only 31% of youth were involved in education or work 1 year after reentry to the community [29]. The failure to reintegrate poses a significant risk factor for recidivism.

There is limited research evaluating treatment programs for justice-involved transitional age youth and there are few programs specifically designed for this population. Most of these programs rely heavily on parent and family involvement. Multisystemic therapy (MST) has been modified to address the needs of TAY, and there have been some promising pilot studies of programs such as MST for Emerging Adults (MST-EA) and Family Integrated Transitions [30]. Both of these programs have demonstrated a reduction in recidivism, and TAY participating in MST-EA also showed a decrease in mental health symptoms. Further research is needed to verify these results and to better understand what modifications in programming are most effective for this population [31].

Another promising approach has been extending foster care for transitional age youth past 18 years old to provide additional family support and financial assistance. One federal initiative is the John H. Chafee Foster Care Independence Program which provides federal dollars to support the transition to independent living. States can use funding for housing, education, vocational training, mentorship, and preventative health activities [32].

Programs that support reentry after detention or out-of-home placement have also shown some promising results, including reduced recidivism rates. The Boston Reentry Initiative (BRI) is designed to decrease recidivism rates among high-risk, violent youth. The program uses individualized reentry plans to address housing, employment, mental health, and substance abuse needs. According to https://youth.gov/youth-topics/preventing-youth-violence/forum-communities/boston/reentry-initiative, recently incarcerated inmates are screened and subsequently selected for eligibility. The program is characterized by a monthly panel of stakeholders that offer services to BRI participants as a united front – both for "life-changing opportunities" and for "severe and swift consequences for reoffending." The program also requires frequent meetings with a mentor, and case management reentry teams often follow participants for 12–18 months post-release to support individual transition plans of community reentry. The program is estimated to have reduced recidivism by 30% [33]. Another promising program is the Multidimensional Family Therapy-Detention to Community program for substance-using juveniles in justice facilities or those who are in the pre-detention phase. Like other MST programs, this intervention relies heavily on family involvement [34]. The minimum treatment dose includes 6 hours per month for the families and 4 hours per month for the individual. Local program commitment to sustainability and availability of post-detention community mental health and substance abuse treatments may be challenging.

Improving outcomes for justice-involved TAY is important and will require several things. First, more needs to be done to address structural issues which create barriers to accessing housing, education, and much needed substance abuse and mental health treatment. This is a widespread problem that will require both federal and state leadership and commitment of resources to solve. There is also a dearth of information on what works best for this population, and more research focused on interventions targeting their specific needs will guide the development of best practices.

Evolution of Developmental Concepts

Transitional age youth are in a stage of life when important decisions are made in the pursuit of identified goals. Characteristics and values unique to the individual evolve during the transitional age, leading to informed decisions based on experiences and values [31]. As noted by Embrett, critical factors for transition include the development of skills to manage relationships, school, or vocational training [5]. Students attending community college may experience stress during their transition to a new educational, cultural, and social setting. Many community colleges promote wellness programs to provide support to help the student navigate the transition [35]. Psychiatrists working with TAY must identify individual strengths while helping with the management of mental health issues, all within the context of understanding the unique demands and resources in the various trajectories chosen by their patients.

During the early 2000's, there was a notable shift in the understanding of youth development by researchers from a focus on problematic behaviors ("deficit"-emphasized perspective) to recognition of an interplay of genetics, social environment, resources, and relationships [31]. Several researchers focused on the critical characteristics necessary for American youth to effectively develop in order to gain a greater understanding of these developmental factors. Note that the theory does not assume that the adolescent does not have problems but rather assumes that characteristics that contribute to effective problem-solving can help with the management of these challenges [36]. This work provided a basic framework for afterschool programs and other community-based initiatives aimed at promoting positive youth development. Positive youth development has been described using multiple terms, each focused on various concepts involving bidirectional engagement with the community and how community resources can be leveraged for optimal cultivation of skills that will lead to a productive life [26]. During the 1990s and beginning of the 2000s, youth development was conceptualized in a more optimistic way than in the previous decades. Focus shifted to an understanding of the plasticity of the brain in response to environmental stressors rather than the belief that behavior is genetically predetermined [25].

Lerner et al. designed a longitudinal study of fifth graders to assess potential benefits of positive youth development as it relates to what they call the "5 Cs." These are divided into behaviors that are "functionally valued" across development (competence, character, and connection) and behaviors that are "structurally valued" across development (contribution to self and contribution to family). The initial study included questionnaires completed by 1700 fifth graders (47.2% male) and 1117 parents (82.5% mothers, 13.9% fathers, 0.2% foster parents) from 57 schools (89.5% public schools). Participants were from all areas of the USA with 57.9% European American, 18% Latino, 8.1% African American, and 4.1% Native American [22]. The study conducted an annual assessment of adolescents over an 8-year span. The identified goal of the study was to follow participants from the 5th through the 12th grade [37]. The model proposes that adolescents can learn effective coping skills throughout development by building on internal strengths and effectively engaging with people and resources. Components of the system include resources embedded in daily life as experienced within the family, school, or neighborhood [18, 38] (Table 17.1).

Positive youth development is reported to be an effective approach to work with the general adolescent population, although the literature on

Table 17.1 Clinical application: identifying characteristics of positive youth development.

The 5 Cs [22]	Primary developmental areas	Potential questions for providers to ask
Competence	Academic, athletic, extracurricular activities	What are you most proud of? What are you best at? What are some things you struggle with? How do you feel like you are performing academically and athletically? How do you feel like you are performing in other extracurricular activities?
Confidence	Academic, athletic, extracurricular activities, social	Is there anything you feel vulnerable about? Have you ever used any substances to perform better academically or athletically? How do you feel about your ability to achieve academically or athletically? How comfortable are you in social situations?
Connection	Social (friendships and romantic relationships), academic, intrafamilial, community	How connected do you feel to your friends? How connected do you feel to your romantic partner? Do you feel like you fit in at your school? Do you feel connected to your community? Do you feel like an included and valued member of your family?
Character	Moral/ethical	What does it mean to you to have integrity? What are the things you value most in life? What characteristics do you value in others? What characteristics do you value in yourself?
Caring	Empathy, sympathy, emotional intelligence, compassion	Who do you care about most in your life? Who is the person in your life who you believe cares about you the most? How well do you think you can read the emotions of those around you?
Contribution (the sixth "C") [39]	Social (friendships, intimate relationships, family), community, society	What do you believe to be your purpose in life? What do you believe you have contributed to society thus far? What do you hope to contribute to society in the future?

positive psychology identifies some controversy regarding the concepts of positive versus negative emotions and behaviors. Positive psychology is a strength-based field developed to facilitate a state of well-being and healthy functioning. Researchers study life experiences with a focus on positive events rather than psychopathology; they explore the presence of "positive individual traits" and attempt to understand the role of institutions in the development of positive experiences [40]. The initial focus was on "normal," but there is increasing effort to apply the concepts to work with individuals dealing with adversity or mental illness [41]. Studies have demonstrated some benefit of "positive psychotherapy" for depression, suicidal ideation, and substance use disorders, but these studies are difficult to quantify and need more in-depth cultural understanding. One meta-analysis (English language studies not limited to TAY) found that positive psychology interventions improved well-being and ameliorated depression [42]. Development of effective coping skills during adolescence may allow TAY to function optimally during a time of increased autonomy.

Providing further information about working with TAY, Narendorf et al. did a qualitative study of uninsured young adults seeking emergency psychiatric care. The study included 55 individuals aged 18–25 years, 45% female, 27% White, 27% Black, 20% Hispanic, and 20% multiracial. Participants completed a structured questionnaire and participated in a semi-structured interview to provide information on their experiences with past mental health services. Patients primarily noted the importance of clinicians whom they consider competent based upon provider communication regarding the rationale for treatment decisions. However, they also stressed the value of having a positive relationship with their mental health provider and feeling respected by others [24].

Conclusion

This book examines aspects of mental healthcare during the critical period of transition from adolescence to adulthood. In the vignette descriptions, we see different kinds of struggles in navigating this life stage and how each individual, working with their psychiatrist, was able to find a path toward young adulthood.

To continue to advance our understanding of how best to support TAY, we need to understand the mental health needs and resources available to those in school and newly entering the workforce. We also need to research the impact of changing health insurance and socioeconomic status early in adulthood and compare practices for transitioning mental healthcare from adolescence to adulthood in various communities. Research indicates that educating and engaging young adults regarding treatment decisions can empower TAY with mental illness to advocate for their care and engage with providers [24].

Psychiatrists require specific education on the challenges facing TAY with mental illness. CAPs must be aware of individual and cultural bias regarding the expected life trajectory of each TAY after high school and should consider the strengths, barriers, and risk factors facing each individual patient. Training should address these concepts. Training programs should consider opportunities to meet Accreditation Council for Graduate Medical Education (ACGME) training requirements for CAP while also emphasizing the importance of the transition from adolescence to young adulthood. This might include integration into the curriculum of didactic discussion with clinical services specifically dedicated to transitional issues. Also important is communication between the child and general psychiatry training programs to ensure discussion of transitional needs and barriers. Partnership with juvenile justice systems, local community colleges, and technical schools could provide opportunity for psychiatrists in training to learn more about the unique needs of this population. General psychiatry residencies can also work to prepare their residents to work with TAY through partnership with child and adolescent psychiatry divisions and local educational institutions.

Child and adolescent psychiatrists can play a key role during this developmental stage. Child psychiatrists assess strengths and opportunities for improvement across domains while also helping patients and parents mobilize necessary resources. When done proactively, the CAP can help guide the TAY to optimal achievement of goals for each individual during this transitional stage of life.

References

1. Davis M, Vander SA. The transition to adulthood for youth who have serious emotional disturbance: developmental transition and young adult outcomes. J Ment Health Adm. 1997;24(4):400–27.
2. Mychasiuk R, Metz GA. Epigenetic and gene expression changes in the adolescent brain: what have we learned from animal models? Neurosci Biobehav Rev. 2016;70:189–97.
3. Martel A, Fuchs DC. Transitional age youth and mental illness – influences on young adult outcomes. Child Adolesc Psychiatr Clin N Am. 2017;26(2):xiii–vii.
4. Leebens PK, Williamson ED. Developmental psychopathology: risk and resilience in the transition to young adulthood. Child Adolesc Psychiatr Clin N Am. 2017;26(2):143–56.
5. Embrett MG, Randall GE, Longo CJ, Nguyen T, Mulvale G. Effectiveness of health system services and programs for youth to adult transitions in mental health care: a systematic review of academic literature. Admin Pol Ment Health. 2016;43(2):259–69.
6. Ma J, Baum S. Trends in community colleges: enrollment, prices, student debt, and completion. College Board Research Brief. 2016;4:1–23.
7. Jones T, Berger K. A promise fulfilled: a framework for equitable free college programs. Washington, D.C.: The Education Trust; 2018.
8. Kena G, Hussar W, McFarland J, De Brey C, Musu-Gillette L, Wang X, Zhang J, Rathbun A, Wilkinson-Flicker S, Diliberti M, Barmer A. The condition of education 2016. NCES 2016–144. Washington, DC.: National Center for Education Statistics; 2016.
9. Cassidy M. Why youth unemployment is still a huge problem. The Fiscal Times [Internet]. 2015 Jan 15 [cited 9 Feb 2020]. Available from: https://www.thefiscaltimes.com/Columns/2015/01/09/Why-Youth-Unemployment-Still-Huge-Problem.
10. David H. Skills, education, and the rise of earnings inequality among the “other 99 percent”.
11. Stewart S, Lim DH, Kim J. Factors influencing college persistence for first-time students. J Develop Edu. 2015:12–20.
12. Grimes SK. Underprepared community college students: characteristics, persistence, and academic success. Commun Collage J Res Practice. 1997;21(1):47–56.
13. Vander Stoep A, Weiss NS, Kuo ES, Cheney D, Cohen P. What proportion of failure to complete secondary school in the US population is attributable to adolescent psychiatric disorder? J Behav Health Serv Res. 2003;30(1):119–24.
14. Katz DS, Davison K. Community college student mental health: a comparative analysis. Commun College Rev. 2014;42(4):307–26.
15. Reynolds GM, Shendruk A. Demographics of the US Military. Washington, D.C.: Council on Foreign Relations; 2018.
16. Department of Defense. Medical standards for appointment, enlistment, or induction into the military services. Report No. 6130.03. 2018.
17. Mitchell E. Military issues 1,000 waivers for soldiers with mood disorders: report. Army Times. 27 Apr 2018.
18. Sharp ML, Fear NT, Rona RJ, Wessely S, Greenberg N, Jones N, Goodwin L. Stigma as a barrier to seeking health care among military personnel with mental health problems. Epidemiol Rev. 2015;37(1):144–62.
19. Schulenberg JE, Johnston LD, O'Malley PM, Bachman JG, Miech RA, Patrick ME. Monitoring the future national survey results on drug use, 1975–2017. Vol. II, College Students & Adults Ages. 19–55. Ann Arbor: Institute for Social Research; 2018.
20. Bukstein OG. Challenges and gaps in understanding substance use problems in transitional age youth. Child Adolesc Psychiatr Clinics. 2017;26(2):253–69.
21. Teeters JB, Lancaster CL, Brown DG, Back SE. Substance use disorders in military veterans: prevalence and treatment challenges. Subst Abuse Rehabilitat. 2017;8:69.
22. Elements of access to health care. Content last reviewed June 2018. Agency for Healthcare Research and Quality, Rockville. https://www.ahrq.gov/research/findings/nhqrdr/chartbooks/access/elements.html.
23. Narendorf SC, Wagner R, Fedoravicius N, Washburn M. Prior experiences of behavioral health treatment among uninsured young adults served in a psychiatric crisis setting. Commun Mental Health J. 2017;53(7):782–92.
24. Wasserman GA, McReynolds LS, Ko SJ, Katz LM, Carpenter JR. Gender differences in psychiatric disorders at juvenile probation intake. Am J Pub Health. 2005;95(1):131–7. of Juvenile Just and Delinquency Prevention, Office of Just Programs, U.S. Department of Justice. (2018). Statistical briefing book. Statistics retrieved from: https://www.ojjdp.gov/ojstatbb/structure_process/qa04106.asp and https://www.ojjdp.gov/ojstatbb/structure_process/qa04101.asp.
25. Zajac K, Sheidow AJ, Davis M. Juvenile justice, mental health and the transition to adulthood: a review of service system involvement and unmet needs in the US. Child Youth Serv Rev. 2015;56:139–48.
26. Wasserman GA, McReynolds LS, Ko SJ, Katz LM, Carpenter JR. Gender differences in psychiatric disorders at juvenile probation intake. Am J Public Health. 2005;95(1):131–7.
27. Shufelt JL, Cocozza JJ. Youth with mental health disorders in the juvenile justice system: Results from

a multi-state prevalence study. National Center for Mental Health and Juvenile Justice: Delmar; 2006.
28. Teplin LA, Abram KM, McClelland GM, Washburn JJ, Pikus AK. Detecting mental health disorders in juvenile detainees: Who receives services. Am J Public Health. 2005;95(10):1773–80.
29. Chung HL, Schubert CA, Mulvey EP. An empirical portrait of community reentry among serious juvenile offenders in two metropolitan cities. Crim Justice Behav. 2007;34(11):1402–26.
30. Trupin EJ, Kerns SEU, Walker SC, DeRobertis MT, Stewart DG. Family integrated transitions: a promising program for juvenile offenders with co-occurring disorders. J Child Adolesc Subst Abuse. 2011;20(5):421–36.
31. Davis M, Sheidow AJ, McCart MR. Reducing recidivism and symptoms in emerging adults with serious mental health conditions and justice system involvement. J Behav Health Serv Res. 2014;42:172.
32. Children's Bureau. (June 28, 2012). John H. Chafee Foster Care Independence Program. Retrieved from: https://www.acf.hhs.gov/cb/resource/chafee-foster-care-program.
33. Braga AA, Piehl AM, Hureau D. Controlling violent offenders released to the community: an evaluation of the Boston reentry initiative. J Res Crime Delinq. 2009;46(4):411–36.
34. Liddle HA, Dakof GA, Henderson C, Rowe C. Implementation outcomes of multidimensional family therapy-detention to community: a reintegration program for drug using juvenile detainees. Int J Offender Ther Comp Criminol. 2011;55(4):587–604.
35. Barrington K. How to manage your stress while attending community college [Internet]. Community College Review. 2017 [cited 26 Dec 2019]. Available from: https://www.communitycollegereview.com/blog/how-to-manage-your-stress-while-attending-community-college.
36. Lerner RM, von Eye A, Lerner JV, Lewin-Bizan S, Bowers EP. Special issue introduction: the meaning and measurement of thriving: a view of the issues. J Youth Adolesc. 2010;39(7):707–19.
37. Lerner RM, Lerner JV. The positive development of youth: comprehensive findings from the 4-H study of positive youth development. Washington, D.C.: National; 2013.
38. Lerner RM, Lerner JV, von Eye A, Bowers EP, Lewin-Bizan S. Individual and contextual bases of thriving in adolescence: a view of the issues. J Adolesc. 2011;34(6):1107–14.
39. Sherrod L. Civic engagement as an expression of positive youth development. Approaches Posit Youth Develop. 2007;1:59–74.
40. Duckworth AL, Steen T, Seligman M. Positive psychology in clinical practice. Annu Rev Clinical Psychol. 2005;1:629–51.
41. Schrank B, Brownell T, Tylee A, Slade M. Positive psychology: an approach to supporting recovery in mental illness. East Asian Arch Psychiat. 2014;24(3):95.
42. Sin NL, Lyubomirsky S. Enhancing well-being and alleviating depressive symptoms with positive psychology interventions: a practice-friendly meta-analysis. J Clin Psychol. 2009;65(5):467–87.

18 Digital Media Use in Transitional-Age Youth: Challenges and Opportunities

Paul Weigle, Kristopher Kaliebe, Kristin Dalope, Tracy Asamoah, and Reem Mohamed Abdel Shafi

Key Points

- Today's TAY are distinct from other generations in their habitual engagement with new media technology, decreased risk-taking, and increased rates of depression and anxiety.
- New digital media for entertainment and communication is extensively interwoven into TAY's lives.
- Interactions with digital technologies can engender or exacerbate mental health problems.
- Mental health disorders often drive excessive digital media use, creating a novel symptom profile.
- Mental health providers must assess digital media use, identifying elements of potential risk and harm.
- TAY often engage in social connections online in place of healthier face-to-face interactions.
- Online activities are often preferred by TAY to other means of managing negative affective states.
- TAY engaging excessively in online entertainment often experience worsening symptoms of ADHD, anxiety, or depression.
- Negative and unhealthy sites, such as those endorsing eating-disordered behaviors, self-harm, or suicide, may be particularly appealing to depressed youth.
- Solutions to common media-related problems can include mindful use and utilizing technology applications to track and limit unhealthy use.
- Incorporating new technologies into treatment can augment interventions, improve communication and alliance, and integrate treatment into our patients' lives.

P. Weigle (✉)
Natchaug Hospital, Mansfield Center, CT, USA

K. Kaliebe
USF Health Department of Psychiatry and Behavioral Neurosciences, Tampa, FL, USA
e-mail: kkaliebe@health.usf.edu

K. Dalope
UPMC Children's Hospital of Pittsburgh, Pittsburgh, PA, USA
e-mail: dalopek@upmc.edu

T. Asamoah
Austin, TX, USA

R. M. A. Shafi
Cairns Hospital and Hinterland Service, Cairns, QLD, Australia

V. Chan, J. Derenne (eds.), *Transition-Age Youth Mental Health Care*,
https://doi.org/10.1007/978-3-030-62113-1_18

Clinical Vignette

Jared is a 19-year-old man who presents reluctantly with his parents to an initial outpatient psychiatry evaluation in relation to a suicidal threat he made after an argument with his parents over completing chores. He dropped out of college 3 months before presentation and has become progressively isolated and despondent. In high school, during which he played video games in moderation, Jared was a fair student, and he did well in his first semester of college. However, after the winter break of college, he returned to campus, bringing his powerful "gaming computer." At a friend's advice, Jared started playing Counter-Strike: Global Offensive (CS:GO) – an online competitive first-person shooter game played in teams. In his second semester, his gaming habit quickly consumed over 8 hours per day, to the detriment of sleep, socialization, homework, and study. Ultimately, Jared stopped attending class in college. He experienced a major depressive episode, lost weight, and contemplated suicide. He dropped out, returned home, and made a plan with his mother to get a full-time job. In the ensuing months, he continued to spend most of his waking hours playing CS:GO. He has not pursued a job, has gained 20 lbs., and has left household chores undone. He reports increasing social anxiety, rarely leaves home, and relapsed into depression. On interview, he makes little eye contact and gives minimal answers. His gaze returns regularly to his phone, and when asked why, he states it is to see if a CS:GO teammate has yet responded to his text. Jared admits that this has been the worst year of his life, but notes that he has at least gotten joy from playing CS:GO, which he calls "my coping skill."

Introduction

Tech is everywhere. Modern youth's engagement with media represents, by many measures, the greatest generational divide in history. Today's transitional age youth represent the first generation whose adolescence began in a world of smartphones and contemporary computers, windows to online entertainment and video games. Dubbed "iGen" [130], this cohort born between 1995 and 2012 is defined by their technology habits. Technology has had a transformative effect on how these youth experience the world on a daily basis. This poses new challenges to their health and maturation, with implications for the assessment and treatment of psychiatric disorders. Transitional age youth of today often possess new skill sets, but also lack abilities considered basic in previous generations. Disorders of mental health in youth are interwoven with the media habits and experiences which dominate their lives. Excessive online habits can themselves become pathological, causing dysfunction, representing a distinct mental disorder. Online activities and experiences such as cyberbullying, sexting, and fear of missing out (FOMO) can also have a dramatic impact on mental health. It is vital that mental health practitioners understand the new normal, as well as digital technology's differential impact on psychiatric disorders including depression, anxiety, attention-deficit/hyperactivity disorder (ADHD), and disorders of the autism spectrum. As such, practitioners must adapt the clinical evaluation of transitional age youth to include effects of technology-related mental health issues and disorders and guide patients toward balanced, healthy lives in a world dominated by screens.

Problematic Internet Use

For many adolescents and young adults, regulating digital media use is challenging; smartphones, tablets, laptops, etc., are the gateway for commerce, education, employment, entertainment, information, and socialization [100].

Researchers use a variety of terms and methods when trying to understand digital media use and when it becomes problematic. To date, there are over 60 terms describing the latter. Problematic interactive media use (PIMU) describes when overuse or compulsive use of media (both online and offline) interfere with one's daily life – having a negative impact on personal hygiene, grades, family interactions, emotional and psychological issues, and relationships [87]. PIMU often presents in one of four ways: gaming, social media, pornography, and information-bingeing.

TAY with PIMU may also have coexisting diagnoses of ADHD, ASD, anxiety, depression, eating disorders, and/or substance use [93] Physically, those who have PIMU may have sedentary lifestyles, weight gain, sleep issues [93], neck/back pain, wrist/hand pain, and eye strain.

Problematic Internet use (PIU) is described as the "use of the Internet that creates psychological, social, school and/or work difficulties in a person's life" [9, p. 378]. PIU focuses upon two factors, time on the Internet and what is done on the Internet, and it includes additional ideas beyond addiction (e.g., Internet use that interferes with offline socialization).

Internet addiction focuses on an addiction specific to the Internet, describing core features of addiction such as loss of control while on the Internet or feelings of withdrawal when away from the Internet [120].

Internet gaming disorder is defined in the 2013 revision of *Diagnostic Statistical Manual of Mental Disorders* 5 (DSM-5) as a condition requiring further study, not yet an official diagnosis. Gaming disorder is listed in the *International Classification of Diseases* (ICD-11) as a diagnosis in the 2018 revision.

The figure below (Fig. 18.1) incorporates language from primary care and mental health practitioners to illustrate the relationship between Internet gaming disorder and related phenomena.

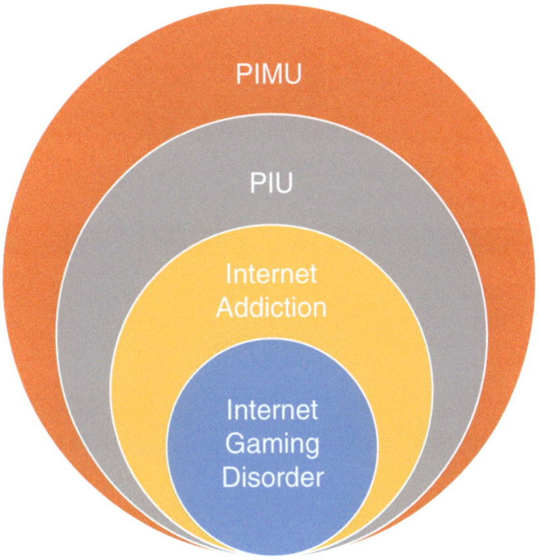

Fig. 18.1 Interrelationship of PIMU, PIU, Internet addiction, and Internet gaming disorders

Table 18.1 compares the definitions of Internet gaming disorder and gaming disorder.

There are over 20 assessment tools that focus on different aspects of problematic use [66]. These tools may measure concepts of addictive behaviors, impulse-control disorders, or behaviors that use the Internet as a medium for other addictive behaviors. Others assess the impact of the use of existing apps [81], or devices like smartphones.

The impact of PIMU/addiction upon TAY may include physical and mental health concerns and decreased success in educational, employment, or social realms – regardless of culture. These behaviors may also have a significant impact upon the family system. For example, TAY who never leave their parents' home may have had a "failure to launch", or a "boomerang" effect may occur if the TAY returns to live at home as a result of PIMU or addiction. In both scenarios, family dynamics may be disrupted, financial stressors increased, and interpersonal conflicts intensified.

The following two tables (Tables 18.2 and 18.3) summarize the current state of research and treatment evidence in therapy and in pharmacological management to address problematic use of digital media. For pharmacological management, the medications listed can be beneficial in treating PIU, which may coexist with one or more comorbid psychiatric diagnoses.

Clinical Vignette

Suzie is a 19-year-old female who has come to see a college counselor, as she is experiencing poor mood and difficulty sleeping. She is studying biomedical sciences and had an argument with a friend about a joint assignment last week. The conflict has escalated, and several other people are involved. She is worried about her reputation and feels excluded, as she is no longer welcome in her former study group. This issue

Table 18.1 Internet gaming disorder and gaming disorder comparison

DSM-5 Internet gaming disorder	ICD-11 gaming disorder
Condition for further study, not an official diagnosis	Diagnosis
Internet-based games	Online or offline video games
Criteria present within 1 year	Criteria present within 1 year
Modifiers of mild, moderate, severe	No modifiers
Repetitive use of Internet-based games, often with other players, that leads to significant issues with functioning	Pattern of gaming behavior (digital gaming or video gaming) which must be of sufficient severity to result in *significant impairment* in family, social, educational, occupational, or other important areas of functioning
5 of 9 criteria (below) needed	**All 3 bolded criteria required**
Preoccupation or obsession with Internet games	**Impaired control over gaming** **Increasing priority given to gaming** over other activities to the extent that gaming takes precedence over other interests and daily activities
Loss of interest in other life activities, such as hobbies	
Lied to others about Internet game usage	
Has lost or put at risk an opportunity or relationship due to Internet games	
Continued overuse of Internet games, even knowing how much they impact their life	**Continuation or escalation of gaming despite the occurrence of negative consequences**
Uses Internet games to relieve anxiety or guilt	No explicit discussion of these topics
Withdrawal symptoms when not playing Internet games	
Tolerance – needs more time playing games	
Tried to stop or decrease playing Internet games, but failed	

Table 18.2 Psychotherapeutic treatment of problematic interactive media use

Therapeutic approach	Details
Acceptance commitment therapy	Accept distress and neutrally engage with emotions
Cognitive behavioral therapy	Identify cognitions, behaviors, and emotions that trigger relapses and focus psychoeducational and coping strategies on the antecedents
Dialectical behavioral therapy	Increase patient's ability to be conscious of experienced feelings, thoughts, and urges so patient can make effective decisions [93]
Digital detoxification	Complete abstinence is promoted for a finite period of time
Family-based/ family therapy	Improve communication and teach family monitoring of digital media use
Motivational interviewing	Evaluation of readiness for change using precontemplation, contemplation, preparation, action, maintenance, and relapse stages
Sports intervention	Sports exercise prescriptions improved PIU [75] Exercise rehabilitation may benefit PIU [60]

has kept her up at night, and she has tried to reason with several people to rejoin the group, to no avail. Her grades are slipping, and she nearly walked into a passing car while simultaneously texting her ex-friend. She has had near misses with traffic like this in the past while using social media on her phone.

Typical Screen Habits and Mental Health Impact

Young adults of this generation come of age with significantly distinct strengths and weaknesses due to individual experiences accumulated in childhood and adolescence. Cross-sectional stud-

Table 18.3 Medication treatment of problematic interactive media use

Medication	Evidence
Atomoxetine	Improved child depression inventory scales [92]
Bupropion	11 patients open-label trial – decreased craving for video games [47]
Citalopram + quetiapine	Case report TAY w/PIU – improvement maintained at 4-month follow-up [19]
Clonazepam + sertraline	Case study of CBT to treat anxiety and Internet addiction reduced both symptomatologies [109]
Escitalopram	Case report of gaming addiction [110] Open-label trial in 19 patients, decreased time online in 11 patients [27]
Fluoxetine	Case report of pornography addiction [26]
Lamotrigine/ fluoxetine	Case report of compulsive sexual behaviors online and offline [112]
Methylphenidate (extended release)	62 children with ADHD, decreased Internet video game use time [46]
Memantine	29 subjects with gambling addiction, open label, 10 weeks decreased gambling behaviors [42]
Naltrexone + sertraline	Case report of Internet sexual addiction, depression, OCD [13]

ies done 15 years apart, in 2000 and in 2015, show a massive increase in daily screen entertainment consumption, to an average of over 6.5 hours per day for adolescents [100, 103]. The average amount of time spent online tripled during this time period, and the average amount of time spent playing video games quadrupled. Taken as a whole, the average transitional age American youth spends about twice as much time engaging in screen entertainment during their teenage years as they spend in school. The extensive time devoted to screens has displaced time traditionally spent in other activities. Generational research indicates that in 2015, adolescents spent significantly less time socializing in person with peers, going out on dates, reading books and magazines, driving, and even sleeping than at any other time in the prior 25 years [130]. However, this time period also saw a significant decrease in adolescent violent crime rates, teen pregnancy, and cigarette and alcohol use. Determining causality is difficult, but it appears that the increase in teen technology habits have displaced both healthy and risky behaviors. Current transitional age youth have less experience with socializing in person (including dating) than any generation before, which is expected to negatively impact their "offline" social skills [130]. Modern youth have also spent less time reading books and magazines for enjoyment, as well as driving, which may impact their education and options for employment as well as social life. Nighttime technology use displaces time spent sleeping, deconditions sleep habits, and increases sleep latency times following video games or other stimulating screen activities. Insufficient sleep is particularly vital to correctly identify and address in psychiatric care, because it strongly predicts depression, anxiety, and suicidality [83]. As a possible protective factor, today's youth also come of age having engaged in fewer experiences with sexual intercourse, pregnancy, interpersonal violence, and drug and alcohol use [130], which may in turn decrease susceptibility to mental disorders such as post-traumatic stress disorder and substance use disorders.

However, there are signs that the current generation is overall less mentally healthy than the last. When compared with young adults who were aged 18–25 years old in the mid-2000s, transitional age youth in the late 2010s are more likely to report specific psychological problems [131]. This relationship is illustrated in Fig. 18.2.

Changing screen habits seems to be the biggest difference between the current and previous generations. Even within the generation of young adults, increased screen habits have been associated with anxiety, depression, psychopathology symptoms, and poor sleep quality [141]. Large systematic reviews of research studies have associated time spent on screen media with depression,

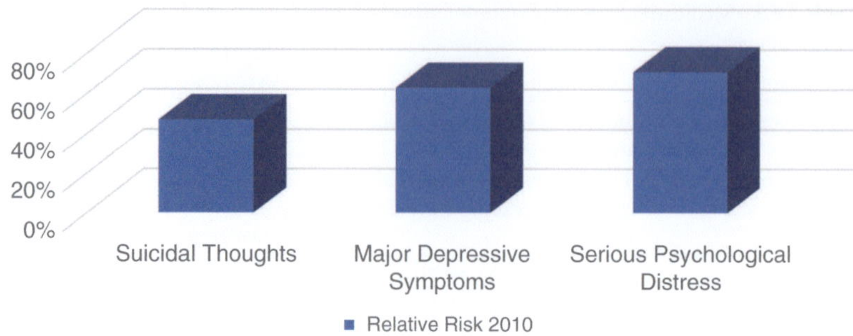

Fig. 18.2 Likelihood of mental health problems in transitional age youth in 2010 as compared to a decade before [131]

psychological distress, behavior problems, low self-esteem, and poor physical fitness, although one review found only a small effect [121].

The amount of screen time youth engage in may be less important than the choices they make regarding quantity and content of use. For example, scrolling social media while in a classroom may distract from learning, while doing so late at night may lead to insufficient sleep.

Advantages and Disadvantages of Online Experiences and Behaviors

Specific online screen habits and experiences have been associated with negative mental health outcomes and warrant particular concern: cyberbullying, sexting, social comparison, FOMO (fear of missing out), violent video game play, and viewing pornography. Cyberbullying is the use of electronic communication to bully another, typically by sending intimidating, humiliating, or threatening messages. Cyberbullying victimization is becoming more common in recent years, and it specifically predicts worsening of depression symptoms over time [67, 77]. Sexting involves sharing sexually explicit photographs or videos via electronic media and is also becoming more common. One survey of young adults found that a majority admitted to having engaged in sexting [122]. Although sexting is not always related to a negative outcome, at greatest risk are females who send a picture for the hopes of starting a new relationship [32]. Sexting has also been associated with depression, anxiety, substance use, and risky sexual behaviors [86, 119]. Social comparison refers to the human tendency to evaluate oneself based on observation of others. This concept can relate to use of various types of media, yet its effects appear particularly powerful via social media, where users often exaggerate or fabricate desirable characteristics in order to compete for "followers," "friends," and "likes." Youth engaging in social comparison are more likely to feel inferior and are significantly more likely to experience depression in relation to social media use [76, 88, 133]. Similarly, FOMO is the feeling of being excluded from experiences one's peers are enjoying. Youth who experience FOMO tend to feel inferior and self-conscious over time [59]. They are more likely to check social media accounts obsessively and to suffer negative consequences of social media use [90]. Similar to engagement with other forms of violent media, violent video game play has been found to increase aggressive thoughts and behaviors in dozens of research studies. Although the effect size is relatively small, it is significant, and may be proportional to the extent of exposure. The mental health implications of watching online pornography are largely unknown, but a significant proportion of young men endorse feeling addicted [43]. These online experiences should be assessed in psychiatric evaluations of youth and addressed in treatment when problematic.

Various habits of screen media engagement appear to confer specific skills and advantages. Regular video game play has been shown to benefit eye-hand coordination, aspects of vision such as detail resolution and contrast sensitivity, visual tracking, mental rotation, task switching, and multitasking.

Social media use may also confer specific benefits and risks to mental health. Social media engagement has been related to increased self-esteem and social support. Youth suffering from depression and anxiety often seek help and support online, typically preferring to socialize online rather than in person. Racial minority and LGBTQ youth, as well as those with niche interests, or learning disabilities, often use social media to connect with like-minded peers and as a result feel less lonely [63]. Some studies indicate that social media engagement in youth may be protective against depression, particularly for those who receive positive feedback and online support and who engage actively, e.g., posting, commenting, and "like-ing." In contrast, other studies have found that social media use by youth who are unpopular, lack self-purpose, and are emotionally invested in their social media image is linked to negative mental health outcomes [12, 136]. Social media use may be riskier for depressed users, who are much more likely to have negative interactions on social media, to feel left out on social media, and to use social media to avoid real-world problems [101]. Youth often disclose suicidal thoughts online rather than in person. Doing so risks delaying needed help, and online discussion about suicide is related to worsening suicidality over time [31, 82].

When compared with previous generations, contemporary transitional age youth have more experience playing video games and engaging on social media. They have considerably less practice with in-person socializing and reading. They are more likely to suffer depression or mental distress, have poorer physical fitness, and have less healthy sleep habits than any time in living memory [130]. These generational differences exist, but generalizations are difficult, due to high variability in individual screen media habits and experiences. Psychiatrists who treat transitional age youth must be able to assess screen habits in patients and their effects on mental health and psychiatric disorders. Providers can guide our patients toward healthier media habits and make use of the unique opportunities computer technology offers for health and recovery.

Assessment and Formulation

Engagement with digital media is an almost universal behavior among TAY across class, sex, and culture. An unheralded level of access to media has shaped youth culture and is an aspect of daily life with multitasking of different media the new norm [95]. An expanding portfolio of evidence demonstrates an impact of digital media use on self-esteem, sleep quality, mood, risk-taking behaviors, and even propensity for accidents [3, 45, 61]. Thus, digital media use bears a role in mediating the risk of depression, anxiety, and self-injurious behavior. There is a need for mental health providers to become attuned to a rapidly shifting digital environment and for psychiatric assessments to reflect this change in youth culture [114]. However, over half of practicing psychiatrists are over 55 years of age and may have less experience with technology than the youth they are evaluating [48]. Professional organizations including the APA and AACAP work to address this practice gap via clinical updates and education about the relevance of digital media within a psychiatric assessment [1, 5].

Considering the type, extent, and impact of digital media use in their lives may be helpful as a broad framework when interviewing the patient. Being aware of the potential for media-related issues within the patient's narrative can help garner pertinent clinical information that may otherwise not be offered.

- *What* digital media does this person use? (number/type of devices, social media, video games)
- *When* do they use digital media? (time of day (night time use, work hours), duration)
- *Why* do they use these forms of media? (entertainment, distraction, boredom, information, communication, anonymity) [61]
- *Impact* – Does the patient feel their media use offers positive, neutral, or negative effects on their functioning? (in addition to objective assessment from the provider including collateral as indicated)

The approach of tailoring questions relevant to each of the assessment domains may be the most intuitive and has been proposed [18]. Psychiatric providers can quickly establish rapport and begin to guide appropriate digital media use by inquiring about digital media use as part of a psychiatric history [18]. The domains can be adapted to consider the influence of digital media within it and be tailored to the patient's presentation.

Screening tools have commonly been used for depression or anxiety, such as the PHQ-9 and GAD-7 [85, 94]. Validated, succinct tools assessing problematic media use are also available and may be a beneficial primer in assessing digital media use. The *Problematic and Risky Internet Use Screening Scale* (*PRIUSS -3*) is a three-question scale that, if positive, can be further evaluated assessing social impairment, emotional impairment, and risky/impulsive Internet use [52]. The *Bergen Social Media Addiction Scale* (*BSMAS*) is another self-report scale that has six items based on the diagnostic criteria of addiction as outlined in the DSM-5: mood modification, conflict, withdrawal, salience, and relapse [3].

Integrating the Clinical History of Media Use into Practice

History of Presenting Illness

This is the initial narrative as to why a patient is coming to seek psychiatric care. This may vary from insomnia to low mood to social problems. Curiosity and exploration as to whether media habits play a role in the chief complaint can be established here. For example, in a case of insomnia or interpersonal conflict, querying about the role of screen media and their perception of its impact may be helpful. Late evening or bedtime screen use can lead to untimely arousal, increased sleep latency, and poor-quality sleep along with suboptimal cognitive and athletic performance the next day [45, 54]. Asking how communication is conducted (e.g., Snapchats that disappear, text messaging, public posts on Facebook or Twitter) helps establish how individuals manage conflict, or if they are a victim and/or perpetrator of cyberbullying [18].

Past Psychiatric and Medical History

TAY access online resources for health-related information and may use mental health applications as their first foray into addressing mental health problems [4]. Asking about applications they utilize and whether they find them beneficial can offer an initial impression as to their treatment preferences [4]. Media use when driving increases risk for accidents and also should be discussed [41, 128].

Social History

TAY are unlikely to differentiate between "real-world" friends and friends they have only ever conversed with online – unless asked [95]. This differentiation offers an opportunity to reflect on the balance between offline and online influences and at times helps establish a diagnosis and illuminate potential risks. Asking about whether a patient uses their phone during work, class, or study is worthwhile as use of smartphones and social media during lectures has a detrimental effect on academic performance [106].

Developmental History

An exploration of how media use evolved, including at what age they started, and how their use was restricted or encouraged by their caregivers can help paint a picture of the nature of their home life and quality of caregiver relationships. Did caregivers provide adequate supervision? Were there arguments about appropriate media use? Did caregivers use screen media predominantly for play, or to soothe them as children? [140]

Safety Assessment

Research has indicated that exposure to NSSI (non-suicidal self-injury) imagery [15] and sexual predators can increase an individual's risk for self-injury or exploitation [99]. Individuals with problematic use, especially with comorbid psychiatric symptoms, are at increased risk of being victim to or engaging in risky behavior such as cyberbullying [115]. A survey among psychiatrically hospitalized youth indicated a positive relationship between problematic Internet use and suicidality [36]. Young people are increasingly communicating distress digitally, particularly to peers [78]. Careful yet overt inquiry and education about exposure to risks and disclosure of suicidality on digital media is necessary here.

Mental Status Examination

A cross-sectional observation of what the patient does with their electronic device during the consultation is useful and can be compared with the narrative obtained [18]. This may vary from keeping it out of sight; setting it on the table; being distracted by it – replying to messages and calls; or using it to communicate with the provider by showing images or texts. This may offer a "teachable moment" whereby the provider can assess and target insight, or as a discussion point when assessing for problematic use.

Formulation

Considering the influence of digital media within each domain of a biopsychosocial framework assists in incorporating its relevance within a summary formulation. The impact of the digital environment youth exist in and have created should be considered within [35]:

- Biological aspects including light exposure, sleep, sedentarism, physical activity, or eating habits [18]
- Psychological aspects: mood including depression, anxiety and FOMO, general sense of well-being [139]
- Social aspects: social supports and the connectedness and similarities between online and offline environments including risks taken

A digital media assessment can help to generate a more holistic and realistic view of the patient with an appropriate management plan tailored to their presentation. This may include intermittent periods of abstinence to reduce stress [129], increased engagement in sports, CBT, or another psychotherapy to target addictive Internet behaviors [87].

Clinical Vignette

Raquel, a freshman at a community college who lived at home, was spending increasing amounts of time alone in her bedroom. Worried about her isolation and moodiness, her mother encouraged her to see a therapist. During the initial meeting, Raquel slumped into a chair, her gaze fixed to the floor. She admitted to habitually coming home after class to confine herself to her bedroom and to spend hours online. Raquel lacked motivation to leave the house or spend time with her family or "offline" friends, preferring connection with her "online-only" friends. Raquel told her therapist that she frequently felt sad and bored but enjoyed watching videos on YouTube. Conflicts often arose with her mother over how much time she has spent online. Raquel dealt with loneliness by further scrolling through the feeds of social media sites, which was often followed by feelings of sadness and hopelessness. Raquel found herself in a cycle of depression and excessive time spent online. Raquel sacrificed sleep and in-person relationships for her activities online. She admitted to frequently updating her status on social media sites and checking responses to her posts, feeling frustrated and disappointed when she received too few "likes," or responses.

Depression and Anxiety

Raquel's story is not uncommon among transitional age youth (TAY). Many struggling with negative mood turn to the Internet for information, entertainment, social connection, and support, often with negative consequences. TAY with moderate to severe depression report a heightened affective response to social media experiences, both positive and negative [101]. Internet devices are immediately available sources of education and feedback. Today's TAY are coming of age at the same time that new digital technologies are emerging as the preferred source of personal expression, entertainment, and information. TAY search online for information about their health conditions as well as to find support from others afflicted with similar issues; 87% of 14- to

22-year-olds access the Internet for health information [101]. However, those dealing with anxiety or depression are vulnerable to certain aspects of digital technology. Compared with peers, anxious and depressed youth prefer socializing online. Internalizing youth often use social media to combat loneliness, but are also more susceptible to cyberbullying and other negative online interactions [11, 96].

Like many of her peers, Raquel's emergence into adulthood coincides with a period of increased autonomy, the emergence of mental illness, and poorly regulated digital technology habits. Major transitions mark this life stage, with TAY typically entering the workforce or college, often moving to a new community in the process. New onset, or exacerbation of existing mental illness, frequently occurs during this time period. Youth now progress through these milestones with the Internet as a constant companion. Although TAY typically seek support and relief from distress online, overdependence on digital technology may lead to ineffective coping skills, increased social isolation, addictive use of social media, and, ultimately, worsening distress.

Young adults who spend the most time online report the highest rates of depression and anxiety [49, 71, 117] as well as suicidal ideation and attempts [60, 78, 113]. Studies of various Internet activities (social media, gaming, blogs, shopping sites, and topic-specific platforms) have found that the highest utilizers of each endorse the most anxiety and depression [79, 89, 125].

TAY endorsing anxiety and depression report more negative interactions online than their peers, a pattern which often worsens the problem. These include:

- Cyberbullying [53] – both perpetrators and victims are significantly more likely to engage in self-harm or suicidal behaviors [105, 132].
- Problematic interactive media use – particularly social media, whether excessive use is intended to manage negative mood states or youth experiencing psychological distress experience greater emotional distress as a result of their use [51, 98, 116, 132, 137].
- Problematic experiences on social media such as attention-seeking behaviors and suffering FOMO [117] – depressed youth spend more time on social media platforms, more frequently checking for reactions to their posts.

Determining causality in the association between Internet habits and psychiatric disorders is complex. The majority of currently published studies utilize cross-sectional designs and are unable to conclude the directionality of the association between Internet habits and psychopathology. However, individuals with excessive and inappropriate Internet use frequently endorse greater rates of depression or anxiety. Youth with internalizing disorders appear to be uniquely vulnerable to the effects of excessive or inappropriate Internet use.

Many TAY prefer to seek information and support for their psychological issues online. A 2018 Hope lab survey found that adolescents and TAY with depression use the Internet for several purposes [101]. TAY often conduct online research as their first step in better understanding their mental health concerns. Websites, blogs, apps, and social networking groups dedicated to mental health issues appeal to many youth with a variety of psychiatric diagnoses. These resources are readily available and can be used anonymously. However, many online resources are not affiliated with a recognized academic or treatment organization and may contain misleading information. Globally accessible platforms allow for youth to connect with individuals experiencing similar problems, who may be better able to understand shared experiences. Used appropriately, the Internet is a powerful tool for TAY to understand and manage their psychiatric symptoms. Supportive family or friends can use similar online tools to engage TAY dealing with such problems.

In planning interventions for TAY dealing with anxiety and depression, special consideration should be given to the role of their online activities. Formal assessment of Internet habits in TAY presenting with depression or anxiety should be part of all initial evaluations. Intensity and frequency of use, platforms used, and other patterns of use can affect anxiety and depression. Understanding patients' online lives will help providers create better-informed treatment interventions. Treatment should include helping TAY identify problematic behaviors and emotional responses related to digital technology, thus reducing or removing unhelpful online behaviors and increasing positive use of technology and other healthy behaviors. The Internet is a powerful educational tool, a source of peer support, and many TAY are receptive to using technology as a component of mental health treatment [38]. The Internet can enable providers who work with TAY to better understand, treat, and support patients.

Clinical Vignette

Aaron, a college freshman, presents to his first appointment with a psychiatrist during his winter break. His parents had insisted that he see a psychiatrist after learning that he had received C's and D's in his first semester. He had been diagnosed with attention-deficit/hyperactivity disorder (ADHD) in third grade by his family doctor, but with treatment had become an A and B letter grade student who was also active in sports. Aaron stares at the floor as the psychiatrist asks about his semester. Aaron insists that he is taking his stimulant daily, but complains of often missing deadlines for assignments, feeling unprepared for tests, and struggling with insomnia. Aaron admits to spending hours, both during and outside of class time, playing a popular multiplayer game. He subscribes to several YouTube channels featuring others playing the game and finds it difficult to turn off his devices to attend to his schoolwork.

Attention-Deficit/Hyperactivity Disorder

It is no surprise that newly-independent Aaron struggled with self-monitoring his Internet habits. TAY with ADHD are particularly susceptible to excessive Internet use and addiction. In such cases, inappropriate and excessive Internet habits further exacerbate physical, psychological, and biological disability. Childhood associations between ADHD and excessive technology use (e.g., causing difficulties with social relationships, sleep, and behavior) persist in transitional years [2, 10]. TAY with insomnia have higher rates of both ADHD and Internet addiction [34]. Those with greater ADHD severity typically have increased social impairment as well as higher levels of state and trait anger, leading to social isolation [107]. Social isolation, in turn, contributes to excessive Internet use, which perpetuates isolation in a vicious cycle. Online activities incorporating high risk or reward, such as gambling and gaming, are particularly habit-forming for those susceptible to addiction. Digital technology is emerging as an important factor in how symptoms of ADHD manifest in TAY.

ADHD, comorbid symptoms, and poorly regulated Internet habits can profoundly impact functioning. TAY and adults with ADHD have higher levels of Internet addiction, a construct recognized worldwide but not yet defined in DSM 5 [49, 69, 124, 135]. Internet use disorders are associated with maladaptive behaviors and negative mood states. Impulsiveness, loneliness, and impaired behavioral inhibition are predictors of Internet addiction among adults with ADHD [70]. Internet gaming disorder is associated with impulsivity and hostility in TAY [142]. Severity of ADHD symptoms is associated with severity of Internet addiction in TAY, particularly so when the Internet is used to help regulate negative emotions [33]. The immediate gratification, fast-paced interfaces, and constantly moving screens may alleviate immediate feelings of boredom [33]. Left unchecked, excessive online behaviors interfere with offline functioning.

Achieving autonomy and independence, key developmental tasks for this age group, are threatened by factors that impair executive functioning skills. A significant proportion of ADHD cases diagnosed in adulthood report an absence of symptoms in childhood, calling into question whether an alternative etiology is responsible for their symptoms [20]. Adults with recent-onset ADHD symptoms are more likely to endorse symptoms of Internet addiction compared to controls [69]. Engagement with video games and other screen media has been linked to deteriorating attention over time [123]. Similarly, gaming disorder has been linked with the development of ADHD symptoms [80]. Although causality is impossible to prove from this data, excessive Internet habits may cause or worsen symptoms of ADHD. When evaluating ADHD, especially for adults with new-onset symptoms, care must be taken to also assess technology habits.

When working with TAY in clinical settings, priorities should include strengthening self-monitoring and self-regulation skills including challenges uniquely impacted by ADHD symptoms and Internet use (e.g., time management, limit setting, need for immediate feedback, problems with sleep and interpersonal relationships). These TAY require strategies to manage these issues to improve their overall functioning. Recognition of the interrelationships between these varied problems will help patients gain insight into their vulnerability to problematic Internet use.

Clinical Vignette

Tony is a 20-year-old male with autism spectrum disorder (ASD) who lives with his family. He was "too high functioning" for vocational rehabilitation services but has not been successful in keeping a job. He doesn't have "real-life" friends; he has "virtual" friends online. When his parents tell him to stop gaming, he throws things; his tablet and controller broke. He learns about sexuality and relationships from online forums, mainstream media, and pornography. He has tried to meet romantic partners via social media but has been unsuccessful.

After Tony and his parents contacted the Office of Vocational Rehabilitation about his employment challenges, he met with a job coach who explained professional interactions in the workplace and via email. He and his family began co-watching movies and programs, and his family taught him which observed behaviors were unreasonable. Tony also joined a social skills group where he made some acquaintances and learned "rules" about appropriate and inappropriate behavior online and offline. They talked about topics like independence, safety, relationships, sexuality, courtship behaviors, consent, pornography, and the law. His therapist also referred him to reliable online resources.

Autism Spectrum Disorder

TAY with autism often find that interactions online are less threatening to navigate [25]. They also have patterns of Internet use that differ from their peers, listed in Table 18.4.

Data demonstrates that TAY with ASD have greater compulsive Internet and video game use, which can lead to fewer opportunities to develop social, academic, and occupational skills and negative impacts for their families. Technology

Table 18.4 Media habits of youth on the autism spectrum

Topics	How youth with ASD differ from peers
General use	More computer use [65]
	Preference for online communication over face-to-face interaction
	Less use of social aspects (email, social media like Facebook, texting)
	Discussion forums: more specific interests and a greater number of interests [55, 56]
	Higher rates of non-social media use (i.e., television and video games)
Online social interactions	More comprehension and control over communication, access to similar others, and the opportunity to express their true selves [37]
	More positive friendships after receiving emails from friends or visiting social networking sites [65]
Employment	Increased social problems – obstacles concerning communication and human interaction in non-autism-specific employment [74]
Gaming	More likely to use mobile phones for games than their peers
	More difficulty disengaging from playing video games, feeling upset when not able to play, getting angry when interrupted from games, and playing longer than intended

can help initiate social interactions with like-minded others, but maintenance of connections with desired friends and romantic partners, knowledge of who is trustworthy, and assessment of appropriate disclosure can be challenging [16]. Benefits and limitations of various low- and high-tech social outlets for this population are listed in Fig. 18.3.

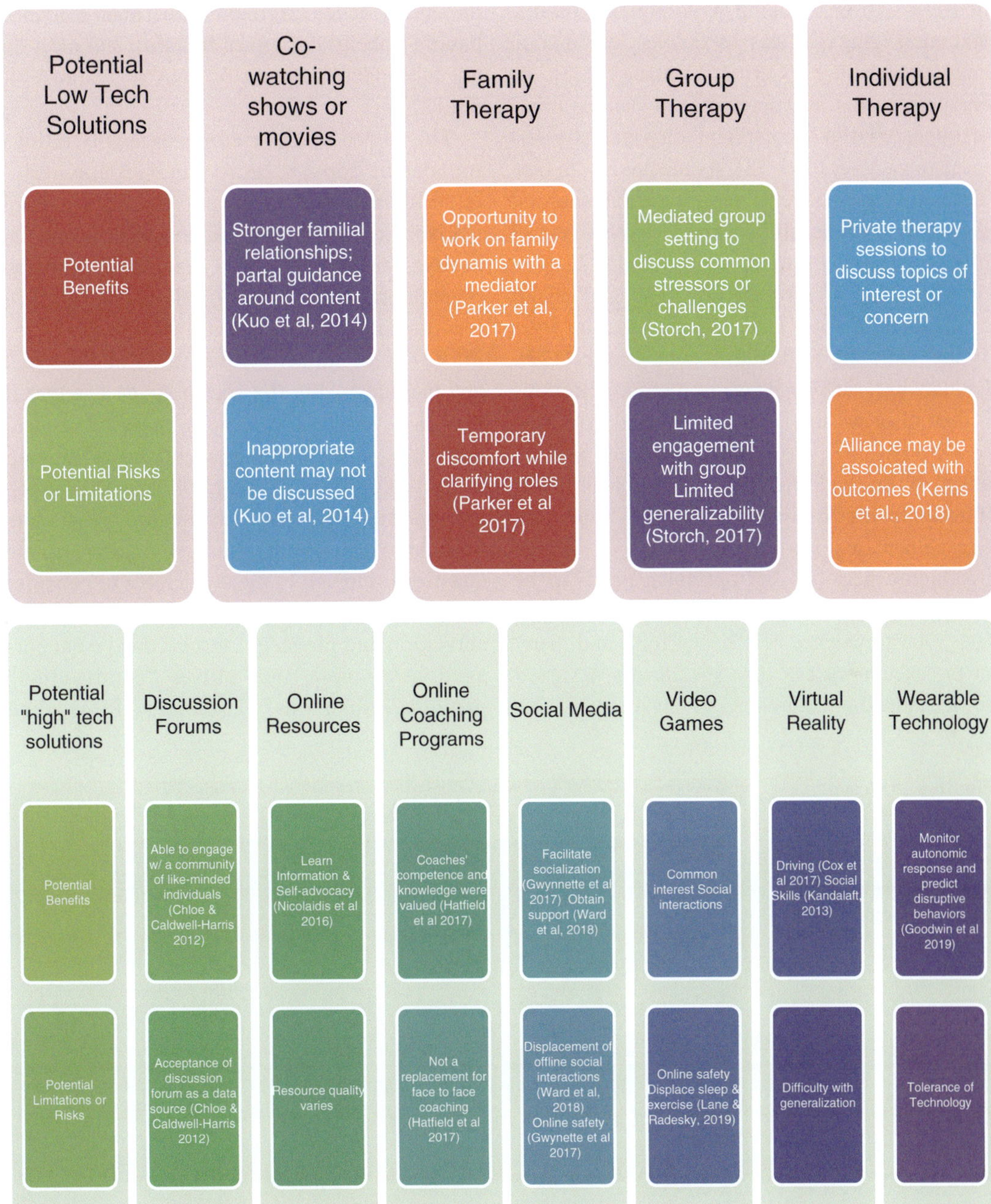

Fig. 18.3 Social outlets for TAY with ASD

Integrating Technology into Treatment

Digital media and related technology are incrementally becoming a part of mental healthcare delivery – from booking appointments online; text messaging services to deliver information and support (e.g., Caring Contacts) [23]; or enabling access to emergent help such as crisis text line, or HIPAA-compliant telepsychiatry services (e.g., VSee) [40, 73]. As mental health burden outstrips current psychiatric resources, digital therapeutic options could play a crucial role in addressing the gap in services [127].

A growing area of interest is mental health applications ("apps"), of which there are over 10,000 claiming to benefit mental health [127]. Patients may already be using these applications in lieu of or to supplement traditional treatment options [91, 97]. Potential advantages include affordability, wide-ranging geographical reach, immediate accessibility in a crisis, improving engagement, and lowering the stigma of seeking psychiatric help [4]. Yet optimism needs to be tempered with caution. The vast majority of apps lack robust evidence of efficacy [68], and many of the exceptions are apps specifically designed for a trial and not commercially available [4, 30, 97]. However, where RCT evidence is available, the results are encouraging [29, 111]. Unfortunately, the rapid development of apps means that their rigorous study is impractical. Practitioners ought to be aware that many apps may be evidence informed (rather than evidence based), unhelpful, or even harmful, and most do not fall under the remit of FDA regulations [4, 68, 127].

The APA does not endorse or supply ratings for specific apps. However, an APA app evaluation model has been published providing guidance to clinicians as to how to examine the utility, suitability, risks (including privacy issues), and benefit of a particular app before recommending it to patients in clinical practice [5, 22]. This model is illustrated in Fig. 18.4 and includes using the app to gauge whether it may add value to specific aspects of clinical care, e.g., stress management, strengthening adaptive coping skills (e.g., the meditation app Headspace) [22], or medication reminders (e.g., MediSafe [108]). Chan et al. also provide questions relevant to these domains to consider before recommending an app [21]. Behavioral activation and physical exercise can be encouraged using apps that utilize "gamification" methods such as Zombies, Run! and

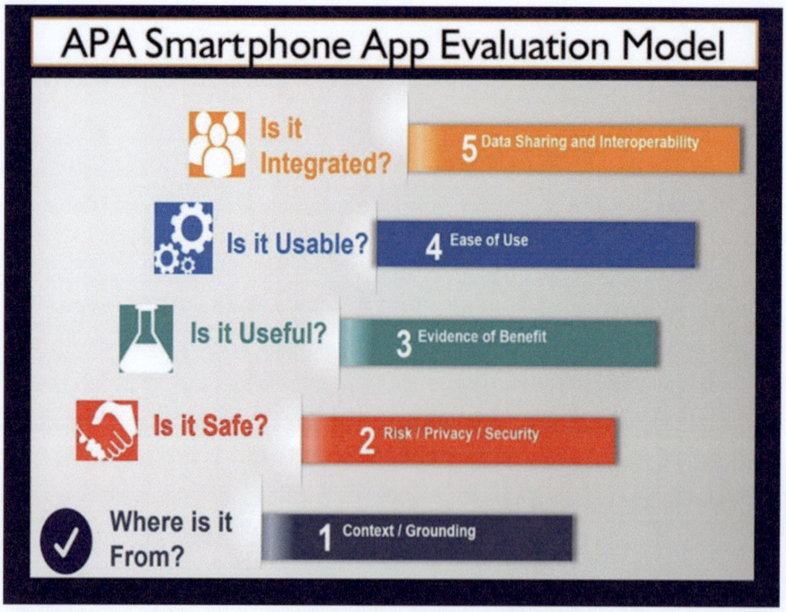

Fig. 18.4 APA app evaluation model [126]. (Adapted APA app evaluation model, reproduced with permission from author)

SuperBetter [7, 104]. The gamelike interface and rewards system have been shown to increase motivation for individuals to reach their goals [22, 84].

Apps engaging in real time or ecological momentary assessment of mood, thoughts, or behavior (e.g., MoodPrism, T2 Mood Tracker) lend themselves well to outpatient care [30, 91]. These may be useful for diagnostic clarification. Apps are perceived positively by youth and can improve patient engagement in treatment [91]. Additional benefits include increasing emotional awareness, reduced subjective experience of depression, a positive "digital placebo effect," and, importantly, limited potential for adverse effects [4, 6, 7, 30]. However, a barrier to clinical use is the inability to incorporate and store app data with current EMR systems [127].

AACAP suggests a few applications, e.g., MY3, which assists users with a readily available safety plan and contact information of supports that they have pre-created for use in times of crisis [1, 72, 127]. However, they are recommended with the proviso that all are utilized in conjunction with a provider [1, 127]. A recent meta-analysis of CBT treatment formats indicated that guided digital self-help was as effective as individual or group based ones for treatment of depression [24]. A burgeoning area is virtual reality exposure therapy via apps such as ZeroPhobia [29]. RCTs have indicated these helpful for an array of anxiety disorders including phobias [17, 29, 58]. CBT-i Coach for insomnia and PTSD Coach, developed by the US Veteran Affairs, have also demonstrated some efficacy [50, 62, 64].

Digital therapeutics are becoming a credible option for treatment, and some app creators are seeking FDA approval as a legitimate treatment option for psychiatric disorders. Recently the FDA approved the app "reSET" for the treatment of substance use disorder (in conjunction with face-to-face treatment) [134]. Other apps that are undergoing FDA approval include Headspace and Akili Interactive Labs' video game for ADHD treatment, for which initial trials yielded positive results [102].

Clinical Vignette

Maria is a 19-year-old female who was living at home while taking classes at the local community college. She had difficulty with making new friends but stayed connected to her high school friends on social media. She did play a couple video games, watch videos, and looked up facts about her favorite topics, but she spent hours on social media instead of doing her schoolwork. After late nights online, she often slept through morning classes. By the time the semester ended, she had regular complaints of neck pain, day and night reversal, and poor grades (C's, D's, and an F).

Maria connected with a therapist and psychiatrist through her college mental health center. She was diagnosed with social anxiety, started on escitalopram, and began the spring semester. She was motivated to see peers in her afternoon classes. With her therapist, she improved her time management – building in time for assignments, physical exercise, eating, and sleeping. Any remaining time before bedtime, she spent at her discretion online. She ended the semester with A's and B's and some acquaintances that she might socialize with over the summer.

Solutions

Higher work- and school-related demands, greater freedom, more opportunities for socializing, and reduced family-related structure and support create increased autonomy and difficult choices for TAY. "On-the-fly" decision-making regarding media engagement is a poor strategy due to its high cognitive demands, poor prioritization, susceptibility to impulsive decisions, and the ever-present digital distractions.

For healthy functioning, TAY should adopt a time management approach which prioritizes productive work and essential responsibilities, captures goals, lists important tasks, and schedules events. Tasks requiring sustained attention must often be "chunked," broken up into manageable portions. TAY should cultivate healthy habits incorporating exercise, in-person socializing, creative activities, and routine chores. A consistent work routine is preferable to sporadic expenditures of effort. Creating calendars, setting timers, and making lists help to organize activities.

Many TAY must be taught about the costs of multitasking. Multitasking has not been shown to cause permanent cognitive deficits [8, 118], but it reduces productivity and increases fatigue [57]. The brain's data processing systems truly only focus on one thing at a time, so what appears to be multitasking is actually rapid shifting of attention back and forth. Cognitive energy and efficiency are lost each time the attentional filter changes from one task to another, the costs of which quickly accumulate.

Frequent distractions and interruptions (such as those created by screen media) reduce productivity in much the same way. Each time sustained attention is turned away from active work, efficiency is sacrificed. The extra effort required to shift attention frequently may give "multitasking" TAY the mistaken impression they are working efficiently. Even the mere availability of an inert smartphone within reach creates a distraction significant enough to hinder cognitive performance [138].

Addressing problems of multitasking and frequent interruption are most important for TAY already suffering disorders which interfere with cognitive control and attention, such as depression, anxiety, and ADHD.

Finally, getting sufficient sleep is an essential activity, not a waste of time as many youth believe. TAY are easily caught up in subcultures which discount the benefits of sleep and normalize insufficient sleep habits. Sleep researcher Lauren Hale has suggested the approach of desist, dampen, and dim. This can be understood as (1) *desist* by stopping digital media at least 1 hour prior to bed, (2) *dampen* by avoiding arousing material just prior to sleep, and (3) *dim* by reducing screen light intensity to minimize sleep-disrupting blue light exposure after sunset [44].

Problematic technology use habits are common in TAY, and professionals should assess these problems as well as motivation for change, coping skills, and psychosocial supports before setting treatment goals. Depending on this assessment, either a harm reduction or abstinence-based approach may be appropriate. It may be helpful to reframe unhealthy or problematic digital behaviors as misguided methods to meet one's basic needs such as receiving attention, stimulation, self-expression, affiliation, or control. Matching these needs with alternative, enjoyable, healthy non-digital activities is often the key to an optimal outcome [39]. A lack of mindfulness often plays a role in excessive online engagement [14]. Transitional age youth should be encouraged to notice and tolerate impulses to use their devices. Creating self-awareness represents a good start while other interventions are initiated. Regular media "fasts" (i.e., periods of abstinence), along with scheduling screen-free elements of daily routine, will help prevent relapse and reduce incidents of overuse. A detailed list of dilemmas associated with technology habits and their solutions can be found in Table 18.5.

Table 18.5 Technology-related dilemmas and solutions

Area of concern	Solutions
Privacy – exposure to junk mail, spam, identity theft, account hacking, and ransomware which misappropriate personal information *Safety* – involvement with stalking, cyberbullying, or disputes risking legal problems or retaliation. Vulnerability to distracted driving and walking	Wise sharing of sensitive information, especially that which may attract unwanted attention, create conflict, or alienate others Use platforms, apps, and websites which are transparent regarding data collection and safeguards Use strong privacy settings on video games, apps, and websites
Displacement of movement – lack of physical activity and deconditioning *Repetitive stress injury* – particularly of the neck, back, and eyes. Contracture and weakening of abdominal and back musculature skeleton due to disuse	Increase exercise, consider fitness tracker or monitoring through phone or mobile device Take frequent screen breaks, set timers to cue breaks Engage a full range of movements of every part of the body Use a standing desk or treadmill, walk while listening or conversing on devices, and schedule times to stand

Table 18.5 (continued)

Area of concern	Solutions
Sensory overload – underexposure to nature Loud, distracting, and agitating noises. Noise-induced hearing loss, often caused by excessive headphone volume *Sleep /circadian rhythm disturbance* – underexposure to natural lighting and overexposure to nighttime light, especially blue light	Seek leisure activities which maximize opportunities in green spaces away from urban stressors Honor the importance of sleep Align digital media use with natural circadian rhythms Turn devices off when not in active use Decrease screen brightness settings or use blue light-filtering glasses at night Use eye shades and earplugs to minimize disruptive sensory exposure to nighttime light and background noise
Attention fatigue and difficulty with focus –excessive time with digital media causing ADHD- like symptoms *Lack of productivity* – digital media displacing essential activities such as work or school. Frequent distractions or "multitasking" causing ineffective work or learning	Minimize distractions including multiple active devices, open windows, pop-ups, notifications, or email Prioritize cognitive energy toward important tasks "Chunk" work into manageable intervals, intermixed with breaks for physical activity and creative diversions Manage information flow via a system which helps order goals, organize dataflow, and ensure task completion
Cognitive distortions related to distorted information and false narratives – worsening of emotional and cognitive deficits via media featuring narrow perspectives, negativity, and/or distorted social comparison, or promoting inaccurate, depressogenic, and anxiety-generating schemas	Self-assessment of positive vs. negative emotional valence and behavioral impacts of engagement with various media sources Monitoring influences on rigid or negative thought patterns, cognitive distortions, and avoidance behavior Build awareness of stressors inherent in following news media, marketing manipulations, and divisive rhetoric
FOMO and/excessive social comparison – distress based on anxieties regarding missed social activities, exclusion, and envy Fueled by recognition of a narrowed social life and relationships primarily conducted through digital media	Avoid social media or other digital diversions which increase distress and isolation Self-assess the balance between online and offline relationships Create a practice to be thankful for what you have, rather than what you lack Proactively establish etiquette and expectations in housing or dorms which promotes real-world experiences
Parental over-involvement/infantilizing – digitally enabled enmeshment and related parental overprotection	Establish boundaries regarding levels of family involvement. Consider digital calendars or reminders to schedule contact TAY may need to set limits on overinvolved parents and prioritize the establishment of an independent identity
Online conflict – cyberbullying and digital "drama." Many platforms, especially those with anonymous posting, support negativity, tribalism, or hate. Due to amplification effects and permanency of the online record, hostile interactions can have long-lasting, more profound effects	Understanding that lack of social cues and anonymity in electronic communication exacerbate conflict Careful stewardship of personal digital footprint and reputation When angry, wait 24 h before sending related posts, texts, or email, and consider going offline to engage directly
Identity formation, purpose, and meaning – disconnected "offline" lives lack social bonds and purpose. Lack of meaning is especially painful for those dissatisfied with school or work and those subscribing to popular and consumer culture emphasis on status and wealth	Assess whether digital media habits are building community and positive relationships Constructive risk-taking regarding building identity and contributing to community Seek out creative and social outlets unrelated to work or school

Conclusion

Today's TAY appear different than previous generations, in part due to the technologies interwoven into their lives. They are required to use smartphones, computers, and other digital devices to function in their school, work, family, and social lives. TAY have ready access to unlimited digitally mediated leisure activities and diversions. They lack role models for media habits and must pave a new path navigating complex and tempting digital environments.

A successful launch into adulthood will require effective strategies, including setting realistic limits on digital media use, effectively prioritizing activities, and honoring the importance of sleep, in-person contact, and physical activity. In clinical populations, unhealthy habits are common, including PIU – problematic Internet use. Changing harmful patterns is often difficult, especially in TAY whose habits are engrained over a substantial portion of their lives. A valid assessment of digital activities is complicated because many intermix benefits (e.g., socialization, learning, and stimulation) with unhealthy patterns that compromise other aspects of life.

Mental health providers working with transitional age youth must assess the quantity, quality, and impact of their digital media habits. Asking the right questions regarding Internet use is vital to gathering the essential information. Thankfully, screening tools can help simplify and standardize such assessments, as can digital devices themselves.

For example, a quick smartphone assessment notes frequently used apps, notification settings, total screen time, and daily steps walked. With little effort and expense, such important data can be gathered, as well as time spent on apps or games. Smart devices can track physiological measures such as blood pressure, medication adherence, or sleep. In the near future, digital devices could routinely and automatically download directly into electronic medical records, easing the identification and tracking of relevant health patterns and simplifying treatment plans.

For TAY, digital media-related issues are often important enough to warrant a substantial component of the biopsychosocial formulation. An ever-expanding range of apps, online treatment, and emerging uses for virtual reality efficiently augment traditional care. Digital technologies can enable patients to learn clinically relevant information and track mood states and could prompt patients, thereby increasing medication compliance, or completion of psychotherapy "homework" assignments.

Thus the paradox of growing up digital is constantly evolving, creating new challenges and opportunities. Youth benefit from virtually unlimited information, the ability to track one's own habits and enhance personal relationships with improved communication. Yet, simultaneously, they suffer far more distractions; receive less trustworthy information, with online acquaintances replacing friendships; and have powerful enticements to establish unhealthy or self-destructive digital behaviors.

To quote Dickens: "it was the best of times, it was the worst of times, it was the age of wisdom, it was the age of foolishness" [28]. Today's digitally native TAY enjoy many positive trends with regard to safety, health, and quality of life. However their generation must contend with an epidemic of depression, anxiety, and suicidality. TAY face unprecedented challenges related to their digital media devices, yet they wield powerful new tools capable of enhancing their lives. Mental health providers who have stood witness to these trends and are well-informed are capable of providing practical solutions to new versions of timeless challenges inherent in emerging into adulthood during extraordinary times.

References

1. AACAP. Resources for Youth. 2019. https://www.aacap.org/AACAP/Families_and_Youth/Resource_Centers/Depression_Resource_Center/Resources_for_Youth_Depression.aspx.
2. Agnew-Blais JC, Polanczyk GV, Danese A, Wertz J, Moffitt TE, Arseneault L. Evaluation of the persistence, remission, and emergence of attention-deficit/hyperactivity disorder in Young adulthood. JAMA Psychiat. 2016;73(7):713–20.
3. Andreassen CS, Pallesen S, Griffiths MD. The relationship between addictive use of social media, narcissism, and self-esteem: findings from a large national survey. Addict Behav. 2017;64:287–93.
4. Anthes E. Mental health: There's an app for that. Nature. 2016;532(7597):20–3.
5. APA. App evaluation model. https://www.psychiatry.org/psychiatrists/practice/mental-health-apps/app-evaluation-model. Accessed 15 Jul 2019.
6. Bakker D, Rickard N. Engagement in mobile phone app for self-monitoring of emotional wellbeing predicts changes in mental health: MoodPrism. J Affect Disord. 2018;227:432–42.
7. Bakker D, Kazantzis N, Rickwood D, Rickard N. Mental health smartphone apps: review and evidence-based recommendations for future developments. JMIR Men Health. 2016;3(1):e7.

8. Baumgartner SE, van der Schuur WA, Lemmens JS, te Poel F. The relationship between media multitasking and attention problems in adolescents: results of two longitudinal studies. Hum Commun Res. 2018;44(1):3–30.
9. Beard KW, Wolf EM. Modification in the proposed diagnostic criteria for internet addiction. Cyberpsychol Behav. 2001;4(3):377–83.
10. Becker SP, Lienesch JA. Nighttime media use in adolescents with ADHD: links to sleep problems and internalizing symptoms. Sleep Med. 2018;51:171–8.
11. Bonetti I, Campbell M, Gilmore L. The relationship of loneliness and social anxiety with Children's and Adolescents' online communication. Cyberpsychol Behav Soc Netw. 2009;13(3):279–85.
12. Booker C, Kelly Y, Sacker A. Gender differences in the associations between age trends of social media interaction and well-being among 10-15 year olds in the UK. BMC Public Health. 2018;18(1):321.
13. Bostwick JM, Bucci JA. Internet sex addiction treated with naltrexone. Mayo Clin Proc. 2008;83(2):226–30.
14. Brewer J. Mindfulness training for addictions: has neuroscience revealed a brain hack by which awareness subverts the addictive process? Curr Opin Psychol. 2019;28:198–203.
15. Brown RC, Fischer T, Goldwich AD, Keller F, Young R, Plener PL. Cutting: non-suicidal self-injury (NSSI) on Instagram. Psychol Med. 2018;48(2):337–46.
16. Burke M, Kraut R, Williams D. Social use of computer-mediated communication by adults on the autism spectrum. In: Proceedings of the 2010 ACM conference on computer supported cooperative work. ACM. 2010. pp. 425–434.
17. Carl E, Stein AT, Levihn-Coon A, et al. Virtual reality exposure therapy for anxiety and related disorders: a meta-analysis of randomized controlled trials. J Anxiety Disord. 2019;61:27–36.
18. Carson NJ, Gansner M, Khang J. Assessment of digital media use in the adolescent psychiatric evaluation. Child Adolesc Psychiatr Clin N Am. 2018;27(2):133–43.
19. Carta MG, Zairo F, Mellino G, Hardoy MC. Add-on quetiapine in the treatment of major depressive disorder in elderly patients with cerebrovascular damage. Clin Pract Epidemiol Ment Health. 2007;3:28.
20. Caye A, Rocha TB, Anselmi L, Murray J, Menezes AM, Barros FC, Gonçalves H, Wehrmeister F, Jensen CM, Steinhausen HC, Swanson JM, Kieling C, Rohde LA. Attention-deficit/hyperactivity disorder trajectories from childhood to Young adulthood: evidence from a birth cohort supporting a late-onset syndrome. JAMA Psychiat. 2016;73(7):705–12.
21. Chan S, Torous J, Hinton L, Yellowlees P. Towards a framework for evaluating Mobile mental health apps. Telemed J E Health. 2015;21(12):1038–41.
22. Chandrashekar P. Do mental health mobile apps work: evidence and recommendations for designing high-efficacy mental health mobile apps. mHealth. 2018;4:6.
23. Comtois KA, Kerbrat AH, DeCou CR, et al. Effect of augmenting standard care for military personnel with brief caring text messages for suicide prevention: a randomized clinical trial. JAMA Psychiat. 2019;76(5):474–83.
24. Cuijpers P, Noma H, Karyotaki E, Cipriani A, Furukawa TA. Effectiveness and acceptability of cognitive behavior therapy delivery formats in adults with depression: a network meta-analysis. JAMA Psychiat. 2019; 76(7): 700–7.
25. Davidson J. Autistic culture online: virtual communication and cultural expression on the spectrum. Soc Cult Georg. 2008;9(7):791–806.
26. De Sousa A. Fluoxetine in the management of pornography addiction. Indian J Ment Health. 2016;3(3):372–4.
27. Dell'Osso B, Hadley S, Allen A, Baker B, Chaplin WF, Hollander E. Escitalopram in the treatment of impulsive-compulsive internet usage disorder: an open-label trial followed by a double-blind discontinuation phase. J Clin Psychiatry. 2008;69(3):452–6.
28. Dickens C, Simon S. A tale of two cities. New York: Vintage Books; 1990.
29. Donker T, Cornelisz I, van Klaveren C, et al. Effectiveness of self-guided app-based virtual reality cognitive behavior therapy for acrophobia: a randomized clinical trial. JAMA Psychiat. 2019;76(7):682–90.
30. Dubad M, Winsper C, Meyer C, Livanou M, Marwaha S. A systematic review of the psychometric properties, usability and clinical impacts of mobile mood-monitoring applications in young people. Psychol Med. 2018;48(2):208–28.
31. Dunlop S, More E, Romer D. Where do youth learn about suicides on the internet, and what influence does this have on suicidal ideation? J Child Psychol Psychiatry. 2011;52(10):1073–80.
32. Englander E. Risky business: talking with your patients about Cyberbullying and sex. Child Adolesc Psychiatr Clin N Am. 2018;27(2):287–305.
33. Evren B, Evren C, Dalbudak E, Topcu M, Kutlu N. Relationship of internet addiction severity with probable ADHD and difficulties in emotion regulation among young adults. Psychiatry Res. 2018;269:494–500.
34. Evren B, Evren C, Dalbudak E, Topcu M, Kutlu N. The impact of depression, anxiety, neuroticism, and severity of internet addiction symptoms on the relationship between probable ADHD and severity of insomnia among young adults. Psychiatry Res. 2019;271:726–31.
35. Finkelhor D. Commentary: cause for alarm? Youth and internet risk research--a commentary on Livingstone and Smith (2014). J Child Psychol Psychiatry. 2014;55(6):655–8.
36. Gansner M, Belfort E, Cook B, et al. Problematic internet use and associated high-risk behavior in an adolescent clinical sample: results from a survey of

psychiatrically hospitalized youth. Cyberpsychol Behav Soc Netw. 2019;22(5):349–54.
37. Gillespie-Lynch K, Kapp SK, Shane-Simpson C, Smith DS, Hutman T. Intersections between the autism Spectrum and the internet: perceived benefits and preferred functions of computer-mediated communication. Intellect Dev Disabil. 2014;52(6):456–69. https://doi.org/10.1352/1934-9556-52.6.456.
38. Gitlow L, Janney B, Lemery C, McDonald J, McGinley B, Rabideau K. How college students diagnosed with anxiety disorders and/or depression use everyday technology. Disabil Rehabil Assist Technol. 2018;14:1–8.
39. Godley MD, Godley SH, Dennis ML, Funk RR, Pasetti LL, Petry NM. A randomized trial of assertive continuing care and contingency management for adolescents with substance use disorders. J Consult Clin Psychol. 2014;82(1):40–51.
40. Gonzales R, Douglas Anglin M, Glik DC. Exploring the feasibility of text messaging to support substance abuse recovery among youth in treatment. Health Educ Res. 2014;29(1):13–22.
41. Gorucu S, Murphy D, Foster D, Hanagriff R, Ewing J. Technology use among youth while operating farm equipment. J Agromedicine. 2018;23(4):305–14.
42. Grant JE, Chamberlain SR, Odlaug BL, Potenza MN, Kim SW. Memantine shows promise in reducing gambling severity and cognitive inflexibility in pathological gambling: a pilot study. Psychopharmacology. 2010;212(4):603–12.
43. Grubbs J, Kraus S, Perry S. Self-reported addiction to pornography in a nationally representative sample: the roles of use habits, religiousness, and moral incongruence. J Behav Addict. 2019;8(1):88–93.
44. Hale LE. Digital media and sleep health among adolescents: Does sleep mediate the association between screen time and depressive symptoms? Poster presented at: the 66th Annual Meeting of the American Academy of Child and Adolescent Psychiatry, 2019 October 14–19; Chicago, IL.
45. Hale L, Kirschen GW, LeBourgeois MK, et al. Youth screen media habits and sleep: sleep-friendly screen behavior recommendations for clinicians, educators, and parents. Child Adolesc Psychiatr Clin N Am. 2018;27(2):229–45.
46. Han DH, Lee YS, Na C, Ahn JY, Chung US, Daniels MA, Haws CA, Renshaw PF. The effect of methylphenidate on Internet video game play in children with attention-deficit/hyperactivity disorder. Compr Psychiatry. 2009;50(3):251–6.
47. Han DH, Hwang JW, Renshaw PF. Bupropion sustained release treatment decreases craving for video games and cue-induced brain activity in patients with Internet video game addiction. Exp Clin Psychopharmacol. 2010;18(4):297–304.
48. Hawryluk. Bulletin HMT. Supply of psychiatrists shrinks. 2016. Accessed 18 Jul 2019.
49. Ho R, Zhang M, Tsang T, Toh A, Pan F, Lu Y, Cheng C, Yip P, Lam L, Lai C-M, Watanabe H, Mak K-K. The association between internet addiction and psychiatric co-morbidity: a meta-analysis. BMC Psychiatry. 2014;14:183.
50. Horsch CH, Lancee J, Griffioen-Both F, et al. Mobile phone-delivered cognitive Behavioral therapy for insomnia: a randomized waitlist controlled trial. J Med Internet Res. 2017;19(4):e70.
51. Hussain Z, Griffiths MD. Problematic social networking site use and comorbid psychiatric disorders: a systematic review of recent large-scale studies. Front Psych. 2018;9:686.
52. Jelenchick LA, Eickhoff J, Christakis DA, et al. The problematic and risky internet use screening scale (PRIUSS) for adolescents and Young adults: scale development and refinement. Comput Hum Behav. 2014;35:171–8.
53. John A, Glendenning AC, Marchant A, Montgomery P, Stewart A, Wood S, Lloyd K, Hawton K. Self-harm, suicidal behaviours, and cyberbullying in children and Young people: systematic review. J Med Internet Res. 2018;19;20(4):129.
54. Jones JJ, Kirschen GW, Kancharla S, Hale L. Association between late-night tweeting and next-day game performance among professional basketball players. Sleep Health. 2019;5(1):68–71.
55. Jordan CJ, Caldwell-Harris CL. Understanding differences in Neurotypical and autism spectrum special interests through internet forums. Intellect Dev Disabil. 2012a;50(5):391–402. https://doi.org/10.1352/1934-9556-50.5.391.
56. Jordan CJ, Caldwell-Harris CL. Understanding differences in neurotypical and autism spectrum special interests through internet forums. Intellect Dev Disabil. 2012b;50(5):391–402. https://doi.org/10.1352/1934-9556-50.5.391.
57. Junco R, Cotten SR. No a 4 U: the relationship between multitasking and academic performance. Comput Educ. 2012;59(2):505–14.
58. Kampmann IL, Emmelkamp PM, Hartanto D, Brinkman WP, Zijlstra BJ, Morina N. Exposure to virtual social interactions in the treatment of social anxiety disorder: a randomized controlled trial. Behav Res Ther. 2016;77:147–56.
59. Keracher M. #StatusofMind [Internet]. Rsph.org.uk. 2019 [cited 19 July 2019]. Available from: https://www.rsph.org.uk/our-work/campaigns/status-of-mind.html.
60. Kim HJ. Exercise rehabilitation for smartphone addiction. J Exerc Rehabil. 2013;9(6):500–5.
61. Kim HJ, Min JY, Kim HJ, Min KB. Accident risk associated with smartphone addiction: a study on university students in Korea. J Behav Addict. 2017;6(4):699–707.
62. Koffel E, Kuhn E, Petsoulis N, et al. A randomized controlled pilot study of CBT-I coach: feasibility, acceptability, and potential impact of a mobile phone application for patients in cognitive behavioral therapy for insomnia. Health Informatics J. 2018;24(1):3–13.
63. Korchmaros J, Ybarra M, Mitchell K. Adolescent online romantic relationship initiation: differences

by sexual and gender identification. J Adolesc. 2015;40:54–64.
64. Kuhn E, van der Meer C, Owen JE, et al. PTSD coach around the world. mHealth. 2018;4:15.
65. Kuo MH, Orsmond GI, Coster WJ, Cohn ES. Media use among adolescents with autism spectrum disorder. Autism. 2014;18(8):914–23.
66. Kuss DJ, Lopez-Fernandez O. Internet addiction and problematic internet use: a systematic review of clinical research. World J Psychiatry. 2016;6(1):143–76. https://doi.org/10.5498/wjp.v6.i1.143. eCollection 2016 Mar 22.
67. Landoll R, La Greca A, Lai B, Chan S, Herge W. Cyber victimization by peers: prospective associations with adolescent social anxiety and depressive symptoms. J Adolesc. 2015;42:77–86.
68. Larsen ME, Huckvale K, Nicholas J, et al. Using science to sell apps: evaluation of mental health app store quality claims. NPJ Dig Med. 2019;2:18.
69. Leménager T, Hoffmann S, Dieter J, Reinhard I, Mann K, Kiefer F. The links between healthy, problematic, and addicted internet use regarding comorbidities and self-concept-related characteristics. J Behav Addict. 2018;7(1):31–43.
70. Li W, Zhang W, Xiao L, Nie J. The association of internet addiction symptoms with impulsiveness, loneliness, novelty seeking and behavioral inhibition system among adults with attention-deficit/hyperactivity disorder (ADHD). Psychiatry Res. 2016;243:357–64.
71. Lin LY, Sidani JE, Shensa A, Radovic A, Miller E, Colditz JB, Hoffman BL, Giles LM, Primack BA. Association between social media use and depression among U.S. young adults. Dep Anx. 2016;33(4):784–94.
72. Link2 Health Solutions I. https://my3app.org/. Accessed 15 Jul 2019.
73. Lopez WM, Lustig SL. Telepsychiatry: watching your back while staying in the black. Psychiatr Times. 2015;32(8):41–4.
74. Lorenz T, Frischling C, Cuadros R, Heinitz K. Autism and overcoming job barriers: comparing job-related barriers and possible solutions in and outside of autism-specific employment. PLoS One. 2016;11(1):e0147040.
75. Lui J, Nie J, Wang Y. Effects of group Counseling programs, cognitive Behavioral therapy, and sports intervention on internet addiction in East Asia: a systematic review and meta-analysis. Int J Environ Res Public Health. 2017;14(12):1470.
76. Lup K, Trub L, Rosenthal L. Instagram #Instasad?: exploring associations among Instagram use, depressive symptoms, negative social comparison, and strangers followed. Cyberpsychol Behav Soc Netw. 2015;18(5):247–52.
77. Machmutow K, Perren S, Sticca F, Alsaker F. Peer victimisation and depressive symptoms: can specific coping strategies buffer the negative impact of cybervictimisation? Emot Behav Diffic. 2012;17(3–4):403–20.
78. Marchant A, Hawton K, Stewart A, Montgomery P, Singaravelu V, Lloyd K, Purdy N, Daine K, John A. A systematic review of the relationship between internet use, self-harm and suicidal behaviour in young people: the good, the bad and the unknown. PLoS One. 2017;12(8):e0181722. Erratum in: PLoS One. 2018;13(3)
79. Marino C, Gini G, Vieno A, Spada MM. The associations between problematic Facebook use, psychological distress and well-being among adolescents and young adults: a systematic review and meta-analysis. J Affect Disord. 2018;226:274–81.
80. Marmet S, Studer J, Grazioli VS, Gmel G. Bidirectional associations between self-reported gaming disorder and adult attention deficit hyperactivity disorder: evidence from a sample of Young Swiss men. Front Psych. 2018;11(9):649.
81. Martinez-Pecino R, Garcia-Gavilan M. Likes and problematic Instagram use: the moderating role of self-esteem. Cyberpsychol Behav Soc Netw. 2019;22(6):412–6. https://doi.org/10.1089/cyber.2018.0701. Epub 2019 May 20
82. Masuda N, Kurahashi I, Onari H. Suicide ideation of individuals in online social networks. PLoS One. 2013;8(4):e62262.
83. Matamura M, Tochigi M, Usami S, Yonehara H, Fukushima M, Nishida A, Togo F, Sasaki T. Associations between sleep habits and mental health status and suicidality in a longitudinal survey of monozygotic twin adolescents. J Sleep Res. 2014;23(3):292–6.
84. Moran MJ, Coons JM. Effects of a smart-phone application on psychological, physiological, and performance variables in college-aged individuals while running. Int J Exerc Sci. 2015;8(2):1.
85. Moreno MA, Arseniev-Koehler A, Selkie E. Development and testing of a 3-item screening tool for problematic internet use. J Pediatr. 2016;176:167–72.e161
86. Mori C, Temple J, Browne D, Madigan S. Association of Sexting with Sexual Behaviors and Mental Health among Adolescents. JAMA Pediatr. 2019;73(8):770–9.
87. Nereim C, Bickham D, Rich M. A primary care pediatrician's guide to assessing problematic interactive media use. Curr Opin Pediatr. 2019;31(4):435–41.
88. Nesi J, Prinstein M. Using social Media for Social Comparison and Feedback-Seeking: gender and popularity moderate associations with depressive symptoms. J Abnorm Child Psychol. 2015;43(8):1427–38.
89. Nie J, Zhang W, Liu Y. Exploring depression, self-esteem and verbal fluency with different degrees of internet addiction among Chinese college students. Compr Psychiatry. 2017;72:114–20.
90. Oberst U, Wegmann E, Stodt B, Brand M, Chamarro A. Negative consequences from heavy social networking in adolescents: the mediating role of fear of missing out. J Adolesc. 2017;55:51–60.
91. Palmier-Claus JE, Rogers A, Ainsworth J, et al. Integrating mobile-phone based assessment for psy-

chosis into people's everyday lives and clinical care: a qualitative study. BMC Psychiatry. 2013;13:34.
92. Park JH, Lee YS, Sohn JH, Han DH. Effectiveness of atomoxetine and methylphenidate for problematic online gaming in adolescents with attention deficit hyperactivity disorder. Hum Psychopharmacol. 2016;31(6):427–32.
93. Pluhar E, Kavanaugh JR, Levinson JA, Rich M. Problematic interactive media use in teens: comorbidities, assessment, and treatment. Psychol Res Behav Manag. 2019;12:447–55.
94. Plummer F, Manea L, Trepel D, McMillan D. Screening for anxiety disorders with the GAD-7 and GAD-2: a systematic review and diagnostic metaanalysis. Gen Hosp Psychiatry. 2016;39:24–31.
95. Poyntz SR, Pedri J. Youth and media culture. Oxford University Press; 2018. Available at https://doi.org/10.1093/acrefore/9780190264093.013.75
96. Prizant-Passal S, Shechner T, Aderka I. Social anxiety and internet use - a meta-analysis: what do we know? What are we missing? Comput Hum Behav. 2016;62:221–9.
97. Radovic A, Vona PL, Santostefano AM, Ciaravino S, Miller E, Stein BD. Smartphone applications for mental health. Cyberpsychol Behav Soc Netw. 2016;19(7):465–70.
98. Raudsepp L, Kais K. Longitudinal associations between problematic social media use and depressive symptoms in adolescent girls. Prev Med Rep. 2019;21:15.
99. Reid D, Weigle P. Social media use among adolescents: benefits and risks. Adolesc Psychiatry. 2014;4(2):73–80.
100. Rideout V. The common sense census: media use by tweens and teens | common sense media [Internet]. Commonsensemedia.org. 2019 [cited 19 July 2019]. Available from: https://www.commonsensemedia.org/research/the-common-sense-census-media-use-by-tweens-and-teens.
101. Rideout V, Fox S, Well Being Trust. Digital health practices, social media use, and mental well-being among teens and young adults in the U.S. articles, Abstracts, and Reports. 2018; 1093.
102. Rijcken C. Chapter 15 - digital therapeutic mangroves. In: Rijcken C, editor. Pharmaceutical care in digital revolution. Academic Press; 2019:169–179.
103. Roberts D. Kids & media @ the new millennium. Menlo Park CA: Henry J. Kaiser Family Foundation; 1999. Available at https://www.kff.org/wp-content/uploads/2013/01/kids-media-the-new-millennium--report.pdf.
104. Roepke AM, Jaffee SR, Riffle OM, McGonigal J, Broome R, Maxwell B. Randomized controlled trial of SuperBetter, a smartphone-based/internet-based self-help tool to reduce depressive symptoms. Games Health J. 2015;4(3):235–46.
105. Rosenthal S, Buka S, Marshall B, Carey K, Clark M. Negative experiences on Facebook and depressive symptoms among Young adults. J Adolesc Health. 2016;59(5):510–6.
106. Rozgonjuk D, Saal K, Taht K. Problematic smartphone use, deep and surface approaches to learning, and social media use in lectures. Int J Environ Res Public Health. 2018;15(1):92.
107. Sacchetti GM, Lefler EK. ADHD symptomology and social functioning in college students. J Atten Disord. 2017;21(12):1009–19.
108. Santo K, Richtering SS, Chalmers J, Thiagalingam A, Chow CK, Redfern J. Mobile phone apps to improve medication adherence: a systematic stepwise process to identify high-quality apps. JMIR Mhealth Uhealth. 2016;4(4):341–4.
109. Santos V, Nardi AE, King AL. Treatment of internet addiction in patient with panic disorder and obsessive compulsive disorder: a case report. CNS Neurol Disord Drug Targets. 2015;14(3):341–4.
110. Sattar P, Ramaswamy S. Internet gaming addiction. Can J Psychiatr. 2004;49(12):869–70.
111. Schlosser DA, Campellone TR, Truong B, et al. Efficacy of PRIME, a Mobile app intervention designed to improve motivation in Young people with schizophrenia. Schizophr Bull. 2018;44(5):1010–20.
112. Schupak C. Case report: lamotrigine/fluoxetine combination in the treatment of compulsive sexual behavior. Prog Neuro-Psychopharmacol Biol Psychiatry. 2007;31(6):1337–8. Epub 2007 Apr 25
113. Sedgwick R, Epstein S, Dutta R, Ougrin D. Social media, internet use and suicide attempts in adolescents. Curr Opin Psychiatry. 2019;32(6):534–41.
114. Shafi RMA, Romanowicz M, Croarkin PE. SwitchedOn: a call for assessing social media use of adolescents. Lancet Psychiatry. 2018;5(11):e27.
115. Shah J, Das P, Muthiah N, Milanaik R. New age technology and social media: adolescent psychosocial implications and the need for protective measures. Curr Opin Pediatr. 2019;31(1):148–56.
116. Shensa A, Escobar-Viera CG, Sidani JE, Bowman ND, Marshal MP, Primack BA. Problematic social media use and depressive symptoms among U.S. young adults: a nationally-representative study. Soc Sci Med. 2017;182:150–7.
117. Shensa A, Sidani J, Dew M, Escobar-Viera C, Primack B. Social media use and depression and anxiety symptoms: a cluster analysis. Am J Health Behav. 2018;42(2):116–28.
118. Shih S-I. A null relationship between media multitasking and Well-being. PLoS One. 2013;8(5):e64508.
119. Smith L, Liu B, Degenhardt L, Richters J, Patton G, Wand H, et al. Is sexual content in new media linked to sexual risk behaviour in young people? A systematic review and meta-analysis. Sex Health. 2016;13(6):501.
120. Spada MS. An overview of problematic internet use. Addict Behav. 2014;39(1):3–6.
121. Stiglic N, Viner R. Effects of screentime on the health and Well-being of children and adolescents: a systematic review of reviews. BMJ Open. 2019;9(1):e023191.

122. Strohmaier H, Murphy M, DeMatteo D. Youth sexting: prevalence rates, driving motivations, and the deterrent effect of legal consequences. Sex Res Soc Policy. 2014;11(3):245–55.
123. Swing E, Gentile D, Anderson C, Walsh D. Television and video game exposure and the development of attention problems. Pediatrics. 2010;126(2):214–21.
124. Tateno M, Teo AR, Shirasaka T, Tayama M, Watabe M, Kato TA. Internet addiction and self-evaluated attention-deficit hyperactivity disorder traits among Japanese college students. Psychiatry Clin Neurosci. 2016;70(12):567–72.
125. Thorisdottir I, Sigurvinsdottir R, Asgeirsdottir B, Allegrante J, Sigfusdottir I. Active and passive social media use and symptoms of anxiety and depressed mood among Icelandic adolescents. Cyberpsychol Behav Soc Netw. 2019;22(8):535–42.
126. Torous J. Evaluating smartphone health apps: 5 key step. 2017. https://www.psychiatrictimes.com/telepsychiatry/evaluating-smartphone-health-apps-5-key-steps.
127. Torous J, Luo J. Mental health apps: what to tell patients. Curr Psychiatr Ther. 2018;17:21–5.
128. Truelove V, Freeman J, Davey J. "I Snapchat and drive!" a mixed methods approach examining snapchat use while driving and deterrent perceptions among young adults. Accid Anal Prev. 2019;131:146–56.
129. Turel O, Cavagnaro DR, Meshi D. Short abstinence from online social networking sites reduces perceived stress, especially in excessive users. Psychiatry Res. 2018;270:947–53.
130. Twenge JM. iGen: why today's super-connected kids are growing up less rebellious, more tolerant, less happy— and completely unprepared for adulthood (and what this means for the rest of us). New York: Atria Books; 2017.
131. Twenge J, Cooper A, Joiner T, Duffy M, Binau S. Age, period, and cohort trends in mood disorder indicators and suicide-related outcomes in a nationally representative dataset, 2005–2017. J Abnorm Psychol. 2019;128(3):185–99.
132. Vannucci A, Flannery K, Ohannessian C. Social media use and anxiety in emerging adults. J Affect Disord. 2017;207:163–6.
133. Vogel E, Rose J, Okdie B, Eckles K, Franz B. Who compares and despairs? The effect of social comparison orientation on social media use and its outcomes. Personal Individ Differ. 2015;86:249–56.
134. Waltz E. Pear approval signals FDA readiness for digital treatments. Nat Biotechnol. 2018;36(6):481–2.
135. Wang BQ, Yao NQ, Zhou X, Liu J, Lv ZT. The association between attention deficit/hyperactivity disorder and internet addiction: a systematic review and meta-analysis. BMC Psychiatry. 2017;17:260.
136. Wardeiner A, Palaganas C, Londrico D, Candow L. The relationship between social media use and negative mental health outcomes. [conference presentation] 2017 Cleveland State Univerity, Cleveland; United States. http://www.gupiaozenmewan.net/sites/default/files/20%20B.pdf.
137. Weinstein A, Dorani D, Elhadif R, Bukovza Y, Yarmulnik A, Dannon P. Internet addiction is associated with social anxiety in young adults. Ann Clin Psych. 2015;27(1):4–9.
138. Wilmer HH, Sherman LE, Chein JM. Smartphones and cognition: a review of research exploring the links between mobile technology habits and cognitive functioning. Front Psychol. 2017;8:605.
139. Wolniewicz CA, Tiamiyu MF, Weeks JW, Elhai JD. Problematic smartphone use and relations with negative affect, fear of missing out, and fear of negative and positive evaluation. Psychiatry Res. 2018;262:618–23.
140. Wooldridge MB, Shapka J. Playing with technology: mother–toddler interaction scores lower during play with electronic toys. J Appl Dev Psychol. 2012;33(5):211–8.
141. Wu X, Tao S, Zhang Y, Zhang S, Tao F. Low physical activity and high screen time can increase the risks of mental health problems and poor sleep quality among Chinese college students. PLoS One. 2015;10(3):e0119607.
142. Yen JY, Liu TL, Wang PW, Chen CS, Yen CF, Ko CH. Association between internet gaming disorder and adult attention deficit and hyperactivity disorder and their correlates: impulsivity and hostility. Addict Behav. 2017;64:308–13.

19 Reproductive Health and Pregnancy in Transitional-Age Youth

Liwei L. Hua and Lois Flaherty

Key Points

- Rate of unintended pregnancy in a population is a measure of public health.
- Transitional age youth have the highest rates of unintended pregnancy: women 20–24 years of age, followed by young women 15–19 years of age and 25–29 years of age.
- Factors contributing to unintended pregnancy include nonuse or inconsistent use of contraception, minority status, adverse life experiences, and substance use.
- Protective factors include positive attitude toward contraception, high-esteem, and having health insurance.
- Unplanned pregnancy has an impact on both mother and child, including upon prenatal care, breast-feeding, and mother-child relationship.
- Unintended pregnancy can also affect mental health. Women should be screened for psychiatric disorders, including depression, anxiety, and substance use, and treated accordingly.
- College and graduate school offer unique opportunities to orient students on safe sex practices and protective strategies in the context of alcohol/substance use.
- Special populations that could benefit from increased screening and attention include those who have intellectual and developmental disabilities and autism spectrum disorder (ASD), those with a history of foster care placement, as well as the lesbian, gay, bisexual, transgender, and questioning (LGBTQ) population.
- Formal policies to better educate and protect children, adolescents, and transitional age youth could help to decrease risky sexual behavior and unintended pregnancy.

Introduction

Transitional age youth are those youth between late adolescence (15–16 years old) and early adulthood (24–26 years old). During this period, transitional age youth are responsible for achieving self-sufficiency, attaining higher levels of education and employment, and negotiating relation-

L. L. Hua (✉)
Catholic Charities of Baltimore, Millersville, MD, USA

L. Flaherty
Harvard University and Cambridge Health Alliance, Cambridge, MA, USA

V. Chan, J. Derenne (eds.), *Transition-Age Youth Mental Health Care*,
https://doi.org/10.1007/978-3-030-62113-1_19

ships with families, friends, and romantic partners [88]. This is an incredible responsibility to undertake during a period when their brains have not fully developed and they are still in the process of maturing and learning to control their impulses. Taking all this into consideration, it stands to reason that while navigating relationships, sometimes through sexual exploration, pregnancy, whether intended or unintended, can occur.

Intended pregnancies are those that occur to women at the desired time (or later) or to women who are indifferent toward the pregnancy. Unintended pregnancies are defined as pregnancies that were not wanted at all or were mistimed (not wanted at time of conception) [86]. Statistics on unintended pregnancies are used to study the fertility of populations and determine needs for reproductive health care. Unintended pregnancy is an indicator of population health since both mothers and children are at increased risk for poorer mental and physical health as a result [62]; reducing unintended pregnancies is one avenue to improving public health [41].

In the United States' National Survey of Family Growth (2006–2010), 77% of pregnancies occurring in women 15–19 years old were unintended, and 50% of pregnancies in women 20–24 years old were unintended [94]. Using data from the National Survey of Family Growth, Finer et al. calculated that 6.1 million pregnancies occurred in the United States in 2011, with 45% of them being unintended (51% in 2008). Forty-two percent of unintended pregnancies, not including miscarriages, ended in abortion [41]. More recent data from the Centers for Disease Control and Prevention (CDC) show a 32.6% decrease in abortion rate from 2012 to 2016 for women 15–19 years old and an 18% decrease for women 20–24 years old [69]. Women who were cohabiting but not married had about four times the rate of unintended pregnancy as those who were married [41]. In 2011, the rate of unintended pregnancy decreased in every demographic [41]. Between 2008 and 2012, the rate of contraceptive use increased. Use of long-acting contraception, in particular intrauterine devices (IUDs), also increased [41]. Nonetheless, per Guzzo, 18% of unmarried women in their 20s did not use contraception at last sex [56].

The highest rate of unintended pregnancy occurred in women 20–24 years of age, with women 15–19 years old and 25–29 years next [41]. Generally, rates of unintended pregnancy decrease with age. However, because estimates of pregnancies usually include all women, and because a lower proportion of adolescents are sexually active, the estimated rate of unintended pregnancy of adolescent females ends up being low. If the rate of unintended pregnancy of only sexually active adolescents 15–19 years old were calculated, it would be much higher than that of women 20–24 years old [38, 53]. Married women had lower rates of unintended pregnancy, and unmarried, cohabiting women had four times the rate of unintended pregnancy as married women [41]. Finer et al. also found an inverse association between income and education level and rate of unintended pregnancy. In addition, there were racial and ethnic disparities in rates of unintended pregnancy, even controlling for income, although overall, rates for these groups decreased as well [41]. Namely, poor, Black, and Hispanic women and girls had higher rates of unintended pregnancy.

Risk Factors Contributing to Unintended Pregnancy

Factors in Contraceptive Use

Nonuse or inconsistent use of contraceptives and change in the frequency and the type of contraception used, as well as using less effective methods of contraception, are risk factors for unintended pregnancy [40, 77]. Lack of knowledge about the risks of unprotected sex and what is involved in effective contraception is also an important contributor to unintended pregnancy. These factors are intricately intertwined with social and cultural factors, especially minority and socioeconomic status.

Minority Status

Of all the unintended pregnancies that occur in the United States (almost half of all pregnancies), the highest proportions occur in racial/ethnic minorities and adolescents [21]. Black and

Hispanic women are more likely to have an unintended pregnancy than White women. Women who earn incomes that are less than the federal poverty line are also more likely to experience an unintended pregnancy than women living at 200% or more of the poverty line [39].

Black and Hispanic women who were at higher risk of having an unintended pregnancy were less likely to use contraception than White women and, if they did, were more likely to have a contraception failure if they did use it [44, 122]. Hispanic young women (18–29-year-olds surveyed) were more likely to report that they did not think they would get pregnant upon having sex [77]. Young Black women were more likely to report fear of adverse effects of contraception. One study of Hispanic women found that incorrect beliefs about how different contraceptives worked resulted in using less effective forms of contraception or cessation of use of contraceptives [51].

Using data from the 2009 National Survey of Reproductive and Contraceptive Knowledge, Craig et al. found that Hispanic women who were born in other countries knew less about contraception than US-born Hispanic women. It is unclear why this is true, but one could hypothesize that strong religious faith or perhaps decreased emphasis on comprehensive sexual education in school could play a role. In the Craig study, Hispanic women generally had the least knowledge, followed by Black women; however, Black women's knowledge of contraception was only slightly lower than that of White women [21]. Many have pointed out how the legacy of forced sterilization of African Americans has made Black women distrustful of contraception (e.g., see [118]).

When looking at age, comparing adolescents and young adults, teenagers generally had lower awareness of the different types of contraception than adults, especially long-acting reversible contraception (the intrauterine device and the implant) [21]. This points to the importance of health-care providers taking the time to explain the different types of contraception methods, including barrier and long-acting reversible contraception.

A study using data from the National Survey of Reproductive and Contraceptive Knowledge found that although White and Black women were similar, Hispanics and teenagers (18–19 years old) had lower awareness of types of contraception and knowledge about specific methods of contraception than White women and young adults (20–29 years old). Hispanics who had immigrated to the United States had even less knowledge [21].

Discrimination experienced by socially disadvantaged women affects mental and physical health and is associated with health disparities, including unplanned pregnancy [58, 128, 132]. A longitudinal population-based cohort study of women aged 18–20 years old was conducted to examine the relationship between social discrimination, mental health, and pregnancy. Perception of moderate/high discrimination was most strongly predicted by pregnancy during adolescence [58]. This study also found that the relationship between discrimination and risk of pregnancy was similar for both socially advantaged and disadvantaged women; in addition, race and socioeconomic status also did not predict discrimination. Employment and enrollment in college seemed to be protective against discrimination [58].

Adolescents' Attitudes and Understanding

Personal beliefs/expectations and the partner's desire to use contraception can also contribute to unintended pregnancy. Kornides et al. reported that non-Hispanic black young adults were more likely to worry that contraception had side effects and would decrease sexual desire [77].

If a partner says that they prefer not to use contraception, a woman's decision to use contraception may be swayed [77]. Craig and colleagues found that Black and Hispanic women were more likely to think that birth control was the responsibility of the woman [21]. Involving the partner in the decision to use contraception and in deciding which method to use could therefore be a point for advocacy to increase use of effective contraception in the future. In a study using data from the National Survey of Reproductive and Contraceptive Knowledge, Black and Hispanic women were more likely to believe that the woman bears the onus of contraception alone [21]. This belief could negatively affect contraceptive use, especially given that women may be more likely to use contraception when the decision is discussed with their sexual partner [21].

Adolescent attitudes toward contraception and understanding of condom use and reproduction, in addition to having immediate outcomes, also have important long-term consequences; they are predictive of adult contraceptive use [56]. This finding supports comprehensive sex education in adolescence, which would then have a higher likelihood of being applied through adulthood.

Adverse Life Experiences

Adverse life experiences are also risk factors for unintended pregnancy. Experiencing violence, discrimination, and/or economic hardship during childhood and early adolescence is associated with difficulties in later adolescence and early adult life, including tobacco, substance and alcohol use, depression, suicide, obesity, social/family conflict, decreased education achievement, fewer work opportunities, delinquency, running away, violence, homelessness, and incarceration [60, 115]. In a study of adolescents 14–17 years old, it was found that adolescents with a history of childhood maltreatment were more likely to engage in risky sexual behaviors, relationships with "risky" peers, and substance use, and to demonstrate more psychological dysregulation and behavioral issues and have poorer relationships with parents [101]. ACEs are also associated with increased risk of younger age at first sexual activity, multiple sexual partners, sexual violence, and history of multiple abortions [3, 30, 101].

Both sexual and physical abuse contribute to risky sexual behaviors [1, 131]. An Australian longitudinal study found an association between sexual abuse, physical abuse, emotional abuse, and neglect and early age at first sexual intercourse [1]. Neglect predicted multiple sexual partners in both males and females. A history of multiple incidents of maltreatment in childhood significantly predicted earlier sexual activity. All types of childhood maltreatment predicted risky sexual behaviors in both males and females and a higher number of pregnancies in youth. Past emotional abuse was associated with future miscarriage [1]. Dietz et al. demonstrated an association between psychological and physical abuse and unintended first pregnancy among adult women [30]. Noll and Shenk reported that past history of sexual abuse increased adolescent childbirth by 2.74-fold, while neglect increased odds by 3.14-fold [100].

These risks extend to males as well as females. Adolescent males who have a history of sexual abuse are more likely to have multiple sexual partners, less likely to use any form of birth control, and more likely to have used alcohol or drugs prior to sex [115]. Anda et al. demonstrated that each ACE exposure in young men was associated with higher risk of impregnating a sexual partner in adolescence [3]. In a cohort study using data from the National Longitudinal Study of Adolescent to Adult Health, increased ACE exposure that occurred in childhood and adolescence was associated with higher risk of unintended first pregnancy in young women [60]. They also found that different levels of ACE scores contributed to different levels of risk for unintended pregnancy in different sociodemographic groups of women [60].

Women who report physical violence or history of sexual victimization are more likely to report ineffective use of contraception (withdrawal method or inconsistent use of condoms/oral contraceptives during their last sexual encounter) [112]. In a study of young urban (primarily minority) women in Philadelphia, authors examined the relationship between violence and psychological factors and the use of contraception [99]. Although there was some limitation in the generalizability of the findings, exposure to childhood sexual violence was strongly, significantly, and positively associated with ineffective contraception use. Low self-esteem at baseline was also significantly related to ineffective contraception use at follow-up.

In one study, adolescent females 14–17 years old who had experienced sexual abuse, physical abuse, or neglect within the prior year were assessed until 19 years old and were found to be twice as likely to become pregnant as their non-abused peers [100]. Birth rates were highest in females who had experienced sexual abuse and neglect [100]. In addition, pregnant or parenting adolescents themselves may be at higher risk of experiencing or perpetrating intimate partner violence (IPV) [117]. Silverman et al. noted that dating violence was twice as likely to occur in adolescents who had experienced pregnancy in the last year versus those who had not (Silverman 2004). A study of postpartum adolescent mothers indicated that adolescent mothers reported IPV at a rate of 67.6% in the 18 months following delivery. Intimate partner violence has also been found to be associated with depression through time [49, 83]. Depression in the adolescent mother can also be associated with mental and behavioral health issues in the offspring [52].

Adolescent Sexual Behavior

Adolescent sexual behaviors are predictive of young adult outcomes with respect to reproductive health, including unintended pregnancy, sexually transmitted disease diagnosis, and number of sexual partners in the past year [119]. The most common risk factor found in this study was having two or more sexual partners in adolescence. Other risk factors included having had a nonmonogamous relationship, having had a casual "hookup" or "one-night stand," inconsistent contraceptive use, and not discussing contraception with partner prior to sex. This risk was cumulative [119].

More recent literature also suggests that use of technology such as sexting increases the likelihood of sexually risky behavior, including unprotected sex, more sexual partners, sexually transmitted infections (STIs), and having sex in the context of alcohol and substance use [7]. These are all factors that increase risk for unintended pregnancy as well.

Substance Use

Substance use is another risk factor for unintended pregnancy. Excessive alcohol consumption, which has been increasing among college women, is associated with increased levels of sexual activity and higher likelihood of risky sexual behaviors, such as engaging in unprotected sex or "casual" sex [92]. In 2001, 2% of full-time 4-year college students (18–24 years old) were victims of sexual abuse by another drinking college student [64].

To attempt to understand this increase, there has been more recent interest in motivation for the consumption of alcohol. A SAMHSA report indicates that 9.4% of adolescents 12–17 years old had used alcohol in the past month, and 57.75% of young adults aged 18–25 years old had done so [126]. The four most common reasons for alcohol consumption are social, enhancement of positive mood, coping with negative emotions, and conformity [17]. Social and enhancement motivations appear to be more relevant to college-aged students as reasons for drinking alcohol. As first-year students enter college, they navigate new friendships and other intimate relationships, often in the setting of parties with alcohol. Conformity motivation is drinking to "fit in." Coping-motivated alcohol intake is more associated with negative consequences and eventual problem drinking. It does not seem to be associated with risky sexual behavior [74, 79].

A study of sexual experience and alcohol consumption in first-year college females demonstrated that freshmen who were sexually experienced upon starting college were more likely to drink in greater quantities and more frequently than did peers who were sexually inexperienced. Coping-related drinking, regardless of alcohol intake and sexual status, was found to be a significant risk factor for college freshman women [79].

Gender, race, and age should also be considered in examining the relationship between alcohol use and risky sexual behavior. One study showed that African American females in college have less positive expectancy of alcohol use than do Hispanic females and White females. Older men in college engaged in more binge drinking and had more sexual partners in the past year [110].

In a case control study using data from the Pregnancy Risk Assessment Monitoring System from 1996 to 1990, 45% of women (median age 26 years old) reported that their pregnancy was unintended, and 14% reported binge drinking prior to conception [96]. Women reporting unintended pregnancies were significantly more likely to have engaged in binge drinking. In addition, as the number of binge drinking episodes increased prior to conception, the proportion of women who had unintended pregnancies rose.

Women in this study who experienced unintended pregnancy were likely to be younger, unmarried, non-White, and less educated. These women were also less likely to have health insurance and more likely to have Medicaid, smoke tobacco, and be exposed to physical violence prior to conception [96]. Smoking and experiencing physical abuse were also associated with unintended pregnancy in White people but not in Black people [96].

A study of undergraduate alcohol use associated with sexual activity found that single undergraduates had a higher association of heavy alcohol use with same-day sexual intercourse [73]. The authors also found that intoxication with alcohol was associated with decreased use of condoms, although marijuana intoxication was not. In addition, although undergraduates who were alcohol- or marijuana-intoxicated were more likely to have same-day sex, most unprotected sex against STIs occurred in sober partners in committed relationships. Therefore, counseling of couples on use of condoms to protect against STIs when getting refills for prescription contraception to protect against pregnancy could be helpful [73].

Some alcohol protective behavioral strategies (PBS), which are aimed at harm reduction to either reduce intake or decrease risk of harm while drinking, have been shown to be helpful. Moorer et al. reported that college women seem to use serious harm reduction strategies more than they use controlled consumption strategies [92]. Discussion of serious harm reduction strategies, such as keeping one's drink close and going home with a friend, may be considered as a universal addition for orientation classes during freshman year of college.

Protective Factors Against Unintended Pregnancy

Attendance at religious services is thought to be a protective factor against unintended pregnancy, although some research has found that women who attend religious services may actually be at higher risk of pregnancy due to not using contraception. One study of college students at a large university in the "Bible Belt" examined the association of alcohol consumption, religious conviction, and risky sexual behavior. In their sample of 210 students, about 40% said they had used alcohol to enhance sexual experiences, and about 70% reported they were less likely to use condoms if they drank alcohol prior to sexual activity [105]. Women who had stronger religious beliefs generally drank less alcohol and were not as likely to engage in sexually risky behavior as their female peers with weaker religious beliefs. For college men, religious conviction had no association with sexual behavior or alcohol consumption [105].

In addition, positive attitude toward contraception can be a protective factor in preventing unintended pregnancy, as well as having instructions on options and proper use of contraception [77, 109]. Having private insurance that covers contraception has been shown to be a protective factor against unintended pregnancy [6, 77]. Satisfaction with one's contraception also leads to more consistent use during sexual encounters [34].

Interestingly, in a recent study of college age women 18–24 years old, high self-esteem was found to be associated with more consistent use of contraception. In addition, confidence, a sense of independence, and life satisfaction were also positively related to consistent use of contraception, whereas symptoms of depression and use of marijuana were associated with inconsistent use of contraception [93].

Impact of Unplanned Pregnancy

Research indicates that women with unplanned pregnancy start receiving prenatal care later than women with intended pregnancies [23, 71, 86].

Initiating prenatal care early is associated with a healthy birth weight [86, 103]. There appears to be a relationship between unintended pregnancy and prematurity and low birth weight; however, the relationship is likely to be moderated through smoking, drinking, poor diet, and decreased vitamin intake [86].

There seems to be an increased risk for postpartum depression in mothers who have unintended pregnancies. There is also increased risk to the mother for experiencing physical abuse during the pregnancy [86]. In addition, there is decreased likelihood of breast-feeding after pregnancy [23, 33, 86].

Children born from unintended pregnancies are at risk for poor physical and mental health, decreased school performance, and less close mother-child relationships. Mothers with unintended pregnancies have been shown to be more likely to use corporal punishment; one study indicated that children born of unwanted pregnancies were more likely to be physically abused as well [86]. In addition, children born of unintended pregnancy have been found to demonstrate problematic physical behaviors and poor educational outcomes. These children have also been shown by some to be less well-adapted in childhood, have lower self-esteem in their early 20s, and experience depression and/or involvement in psychiatric care in their late 20s/early 30s [25, 86].

Mental Health

Depression during pregnancy is the greatest risk factor for developing postpartum depression. It is associated with higher risk of preterm birth, decreased birth weight, and behavioral issues, such as increased fussiness or less reactivity [82, 120, 121]. Depression is also associated with difficulty forming attachment with the baby, behavioral changes in the infant, and decreased likelihood of breast-feeding. In a review of research on young women 21 years and younger with depression, anxiety, bipolar disorder, and psychosis, Siegel and colleagues found that pregnant and parenting adolescents were more likely to report depressive symptoms than pregnant and parenting older women but not more than non-pregnant or parenting adolescents. This is especially concerning given the known risk of depression to the unborn child and then to later attachment between mother and child and behavioral issues as the child grows [121].

The study by Hall et al., of young women 18–20 years old who wanted to avoid pregnancy, demonstrated that depression and stress at baseline were associated with higher risk for pregnancy [57]. Pregnancy rate was 1.6 times higher in young women with symptoms of stress versus those without. In women with both depression and stress symptoms, pregnancy risk was two times higher than in women who did not have these symptoms [57]. Depression may also be associated with increased risk of alcohol and substance use in adolescent mothers, as well as with rapid repeat childbirth [5, 18, 26]. Corcoran also demonstrated that conduct problems in youth are also associated with higher risk for pregnancy in young adulthood, in addition to repeat childbearing [20].

Another study based on data from the National Longitudinal Study of Adolescent to Adult Health found that moderate to severe symptoms of depression were associated with increased risk of experiencing an unintended first pregnancy [59]. Depression increased the risk of pregnancy in minority adolescents and young women but not White women. Depression also increased risk of pregnancy in women with income levels of $0–$19,999 and $20,000–$49,000 but not above. In addition, depression increased pregnancy risk in women less than 20 years old but decreased the risk in women greater than 24 years old [59]. This group also found that moderate to severe stress symptoms, as well as depressive symptoms to a lesser extent, in 18–19-year-olds were associated with increased nonuse and misuse of contraception, likelihood of using less effective methods of contraception, sexual activity, and unintended pregnancy over a year of follow-up [59].

A retrospective cohort study using data from the Rhode Island Pregnancy Risk Assessment Monitoring System from 2004 to 2008 found that adolescents and young adults had a higher likelihood of reporting a depression diagnosis before their most recent pregnancy [102]. Twenty- to twenty-four-year-olds had the highest rate of prenatal depression. Prenatal depression decreased with age. In addition, adolescents and young adult mothers were more likely to experience postpartum depression. This also decreased with age [102]. Risk factors found in this study to be associated with postpartum depression include smoking and drinking pre-pregnancy, infant being alive, infant living with mother, stressors, and decreased social support [102].

Not only do adolescents/young women (15–19 years old) with mental health disorders, including affective and psychotic disorders, have multiple risk factors that are associated with pregnancy, but one large Canadian study indicated that they have a higher fertility rate than adolescents with no mental illness as well [130].

It is also important to consider the risk of maternal depression to children's mental health. Depression during pregnancy is associated with poor nutrition, delayed or inadequate prenatal care, increased substance use, preeclampsia, low birth weight, preterm delivery, postpartum depression, and suicide [50, 90, 95]. Infants of depressed mothers seem to be more irritable, less active, and less attentive, with less facial expression and increased likelihood of developmental delay. The relationship between mother and infant is also often impaired [27, 35, 95]. Toddlers and preschoolers of mothers with depression present with increased likelihood of poorer cognitive functioning, as well as increased likelihood of responding negatively when someone is friendly, and decreased likelihood of engaging in creative play independently. School-aged children, as well as adolescents, of mothers with depression have a higher chance of having ADHD and depression, as well as adolescents. They are also at higher risk for anxiety and conduct disorders [76, 133].

Currently, the recommendation is that antenatal and postpartum mild to moderate depression first be treated with cognitive behavioral therapy or interpersonal therapy. If depression does not improve, medication, with SSRIs as first-line choice, should be used at lowest effective dose in combination with therapy. If depression is more severe, the antidepressant may be started in conjunction with evidence-based therapy [90].

With regard to treatment for depression, given that TAY span about 15 years old to 24 years old, it is important to take into consideration that for part of this age group, the only Food and Drug Administration (FDA)-approved first-line pharmacological treatments for major depression are fluoxetine and escitalopram, and that for this entire age group, there is a black box warning for possible increased suicidal ideation with antidepressant treatment. These concerns need to be balanced with risks to both mother and unborn child and infant if depression is not treated. Informed consent with full understanding of risks needs to be given after partnered decision-making between the patient and the physician.

College/Graduate School-Related Concerns

The American College Health Association-National College Health Assessment (ACHA-NCHA), a nationally recognized research survey with the participation of multiple US college institutions and participation from tens of thousands of students, reported that about 65% of college students engaged in sexual intercourse in 2018 and 1.1% experienced pregnancy [2]. College-aged students are at particularly high risk of engaging in risky sexual behaviors, including sex with multiple and or unknown partners, inconsistent use of condoms, and not discussing risk-relevant topics prior to having sex, such as use of protection against pregnancy and any existing sexually transmitted infections [75]. As these risky sexual behaviors in college put students at risk of consequences such as assault, STI, unintended pregnancy, and psychological distress, it is important to consider other risk factors that contribute to engaging in these behaviors [119].

"Hookups" refer to sexual encounters between partners who are not romantically involved and who do not expect any sort of relationship commitment after the initial hookup. "Hooking up" appears to be common in college students, with a 2012 review indicating that the lifetime prevalence rates in college students were 60–80% [46]. One study of college students found a hookup rate of approximately 55% within the past year [80]. A longitudinal study of almost 500 first-year female undergraduate students (between 18 and 25 years of age) from a private university found that hookups were correlated with experiencing symptoms of depression [37]. Hookups also appeared to increase the risk of sexual victimization and to predict sexually transmitted infections [37].

In addition to being associated with high-risk behavior generally, alcohol use is linked to casual sexual encounters [70]. Two-thirds to three-quarters of college students report alcohol intake prior to hooking up, and both male and female college students state that there is a higher likelihood of hooking up as opposed to more traditional romantic interactions if they have had alcohol prior [36, 47]. They also report more alcohol intake during the hookup. In addition, results from Fielder's study demonstrated that no one used condoms during last oral sex, and 31% did not use condoms during vaginal sex, which increases risk of sexually transmitted infections, as well as unintended pregnancy [36].

According to the National Campaign to Prevent Teen and Unplanned Pregnancy [125], unplanned births are responsible for about 10% of female dropouts from community college and 7% of community college student dropouts overall. In addition, an estimated 61% of community college students who have children during college do not complete their college education [125]. Those students who do not drop out of college after having a child are likely to carry a heavy burden, including having to study and maintain good grades while caring for a child, as well as obtaining childcare for their children when they are in school. The National Campaign recommends that colleges integrate information on unplanned pregnancy into student support services, such as student orientation, and into some required freshman classes. It also recommends providing resources about unplanned pregnancy to students and helping all students connect with student health services and access to contraception. Some state and private colleges/universities also have information on their online student health and counseling service websites. The American Academy of Community Colleges and the National Campaign to Prevent Teen and Unplanned Pregnancy partnered to write the report Making it Personal: How Pregnancy Planning and Prevention Help Students Complete College, which can be a helpful resource. This resource focuses mainly on three ways to create more awareness on pregnancy prevention: by integrating information into the curriculum, implementing college success courses, and posting online resources [106].

Online Information for graduate students can also be helpful with regard to unplanned pregnancy. As an example, the University of Nebraska webpage on Pregnancy and Parenting in Graduate School (https://www.unl.edu/gradstudies/connections/pregnancy-and-parenting-graduate-school) discusses positive and more challenging aspects of being pregnant in graduate school and encourages planning ahead (including letting thesis/dissertation advisors know as soon as possible).

Special Populations

Intellectual and Developmental Disabilities

A common misconception is that people with intellectual and developmental disabilities (IDD) are more likely to be "asexual." As such, less emphasis may be placed on this population receiving sexual education in a way they can understand or receiving appropriate counseling from care providers [43]. This can potentially lead to consequences such as rape, infection, or unintended pregnancy while adolescents/young adults with IDD try to navigate their sexual development on their own, as studies indicate that they are likely to be just as sexual as their peers [43]. They are also more likely to have a history of sexual victimization [29]. A review of literature on contraception and adolescents with disabilities indicated that contraception can help with treatment of gynecological conditions as well as prevent unwanted pregnancy [29], although ethical issues, such as autonomy and justice, are relevant.

A study in the United Kingdom found that women with ID have less understanding of sexual health and reproduction; they are also less likely to use contraception [4]. In a Swedish study, women with intellectual disability who gave birth were more likely to be teenagers, obese, and single compared to women who did not have intellectual disability [65]. Women with ID had a higher likelihood of preterm birth, requiring a C-section and being discharged to somewhere other than their own home [65]. Women with IDD who give birth are more likely to be less than 25 years old [9]. Rapid repeat pregnancies were more common in women with intellectual and developmental disabilities, but this seemed to be mediated in part by social, health, and health-care disparities [9].

Autism Spectrum Disorder (ASD)

As in individuals with intellectual disability, it was long believed that individuals with autism were not interested in romantic relationships or sexuality. More recent research has indicated that this is untrue and that individuals with autism do engage in romantic relationships and sexual activity [61, 89]. Youth with autism are more vulnerable to abuse and sexual exploitation [10, 66]. Some research indicates that individuals with ASD may have a higher likelihood of engaging in risky sexual behavior and experiencing victimization [10, 61]. Approximately 42–69% of individuals with autism (compared to 8% of their peers without autism) report that they are attracted to members of the same sex or identify as sexual minorities [11, 28, 61, 104]. When comparing parent reports of the sexual knowledge and experiences of their young adult children with ASD to the young adult reports, the young adults themselves reported more typical sexual behaviors and sexual victimization than what their parents reported [61]. Although parents were likely to be accurate when describing the asexuality or heterosexuality of their young adult children, they were less likely to be aware if their child had a same-sex attraction [61]. This study also indicated that family sexual communication and overall information on sex would be helpful to these young adults with ASD and hopefully decrease likelihood of risky sexual behavior and victimization.

Interviews of those who care for young adults with ASD indicate that sexuality is not a topic often brought up by health-care providers, other than to discuss hygiene [61]. Research indicates that traditional sex education is not as effective for individuals with ASD, and so alternative ways of delivering this information, including more personalized communication through parents/caretakers, should be considered [61]. A study of family sexual communication in adolescent girls with ASD indicated that parents generally discussed basic information such as privacy, caution for sexual abuse, menstruation, and hygiene, whereas they often left out information on relationship, sex, and sexuality, particularly in females with low intellectual functioning [66]. Although the average age of females in this study was 14 years old, it is relevant in that parents did report a need for improved guidance on how to discuss these topics with their children/adolescents with ASD [66].

Two studies of pregnancy in women with autism found they had increased difficulty with sensory processing, adapting to changes associated with pregnancy, and communicating with their health-care providers [113]. In one Swedish national cohort study, pregnant women with autism had a higher chance of preterm birth, especially medically indicated preterm birth [123]. They also tended to be younger than the control group (pregnant women without autism). Authors also indicated that due to high likelihood of comorbidities with other issues, such as epilepsy/seizure disorder and ADHD, pregnant women with a diagnosis of ASD may warrant a higher degree of monitoring [123].

One helpful webpage with multiple resources for sexuality education in youth with disability or chronic illness, including intellectual disability and ASD, is https://www.parentcenterhub.org/sexed/.

Young People with a History of Foster Care

Youth in foster care often have an accumulation of risk factors for adolescent pregnancy, including a history of maltreatment, poverty, low parental education, and family disruption [15]. A study of 215 young adults (ages 18–22 years old) with a history of foster care and rates of pregnancy and parenthood indicate that by 21 years of age, 49% of young women had become pregnant, and 33% of young men had gotten someone pregnant [15]. A study in California (CalYOUTH Study) and in the Midwest (the Midwest Study) followed youth who had been emancipated from foster care into adulthood. In both studies, approximately one-third of women reported they were pregnant at 18 years old; by 19 years old, this had increased to half of these women [31]. Adolescent mothers in foster care also have a higher risk of having a rapid repeat pregnancy, defined as within 24 months [19, 42].

Young adults who have experienced foster care are less likely to graduate from high school, or earn their GED, and are also more likely to experience homelessness at least once before 26 years old [19, 32]. These outcomes can be worse when further compounded with pregnancy. Less is known about men with a history of foster care, but they seem at higher likelihood of impregnating someone in adolescence. Combs et al. found that young adults with a history of foster care (between 9 and 11 years old) had a similar likelihood of pregnancy (women and men) as young adults who were emancipated from foster care [15]. Authors also found that women were more likely to be raising the children and that men supported their children financially. In addition, having a child was associated with attaining a lower education level, having less employment (specific to women), not having a savings or checking account, and experiencing homelessness [15].

A study in California (CA) found that 35% of adolescents in foster care gave birth by age 21 years [108]. By race, average birth rates by age 21 years old were 43.1% for Hispanic young adults, 33.0% for Black young adults, and 29.4% for White young adults [108]. With federal legislation that extends foster care to beyond 18 years old, efforts in CA are being made to design programs to prevent pregnancy and also provide more supports to young parents. One recent national study also found that living in a state with a higher proportion of housing-burdened, low-income renters increased the risk of substance abuse and childbirth for adolescents leaving foster care. Participants were interviewed at 17 years old and 19 years old. This study recommended considering increased financial and housing supports for young adults transitioning out of foster care, as well as extending foster care to 19 years old, to mitigate homelessness, substance abuse, incarceration, and pregnancy [107].

Lesbian Gay Bisexual Transgender Queer/Questioning

Young women who identify as sexual minorities are about twice as likely as young women who identify as heterosexual to experience pregnancy in adolescence (prior to 20 years of age) [14, 84]. Earlier age at sexual initiation is thought to be one risk factor [13]. Sexual minority young women are reportedly more likely to engage in vaginal intercourse with males at younger ages, to have sexual intercourse more frequently with men, to be under the influence of drugs or alcohol during sex, and to have higher rates of coerced sex as compared to their heterosexual peers [48, 114, 116, 127].

Using data from the Growing Up Today Study (GUTS), compared with women who identified as "completely heterosexual," sexual minorities (bisexual and lesbian) experienced more bullying (victimization and perpetration), more maltreatment in childhood, and greater gender nonconformity [13]. Women who identified themselves as sexual minorities, particularly bisexual persons, were at a higher likelihood of adolescent pregnancy compared to women who identified as heterosexual. This higher likelihood was explained in part by their experiences of bullying and childhood maltreatment. Among sexual minorities, earlier age of sexual minority developmental milestones (such as age at first experiencing same gender attraction, age at first engagement in same-gender sexual behavior, age at first identifying as a sexual minority) was also a significant risk factor for adolescent pregnancy [13, 72]. Another study of transitional age women from 15 to 20 years old, using data from the 2006–2010 National Survey of Family Growth, found that both bisexual and lesbian women were younger at heterosexual sexual debut and had more male and female partners. They were also more likely to report being forced into having sex than heterosexuals. In addition, young women identifying as bisexual reported the earliest initiation of sexual intercourse, the highest numbers of male sexual partners, highest use of emergency contraception, and the greatest frequency of termination of pregnancy [127].

A study of unintended pregnancies in sexual minority women (ages 18–44 years with average age of 25 years) also supported the finding that sexual minority women were more likely to have unintended pregnancies than their heterosexual peers. This finding appeared to be driven specifically by women who identified themselves as heterosexual with same-sex attractions, mediated by a higher number of male sex partners [62].

Contraception

Contraception has had an important role in decreasing the rate of unintended pregnancy and transmission of STI. It is important that transitional age youth recognize the different types of contraception available and are aware of the choices that might be most effective for them. See Table 19.1 for general methods of contraception. Decision-making can include a discussion with the primary care doctor, the gynecologist, and the partner. Table 19.1 summarizes contraception methods, described further in the chapter.

Barrier Methods

Barrier methods are removable and prevent sperm from entering the uterus. These include condoms (male and female), contraceptive sponges, spermicides, diaphragms, and cervical caps [97]. Unlike other forms of contraception (besides abstinence), only condoms can protect from both

Table 19.1 Methods of Contraception

Barrier	Hormonal (short-acting)	Long-acting reversible contraception (LARC)	Emergency contraception (EC)	Sterilization	Other methods
Male condom	Combined oral contraceptive pills	Implants	Ulipristal	Tubal ligation	Abstinence
Female condom	Contraceptive patch	Intrauterine device (IUD)	Levonorgestrel	Vasectomy	Withdrawal
Contraceptive sponges	Vaginal ring		Copper IUD	Sterilization implant	Fertility awareness
Spermicide	Transdermal contraceptive patch				
Diaphragm	Progestin-only injectable contraception				
Cervical caps					

unintended pregnancy and sexually transmitted infection. The CDC reports that women ages 15–24 years old are at highest risk for sexually transmitted infection [12]. Condoms are some of the most used contraceptives [16, 87]; the ACHA-National College Health Assessment of 2018 reported that more than 61% of college students used condoms when they did use contraception [2]. For both men and women, younger age and greater concern for HIV infection were associated with increased use of condoms [110].

A study using data from the 2006–2010 National Survey of Family Growth found that a high percentage of young adults 15–24 years old felt that using a male condom during sexual intercourse would decrease arousal and enjoyment of sex and were therefore unlikely to use one. These negative perceptions of the effect of condom use on pleasurable sexual experience appeared to outweigh other reasons for not using condoms, including sociodemographic, psychosocial, or sexual history factors [63].

Hormonal Methods

Hormonal methods include short-acting and combination hormonal methods to decrease the risk of pregnancy by regulation or stopping ovulation. Short-acting methods include injectable birth control and progestin-only pills. Combination hormonal methods include combined oral contraceptives, the contraceptive patch, and the vaginal ring [97]. Combined oral contraceptive pills are the most popular forms of contraception in adolescence [16, 87].

Long-Acting Reversible Contraception (LARC)

The most effective form of contraception, other than abstinence, is long-acting reversible contraception (LARC), which includes implants and intrauterine devices (IUDs) [97]. LARC, while very effective for pregnancy prevention, is underutilized. Logan et al. [87] assessed LARC use in college-aged women and found that while 44% of women used contraception at last sexual encounter, only 2.5% of women used LARC (and 90% of these used an intrauterine device).

LARC is also highly recommended for adolescents parents within 8 weeks of birth to decrease the chances of rapid repeat pregnancy/childbirth, which can affect both parents and their children negatively [22, 124].

Emergency Contraception (EC)

Emergency contraception is used after sexual intercourse to decrease the risk of pregnancy. These consist of hormonal emergency contraceptive pills (ulipristal and levonorgestrel) and the copper intrauterine device [129]. In a 2013 CDC reports on use of emergency contraception in women ages 15–44 years from 2006 to 2010, use was about 11%, up from 4% in 2002. For age groups 15–19 years of age, 14% of sexually experienced women had used EC, and for age groups 20–24 years old, 23% of sexually experienced women had used EC [24]. The ACHA-NCHA of 2018 reported that almost 15% of sexually active college students used emergency contraception [2] in the last 12 months.

Although studies indicate that adolescents are more likely to use EC if they have already been prescribed it, surveys indicate that most pediatricians do not prescribe it or provide education about it. Levonorgestrel has been approved for over-the-counter sales since 2013; however, due to cost or lack of availability from the pharmacy, access can be limited.

Sterilization

Sterilization is a permanent, usually nonreversible, form of contraception that must be performed by a health-care provider. Sterilization consists of tubal ligation, vasectomy, and sterilization implant. This is less common in adolescents and young adults [16] who may be planning childbearing in the future.

Other Methods

Additional methods that are used to avoid pregnancy are abstinence, withdrawal (withdrawing of penis prior to ejaculation), and periodic abstinence, or fertility awareness (avoiding sexual intercourse during period around ovulation) [16].

Improving Knowledge

Lack of knowledge about effective contraceptive use is widespread among transitional age youth and young adults. Not only is this one of the main factors impeding effective use; it is also—at least in theory—the most easily addressed.

A 2009 telephone survey of 1800 unmarried women and men aged 18–29 years old studied the association between "contraceptive knowledge, norms and attitudes, and selected risky contraceptive behaviors." Contraceptive methods queried were the condom, oral contraceptive pills (OCPs), injectable contraception, and intrauterine device. In this study, 25% of survey respondents were 18–19 years old, and about 40% were 20–24 years old. The study found that about 60% of men and 25% of women had low scores for contraceptive knowledge. However, for every correct response on the contraceptive knowledge scale by women, there was a 9% decrease in the odds of expecting to have unprotected sex in the next 3 months. Additionally, for women, every correct answer increased the odds that they were using hormonal or long-acting reversible contraception by 17%. For women who were in a relationship, the odds of their using no contraception were reduced by 17% [45]. About 20% of men and women thought the likelihood of a side effect was high with hormonal or long-acting forms of contraception. A high percentage of young adults in this survey accepted norms that it was acceptable for an unmarried woman to be pregnant and that every pregnancy is a blessing. An even higher percentage agreed that their friends felt that using birth control was important. With regard to attitudes, about 21–29% of respondents felt it was a "hassle" to use condoms every time one had sex, while about 40% felt that using contraception did not really matter. About 70% of women were committed to avoiding pregnancy, and approximately 45% of men were. In addition, about 43% of men said they were somewhat or extremely likely to engage in unprotected sex in the next 3 months; 34% of men responded that their partners were using hormonal or long-acting contraception. For women, about 30% stated they were likely to have unprotected sex in the next 3 months, and 54% were using hormonal or long-acting form of contraception. Approximately 43% of women who used contraception say they used their method inconsistently. Authors of this study suggested improved education about side effects of hormonal and long-acting contraception to increase understanding and use of contraception, utilizing the desire to adhere to social norms. They also suggested that education could be improved by spreading messages, such as considering use of birth control as being important to avoid unintended pregnancy and the benefits of using condoms outweighing the "hassles" [45].

Improving Access

Kornides et al. found that affordability, effectiveness, and low side effect profile were the most important determinants of contraceptive use [77]. Lack of insurance is one of the major barriers to accessibility of contraception. States with the highest proportions of uninsured women have higher rates of unintended pregnancy. In fact, health insurance status seems to be a more important factor than racial and ethnic composition of the population [78]. Expansion of state Medicaid services, with more women covered, is associated with decreased rates of unintended pregnancy [78].

Colleges should offer the full spectrum of contraceptive methods while ensuring that women are receiving evidence-based and patient-centered counseling about contraception. Young women should neither be denied LARC methods, nor should they face pressure from providers to use long-acting reversible contraception. Evidence-based approaches include offering all reproductive age women long-acting reversible contraception as one of many contraception options. Patient-centered care supports women's freedom to decide what is right for them while coordinating and tailoring chosen forms of care as appropriate [85].

Implementing Patient-Centered Care

Patient-centered care is a concept that arose out of the consumer movement to incorporate the perspectives of health-care users; it focuses on empowering patients to make informed decisions about their health care in partnership with their health-care professionals [68]. It contrasts with a traditional paternalistic approach, in which the professional is the expert and the patient just a passive recipient of services.

Patient-centered care is particularly appropriate for transitional age youth as it supports their autonomy and respects their ability to make informed decisions, both key developmental tasks of this age period. Rebecca Logan, who has studied college women's use of contraception, has called upon colleges to implement patient-centered care, stating:

> …patient-centered care supports women's freedom to decide what is right for them, while coordinating and tailoring chosen forms of care as appropriate. [85]

Options Counseling

An important part of patient-centered care is options counseling. Options counseling is a term used to describe courses of action so that the young person can make an informed choice. Pediatricians, adolescent medicine specialists, and obstetricians/gynecologists should be consulted for options counseling upon learning of pregnancy. It is important that pregnant adolescent females and young women receive factual and unbiased information on their legal options. The three major options for the pregnant person are continuing the pregnancy to delivery and caring for the infant, continuing the pregnancy to delivery and making a plan for adoption or kinship care, and termination of the pregnancy [67].

If the adolescent or young adult decides to carry the pregnancy to delivery, there should be an immediate referral to a provider that will provide prenatal care. If the adolescent or young adult wants to continue the pregnancy but does not feel she is ready to raise a child, informal kinship care through a private agreement or through the state child welfare system may be arranged. Adoption is another possibility but is less common these days. Women who choose this option are more likely to be women who have completed high school and may have gone through some college or vocational training. The third option is termination of the pregnancy; pediatricians/primary care practitioners should be prepared to objectively and dispassionately discuss this option with medically accurate information on pharmacological and surgical procedures that can be used [67].

Current Policy

The prevention of unintended pregnancy faces many challenges owing to local and national political opposition to comprehensive sex education and availability of contraception and abortion. Changes to the Title X Family Planning Program have gone into effect, which essentially limit the ability to provide comprehensive reproductive health care to women and men. This has resulted in Planned Parenthood and several state health department grantees dropping out of the family planning program. Many states have sought to limit abortion access; some of these cases will be heard by the Supreme Court. The Teen Pregnancy Prevention Program, which had funded evidence-based programs for the prevention of adolescent pregnancy, is now redirecting funds to programs aiming to prevent pregnancy with abstinence-only. In addition, the mandate that employers had to provide access to contraception in employee health plans at no charge is currently being held, while courts come to a final resolution on the legality of the contraception coverage mandate.

On a more positive note, many states allow minors to consent to reproductive health care, 23 states and Washington, D.C., with no conditions and 24 states allowing minors to consent under certain conditions [54]. In addition, 29 states and the District of Columbia allow minors to consent to prenatal care with no conditions; 8 states allow it under certain conditions. In 15 states, the physicians are allowed to inform the parents of their child's pregnancy if the physician feels it is in the best interest of the minor to do so [55].

Practical Advice for Clinicians

As with children and adolescents, it is important to be open to discussing sex and sexuality with transitional age youth. These discussions should occur confidentially in a private setting (with options to include the partner or parents/guardians if preferred by the youth). Sexuality education includes more than just anatomy and physiology; it also includes gender identity, sexual orientation, relationships, sexual activity, sexually transmitted infections, and wishes regarding pregnancy and contraception. All patients, including patients with IDD and ASD, disabilities, and chronic health conditions, should be routinely queried about all of these topics in a manner that is calm and nonjudgmental [8]. Discussions of the role of substance and alcohol use in the context of sexual activity are also important. If a patient is in a relationship, asking about sexual activity; use of contraception, including condom use, stressing that it is the only contraception that can protect from sexually transmitted infections; and intimate partner violence (whether the relationship is healthy and if the patient feels safe) is recommended.

Adolescents who report age younger than 14 years at first sex are more likely to report that the encounter was involuntary compared to adolescents who first had sex between 17 and 19 years old [8]. It is therefore important to screen for sexual trauma, as it is a risk factor for adolescent childbirth. Adolescents who have chronic health conditions and disabilities are at increased risk for sexual victimization, indicating the importance of screening for nonconsensual sexual encounters in this population as well [8].

Confidentiality is extremely important with this group of adolescents/young adults. Confidential health services should be delivered with regard to sexuality, mental health, and substance use. However, in certain situations, such as concern for safety to self or others, suspicion of abuse, and potentially dangerous or risky behavior, confidentiality may be broken. Although a majority of transitional age youth are legally "adults" and able to see a provider on their own, many of them remain on their parents' insurance, so if a parent requested documentation from a particular visit, it would not truly be confidential [126]. It is also important to note that in situations where confidentiality is limited, use of contraception decreases, and risk for pregnancy increases [16, 111].

Conclusion

A comprehensive discussion of reproductive health and unintended pregnancy in transitional age youth is presented in this chapter, with focus on risks and protective factors; vulnerable populations of transitional age youth, including those with intellectual and developmental disabilities, ASD, and LGBTQ; and contraception. It is clear that TAY, who are navigating this complicated transition between adolescence and adulthood and working on formation of romantic and sexual relationships while also managing education and career goals, may be more likely to engage in risky sexual behavior and possible substance use. This combination can increase the likelihood of unintended pregnancy, sexually transmitted infections, and sexual victimization.

This population could benefit from universal sexual education including information on contraception, as well as directed in particular at specific TAY populations. Parental/guardian education is also important, as it can allow parents/guardians to reinforce lessons learned at school and better tailor this information to their children. In addition, sessions that include information on the dangers of risky sexual behavior, including hookups, which could lead to sexually transmitted infections, sexual victimization, and unintended pregnancy are essential components of college orientations. It is also important to give education on the dangers of alcohol/substance intake in combination with risky sexual behavior. In addition to education, ongoing access to and availability of reproductive health care and counseling are important. More formal policy to protect and educate TAY could further decrease unintended pregnancy.

References

1. Abajobir AA, Kisely S, Williams G, Strathearn L, Najman JM. Risky sexual behaviors and pregnancy outcomes in young adulthood following substantiated childhood maltreatment: findings from a prospective birth cohort study. J Sex Res. 2018;55(1):106–19.
2. American College Health Association. National college health assessment. Reference group executive summary. 2018; https://www.acha.org/documents/ncha/NCHA-II_Fall_2018_Reference_Group_Executive_Summary.pdf
3. Anda RF, Chapman DP, Felitti VJ, Edwards V, Williamson DF, Croft JB, Giles WH. Adverse childhood experiences and risk of paternity in teen pregnancy. Obstet Gynecol. 2002;100(1):37–45.
4. Baines S, Emerson E, Robertson J, Hatton C. Sexual activity and sexual health among young adults with and without mild/moderate intellectual disability. BMC Public Health. 2018;18:667.
5. Barnet B, Duggan AK, Wilson MD, Joffe A. Association between postpartum substance use and depressive symptoms, stress, and social support in adolescent mothers. Pediatrics. 1995;96(4 pt 1);659–66.
6. Bearman P, Bruckner H. Power in numbers: peer effects on adolescent girls' sexual debut and pregnancy. In: NCtPT, editor. Washington, DC; 1999.
7. Benotsch EG, Snipes DJ, Martin AM, Bull S. Sexting, substance use, and sexual risk behavior in young adults. J Adolesc Health. 2012;52:307–13.
8. Breuner C, Mattson G, Committee on Adolescence, Committee on Psychosocial Aspects of Child Health. Sexuality education for children and adolescents. Pediatrics. 2016;138(2):e1–e11.
9. Brown HK, Ray JG, Liu N, Lunsky Y, Vigod SN. Rapid repeat pregnancy among women with intellectual and developmental disabilities: a population-based cohort study. CMAJ. 2018;190(32):E949–56.
10. Brown-Lavoie SM, Viecili MA, Weiss JA. Sexual knowledge and victimization in adults with autism spectrum disorders. J Autism Dev Disord. 2014;44(9):2185–96.
11. Byers ES, Nichols S, Voyer SD. Challenging stereotypes: sexual functioning of single adults with high functioning autism spectrum disorder. J Autism Dev Disord. 2013;43(11):2617–27.
12. Centers for Disease Control. Incidence, prevalence, and cost of sexually transmitted infections in the United States. Fact Sheet. 2013. https://www.cdc.gov/std/stats/sti-estimates-fact-sheet-feb-2013.pdf.
13. Charlton BM, Corliss HL, Missmer SA, et al. Reproductive health screening disparities and sexual orientation in a cohort study of US adolescent and young adult females. J Adolesc Health. 2011;49(5):505–10.
14. Charlton BM, Roberts AL, Rosario M, Katz-Wise SL, Calzo JP, Spiegelman D, Austin SB. Teen pregnancy risk factors among young women of diverse sexual orientations. Pediatrics. 2018;141(4):e20172278.
15. Combs KM, Begun S, Rinehart DJ, Taussig H. Pregnancy and childbearing among young adults who experienced foster care. Child Maltreat. 2018;23(2):166–74.
16. Committee on Adolescence. Contraception for adolescents. Pediatrics. 2014;134(4):e1244–56.
17. Cooper ML. Motivations for alcohol use among adolescents: development and validation of a four-factor model. Psychol Assess. 1994;6:117–28.
18. Corcoran J. Teenage pregnancy and mental health. Societies. 2016;6(3):21–9.
19. Courtney ME, Dworsky A, Havlicek J, Perez A, Keller T. Midwest evaluation of the adult functioning of former foster youth: outcomes at age 21. Chicago: Chapin Hall at the University of Chicago; 2007. https://www.chapinhall.org/wp-content/uploads/Midwest-Eval-Outcomes-at-Age-21.pdf
20. Crittenden CP, Boris NW, Rice JC, Taylor CA, Olds DL. The role of mental health factors, behavioral factors, and past experiences in the prediction of rapid repeat pregnancy in adolescence. J Adolesc Health. 2009;44(1):25–32.
21. Craig AD, Dehlendorf C, Borrero S, Harper CC, Rocca CH. Exploring young adults' contraceptive knowledge and attitudes: disparities by race/ethnicity and age. Womens Health Issues. 2014;24(3):e281–9.
22. Damle LF, Gohari AC, McEvoy AK, Desale SY, Gomez-Lobo V. Early initiation of postpartum contraception: does it decrease rapid repeat pregnancy in adolescents? J Pediatr Adolesc Gynecol. 2015;28(1):57–62.
23. D'Angelo DV, Gilbert BC, Rochat RW, Santelli JS, Herold JM. Differences between mistimed and unwanted pregnancies among women who have live births. Perspect Sex Reprod Health. 2002;36(5):192–7.

24. Daniels K, Jones J, Abma J. Use of emergency contraception among women aged 15-44: United States, 2006-2010. NCHS Data Brief. 2013;112:1–7.
25. David HP. Born unwanted, 35 years later: the Prague study. Health Matters. 2006;14(27):181–90.
26. De Genna NM, Cornelius MD, Donovan JE. Risk factors for young adult substance use among women who were teenage mothers. Addict Behav. 2009;34(5):463–70.
27. Deave T, Heron J, Evans J, Emond A. The impact of maternal depression in pregnancy on early child development. BJOG. 2008;115(8):1043–51.
28. Dewinter J, De Graaf H, Begeer S. Sexual orientation, gender identity, and romantic relationships in adolescents and young adults with autism spectrum disorder. J Autism Dev Disord. 2017;47:2927–34.
29. Dickson J, Thwaites A, Bacon L. Contraception for adolescents with disabilities: taking control of periods, cycles and conditions. BMJ Sex Reprod Health. 2018;44:7–13.
30. Dietz PM, Spitz AM, Anda RF, Williamson DF, McMahon PM, Santelli JS, Nordenberg DF, Felitti VJ, Kendrick JS. Unintended pregnancy among adult women exposed to abuse of household dysfunction during their childhood. JAMA. 1999;282(14):1359–64.
31. Dworsky A, Courtney ME. The risk of teenage pregnancy among transitioning foster youth: implications for extending state care beyond age 18. Child Youth Serv Rev. 2010;32:1351–6.
32. Dworsky A, Napolitano L, Courtney M. Homelessness during the transition from foster care to adulthood. Am J Pub Health. 2013;103:S318–23.
33. Dye TD, Wojtowycz MA, Aubry RH, Quade J, Kilburn H. Unintended pregnancy and breast-feeding behavior. Am J Public Health. 1997;87(10):1709–11.
34. Ersek JL, Brunner Huber LR, Thompson ME, Warren-Findlow J. Satisfaction and discontinuation of contraception by contraceptive method among university women. Matern Child Health J. 2011;15(4):497–506.
35. Field T, Diego M, Hernandez-Reif M. Prenatal depression effects on the fetus and newborn: a review. Infant Behav Dev. 2006;29(3):445–55.
36. Fielder RL, Carey MP. Prevalence and characteristics of sexual hookups among first-semester female college students. J Sex Marital Ther. 2010;36:346–59.
37. Fielder RL, Walsh JL, Carey KB, Carey MP. Sexual hookups and adverse outcomes: a longitudinal study of first-year college women. J Sex Res. 2014;51(2):131–44.
38. Finer LB. Unintended pregnancy among U.S. adolescents: accounting for sexual activity. J Adolesc Health. 2010;47(3):312–14.
39. Finer LB, Henshaw SK. Disparities in rates of unintended pregnancy in the United States, 1994 and 2001. Perspect Sex Reprod Health. 2006;38(2):90–6.
40. Finer LB, Zolna MR. Unintended pregnancy in the United States: incidence and disparities, 2006. Contraception. 2011;84(5):478–85.
41. Finer LB, Zolna MR. Declines in unintended pregnancy in the United States, 2008-2011. NEJM. 2016;374(9):843–52.
42. Finigan-Carr NM, Murray KW, O'Connor JM, Rushovich BR, Dixon DA, Barth RP. Preventing rapid repeat pregnancy and promoting positive parenting among young mothers in foster care. Soc Work Pub Health. 2015;30:1–17.
43. Fouquier KF, Camune BD. Meeting the reproductive needs of female adolescents with neurodevelopmental disabilities. JOGNN. 2015;44:553–63.
44. Frost JJ, Singh S, Finer LB. Factors associated with contraceptive use and nonuse, United States, 2004. Perspect Sex Reprod Health. 2007;39(2):90–9.
45. Frost JJ, Lindberg LD, Finer LB. Young adults' contraceptive knowledge, norms and attitudes: associations with risks of unintended pregnancy. Perspect Sex Reprod Health. 2012;44(2):107–16. https://www.guttmacher.org/journals/psrh/2012/05/young-adults-contraceptive-knowledge-norms-and-attitudes-associations-risk
46. Garcia JR, Reiber C, Massey SG, Merriweather AM. Sexual hookup culture: a review. Rev Gen Psychol. 2012;16:161–76.
47. Garcia TA, Litt DM, Davis KC, Norris J, Kaysen D, Lewis MA. Growing up, hooking up, and drinking: a review of uncommitted sexual behavior and its association with alcohol use and related consequences among adolescents and young adults in the United States. Front Psyc. 2019;10:1–16.
48. Garofalo R, Wolf RC, Kessel S, et al. The association between health risk behaviors and sexual orientation among a school-based sample of adolescents. Pediatrics. 1998;101:895e902.
49. Gavin AR, Lindhorst T, Lohr MR. The prevalence and correlates of depressive symptoms among adolescent mothers: results from a 17-year longitudinal study. Women Health. 2011:51(6):525–45.
50. Gelaye B, Rondon M, Araya R, Williams M. Epidemiology of maternal depression, risk factors, and child outcomes in low-income and middle-income countries. Lancet Psychiatry. 2016;3(10):973–82.
51. Gilliam ML, Warden M, Goldstein C, Tapia B. Concerns about contraceptive side effects among young Latinas: a focus-group approach. Contraception. 2004;70(4):299–305.
52. Goodman SH, Rouse MH, Connell AM, Broth MR, Hall CM, Heyward D. Maternal depression and child psychopathology: a meta-analytic review. Clin Child Fam Psychol Review. 2011;14:1–27.
53. Guttmacher Institute. Unintended pregnancy in the United States fact sheet. 2019. https://www.guttmacher.org/fact-sheet/unintended-pregnancy-united-states.

54. Guttmacher Institute. Minors' access to contraceptive services. 2020. https://www.guttmacher.org/state-policy/explore/minors-access-contraceptive-services.
55. Guttmacher Institute. Minors' access to prenatal care. 2020. https://www.guttmacher.org/state-policy/explore/minors-access-prenatal-care.
56. Guzzo KB, Hayford SR. Adolescent reproductive and contraceptive knowledge and attitudes and adult contraceptive behavior. Matern Child Health J. 2018;22(1):32–40.
57. Hall KS, Kusunoki Y, Gatny H, Barber J. The risk of unintended pregnancy among young women with mental health symptoms. Soc Sci Med. 2014;100:62–71.
58. Hall KS, Kusunoki Y, Gatny H, Barber J. Social discrimination, stress, and risk of unintended pregnancy among young women. J Adol Health. 2015;56:330–7.
59. Hall KS, Richards JL, Harris KM. Social disparities in the relationship between depression and unintended pregnancy during adolescence and young adulthood. J Adolesc Health. 2017;60(6):688–97.
60. Hall KS, Beauregard JL, Rentmeester ST, Livingston M, Harris KM. Adverse life experiences and risk of unintended pregnancy in adolescence and early adulthood: implications for toxic stress and reproductive health. Popul Health. 2019;7:1–10.
61. Hartmann K, Urbano MR, Raffaele CT, Qualls LR, Williams TV, Warren C, Kreiser NL, Elkins DE, Deutsch SI. Sexuality in the autism Spectrum study (SASS): reports from young adults and parents. J Autism Dev Disord. 2019;49:3638–55.
62. Hartnett CS, Lindley LL, Walsemann KM. Congruence across sexual orientation dimensions and risk for unintended pregnancy among adult U.S. women. Womens Health Issues. 2017;27(2):145–51.
63. Higgins JA, Wang Y. The role of young adults' pleasure attitudes in shaping condom use. Am J Public Health. 2015;105(7):1329–32.
64. Hingson RW, Zha W, Weitzman ER. Magnitude of and trends in alcohol-related mortality and morbidity among U.S. college students ages 18-24, 1998-2005. J Stud Alcohol Drugs. 2009;16:12–20.
65. Hoglund B, Lindgren P, Larsson M. Pregnancy and birth outcomes of women with intellectual disability in Sweden: a national register study. Acta Obstet Gynecol Scand. 2012;91:1381–7.
66. Holmes LG, Strassberg DS, Himle MB. Family sexuality communication for adolescent girls on the autism spectrum. J Autism Dev Disord. 2019;49:2403–16.
67. Hornberger LL, Committee on Adolescence. Options counseling for the pregnant adolescent patient. Pediatrics. 2017. 140(3). https://pediatrics.aappublications.org/content/140/3/e20172274.
68. International Alliance of Patients' Organizations. What is patient-centered health care? A review of definitions and principles. London: IAPO; 2007.
69. Jatlaoui TC, Eckhaus L, Mandel MG, Nguyen A, Oduyebo T, Peterson E, Whiteman MK. Abortion surveillance – United States, 2016. Surveill Summ. 2019;68(11):1–41. https://www.cdc.gov/mmwr/volumes/68/ss/ss6811a1.htm?s_cid=ss6811a1_w;deliveryName=USCDC_921-DM14137
70. Johnson MD, Chen J. Blame it on the alcohol: the influence of alcohol consumption during adolescence, the transition to adulthood, and young adulthood on one-time sexual hookups. J Sex Res. 2015;52:570–9.
71. Joyce TJ, Kaestner R, Korenman S. The effect of pregnancy intention on child development. Demography. 2000;37(1):83–94.
72. Katz-Wise SL, Rosario M, Calzo JP, Scherer EA, Sarda V, Austin SB. Associations of timing of sexual orientation developmental milestones and other sexual minority stressors with internalizing mental health symptoms among sexual minority young adults. Arch Sex Behav. 2017;46(5):1441–52.
73. Kerr DCR, Washburn IJ, Morris MK, Lewis KAG, Tiberio SS. Event-level associations of marijuana and heavy alcohol use with intercourse and condom use. J Stud Alcohol Drugs. 2015;76:733–7.
74. Kilwein TM, Looby A. Predicting risky sexual behaviors among college student drinkers as a function of event-level drinking motives and alcohol use. Addict Behav. 2018;76:100–5.
75. Kilwein TM, Kern SM, Looby A. Interventions for alcohol-related risky sexual behaviors among college students: a systematic review. Psychol Addict Behav. 2017;31(8):944–50.
76. Kingston D, Kehler H, Austin MP, Mughal MK, Wajid A, Vermeyden L, Benzies K, Brown S, Stuart S, Giallo R. Trajectories of maternal depressive symptoms during pregnancy and the first 12 months postpartum and child externalizing and internalizing behavior at 3 years. PLoS One. 2018;13(4):e0195365.
77. Kornides ML, Kitsantas P, Lindley LL, Wu H. Factors associated with young adults' pregnancy likelihood. J Midwifery Womens Health. 2015;60(2):158–68.
78. Kost K, Finer LB, Singh S. Variation in state unintended pregnancy rates in the United States. Perpsect Sex Reprod Health. 2012;44(1):57–64.
79. LaBrie JW, Kenney SR, Millbury S, Lac A. Sexual experience and risky alcohol consumption among incoming first-year college females. J Child Adolesc Subst Abuse. 2010;20(1):15–33.
80. LaBrie JW, Hummer JF, Ghaidarov TM, Lac A, Kenney SR. Hooking up in the college context: the event-level effects of alcohol use and partner familiarity on hookup behaviors and contentment. J Sex Res. 2014;51:62–73.
81. Leadbeater BJ, Bishop SJ, Raver CC. Quality of mother-toddler interactions, maternal depressive

symptoms, and behavior problems in preschoolers of adolescent mothers. Dev Psychol. 1996;32:380.
82. Lee Y. Early motherhood and harsh parenting: the role of human, social and cultural capital. Child Abuse Negl. 2009;33:625.
83. Lindhorst T, Oxfor M. The long-term effects of intimate partner violence on adolescent mothers' depressive symptoms. Soc Sci Med. 2008;66(6):1322–33.
84. Lindley LL, Walsemann KM. Sexual orientation and risk of pregnancy among New York City high-school students. Am J Public Health. 2015;105(7):1379–86.
85. Logan R. How colleges can improve contraception care and offer a full range of options to students. Cambridge, MA: Scholars Strategy Network; 2018. October 3. Retrieved from https://scholars.org/contribution/how-colleges-can-improve-contraception-care-and-offer-full-range-options-students
86. Logan C, Holcombe E, Manlove J, Ryan S. The consequences of unintended childbearing: a white paper. Child Trends, Inc.; 2007. https://pdfs.semanticscholar.org/b353/b02ae6cad716a7f64ca48b3edae63544c03e.pdf.
87. Logan RG, Thompson EL, Vamos CA, Grines SB, Vasquez-Otero C, Dalem EM. Is long-acting reversible contraceptive use increasing? Assessing trends among U.S. college women, 2008–2013. Matern Child Health J. 2018;22:1639–46.
88. Martel A, Fuchs DC. Transitional age youth and mental illness – influences on young adult incomes. Child Adol Psychiatric Clin. 2017;26(2):xiii–vii.
89. May T, Kang PC, Williams K. Brief report: sexual attraction and relationships in adolescents with autism. J Autism Dev Disord. 2017;47(6):1920–16.
90. McClanahan KK. Depression in pregnant adolescents: considerations for treatment. J Pediatr Adolesc Gynecol. 2009:22(1):59–64.
91. Meyer JL, Gold MA, Haggerty CL. Advance provision of emergency contraception among adolescent and young adult women: a systematic review of literature. L Pedatr Adolesc Gynecol. 2011;24(1):2–9.
92. Moorer KD, Madson MB, Mohn RS, Nicholson BS. Alcohol consumption and negative sex-related consequences among college among women: the moderating role of alcohol protective behavioral strategies. J Drug Educ. 2013;43(4):365–83.
93. Morrison LF, Sieving RE, Pettingell SL, Hellerstedt WL, McMorris BJ, Bearinger LH. Protective factors, risk indicators, and contraceptive consistency among college women. J Obstet Gynecol Neonatal Nurs. 2016;45:155–65.
94. Mosher WD, Jones J, Abma JC. Intended and unintended births in the United States: 1982–2010. Natl Health Stat Report. 2012;55:1–28.
95. Muzik M, Borovska S. Perinatal depression: implications for child mental health. Ment Health Fam Med. 2010;7(4):239–47.
96. Naimi TS, Lipscomb LE, Brewer RD, Gilbert BC. Binge drinking in the preconception period and the risk of unintended pregnancy: implications for women and their children. Pediatrics. 2003;111(5 pt 2):1136–41.
97. National Institute of Health. What are the different types of contraception? 2017. https://www.nichd.nih.gov/health/topics/contraception/conditioninfo/types.
98. Nelson DB, Lepore SJ, Mastrogiannis DS. Childhood sexual violence and consistent, effective contraception use among young, sexually active urban women. Behav Sci. 2015;5:230–46.
99. Nelson DB, Zhao H, Corrado R, Mastrogiannis DS, Lepore SJ. Preventing unintended pregnancy among young sexually active women: recognizing the role of violence, self-esteem, and depressive symptoms on use of contraception. J Women's Health. 2017;26(4):352–9.
100. Noll JG, Shenk CE. Teen birth rates in sexually abused and neglected females. Pediatrics. 2013;131(4):e1181–7.
101. Noll JG, Haralson KJ, Butler EM, Shenk CE. Childhood maltreatment, psychological dysregulation, and risky sexual behaviors in female adolescents. J Pediatr Psychol. 2011;36(7):743–52.
102. Nunes AP, Phipps MG. Postpartum depression in adolescent and adult mothers: comparing prenatal risk factors and predictive models. Matern Child Health J. 2013;17(6):1071–79.
103. Padilla Y, Reichman N. Low birthweight: do unwed fathers help? Child Youth Serv Rev. 2001;23(4/5):427–52.
104. Pecora LA, Mesibov GB, Stokes MA. Sexuality in high-functioning autism: a systematic review and analysis. J Autism Dev Disord. 2016;46:3519–56.
105. Poulson RL, Eppler MA, Sattlewhite TN, Wuensch KL, Bass LA. Alcohol consumption, strength of religious beliefs, and risky sexual behavior in college students. J Am Coll Heal. 1998;46(5):227–32.
106. Prentice M, Storin C, Robinson G. Make it personal: how pregnancy planning and prevention help students complete college. 2012. https://www.gailrobinsonconsulting.com/publications/Make_It_Personal.pdf.
107. Prince DM, Vidal S, Okpych N, Connell CM. Effects of individual risk and state housing factors on adverse outcomes in a national sample of youth transitioning out of foster care. J Adol. 2019;74:33–4.
108. Putnam-Hornstein E, Hammond I, Eastman AL, McCroskey J, Webster D. Extended foster care for transition-age youth: an opportunity for pregnancy prevention and parenting support. J Adol Health. 2016;58:485–7.
109. Raj A, Silverman JG, Amaro H. The relationship between sexual abuse and sexual risk among high school students: findings for the 1997 Massachusetts youth risk behavior survey. Matern Child Health J. 2000;4(2):125–34.
110. Randolph ME, Torres H, Gore-Felton C, Lloyd B, McGarvey EL. Alcohol use and sexual risk behavior among college students: understanding gender

and ethnic differences. Am J Drug Alcohol Abuse. 2009;35(2):80–4.
111. Reddy DM, Fleming R, Swain C. Effect of mandatory parental notification on adolescent girls' use of sexual health care services. JAMA. 2002;288(6):719–4.
112. Rickert VI, Wiemann CM, Harrykissoon SD, Berenson AB, Kolb E. The relationship among demographics, reproductive characteristics, and intimate partner violence. Am J Obstet Gynecol. 2002;187:1002–7.
113. Rogers C, Lepherd L, Ganguly R, Jacob-Rogers S. Perinatal issues for women with high functioning autism spectrum disorder. Women Birth. 2017;30(2):e89–95.
114. Saewyc EM, Bearinger LH, Blum RW, Resnick MD. Sexual intercourse, abuse and pregnancy among adolescent women: does sexual orientation make a difference? Fam Plan Perspect. 1999;31:127e31.
115. Saewyc EM, Magee LL, Pettingell SE. Teenage pregnancy and associated risk behaviors among sexually abused adolescents. Perspect Sex Reprod Health. 2004;36(3):98–105.
116. Saewyc EM, Poon CS, Homma Y, Skay CL. Stigma management? The links between enacted stigma and teen pregnancy trends among gay, lesbian, and bisexual students in British Columbia. Can J Hum Sex. 2008;17:123e39.
117. Saltzman LE, Johnson CH, Gilbert BC, Goodwin MM. Physical abuse around the time of pregnancy: an examination of prevalence and risk factors in 16 states. Maternal Child Health J. 2003;7(1):31–43.
118. Schoen J. Choice & coercion: birth control, sterilization, and abortion in public health and welfare. Chapel Hill: University of North Carolina Press; 2005.
119. Scott M, Wildsmith E, Welti K, Ryan S, Schelar E, Steward-Streng NR. Risky adolescent sexual behaviors and reproductive health in young adulthood. Perspect Sex Reprod Health. 2011;43:110–8.
120. Shaw M, Lawlor DA, Najman JM. Teenage children of teenage mothers: psychological, behavioural and health outcomes from an Australian prospective longitudinal study. Soc Sci Med. 2006;62:2526.
121. Siegel RS, Brandon AR. Adolescents, pregnancy, and mental health. J Pediatr Adolesc Gynecol. 2014;27:138–50.
122. Sundaram A, Vaughan B, Kost K, Bankole A, Finer L, Singh S, Trussel J. Contraceptive failure in the United States: estimates from the 2006-2010 National Survey of family growth. Perspect Sex Reprod Health. 2017;49(1):7–16.
123. Sundelin HEK, Stepphanson O, Hultman CM, Ludvigsson JF. Pregnancy outcomes in women with autism: a nationwide population-based cohort study. Clin Epidemiol. 2018;10:1817–26.
124. Teal SB, Sheeder J. IUD use in adolescent mothers: retention, failure and reasons for discontinuation. Contraception. 2012;85(3):270–4.
125. The National Campaign to Prevent Teen and Unplanned Pregnancy. Unplanned pregnancy among college students and strategies to address it. 2015. https://powertodecide.org/sites/default/files/resources/primary-download/briefly-unplanned-pregnancy-college.pdf.
126. The Society for Adolescent Health and Medicine and the American Academy of Pediatrics. Confidentiality protections for adolescents and young adults in the health care billing and insurance claims process. J Adol Health. 2016;58:374–7.
127. Tornello SL, Riskind RG, Patterson CJ. Sexual orientation and sexual and reproductive health among adolescent young women in the United States. J Adol Health. 2014;54:160–8.
128. Trent M, Dooley DG, Douge J. Section on adolescent health, council on community Pediatrics, committee on adolescence. The impact of racism on child and adolescent health. Pediatrics. 2019;144(2):e20191765.
129. Upadhya KK, Committee on Adolescence. Emergency contraception. Pediatrics. 2019;144(6). https://pediatrics.aappublications.org/content/pediatrics/early/2019/11/14/peds.2019-3149.full.pdf.
130. Vigod SN, Dennis CL, Kurdyak PA, Cairney J, Guttman A, Taylor VH. Fertility rate trends among adolescent girls with major mental illness: a population-based study. Pediatrics. 2014;133(3):e585–91.
131. Werner KB, Cunningham-Williams RM, Sewell W, Agrawal A, McCutcheon VV, Waldron M, Heath AC, Bucholz KK. The impact of traumatic experiences on risky sexual behaviors in black and white young adult women. Womens Health Issues. 2018;28(5):421–9.
132. Williams DR. Race, socioeconomic status, and health. The added effects of racism and discrimination. Ann N Y Acad Sci. 1999;896:173–88.
133. Wu V, East P, Delker E, Blanco E, Caballero G, Delva J, Lozoff B, Gahagan S. Associations among mother's depression, emotional and learning-material support to their child, and children's cognitive functioning: a 16-year longitudinal study. Child Dev. 2019;90(6):1952–68.

20 Sexual and Gender Minorities (SGM)/(LGBTQ+) Transitional-Age Youth (TAY): Proclaiming Integrity, Legitimacy, and Certainty in the 2020's

Timothy Van Deusen

Key Points

- Healthcare providers should know there is no medically valid evidence that gender identity and sexual orientation can be altered through therapy and that attempting this may lead to decreased self-esteem, homelessness, depression, and suicidality.
- Delivering affirming care, free from heteronormative assumptions, by asking patients their chosen name and personal pronouns allows patients to speak openly about their health concerns leading to a trusting doctor-patient relationship.
- Physical and mental health issues such as substance use disorders, suicide, sexually transmitted infections (STI), unplanned pregnancy, and homelessness are all more common among SGM transitional age youth compared to same-age peers.
- Although SGM transitional age youth are vulnerable and experience health disparities, many are resilient and adapt to living in a society constantly faced with heteronormative adversity.
- A large survey of transgender adults (mean age, 23 years), who received pubertal suppression drugs as adolescents during treatment, had a lower odds of lifetime suicidal ideation compared to those who had no puberty blockers as adolescents in the course of their transgender care.
- Same-sex marriage became a federal law in 2015, but most laws protecting SGM people are at the state and local level. There are currently no federal legal protections for SGM regarding employment or housing.

Introduction

The term "sexual and gender minority" (SGM) encompasses a variety of gender and sexual identities and expressions that differ from the majority (e.g., lesbian, gay, bisexual, transgender, questioning (LGBTQ+), as well as the "plus sign" capturing identities and expressions that defy discrete labels (e.g., queer, gender non-conforming)). The abbreviations LGBT and

T. Van Deusen (✉)
Department of Psychiatry, Yale University School of Medicine, New Haven, CT, USA
e-mail: Timothy.vandeusen@yale.edu

V. Chan, J. Derenne (eds.), *Transition-Age Youth Mental Health Care*,
https://doi.org/10.1007/978-3-030-62113-1_20

LGBTQ are frequently used in the medical literature and lay press. Sexual orientation and identity may be fluid during adolescent and TAY development. Adolescents may have same-sex attractions and fantasies but do not identify as gay, while self-identified gay teens may be sexually inexperienced. Moreover, transgender youth may express their sexual orientation as heterosexual, gay, or bisexual. (For a complete glossary of terms, please refer to Table 20.1.)

Surveying the prevalence of SGM Americans using a Pew Research Center phone survey of a random, nationally representative group of 35,031 US citizens, Smith (2015) found that 5% of men and women identified as lesbian, gay, or bisexual . The largest population-based survey in the United States on sexual orientation was conducted in 2012, which showed that 3.4% of the

Table 20.1 Glossary of terms (hrc.org)

Ally | A person who is not LGBTQ but shows support for LGBTQ people and promotes equality in a variety of ways
Androgynous | Identifying and/or presenting as neither distinguishably masculine nor feminine
Asexual | The lack of a sexual attraction or desire for other people
Biphobia | Prejudice, fear, or hatred directed toward bisexual people
Bisexual | A person emotionally, romantically, or sexually attracted to more than one sex, gender, or gender identity though not necessarily simultaneously, in the same way or to the same degree
Cisgender | A term used to describe a person whose gender identity aligns with those typically associated with the sex assigned to them at birth
Closeted | Describes an LGBTQ person who has not disclosed their sexual orientation or gender identity
Coming out | The process in which a person first acknowledges, accepts, and appreciates their sexual orientation or gender identity and begins to share that with others
Gay | A person who is emotionally, romantically, or sexually attracted to members of the same gender
Gender dysphoria | Clinically significant distress caused when a person's assigned birth gender is not the same as the one with which they identify. According to the American Psychiatric Association's *Diagnostic and Statistical Manual of Mental Disorders* (DSM), the term – which replaces gender identity disorder – "is intended to better characterize the experiences of affected children, adolescents, and adults"

Table 20.1 (continued)

Gender-expansive | Conveys a wider, more flexible range of gender identity and/or expression than typically associated with the binary gender system
Gender expression | External appearance of one's gender identity, usually expressed through behavior, clothing, haircut, or voice and which may or may not conform to socially defined behaviors and characteristics typically associated with being either masculine or feminine
Gender-fluid | According to the *Oxford English Dictionary*, a person who does not identify with a single fixed gender; of or relating to a person having or expressing a fluid or unfixed gender identity
Gender identity | One's innermost concept of self as male, female, a blend of both, or neither – how individuals perceive themselves and what they call themselves. One's gender identity can be the same or different from their sex assigned at birth
Gender non-conforming | A broad term referring to people who do not behave in a way that conforms to the traditional expectations of their gender, or whose gender expression does not fit neatly into a category
Genderqueer | Genderqueer people typically reject notions of static categories of gender and embrace a fluidity of gender identity and often, though not always, sexual orientation. People who identify as "genderqueer" may see themselves as being both male and female, as neither male nor female, or as falling completely outside these categories
Gender transition | The process by which some people strive to more closely align their internal knowledge of gender with its outward appearance. Some people socially transition, whereby they might begin dressing and using names and pronouns and/or be socially recognized as another gender. Others undergo physical transitions in which they modify their bodies through medical interventions
Homophobia | The fear and hatred of or discomfort with people who are attracted to members of the same sex
Intersex | An umbrella term used to describe a wide range of natural bodily variations. In some cases, these traits are visible at birth, and in others, they are not apparent until puberty. Some chromosomal variations of this type may not be physically apparent at all
Lesbian | A woman who is emotionally, romantically, or sexually attracted to other women
LGBTQ | An acronym for "lesbian, gay, bisexual, transgender, and queer"
Living openly | A state in which LGBTQ people are comfortably out about their sexual orientation or gender identity – where and when it feels appropriate to them

Table 20.1 (continued)

Non-binary I An adjective describing a person who does not identify exclusively as a man or a woman. Non-binary people may identify as being both a man and a woman, somewhere in between, or as falling completely outside these categories. While many also identify as transgender, not all non-binary people do
Outing | Exposing someone's lesbian, gay, bisexual, or transgender identity to others without their permission. Outing someone can have serious repercussions on employment, economic stability, personal safety, or religious or family situations
Pansexual | Describes someone who has the potential for emotional, romantic, or sexual attraction to people of any gender though not necessarily simultaneously, in the same way or to the same degree
Queer | A term people often use to express fluid identities and orientations. Often used interchangeably with "LGBTQ"
Questioning | A term used to describe people who are in the process of exploring their sexual orientation or gender identity
Same-gender loving | A term some prefer to use instead of lesbian, gay, or bisexual to express attraction to and love of people of the same gender
Sex assigned at birth I The sex (male or female) given to a child at birth, most often based on the child's external anatomy. This is also referred to as "assigned sex at birth"
Sexual orientation | An inherent or immutable enduring emotional, romantic, or sexual attraction to other people
Transgender | An umbrella term for people whose gender identity and/or expression is different from cultural expectations based on the sex they were assigned at birth. Being transgender does not imply any specific sexual orientation. Therefore, transgender people may identify as straight, gay, lesbian, bisexual, etc.
Transphobia | The fear and hatred of, or discomfort with, transgender people

121,290 respondents age 18 years and older identified as LGBT. When looking at young adults age 18–29 years, 8.3% women and 4.6% men identified as LGBT. The 2015 CDC Youth Risk Behavior Surveillance System (YRBSS) [1] found that 11% of US high school students reported a sexual identity other than heterosexual (2% gay or lesbian, 6% bisexual, 3% not sure) and 6% reported same-sex sexual behavior. Of these youth with same-sex experience, 61% identified as gay, lesbian, or bisexual, and 14% were not sure.

SGM Identity Development

Many SGM adolescents and TAY may experience struggles with their sexual and gender identity. It is quite common for them to experience internalized sexual prejudice (homophobia and transphobia), in which negative attitudes toward homosexuality and/or transgenderism are adopted toward oneself, leading to self-loathing. SGM youth can also manifest sexual prejudice externally, leading to the mistreatment of others who they perceive as sexual minorities. Both externalized and internalized sexual prejudice may lead teens and young adults to avoid sexual activity or adopt heterosexual activity.

Children as young as 2 years learn to label themselves and other children as a boy or a girl, and by age 4–5 years, they are able to understand that gender is a stable and lasting aspect of their identity [2]. Boys and girls have group differences in toy preference by as early as 12 months [3]. Some children experience not only gender non-conformity but also discomfort with their biological sex and therefore wish to be or are comforted by being perceived as the opposite sex (i.e., gender discordance). Many categories of gender discordance with developmental trajectories have been described. The differences are based on whether discordance begins in childhood, adolescence, or adulthood or is transient or persistent and whether individuals develop a same-sex or heterosexual orientation after transitioning to the opposite gender. Follow-up studies of prepubertal boys with gender discordance showed that cross-gender wishes usually fade over time with only 2–11% continuing into adulthood [4, 5]. A follow-up study of the natural histories of prepubertal girls with gender identity disorder (DSM-IV) reported that 12% of the young women had persistent gender dysphoria (DSM-5) as young adults and 1/3 to 1/2 identified as gay [6].

Children referred for assessment due to gender non-conformity may demonstrate gender nonconforming behaviors at a very young age, sometimes as early as 3 years [7]. Other persons may disclose a transgender identity later in adolescence or adulthood, without a history of gender non-conformity in early childhood [8, 9]. Young children who are gender non-conforming or who identify as transgender may or may not continue to identify as transgender as adolescents and adults. In fact, there is evidence to suggest that for a majority of young children with cross-gender identity, this identity does not persist into adolescence [10]. At the time of puberty, their transgender identity may desist and perhaps evolve into a gay or lesbian sexual orientation [10, 11]. However, those who have persistence of transgender identity and/or worsening of gender dysphoria in puberty are thought to be much less likely to identify as cisgender through adolescence. Clinicians can use signs of worsening gender dysphoria at the onset of puberty as a diagnostic tool for persistent transgender identity and as a criterion for eligibility for medical intervention [12]. If these feelings present in adolescence, they usually persist into adulthood, leading to life-long efforts to become the opposite sex through cross-dressing, grooming, or sex reassignment through hormones or surgery [13]. Certainty about sexual orientation and identity – both gay and straight – increases with age, suggesting "an unfolding of sexual identity during adolescence, influenced by sexual experience and demographic factors" [14]. Although it may be difficult to tell on which developmental path a particular adolescent is at a given moment, a consistently same-sex pattern of fantasy, arousal, and attraction suggests a developmental path toward same-sex orientation in adulthood. Retrospectively, many gay men and lesbians report same-sex erotic attraction from youth onward [15].

Minority Stress

Minority stress theory (Meyer 2003) [15] explains that health disparities experienced by SGM people will chronically cause social stress due to negative social attitudes and prejudice. Internalized homophobia refers to inwardly directing society's negative attitudes toward homosexuality, and perceived stigma is the extent that SGM people sense that people in the wider population hold negative attitudes toward homosexuality (e.g., homophobic abuse, exclusion, and discrimination) [16]. These stressors are said to have an additive effect on general psychosocial stressors and can negatively affect an individual's coping mechanisms. They may increase the susceptibility of same-sex-attracted people to develop problems with mental health and substance use [17]. Meyer (2003) concludes that gay men with high levels of minority stress are two times more likely to suffer from distress affecting their mental and physical health [15]. Lesbian, gay, bisexual, and other same-sex-attracted young people have been shown to be at a higher risk of mental health problems, including depression, anxiety, suicidality, and substance abuse, compared to their heterosexual peers. An online survey [18] in Sydney, Australia, recruited 254 same-sex-attracted TAY ages 18–25 years (254 women and 318 men) and found that internalized homophobia, perceived stigma, and experienced homophobic physical abuse were associated with higher levels of psychological distress and suicidal thoughts in the previous month. Perceived stigma and homophobic physical abuse were associated with reporting a lifetime suicide attempt, but the association between minority stress and substance use was inconsistent [18].

The concept of minority stress is not based on one congruous theory but is inferred from several social and psychological theoretical orientations. Hatzenberger et al. propose that sexual minorities confront increased stress exposure resulting from stigma which increases emotion dysregulation, social/interpersonal problems, and cognitive processes which facilitate the relationship between stigma-related stress and psychopathology [16]. They also found that sexual minorities are at increased risk for multiple mental health burdens compared with heterosexuals [16]. According to the National Coalition of Anti-Violence Programs (NCAVP) [19], LGBTQ individuals who also identify as racial and/or ethnic minorities represented 79% of anti-LGBTQ hate-related homicides in the United States, of which 14% were Latinx. Of the total survivors of anti-LGBTQ hate crimes, 29% were Latinx. These figures are likely to underestimate the true incidences because the NCAVP bases its statistics only on cases for which it can confirm the identity characteristics of the victim. NCAVP also reports that LGBTQ Latinx individuals were more likely to experience online harassment, to be threatened, to experience robbery, and to experience violence by their employers [20].

SGM youth are at high risk for school victimization. In a 2011 national survey of 8584 LGBT students aged 13–20 years, 71–85% reported hearing sexual prejudicial remarks (e.g., "dyke"; "faggot"; "that's so gay") [21]. In the same study, 57% reported hearing such remarks from a teacher or staff member, 64% felt unsafe at school because of their sexual orientation, and 38% were physically harassed (e.g., pushed), while 18% were physically assaulted (e.g., punched, kicked, or hit with a weapon). The 8th biennial 2013 National School Climate Survey by the Gay, Lesbian, and Straight Education Network (GLSEN) [22] revealed that hostile school climates negatively affect educational success. LGBT students who experienced victimization and discrimination showed lower GPAs than students who had not (2.8 vs. 3.3) and were less likely to plan for college (92% vs 96%). School victimization has been linked to compromised academic achievement and school absenteeism, aggressive behavior, compromised emotional health, and suicidal ideation, substance use, delinquency, and aggression, particularly for boys [23]. Affecting attendance, 30% of these kids missed at least one school day per month because they felt unsafe [24]. School climate for LGBT youth was improved in schools with extracurricular gay-straight alliance groups [22] (see Table 20.2). SGM adolescents suffer higher rates of parental abuse and polyvictimization than their heterosexual peers. The Human Rights Campaign [25] polled 10,000 youth ages 13–17 years in 2012; 26% reported family rejection after coming out, 21% reported being bullied at school, and 18% were fearful for being "out." Some findings indicate that gender nonconformity in children accounts for at least a portion of the disparities in abuse. For example, Roberts (2012) found that gender non-conformity prior to age 11 years partly accounted for greater rates of child abuse and later rates of PTSD in early adulthood, both among children who identify as heterosexual and children who have a minority sexual orientation [26].

Table 20.2 School bullying and SGM youth

Nearly 60% youth have no protections from bullying in school
71.5% of US school districts have anti-bullying policies, but only 42.6% include sexual orientation, and only 14.1% include gender expression
Having strict anti-bullying policies and gay-straight alliances in place for 3 or more years significantly reduced suicidal thoughts and attempts according to a 2014 study
Only 10% of youth report that their school has a policy which includes SGM protections

Healthcare: Medical and Mental Health

According to the Dane County Youth Assessment Surveys in 2008–2009, multiple factors accounted for unsafe sexual behaviors in LGBT youth, including earlier age of first sexual encounter, increased number of known and anonymous sexual partners, lack of education on safe sex practices, ineffective use of condoms, and inadequate perception of sexually transmitted infection (STI) acquisition and testing [27]. One study on LGBTQ adolescents found that only 35% of the respondents had disclosed their sexual orientation or gender identity to their healthcare provider, with bisexual youth disclosing at lower rates (Meckler et al. 2006) [28]. Intrapersonal factors impacting disclosure may be especially pertinent among TAY, who may still be navigating and defining their identities and who may be more selective about disclosure. Also, sociodemographic characteristics of the patient, such as race and income, have been associated with nondisclosure among men who have sex with men (MSM), with African American and/or low-income individuals being less likely to disclose their sexual orientation to providers [28]. These findings suggest that rates of disclosure may vary, not only between different identity groups within the LGBTQ community but also based on racial/ethnic identity and socioeconomic status.

Another factor in LGBT health disparities is discriminatory treatment in healthcare settings. Surveys of both patients [29] and providers [30] reveal that LGBT people experience prejudicial treatment in clinical settings and that some providers exhibit anti-LGBT bias. As a result, many LGBT patients report culturally incompetent care or avoid visiting healthcare facilities for fear of receiving substandard care [30]. The lack of LGBT-inclusive cultural competency and clinical training for providers contributes to their widespread failure to discuss SGM issues with their patients, perpetuating invisibility of LGBT patients in clinical settings. SGM data collection is a key component of enhancing the ability of patients and providers to engage in meaningful dialogue in the exam room and to promote the provision of high-quality care for LGBT people [31]. Patient-provider discussions about SGM issues can facilitate a more accurate assessment of patient self-reported health and risk behaviors [32]. These open communications at clinics and hospitals are especially important, where LGBTQ youth find it difficult to share their sexual identities with their clinicians, and the lack of communication is responsible for the poor therapeutic alliance, poor illness-related education, inadequate scheduled screening for communicable diseases, and inadequate interventions to prevent STIs [33].

Sexually Transmitted Illnesses (STIs)

SGM youth are more likely to engage in high-risk sexual behaviors leading to an increased incidence of STIs (sexually transmitted illnesses), e.g., syphilis, human papillomavirus (HPV) infections, and hepatitis in MSM [26]. The rates of gonorrhea, chlamydia, and HIV are two times as high in sexual minority youth compared to those in heterosexual men [34]. In 2016, the Centers for Disease Control and Prevention (CDC) [35] reported that new HIV diagnoses in the United States totaled 37,832 and that youth ages 13–24 years old accounted for 7807 (21%) of them. Most new HIV infections among youth occur among young men who have sex with men (YMSM), gay and bisexual men, with young black/African American and Hispanic/Latinx gay and bisexual men especially affected. Many of these youth do not know they are infected. Alcohol, methamphetamine, and other drug use are common among YMSM and can lead to risky sexual behavior resulting in STIs. Youth who developed HIV as children or adolescents tend to form close attachments to their adolescent care team and may have difficulty transitioning to adult care. Adolescent providers have stressed the importance of matching these patients with adult clinics that are comfortable treating LGBTQ+ young people [34].

Health Outcomes

Transgender or non-conforming (TGNC) youth report poor health outcomes compared to their cisgender peers. The 2016 Minnesota Student Survey of 80,000 9th and 11th graders, 2.7% who identified as TGNC found that nearly 2/3 of TGNC students reported their health as poor, fair, or good versus very good or excellent, compared to 1/3 of cisgender students [36].

Other studies in children as young as 3–9 years old have found higher prevalence of anxiety and attention-deficit/hyperactivity disorder (ADHD) in TGNC youth [34]. The 2015 CDC Youth Risk Behavior Surveillance System (YRBSS) determined that 9% of American high schoolers attempted suicide in 2014. Rates of suicidal thoughts and suicide attempts of LGB youth were three to four times that of the general population. In one study of youth who identify as LGBTQ, 45% had experienced suicidal thoughts, and 35% had attempted suicide [37]. The developmental period following same-sex experience but before self-acceptance as gay may be one of especially elevated safety risks. Suicidal thoughts, depression, and anxiety are especially high among gay males who displayed gender non-conforming behavior as children. A study of 224 white and Latinx self-identified LGB young adults who reported high levels of family rejection during adolescence showed that they were 8.4 times more likely to report having attempted suicide, 5.9 times more likely to report depression, 3.4 times more likely to use illegal drugs, and 3.4 times more likely to engage in unprotected sex than those who reported no or low levels of family rejection [38].

Given the high prevalence of HIV transmission among MSM, adolescent gay males are at high risk for HIV, as well as other STIs. Young bisexual and lesbian women, not factoring in race or ethnicity, are twice as likely to have a teen pregnancy than their heterosexual peers, and depression in adolescence may be more predictive of subsequent unintended pregnancy than depression at young adult ages [39]. Poor safe sex practices (i.e., no contraception) may be a result of low motivation to use protection secondary to low self-esteem, shame, or guilt about same-sex attraction.

Substance Use and Dependence

Rates of drug use among SGM youth are higher than those of their heterosexual peers [40, 41]. For example, 56% of high school youth who identify as bisexual report past-month alcohol use, compared to 38% of their peers who identify as heterosexual [39]. Lifetime prevalence rates for heroin, inhalants, steroids, cocaine, and MDMA/ecstasy use are also higher among sexual minority high school youth compared to heterosexual youth. Sexual minority youth likely engage in drug use for the same reasons as their heterosexual peers, including prevailing peer and social influences. However, sexual minority youth must also contend with negative reactions to their minority status and a concomitant lack of social support from family, peers, and others [42]. Although drug abuse prevention programs focus on such risk factors as peer and social influences and stress, these programs largely assume a heterosexual audience [43, 44].

Substance use disorders, suicide, STIs, unplanned pregnancy, and homelessness are all more common among sexual minority youth [43]. Estimated prevalence rates of drug and alcohol abuse among LGBTQ people are 20–30%, compared to 9% in the general population [44, 45]. The odds of substance use for LGB youth were, on average, 190% higher than for heterosexual youth and substantially higher within some subpopulations of LGB youth: 340% higher for bisexual youth and 400% higher for females [44, 45]. Substances may be utilized in response to peer pressure in order to gain acceptance and to relieve emotional distress related to the effects of bullying, exclusion from support networks (e.g., friends, family), or internalized sexual prejudice or due to increased exposure to substances at venues where one's identity is being explored (e.g., night clubs) [46, 47]. Anabolic steroid (AAS) abuse is six times higher in gay males compared to straight adolescent males. Substantial sexual orientation health disparities exist in regard to the prevalence of AAS use, with sexual minority males reporting a lifetime rate of 21% compared to 4% for heterosexual adolescent males, over five times the rate [48].

Depression and Suicide

It has been shown that adolescents and TAY who receive gender-affirming care, including puberty blockers and hormonal therapy, have lower rates of suicidal attempts and depression. Turban et al. (2020) completed a large cross-sectional survey of 20,619 transgender adults ages 18–36 years (mean age of 23, 45% assigned male at birth) which showed that those who received pubertal suppression drugs as adolescents had a lower odds of lifetime suicidal ideation compared to those who had no puberty blockers as adolescents in the course of their transgender care [49]. Also, self-reported peer victimization (for males and females), as well as parental rejection (for females/bisexuals), mediated the association between sexual orientation and depressive symptoms. Cross-sectional studies have found higher levels of depressive symptoms for LGB people, in comparison to heterosexuals, in adolescence

[50] as well as adulthood [51, 52]. Longitudinal studies on the topic are scarce, with exceptions relying largely on data from the National Longitudinal Study of Adolescent to Adult Health (Add Health) [53–55]. These studies found that, compared to heterosexual youth, same-sex- or bisexually attracted youth experienced elevated levels of depressive symptoms in late adolescence (age 16 years), which persisted into young adulthood (age 29 years). However, some empirical evidence suggests the contrary: that black sexual minority male youth report better psychological health (fewer major depressive episodes and less suicidal ideation and alcohol abuse or dependence) than their white sexual minority male counterparts [56]. A community sample of SGM TAY ages 16–20 years revealed that nearly 33% of participants met the diagnostic criteria for a mental disorder and/or reported a suicide attempt in their lifetime [57]. When comparing these findings to mental health diagnosis rates in the general population, about 18% of lesbian and gay youth participants met the criteria for major depressive disorder (MDD) and 11.3% for PTSD in the previous 12 months. Of the LGBT sample, 31% recounted suicidal behavior at some point in their life. National baseline rates for these diagnoses and behaviors among youth are 8.2% (MDD), 3.9% (PTSD), and 4.1% (suicidal behavior) [58, 59]. Much of what has been learned scientifically about sexual orientation and gender development in the last generation has occurred in parallel with societal changes in attitudes toward sexual orientation and gender roles. Biological, psychological, and social influences have been discussed in the literature over the past five decades with the leading theories shifting dramatically over that time.

Biological Aspects

The neurohormonal theory suggests that prenatal sex hormone levels influence development of gender role behavior in childhood and sexual orientation in adults. While sex hormone levels during fetal development may influence childhood gender variance and adult sexual orientation, neither same-sex attraction nor gender variance is an indication for endocrine, genetic, or any other special medical evaluation. There is evidence of genetic influence on gender role in childhood and sexual orientation in adulthood from family, twin, and molecular studies. Bailey et al. (1993) and colleagues found that, among gay males, 52% of monozygotic co-twins were gay compared to 22% of dizygotic twins and 11% of adoptive brothers. There is little data on differences in neuroanatomy [60]. Some research studies have tested the hypothesis that sexual minority identity, in and of itself, is linked to atypical patterns of cortisol levels. Studies that have looked at diurnal slopes and acute reactivity of cortisol have generally not found that self-identified LGB individuals differ in their diurnal cortisol patterns from heterosexual individuals [61, 62]. Research questions that propose to address social group differences (e.g., LGB vs heterosexual) based on the endorsement of a single categorical social construct (e.g., sexual orientation) do not account for the *diversity of individuals within those groups*. Conversely, some researchers have reported differences when accounting for the dual categories of sexuality and gender. For example, lesbian and bisexual women showed higher and prolonged cortisol elevation to an experimental induction of acute social stress when compared to heterosexual women, but gay and bisexual men showed lower cortisol levels than heterosexual men throughout the duration of the stressor [63]. One possible way to investigate these findings might be to look at the *multiple forms of oppression* these individuals experience at the intersections of sexual orientation and gender. Understanding the tightly interwoven associations between the social constructs of sexuality and gender requires examining the shared and unique lived experiences of LGBTQ and heterosexual individuals [64].

Psychological Factors

The last decade of research on LGBTQ youth has seen a gradual expansion from its focus on risk to the resources associated with resilience, "positive adaptation in the context of risk or adversity," e.g., race and poverty [65]. The inclusion of sexual and gender diversity as a source of adversity is relatively new in resilience research, and the dearth of studies does not spell out what adversities their study participants commonly experienced. Asakura et al. (2019) posit that LGBTQ youth might experience their everyday realities differently from their cisgender, heterosexual peers, and it might be rash to transfer knowledge of youth resilience in general to SGM youth. They surveyed a gender and racially diverse group of 16- to 24-year-olds about their life "stressors" to define their "resilience" [66]. All participants rejected the normative definitions of positive adaptation such as the "absence of psychopathologies" and "school success" and instead used the phrases "still struggling," "battling through," and "having your head above water." Overall, this qualitative study adds to research on risk and resilience by conceptualizing hetero-cis-normativity as a source of adversity and echoes the need for continued resources and further research (Asakura K et al. 2019) [66].

A similar qualitative study that explored the resilience of 13 transgender youth of color found that, despite experiencing racism and prejudice, the participants were often able to use social media to assert their identities and counter negative representations (Singh 2012) [67].

The distance created by online communication may also help to buffer the negative content LGBTQ youth encounter and provide opportunities for personal advocacy. For example, insults may feel less threatening to youth who can respond to them from the safety of their homes. Encountering negativity online may actually allow young people to develop and practice skills such as buffering, deflecting, or resisting homophobia and heterosexism [68]

For those raised in Evangelical Christian families, "coming out" may create a new psychological stressor, and for many, it can result in being ostracized by family members who believe that LGBTQ people are "sick, or sinners," who "should not marry, raise a family, or adopt children." A good number of these youth have been pressured to undergo "conversion therapy" or "sexual orientation change efforts" (SOCE), which entails aversive methods such as electric shocks, delivered when aroused by same-sex photographs, in order to change their sexual orientation or gender identity to heteronormative accepted standards. The youth exposed to this practice have suffered serious psychiatric disorders such as PTSD, depression, anxiety, and suicide. Attempts to change sexual orientation during adolescence are associated with elevated young adult depressive symptoms and suicidal behavior and with lower levels of young adult life satisfaction, social support, and socioeconomic status. Ryan (2020) interviewed 245 LGBT young adults ages 21–25 years, and more than half reported some form of attempt by their parents and caregivers to change their sexual orientation during adolescence. Thus SOCE is associated with multiple domains of functioning that affect self-care, well-being, and adjustment [38, 69]. The American Academy of Child and Adolescent Psychiatry (AACAP) Policy finds "no evidence to support the application of any therapeutic intervention operating under the premise that a specific sexual orientation, gender identity, and/or gender expression is pathological." Furthermore, based on the scientific evidence, the AACAP asserts that such "conversion therapies" (or other interventions imposed with the intent of promoting a particular sexual orientation and/or gender as a preferred outcome) lack scientific credibility and clinical utility. Additionally, there is evidence that such interventions are harmful. As a result, "conversion therapies" should not be part of any behavioral health treatment of children and adolescents. Table 20.3 lists 20 states that have laws banning conversion therapy (hrc.org).

However, according to the Williams Institute at the UCLA School of Law, an estimated 20,000 LGBT youth (ages 13–17 years) will receive con-

Table 20.3 Twenty states have laws banning the practice of "conversion therapy" (including Washington, D.C., and Puerto Rico)

Massachusetts	Vermont	New Hampshire	Connecticut	Rhode Island
Maine	New York	New Jersey	Delaware	Maryland
Virginia	Illinois	California	Washington	Oregon
Nevada	New Mexico	Colorado	Hawaii	Utah

version therapy from a licensed healthcare professional before they reach the age of 18 years in other states [70].

Social Impacts

A 2014 Williams Institute study looked at the economic impact of SGM rights in 39 countries and 39 emerging economies around the world. They learned that the exclusion of LGBTQ people caused economic harm such as decreased productivity, lost labor time, underinvestment in human capital, and the inefficient allocation of human resources through hiring practices and education. The study also showed that expansion of SGM rights was correlated with higher per capita income and higher levels of well-being for everyone [71].

It is estimated that there are 1.6–2 million homeless youth in the United States and that 20–40% are LGBT. Given that LGBT youth comprise less than 10% of the general adolescent population, a disproportionate number of LGBT youth are displaced from their homes. Homeless sexual minority youth report high rates of substance abuse, suicide attempts, risky sexual behaviors (prostitution, unprotected intercourse), and sexual victimization [72]. Homelessness is one of the most common drivers of youth engagement in survival sex [73, 74]. Nationally, estimates of the proportion of runaway and homeless youth involved in survival sex range from 10% to as high as 50% [74]. Seeking refuge in shelters may perpetuate discrimination; many youth report maltreatment in this setting.

Recent research suggests differences in child welfare experiences for sexual minority youth. LGBTQ youth in foster care, when compared to their heterosexual peers, experience a higher number of child welfare placements and longer lengths of stay [75, 76]. The social stigma and discrimination combined with differences in child welfare experiences suggests that LGBTQ youth in foster care have an increased vulnerability for substance use and misuse. The rationale for a detailed focus on sexual minority youth stems from the likelihood that their young adulthood lives may be compromised as a result of factors related to representing a "largely invisible population within child welfare systems" [77]. Moreover, though the state of research on sexual minority youth during their involvement with child welfare is deemed "growing yet still insufficient" [78], research on their lives immediately following emancipation is virtually non-existent [79]. Spiegel et al. (2016) [80] studied information from the Chafee Act and the Children's Bureau 2011 Information Memorandum and data from one site of the Multi-Site Evaluation of Foster Youth Programs (MEFYP) study. They found that compared to same-age heterosexual peers, sexual minority TAY demonstrate significantly lesser functioning in education, employment, housing stability, and financial matters. They were more likely to experience financial hardships and indicate that they were "struggling to make it." SGM TAY were less likely to be "financially stable" or to have bank accounts and were more likely to use public assistance. For related functional well-being indicators, sexual minority youth were less likely to have high school diplomas/GEDs and work experience and more likely to experience homelessness compared to their heterosexual counterparts [80]. Services and programs for youth in care should be designed to address substance use and misuse prevention, housing stability, and independent living preparation needs unique to the youth and should address needs of sexual minority youth.

LGBQ Discrimination in the Workplace Scholars have documented a variety of disproportionate barriers to employment and discriminatory practices in the workplace against LGBQ individuals. Several studies matched résumés or job candidates on skill level but altered one key characteristic: implied sexual orientation. In all these studies, compared to the heterosexual job candidates, the LGBTQ job candidate received fewer interview invitations and was deemed less qualified for the position [81]. Furthermore, LGBTQ employees are vulnerable to direct and indirect forms of victimization in the workplace, such as being passed up for promotions or terminated from their position as well as experiencing verbal or physical harassment, derogatory comments, and discriminatory attitudes [83-86]. One policy report released in 2007 claims that anywhere between 7% and 41% of LGBQ people surveyed had been either physically or verbally abused in the workplace or had their property vandalized at work [81].

Higher Education: College Campus Life

Approximately 10% of colleges and universities (320 campuses) have at least 1 paid professional staff or graduate assistant directing LGBT resources [87]. There has been a steady growth in the number of established LGBTQ centers at institutions of higher education since 1971, when the first dedicated space at the University of Michigan opened to serve gay and lesbian students [88] in varying degrees, and eventually inclusive of all SGMs. Data from the University of Wisconsin's HOPE Lab survey, entitled "Still Hungry and Homeless in College," reveals that transgender and non-binary students are more likely to face food and housing insecurity and homelessness, at rates significantly higher than their cisgender peers. Their findings are based on a survey of 43,000 students at 66 institutions in 20 states and the District of Columbia [89]. It includes more than 20,000 students at 35 4-year colleges and universities, as well as students at community colleges. LGB respondents faced higher risks of basic need insecurity compared to heterosexual students – with bisexual students at the highest risk of this group. Nearly 50% of bisexual respondents experienced food and/or housing insecurity, and over 20% bisexual community college students have experienced homelessness. Researchers think that these disparities seen in SGM students are linked to lower levels of family and financial support. These results are consistent with data recently released by Chapin Hall at the University of Chicago [90], which found that LGBTQ young adults had a 120% higher risk of reporting homelessness compared to youth who identified as heterosexual and cisgender. Colleges face increasing numbers of students with mental health problems [91]. Despite having access to campus services, only half of college students with mental health problems use supports [92, 93].

Culture and Religion

Many adolescents and young adults have internal conflicts related to their religious upbringing because some religions are not accepting of LGBT people. Others are all inclusive (i.e., accepting of people regardless of race, culture, gender, and sexual orientation). Adolescents may be justifiably reluctant about "coming out" to families who may engage in rejecting behaviors based on their own religious and/or cultural beliefs. Latino, immigrant, religious, and low-socioeconomic status families appear to be less accepting, on average, of LGBT adolescents. It appears that it is not the sexual orientation or gender identity of the adolescents themselves but the characteristics of their families (their ethnicity, immigration and occupation status, and religious affiliation) that seem to make a difference in distinguishing between those that score high versus low on acceptance of their LGBT children [38]. In certain situations, healthcare providers should be cautious about recommending open conversations at home and instead should guide the patient to people and organizations that may be useful sources of education and support (see Resources section below). While a small number of religious denominations have become more affirming of same-sex sexuality, the religious context remains challenging for some sexual minorities. The presupposition and normative standard of heterosexuality is salient and often unchallenged within Western society, and it can be reinforced within Christian religious contexts. Sexual minority individuals within these settings may be exposed to negative and condemning denominational teachings regarding their sexual attractions and behavior. This may lead to heightened frustration and confusion regarding their own values related to sexual behavior, attractions, faith, family, and the afterlife.

Dahl et al. (2012) did a qualitative study looking into the positive and negative experiences of sexual minority adolescents and young adults coming out within a Christian religious context [94]. Sexual minority adolescents and young adults are presumed to be going through the process of identity negotiation [95] and, as such, can provide more current information regarding their experiences. Researchers have highlighted the importance of context when considering the developmental experiences of sexual minorities, individuals who identify as lesbian, gay, bisexual, transgender, or queer (LGBTQ) or use another label of personal meaning [96]. One context, and a major socializing force in the United States, is religion. Seventy-six percent of Americans report a Christian religious affiliation, and approximately 4% of Americans describe a religious affiliation other than Christianity [97]. As such, developmental processes can be complicated for sexual minorities attempting to negotiate their sense of identity within Christian religious contexts [95, 97]. Research has also examined the relationship between sexual minority religiosity and substance use. These studies [98] found religious commitment associated with lowered levels of binge drinking, substance use, and risky sexual behavior in male gay and bisexual adolescents but not female lesbian and bisexual youth.

Federal and State Law Protections

The Human Rights Campaign (hrc.org), founded in 1980, is the largest advocacy group in the United States fighting for LGBTQ legal protections at the federal and state level. Family Equality Council (familyequality.org) connects, supports, and represents the three million parents who are lesbian, gay, bisexual, transgender, and queer in this country and their six million children. They work to ensure equality for LGBT families by building community, changing hearts and minds, and advancing social justice for all families. The Lambda Legal Defense and Education Fund is the largest legal organization in the United States. Since 1973, the staff has worked to secure civil rights for gays, lesbians, and persons with HIV via education, public policy work, and litigation.

After years of lawsuits in district, federal, and the Supreme Court, same-sex marriage became a federal law in 2015. However most laws protecting LGBTQ people are at the state and local level. There are currently no federal legal protections for SGM regarding employment or housing. This means that one can be fired or evicted for being a SGM individual. Section 1557 of the Patient Protection and Affordable Care Act ("ACA") provides that individuals may not be excluded on the basis of race, sex, age, or disability from participation in, be denied the benefits of, or be subjected to discrimination under any health program or activity that receives federal financial assistance. However, the current administration has implemented a "proposed rule," which re-interprets Section 1557 to remove protections against discrimination based on gender identity and will most likely be challenged in the courts. The Equality Act, passed by the US House of Representatives on May 17, 2019, and gaining momentum in the Senate, would amend existing civil rights law – including the Civil Rights Act of 1964, the Fair Housing Act, the Equal Credit Opportunity Act, the Jury Selection and Services Act, and several laws regarding employment with the federal government to explicitly include sexual orientation and gender identity as protected characteristics (HRC.ORG).

Summary

SGM TAY face multiple challenges on a daily basis, and most have experienced minority stress during their child, adolescent, and transitional age development increasing their risk of depression, substance abuse, and suicide. Many have also encountered job discrimination leading to unemployment and disillusionment, lower earned incomes, and higher rates of homelessness compared to their cisgender, heterosexual peers. Many SGMs have been rejected by their families because of their identities and sexual orientation, forcing them into homelessness and sexual survival behaviors. Their rates of life-threatening STIs outnumber their same-age non-SGM peers. Those SGMs who do attend college tend to select schools that are welcoming and that have LGBTQ centers on campus, providing support and a sense of community. Those who have religious beliefs but are banned from their own religious houses of worship can discover the many faiths that are inclusive of all genders and sexual orientation. The SGM TAY community is quite diverse and is represented by members of all cultures, races, and religions. More research is needed to understand the intersectionality of their similarities and differences which can improve care.

References

1. Youth Risk Behavior Surveillance System (YRBSS).
2. Kohlberg LA. A cognitive-developmental analysis of children's sex role concepts and attitudes. In: Maccoby E, editor. The development of sex differences. Stanford: Stanford University; 1966. p. 82–173.
3. Fausto-Sterling A. The dynamic development of gender variability. J Homosex. 2012;59(3):398–421.
4. Green R. The "Sissy-Boy Syndrome" and the development of homosexuality, vol. 63. New Haven: Yale University Press; 1987.
5. Zucker KJ, Bradley SJ. Gender identity disorder and psychosexual problems in children and adolescents. New York: Guilford Press; 1995.
6. Smith YL, van Goozen SH, Cohen-Kettenis PT. Adolescents with gender identity disorder who were accepted or rejected for sex reassignment surgery: a prospective follow-up study. J Am Acad Child Adolesc Psychiatry. 2001;40:472–81.
7. Rosenthal SMJ. Approach to the patient: transgender youth: endocrine considerations. Clin Endocrinol Metab. 2014;99(12):4379–89.
8. Gooren LJ. Care of transsexual persons. N Engl J Med. 2011;364(13):1251–7.
9. Drummond KD, et al. A follow-up study of girls with gender identity disorder. Dev Psychol. 2008;44(1):34–45.
10. Wallien MS, et al. Cross-national replication of the gender identity interview for children. J Pers Assess. 2009;91(6):545–52.
11. AACAP Official Action Journal Of The American Academy Of Child & Adolescent Psychiatry. 2012;51(9). 961www.jaacap.org.
12. Remafedi G, Resnick M, Blum R, Harris L. Demography of sexual orientation in adolescents. Pediatrics. 1992;89:714–21.
13. Shechner T. Gender identity disorder: a literature review from a developmental perspective. Isr J Psychiatry Relat Sci. 2010;47(2):132.
14. Bell AP, Weinberg MS, Hammersmith SK. Sexual preference: its development in men and women. Bloomington: Indiana University Press; 1981.
15. Meyer IH. Prejudice, social stress, and mental health in lesbian, gay, and bisexual populations: conceptual issues and research evidence. Psychol Bull. 2003;129(5):674–97. Meyer I. J Health Soc Behav. 1995;36(March):38–56.
16. Hatzenbuehler ML. How does sexual minority stigma "get under the skin"? A psychological mediation framework. Psychol Bull. 2009;135(5):707–30.
17. Lea T, et al. Minority stress in lesbian, gay, and bisexual young adults in Australia: associations with psychological distress, suicidality, and substance use. Arch Sex Behav. 2014;43:1571–8.
18. Sydney online survey.
19. National Coalition of Anti-Violence Programs (NCAVP, 2017).
20. Parra L, Hastings P. Challenges to identity integration indirectly link experiences of heterosexist and racist discrimination to lower waking salivary cortisol in sexually diverse latinx emerging adults. Front Psychol. 2020;11:228.
21. Woodford MR, et al. "That's so gay!" examining the covariates of hearing this expression among gay, lesbian, and bisexual college students. J Am Coll Heal. 2012;60:429–34.
22. The 2013 National School Climate Survey.
23. Robinson JP, Espelage DL. Peer victimization and sexual risk differences between lesbian, gay, bisexual, transgender, or questioning and non-transgender heterosexual youths in grades 7–12. Am J Public Health. 2013;103:1810–9.
24. Hafeez H, Zeshan M, Tahir MA, et al. Health care disparities among lesbian, gay, bisexual, and transgender youth: a literature review. Cureus. 2017;9(4):e1184.
25. Human Rights Campaign (hrc.org).

26. Roberts A. Childhood gender nonconformity: a risk indicator for childhood abuse and posttraumatic stress in youth. Pediatrics. 2012;129(3):410.
27. Russell ST, Fish JN. Mental health in lesbian, gay, bisexual, and transgender (LGBT) youth. Annu Rev Clin Psychol. 2016;12:465–87.
28. Meckler GD, Elliott MN, Kanouse DE, Beals KP, Schuster MA. Nondisclosure of sexual orientation to a physician among a sample of gay, lesbian, and bisexual youth. Arch Pediatr Adolesc Med. 2006;160:1248–54.
29. Petroll AE, Mosack KE. Physician awareness of sexual orientation and preventive health recommendations to men who have sex with men. Sex Transm Dis. 2011;38:63.
30. Smith D, Mathews W. Physicians' attitudes toward homosexuality and HIV: survey of a California medical society-revisited (PATHH-II). J Homosex. 2007;52(3–4):1–9. [PubMed].
31. Makadon H. Ending LGBT invisibility in health care: the first step in ensuring equitable care. Cleve Clin J Med. 2011;78:220–4. [PubMed].
32. Klitzman R, Greenberg J. Patterns of communication between gay and lesbian patients and their health care providers. J Homosex. 2002;42(4):65–75. [PubMed].
33. Benson PA, Hergenroeder AC. Bacterial sexually transmitted infections in gay, lesbian, and bisexual adolescents: medical and public health perspectives. Semin Pediatr Infect Dis. 2005;16:181–91.
34. Dowshen N, D'Angelo L. Health care transition for youth living with HIV/AIDS. Pediatrics. 2011;128(4):762–71.
35. Center of Disease Control's HIV Surveillance Report: Diagnoses of HIV infection in the United States and dependent areas, 2018; vol. 30 pdf icon.
36. Baams L. Disparities for LGBTQ and gender nonconforming adolescents. Pediatrics. 2018;141(5):e20173004.
37. YRBSS.
38. Ryan C, et al. Family rejection as a predictor of negative health outcomes in white and latino lesbian, gay, and bisexual young adults. Pediatrics. 2009;123:346. https://doi.org/10.1542/peds.2007-3524.
39. Charlten B, et al. Teen pregnancy risk factors among young women of diverse sexual orientations. Pediatrics. 2018;141:4.
40. Marshal MP, Friedman MS, Stall R, et al. Sexual orientation and adolescent substance use: a meta-analysis and methodological review. Addiction. 2008;103:546e56.
41. Corliss HL, Rosario M, Wypij D, et al. Sexual orientation and drug use in a longitudinal cohort study of U.S. adolescents. Addict Behav. 2010;35:517e21.
42. Kann L, Olsen EO, McManus T, et al. Sexual identity, sex of sexual contacts, and health-risk behaviors among students in grades 9–12: youth risk behavior surveillance, selected sites, United States, 2001-2009. MMWR Surveill Summ. 2011;60:1e133.
43. Goldbach JT, Tanner-Smith EE, Bagwell M, Dunlap S. Minority stress and substance use in sexual minority adolescents: a meta-analysis. Prev Sci. 2014;15:350e63.
44. Hatzenbuehler ML. How does sexual minority stigma "get under the skin"? A psychological mediation framework. Psychol Bull. 2009;135:707e30.
45. Rosario M, Schrimshaw EW, Hunter J. A model of sexual risk behaviors among young gay and bisexual men: Longitudinal associations of mental health, substance abuse, sexual abuse, and the coming-out process. AIDS Educ Prev. 2006;18:444e60.
46. Adelson SL, Stroeh OM, Ng YKW. Development and mental health of lesbian, gay, bisexual, or transgender youth in pediatric practice. Pediatr Clin N Am. 2016;63(6):971–83.
47. Li G, Kung KTF, Hines M. Childhood gender-typed behavior and adolescent sexual orientation: a longitudinal population-based study. Dev Psychol. 2017;53(4):764–77.
48. Blashill AJ, Safren SA. Sexual orientation and anabolic-androgenic steroids in U.S. adolescent boys. Pediatrics. 2014;133(3):469–75.
49. Turban JL, et al. Pubertal suppression for transgender youth and risk of suicidal ideation. Pediatrics. 2020;145:2.
50. Marshal MP, Dietz L, Friedman M, Stall R, Smith H, McGinley J, et al. Suicidality and depression disparities between sexual minority and heterosexual youth: a meta- analytic review. J Adolesc Health. 2011;49(2):115–23.
51. Institute of Medicine. The health of lesbian, gay, bisexual, and transgender people: building a foundation for better understanding. 2011. http://www.iom.edu/Reports/2011/The-Health-of-Lesbian-Gay-Bisexual-and-Transgender-People/Report-Brief.aspx.
52. Meyer IH. Prejudice, social stress, and mental health in lesbian, gay, and bisexual populations: conceptual issues and research evidence. Psychol Bull. 2003;129(5):674–97.
53. Fish JN, Pasley K. Sexual (minority) trajectories, mental health, and alcohol use: a longitudinal study of youth as they transition to adulthood. J Youth Adolesc. 2015;44(8):1508–27.
54. Marshal MP, Dermody SS, Cheong J, Burton CM, Friedman MS, Aranda F, Hughes TL. Trajectories of depressive symptoms and suicidality among heterosexual and sexual minority youth. J Youth Adolesc. 2013;42(8):1243–56.
55. Needham BL. Sexual attraction and trajectories of mental health and substance use during the transition from adolescence to adulthood. J Youth Adolesc. 2012;41(2):179–90.
56. Burns MN, Ryan DT, Garofalo R, Newcomb ME, Mustanski B. Mental health disorders in young urban sexual minority men. J Adolesc Health. 2015;56:52–8.

57. Mustanski BS, Garofalo R, Emerson EM. Mental health disorders, psychological distress, and suicidality in a diverse sample of lesbian, gay, bisexual, and transgender youths. Am J Public Health. 2010;100:2426–32.
58. Kessler RC, Avenevoli S, Costello J, Georgiades K, Green JG, et al. Prevalence, persistence, and sociodemographic correlates of DSM-IV disorders in the National Comorbidity Survey Replication adolescent supplement. Arch Gen Psychiatry. 2012;69:372–80.
59. Nock MK, Green JG, Hwang I, McLaughlin KA, Sampson NA, et al. Prevalence, correlates, and treatment of lifetime suicidal behavior among adolescents. JAMA Psychiat. 2013;70:300–10.
60. Bailey JM, et al. Heritable factors influence sexual orientation in women. Arch Gen Psychiatry. 1993;50:217–23.
61. Austin SB, et al. Sexual orientation and diurnal cortisol patterns in a cohort of U.S. young adults. Psychoneuroendocrinology. 2016;69:197–208.
62. Juster RP, Lupien SJ. Chronic stress and allostatic load. In: Handbook of clinical gender medicine. Basel: Karger AG; 2012. p. 70–81.
63. Juster RP, et al. Sexual orientation modulates endocrine stress reactivity. Biol Psychiatry. 2015;77(7):668–76.
64. Parra AP, Hastings PD. Integrating the neurobiology of minority stress with an intersectionality framework for LGBTQ-latinx populations. New Dir Child Adolesc Dev. 2018;161:91–108.
65. Masten A. Global perspectives on resilience in children and youth. Child Dev. 2014;85(1):6–20.
66. Asakura K. Extraordinary acts to "show up": conceptualizing resilience of LGBTQ youth. Youth Soc. 2019;51(2):268–85.
67. Singh AA. Transgender youth of color and resilience: negotiating oppression and finding support. Sex Roles. 2012;68:690–702.
68. Craig S, et al. Media: a catalyst for resilience in lesbian, gay, bisexual, transgender, and queer youth. J LGBT Youth. 2015;12(3):254–75. https://doi.org/10.1080/19361653.2015.1040193.
69. Ryan C, et al. Parent-initiated sexual orientation change efforts with LGBT adolescents: implications for young adult mental health and adjustment. J Homosex. 2020;67(2):159–73.
70. Mallory C, Brown T, Conron KJ. Conversion therapy and LGBT youth. The Williams Institute, UCLA School of Law. January 2018. https://williamsinstitute.law.ucla.edu/wp-content/uploads/Conversion-Therapy-LGBT-Youth-Jan-2018.pdf.
71. Deschamps D, Singer B. LGBTQ STATS. New York: The New Press; 2017.
72. Greeno EJ, Lee BR, Tuten M, et al. Prevalence of substance use, housing instability, and self-perceived preparation for independence among current and former foster youth. Child Adolesc Soc Work J. 2019;36:409–18.
73. Martin-Storey A. Gender, sexuality, and gender nonconformity: understanding variation in functioning. Child Dev Perspect. 2016;10(4):257–62.
74. Kosciw JG, et al. Reflecting resiliency: openness about sexual orientation and/or gender identity and its relationship to well-being and educational outcomes for LGBT students. Am J Community Psychol. 2015;55:167–78.
75. Kosciw JG, et al. Promising strategies for prevention of the bullying of lesbian, gay, bisexual, and transgender youth. Prev Res. 2012;19(3):10+.
76. Russell ST, Toomey RB, Ryan C, Diaz RM. Being out at school: the implications for school victimization and young adult adjustment. Am J Orthopsychiatry. 2014;84:635–43.
77. Elze D. LGBT youth and their families. In: Mallon GP, Hess PM, editors. Child welfare for the twenty-first century: a handbook of practices, policies, and programs. New York: Columbia University Press; 2014. p. 158–78.
78. Institute of Medicine and National Research Council, 2013.
79. Gallegos A, et al. Exploring the experiences of LGBTQ adolescents in foster care. J Social Work. 2011;14:226–36.
80. Shpiegel S, et al. Functional outcomes among sexual minority youth emancipating from the child welfare system. Child Youth Serv Rev. 2016;61:101–8.
81. Holman GH. Theoretical extensions of minority stress theory for sexual minority individuals in the workplace: a cross-contextual understanding of minority stress processes. J Fam Theory Rev. 2018;10:165–80.
82. Dank M, et al. Locked in: interactions with the criminal justice and child welfare systems for LGBTQ youth, YMSM, and YWSW who engage in survival sex. College of William & Mary Law School, William & Mary Law School Scholarship Repository. 2015.
83. Sue DW. Microaggressions in everyday life: race, gender, and sexual orientation. Hoboken: Wiley; 2010.
84. Embrick DG, Walther CS, Wickens CM. Working class masculinity: keeping gay men and lesbians out of the workplace. Sex Roles. 2007;56:757–66.
85. Herek G. Confronting sexual stigma and prejudice: theory and practice. J Soc Issues. 2009;63(4):905–25.
86. Badgett MVL, Lau H, Sears B, Ho D. Bias in the workplace: consistent evidence of sexual orientation and gender identity discrimination. Williams Institute of UCLA. 2007.
87. Consortium of higher education LGBT resource professionals [the Consortium], 2017.
88. Marine SB, Nicolazzo Z. Names that matter: exploring the tensions of campus LGBTQ centers and trans* inclusion. J Divers High Educ. 2014;7(4):265–81.
89. Still Hungry and Homeless in College, Hope Lab, U-W, 2018.

90. University of Chicago, Chapin Hall Survey.
91. Gallager RP. National Survey of Counseling Center Directors, 2010. Available at www.collegecounseling.org/pdf/2010_survey.pdf.
92. Eisenberg D, Hunt J, Speer N, et al. Mental health service utilization among college students in the United States. J Nerv Ment Dis. 2011;199:301–8.
93. National Alliance on Mental Illness. College students speak: a survey report on mental health. Available at www.nami.org/collegesurvey.
94. Dahl AL, et al. LGBTQ adolescents and young adults raised within a Christian religious context: Positive and negative outcomes. J Adolesc. 2012;35(6):1611–8.
95. D'Augelli AR. Developmental and contextual factors and mental health among lesbian, gay and bisexual youths. In: Omoto AM, Kurtzman HS, editors. Sexual orientation and mental health: examining identity and development in lesbian, gay and bisexual people. Washington, DC: American Psychological Association; 2006. p. 37–53.
96. Statistical Abstract of the United States, 2011.
97. Rosario M, Yali AM, Hunter J, Gwadz MV. Religion and health among lesbian, gay and bisexual youths: an empirical investigation and theoretical explanation. In: Omoto AM, Kurtzman HS, editors. Sexual orientation and mental health: examining identity and development in lesbian, gay and bisexual people. Washington, DC: American Psychological Association; 2006. p. 117–40.
98. Rostosky SS, Danner F, Riggle ED. Religiosity as a protective factor against heavy episodic drinking in heterosexual, bisexual, gay and lesbian young adults. J Homosex. 2010;57:1039–50.

Resources

Resources for LGBTQ youth from the Harvey Milk School at the Hetrick Martin Institute. www.hmi.org

Gay Straight Alliance Network, provides information for youth activism. www.gsanetwork.org

Parents, Friends, and Families of Lesbians and Gays, support organization. www.pflag.org

Gay, Lesbian and Straight Education Network, supports school climate. www.glsen.org

Lesbian and Gay Child and Adolescent Psychiatric Association, includes extensive list of resources for adolescents, parents, and providers. www.lagcapa.org

Association for Gay and Lesbian Psychiatrists, information for patients and providers. www.aglp.org

Child Welfare League of America, information for LGBT youth in foster care or juvenile justice. www.cwla.org

Gay Lesbian Medical Association, resources for patients, families, and providers. www.glma.org

World Professional Association for Transgender Health, information and advocacy resource. www.wpath.org

GLBT National Youth Talkline 1-800-246-PRIDE (7743) (serving youth through age 25).

Video and social media messages of hope for LGBT youth. www.itgetsbetter.org

Information related to bullying of LGBT youth. www.stopbullying.gov/at-risk/groups/lgbt/

LGBTQ laws and protections by state. http://www.lgbtmap.org/equality-maps/conversion_therapy

Fenway Health, health center with focus on LGBT care, research, education, and advocacy. http://fenwayhealth.org/the-fenway-institute/

The Trevor Project, trevorproject.org

Diversity and Culture

21

Sarah H. Arshad, Jaclyn Datar Chua,
Lauren P. Baker, and Cheryl S. Al-Mateen

Key Points

- The population of the United States is becoming more diverse.
- Healthcare disparities and poorer mental health outcomes are disproportionately faced by minorities and people from lower socioeconomic backgrounds.
- There continues to be stigma against seeking evaluation or treatment for mental healthcare.
- Understanding patients' cultural identities and backgrounds is paramount to conducting mental health evaluations and treating patients and families. Many transitional age youth continue to rely on their families for support.
- As children transition to adulthood, they are more likely to engage in abstract thinking and identity formation.
- Family and community influences may provide support and/or complications, which could contribute to either resilience or impairment in functioning. These may affect tasks otherwise expected of transitional age youth: gaining financial independence from parents, establishing longer-term relationships, and completing education requirements.
- Different cultural backgrounds can influence how well a youth is able to complete developmental tasks, how involved families expect to remain, and also provide different expectations for these youth.
- According to the Integrative Model of Racial Identity Development, people go through stages from conformity to integrative awareness, which are different for people of color than for White people.
- Intersectionality is a framework to consider how multiple identities interact. Patients should be conceptualized using

S. H. Arshad · J. D. Chua
The Children's Hospital of Philadelphia, Department of Child and Adolescent Psychiatry and Behavioral Sciences, Philadelphia, PA, USA
e-mail: arshads@chop.edu; chuaj1@chop.edu

L. P. Baker
Department of Psychiatry, Child and Adolescent Psychiatry, Virginia Treatment Center for Children, Virginia Commonwealth University Health System, Richmond, VA, USA
e-mail: lauren.p.baker@vcuhealth.org

C. S. Al-Mateen (✉)
Departments of Psychiatry and Pediatrics, Virginia Treatment Center for Children, Virginia Commonwealth University Health System, Richmond, VA, USA
e-mail: cheryl.al-mateen@vcuhealth.org

V. Chan, J. Derenne (eds.), *Transition-Age Youth Mental Health Care*,
https://doi.org/10.1007/978-3-030-62113-1_21

this intersectional framework. Providers must consider how patients' cultural backgrounds affect their symptom presentation in ways specific to the patient's intersectional identity and avoid generalizations.

- Providers should consider acculturation and acculturative stress, especially with immigrants and refugees.
- There have been studies demonstrating implicit and explicit bias in healthcare providers. Bias can also affect health seeking behavior.
- The *Diagnostic and Statistical Manual of Mental Disorders* (DSM-5) has an Outline for Cultural Formulation (OCF) and a Cultural Formulation Interview (CFI) which can help providers obtain important information to make a cultural formulation.

Introduction

The US population is becoming more diverse, and racial and ethnic minorities are soon to collectively become the majority. US Census data predicts that, by 2020, more than half of the children in the nation will be from "minority" racial or ethnic backgrounds and that, by 2044, more than half of the US population will be comprised of minorities. By 2060, almost one in five, or 19%, of the US population will be foreign born [1]. Currently, minority groups and those from lower socioeconomic backgrounds bear the brunt of healthcare disparities in this country, increasing their morbidity and mortality [2]. Specifically, racial and ethnic minorities receive lower-quality healthcare, even when access-related factors are controlled [3]. Social determinants, defined as "the conditions in which people are born, grow, live, work, and age" [4], further divide "certain population subgroups [who] are at higher risk of mental disorders because of greater exposure and vulnerability to unfavorable social, economic, and environmental circumstances" [5] (p. 09). These social determinants of health must be considered when attempting to improve overall health and include socioeconomic status, the stability of family and community systems, immigration, and protective factors such as religiosity and social supports [5]. These determinants are not fully reviewed in this chapter, as they warrant a larger body of work in and of themselves, but are incorporated in the situations of the patients from the sample cases.

In addition to disparities, there continues to be significant discrimination and stigma against mental health care [6]. To help combat disparities, an Institute of Medicine (IOM) report recommends that healthcare professionals receive training in cultural communication [7] given that clinical providers may have a significant role in reducing discrimination and stigma [6]. Additionally, the American College of Physicians' (ACP) 2003 position paper exhorts that all patients, regardless of their cultural identities, deserve equitable, high-quality healthcare and also calls for cultural awareness and sensitivity among providers, a reduction in bias, and training in cultural competency [8]. Studies have demonstrated explicit and implicit bias among providers when considering their patients' personalities as well as patients' abilities to comply with treatment [9].

A patient's cultural background is important in the developmental process of identity formation. Understanding its impact is also vital in their mental health evaluation, treatment planning, and recovery. Providers are charged to practice "cultural competence" [10], which has been defined as "a set of congruent behaviors, attitudes, and policies that come together in a system, agency, or among professionals and enables that system, agency, or those professionals to work effectively in cross-cultural situations" [11] (p. 4). When transitional age youth begin to define themselves by prioritizing their multiple cultural identities, which can create a sense of solidarity with particular groups [12], it becomes especially important for providers to identify and inquire about these associations.

Cultural competence has broadened over time to include the conceptualization of "cultural humility" which adds acknowledgment that culture is not static [13]. It posits that understanding culture requires "a critical consciousness" by considering medical, social, and historical context [14]. In addition, intersectionality theory discusses the interplay between cultural factors and systems and how they can influence beliefs about health and illness [2]. Tools to obtain and conceptualize this information include the Cultural Formulation Interview (CFI) and the Outline for Cultural Formulation (OCF), both found in DSM-5 [15]. This chapter presents these concepts related to culture through clinical case examples of several transitional age youth (TAY).

Cases

Case 1: Maaria, a 17-year-old young woman, currently a junior in high school, is referred by neurology for mental health consultation because she has had a worsening of chronic tension headaches now with migrainous features. She is from an Indian family (parents immigrated to the United States before she was born), and she has an older sister. The patient tells the mental health professional that her sister also "has issues" but that "no one talks about it." The parents are practicing Muslims (mom wears a hijab), but Maaria, who is not identifiably Muslim by her choice of clothing, privately says that she is "taking a break" from religion. She also says that she has experienced some bullying because her family is Muslim. The patient tells the mental health provider that she identifies as bisexual but would never discuss this with her parents. The patient endorses being "very depressed" with passive thoughts of death. When the patient's mother is interviewed, she describes herself as an "overbearing 'Desi' mom" and is most concerned about the patient's declining school performance.

Case 2: "Sam" (Samantha), a 17-year-old youth assigned female gender at birth presenting with depression, confides in the psychiatrist that he identifies as transgender male and that his family does not know. His depressive symptoms began about a year ago and have been getting progressively worse. He lives in a rural area, his father is employed as a construction worker, and his mother is a stay-at-home mom. The family's income intermittently dips below the poverty line, and they require public assistance to meet their basic needs. Sam is the eldest of four children (two brothers and one sister). Sam has been an above-average student, and his family was hoping he would go to college, which would make him the first in the family to achieve this. However, his dream is to pursue a music career full-time, without obtaining a higher education. His family belongs to a conservative Christian church, and he identifies as Christian but believes he would not be supported after his transition. Sam's family does know about his depression, and even though he thinks that medications and therapy would be helpful, the family shares that they will instead pray and turn to the church for help with Sam's depressive symptoms.

Case 3: "Lily" (Lilliana), a 22-year-old woman, presents to a therapist with symptoms of anhedonia, troubles with sleep, lower energy, and guilt. She has had transient periods of feeling sad in the past but has never sought treatment before. A college student majoring in accounting, she is in her final year of college with a 3.8 grade point average. It was a difficult decision for her to pursue higher education instead of working because she and her family are undocumented immigrants from Mexico. She was initially hopeful about being able to apply for citizenship, but this is no longer possible for her. She is persistently concerned about her family's real risk for deportation. She is also worried about her legal status impacting her ability to find a job after graduation. Moreover, she feels a responsibility to contribute to the family's finances. Her parents both work as day laborers, and she has three younger siblings, one of whom chose to work after high school completion to financially support the family. The younger two siblings are still in middle and high school, and they were born in the United States.

Case 4: Becca, a 20-year-old Caucasian woman from a middle-class family, presents to the emergency room with suicidal ideation. She identifies with her Jewish heritage and grew up going to her synagogue regularly and attending camp for Jewish youth over the summers. She is enrolled in the local community college while holding a part-time job doing clerical work at her synagogue. She lives at home with her family and has a supportive friend group. She confides that in the past 6 months, she formed a romantic relationship with a woman but does not want to tell her family. Her fear of rejection, not only by her family but also by her community and peers, has led to increasing symptoms of depression and eventual thoughts that she would rather be dead. Neither Becca, nor anyone in her family, has previously sought mental health treatment.

Case 5: William, a 17-year-old African American cisgender heterosexual male, presents to his family doctor due to anxiety and frequent panic attacks. He has been mostly shy his whole life, preferring to stay inside and play video games. He has experienced mild to moderate heterogeneous anxiety since childhood, where he worried about his academic performance and the safety of his parents. His cognitive ruminations and occasional "nervous stomach" mostly were managed with intermittent supportive therapy. His recent-onset panic attacks began 3 months ago when he was a passenger during a police stop when his mother had a broken headlight. He had his first panic attack while in the car and continues to have recurrent panic episodes triggered by sirens and occasional loud noises (like the doorbell). He had no prior interactions with any law enforcement, but some of his family members were killed by gun violence (not police). He has stopped driving because he is afraid of recurrent panic attacks. His immediate family's socioeconomic status is middle class. Some of his uncles have substance use disorders and have temporarily experienced homelessness.

Case 6: Alice, a 19-year-old woman and an only child who currently lives with her parents, is referred for a mental health evaluation due to frequent tearfulness. Her family immigrated from Korea before she was born. Alice had plans to attend a local college after she graduated high school, but in her senior year, she was diagnosed with leukemia. She had to take a year off to complete chemotherapy treatment, including two bone marrow transplants. She had to lose her ear piercings due to the infection risk. She no longer fits into her previous clothing due to side effects from her medications, which caused her to lose weight overall, including her steroid regimen which changed her body composition. She used to take pride in her appearance and had hopes of becoming a social media influencer as a makeup artist and fashion icon. She no longer feels inspired to do this. Due to her compromised immune state, for 100 days after her bone marrow transplants, she had to remain in relative isolation, which she describes as a very lonely time. Her friends were supportive, but most of them went to college, while she had to stay behind. Her family also accumulated significant financial bills from her treatment as well as caring for her during that time – her parents missed work, parked at the hospital, bought meals, etc. She currently feels "stuck" and purposeless. She wants to apply for a job as well as continue to pursue college, but Alice's parents feel very uncomfortable with her having responsibilities outside of the house. They do not want her to consider living in the residence halls while at college due to fears about her health as well as concerns about the financial costs. They would prefer that she live at home.

Case 7: Jerome is an 18-year-old senior in high school raised in an affluent African American family who presents for a follow-up appointment with his mental health provider. He has sickle cell disease, and after his first hospitalization for acute chest syndrome when he was 14 years old, he also developed an initial adjustment disorder followed by major depressive disorder. He and his family were on board with mental health treatment, and his depression has been previously managed with intermittent therapy and medications. His parents have been slightly more lax in their academic expectations of Jerome because of his numerous hospitalizations for sickle cell crises despite following medical advice to prevent these, especially in his senior year. Both of his parents have doctoral degrees and have high educational expectations for their children. Jerome is the youngest child, with an older brother and sister, both of whom attend Ivy League universities. After his recent birthday, Jerome told his parents he was not planning on attending college immediately but wanted to get involved in political grassroots organizations and social justice activities. His parents had not known he had already attended protests, or that there were a few times he had almost gotten hurt or arrested. They are very upset that he is not applying to college, and they also think he has been more irritable, angry, and depressed in the past year.

Case 8: Adenike is a 21-year-old woman with no past medical or psychiatric history who presents for possible first break of psychosis to the emergency room, and after a medical workup is normal, she is admitted to a psychiatric hospital. She is brought in by her Nigerian-born parents, who are currently going through a marital divorce. Her mom works in retail, and her dad works in the food service industry; both of their employers require strict attendance. This has made it very difficult for them to come to the hospital for daytime meetings with her primary treatment team. Her mom is very concerned that Adenike, who never used to be religious, has been praying more and has been conversing out loud to God. Her dad is adamant that, as a deeply faithful Christian, Adenike has always been devout. He thinks that these behaviors are within normal limits for her, the family, and their church. Adenike's dad believes prayer alone will help her to move forward. She is an only child, and the rest of their immediate family are in Nigeria. The family identifies a local Nigerian community as a source of support.

Case 9: Abraham is a 19-year-old Latinx cisgender man who presents for symptoms of feeling overwhelmed, difficulty getting out of bed, and intermittent stomachaches. His mom is from the Dominican Republic and his dad is from Puerto Rico. He is a middle child – his older brother received a football scholarship to attend college, and he had received some offers as well but opted to forego college. His two younger sisters are both still in middle and high school. He is working at a local electronics store while trying to teach himself graphic design. His parents are conservative Catholics, and while he enjoys some of the cultural traditions from his childhood, he does not believe in God. This has led to some discord between him and his family, and he just learned that his 18-year-old girlfriend is pregnant. He is not sure how he will tell his family, or how he will support his girlfriend and child.

Developmental Considerations for Culture in the Transitional Age

As children transition through adolescence to young adulthood, they undergo evolutions in their thought process. Piaget describes formal operations as the beginning of abstract thinking as teens reason through moral and philosophical issues and thought becomes more logical [16]. Erikson describes adolescence as a time of searching for personal identity by exploring different values with the rise of independence. Youth in this stage begin to consider the place they will take in the "real world," whether it involves continuing education or starting a career, or leaving their parents' home [17]. Additionally, growing into the transitional age, relationships become more intimate (Fig. 21.1).

Through these developmental stages, youth are also "charged" to take ownership over their identities, including gender, race, ethnicity, religion, and sexual orientation, among others. This marks a shift from identity being largely informed by their family and community to increasingly self-selected. However, family and community influences remain factors that may both support and complicate the formation of the TAY's unique identity. As highlighted in many of the sample cases, TAY may wrestle with conflicts between family's culture and their own as it begins to take shape. For example, Maaria, Sam, and Becca each come from different religious and ethnic backgrounds but have similar concerns about family or community acceptance of their gender or sexual identities. There are also concerns about conflict as a consequence of their emerging identities, which could impact other aspects of their lives, including finances and housing (e.g., Maaria lives with her parents; Becca works for her synagogue).

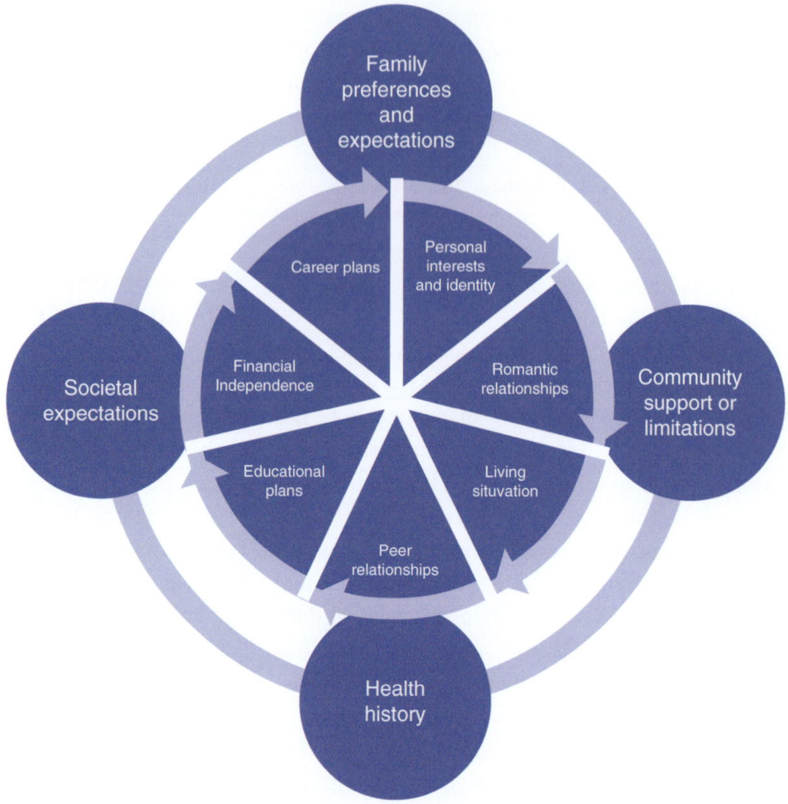

Fig. 21.1 Interplay of personal aspects of TAY individuation and cultural or other factors

While some conflict is part of normal development, significant conflict may impact optimal functioning. A positive sense of ethnic-racial identity is associated with fewer depressive symptoms; internalizing, externalizing, and antisocial behaviors; less substance abuse; and less risky sexual attitudes [18]. It should be similarly considered that having a positive sense of identity also lends itself to psychosocial benefits. Connection with self-identified culture, overall parenting style, and parent response to individuation can also impact mental wellbeing during this time of transition, as highlighted in Fig. 21.2 [19]. Conversely, divergence of ideals between TAY and their parents can negatively impact mental health. One study of migrant families found an increase in suicide rate among female immigrants ages 18–25 years compared to other age groups, with adolescents in this group who took overdoses holding less traditional cultural views than their parents [20].

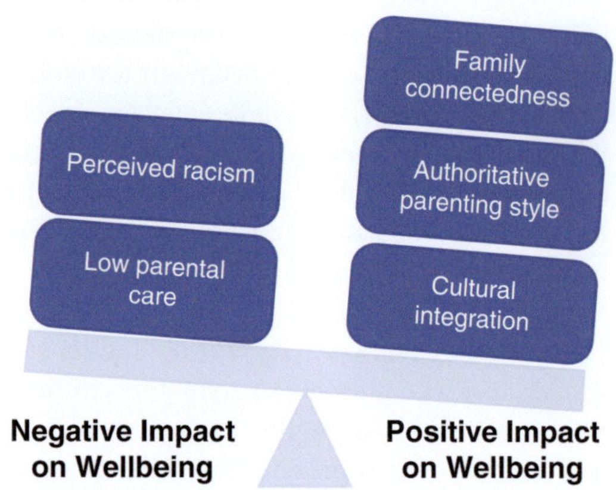

Fig. 21.2 Summary of factors influencing mental wellbeing [19]

A positive sense of identity can provide better grounding as the emerging adult navigates the world with a growing host of responsibilities. Developmental tasks for transitional age youth ages 18–25 years include developing self-identity, emotional and financial independence from parents, management of personal self-care, completion of educational requirements, and establishment of long-term relationships. This may be overwhelming for some TAY, particularly those with known psychiatric disorders [21]. From the cases above, Alice struggles with navigating independence from her family, and Becca is worried about complete financial independence. TAY must navigate whether to pursue higher education, vocational training, getting a job, or a combination thereof. In the case examples, Lily struggles with guilt over having chosen higher education instead of economic employment. Sam and Jerome, who are from very different backgrounds, both struggle with the parental expectation of higher education when they both would like to pursue other ambitions. Abraham is also struggling with establishing financial independence for himself, as well as for his pregnant girlfriend.

In addition, each TAY continues to pursue relationships, intimate and platonic, navigating these over the course of their otherwise changing lives and responsibilities. It is more difficult to predict demographic information (i.e., employment, student, relationship or health insurance status) within this group than in adolescents under 18 years or adults over 25 years. This highlights the great range of opportunities during this developmental stage with high levels of exploration and experimentation and particularly low constraints [22]. De Goede et al. [23] note that "the transition to a vocational career and entering into a satisfying intimate relationship are two important developmental tasks in the lives of youngsters" (p. 15) which are important for their mental health. Strides toward establishment of vocational and relational identity correlate with improved mental wellbeing.

Opportunities during this phase of life are broad and varied but may be restricted by cultural constructs. Cultural background and expectations can either bolster or limit a youth's perceived options [22]. Perceived discrimination, weak ethnic identity, low self-esteem, and increased conflict with family have all been associated with increased psychiatric symptoms and disorders [24]. There may also be different cultural pressures on TAY in different areas of their growing independence (e.g., pressure to pursue higher education over contributing to the family finances, to live independently or within families, to find romantic partners and pursue serious intimate relationships). From the case examples, Lily worries about contributing financially to her family although she is doing well in her last year of college, while Jerome's parents wish he would apply to college when he prefers to focus on social justice efforts. Abraham chooses to work and independently train himself in graphic design over attending college, and he will likely have increasing financial burdens coming soon with his expected child. Alice wants to work or attend school but is discouraged by her parents due to her recent medical problems. Maaria's mom seems to downplay her depression symptoms and focuses instead on her school performance.

Depending on their specific identities and circumstances, this period can be more complex for transitional age youth. Individuals may go through additional developmental processes based on their personal history, identity, and cultural background. Models have been generated to demonstrate the phases of identity formation and acceptance for several such populations including racial or ethnic minorities, individuals with migration histories, gay/lesbian/bisexual individuals, and White/dominant cultural members [25]. For example, Fig. 21.3 highlights the developmental stages of LGB sexuality as described by Garnets and D'Augelli [26]. These developmental tasks are not necessarily completed at specific

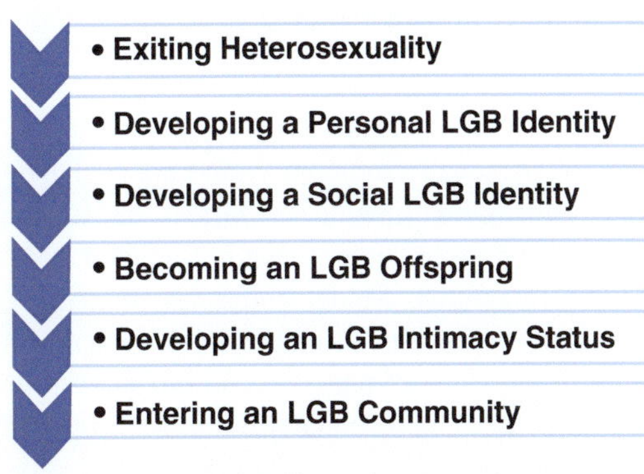

Fig. 21.3 Developmental stages in LGB identity formation [26]

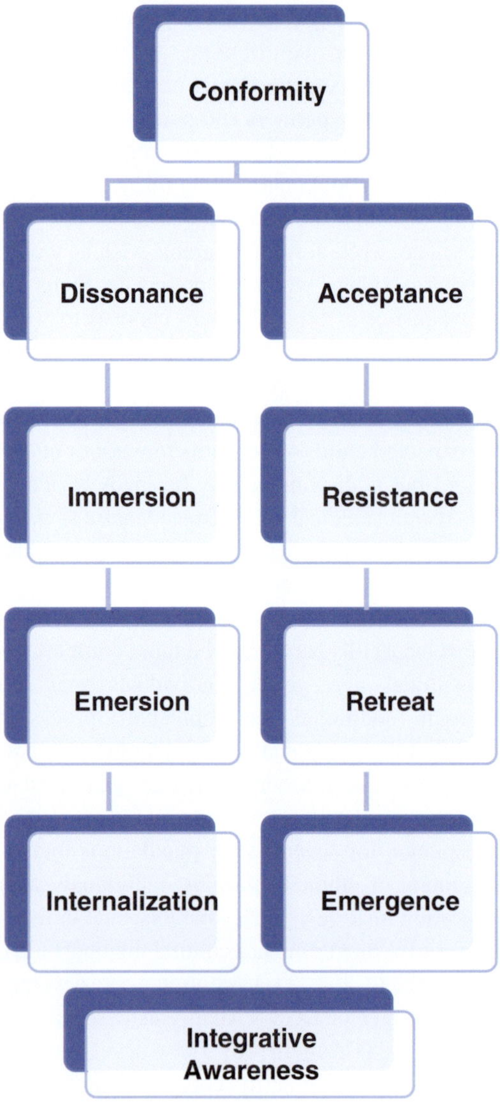

Fig. 21.4 Integrative Model of Racial Identity Development. (Adapted from [34])

stages of life, but occur over time with the influence of personal, community, and societal factors. Hoffman's Integrative Model of Racial Identity Development is shown in Fig. 21.4.

The Integrative Model combines models of identity development in undervalued (people of color in the United States) and dominant (White people in the United States) cultural groups. It represents an integration of many models proposed for specific groups by others including Black Racial Identity Models by both Cross [27] and Helms [28, 29], the White Racial Identity Model by Helms [29, 30], and the Filipino American Identity Development by Nadal [31, 32]. Acculturation [33] and multiracial [32] models are also included.

In the Integrative Model, everyone begins in "conformity" where conscious awareness of one's own race is minimal, and the dominant culture is held as a positive standard. At the next stage, people of color and White people diverge to "dissonance" and "acceptance," respectively, and they remain divergent for the next four stages. In "dissonance," confusion between having upheld dominant cultural norms and a new recognition of the disparities of opportunity emerges. Also, the discovery of racism or acceptance of other biases as reality is at the heart of the dissonance stage. This stage is typically precipitated by a significant event, such as a personal or national trauma. In contrast, acceptance for White people involves some recognition of disparities as "universal struggles" such as "we can't all get the job" or "they must not have been a good enough student to get into that school." These "struggles" are dismissible under the guise of universality or being "the way the world works" and potentially applicable to any person regardless of race (or other minority status). For people of color, "dissonance" is followed by "immersion" – where the disillusionment of "dissonance" leads to anger and frustration that the dominant culture has created and perpetuates the problem. This flows into the next stage, "emersion," where individuals of the underrepresented cultural group affiliate with their own group to avoid the other problematic group. In this model, the parallel two steps for the dominant group are "resistance" and "retreat." Resistance occurs where disparities such as racism are acknowledged as a thing of the past and "reverse racism" against the dominant culture may be touted as the current climate. Reverse racism occurs when a White or majority group person assumes that their own opportunities are limited by systemic or societal responses to racism, for example, the claim that being an ethnic minority makes it "easier" to be accepted to jobs or academic programs and therefore makes it harder for White or majority people to get those coveted positions. "Retreat" begins with realization of the falsehoods of reverse racism beliefs and then moves into feelings of guilt or shame about ongoing disparities for the underrepresented culture. In "retreat," White people can be frustrated toward their own culture for not yet understanding its role in maintaining disparities. The underrepresented group moves out of "emersion" and goes on to "internalization" where their own group's negative qualities come into recognition. The "problem" shifts away from the whole dominant group to the inequalities themselves. In this stage, psychic space opens up to allow more expression of individual identity, for example, recognizing an intersectional identity that is more than race alone.

Coined in 1989, the term "intersectionality" was first used to describe women of color and how their identities both as women and people of color together handicapped them from prominence in both the feminist and civil rights movements [35] and has subsequently grown to encompass the interplay of different identities within one individual. "Intersectionality is a theoretical framework for understanding how multiple social identities such as race, gender, sexual orientation, SES, and disability intersect at the micro level of individual experience to reflect interlocking systems of privilege and oppression (i.e., racism, sexism, heterosexism, classism) at the macro social-structural level" [36] (p. 1267).

The individual within dominant culture makes similar intersectional identity gains in the stage of "emergence" following retreat. They grow to understand the impact of dominant culture privilege in their life and recognize that there is choice in what type of person they want to be within this frame. Hoffman's Integrative Model ends with "integrative awareness" for both groups, where the individual is able to positively identify with their own racial group along with other aspects of their unique identity [34].

TAY may be operating at any stage within this model. Understanding their place within it could be very helpful in conceptualizing their presentation and planning their care [29]. From the case examples, several of the individuals and their families are at different stages of racial identity development. Maaria is "taking a break from religion" and may be in the beginning stage of conformity, where she identifies more with the dominant or majority culture than her family's stated religion. Could William's panic attacks be related to the dissonance stage of racial identity development, where he is realizing that his mother was pulled over for something a White driver might not have been? For Jerome, there is not enough information from the case vignette alone to determine with confidence which stage he is in. His interest in protesting could be fueled by anger at the disparities he sees, and it sounds likely as his parents report he has been irritable and unhappy. This is consistent with the immersion stage. However, with more information from him, we might learn that he has recognized racial disparities but also sees positive and negative features of both his own racial group and the majority group which is more consistent with the stage of internalization. It is also important to understand his parents' stage in this developmental process in order to identify and address tensions in the family related to discrepant stages of racial identity development.

Delayed Adulthood

Family and community cultural values affect youth's journey of identity formation, and TAY's individual identities can both help and hinder them in facing the social and cultural challenges of this developmental period. Some of society's goals and pressures on transitional age youth may differ from past generations. Unfortunately, there are disparities in future trajectories for minority or immigrant TAY experiencing acculturative stress and discrimination. Black and Latinx young adults are less likely than Asian and non-Latinx White peers to be enrolled in post-secondary education, and Black and Latino men are more likely to be incarcerated. The same groups are more likely to start "family building behaviors" such as cohabiting, parenting, and marrying before age 25 years than their peers in other ethnic groups [18]. Although it is an intergenerational gain to obtain higher education degrees, TAY postponing gainful employment have more financial debt [37]. According to Rumbaut [38], up to 60.7% of the second generation of 18- to 24-year-olds remain at home with their parents but have the overall highest educational attainment with up to 34.6% having received a bachelor's degree or higher.

Surveyed ethnic minorities expressed a desire of opportunity for upward social mobility which was influenced by their parents' often low-status work [19]. However, each individual's unique trajectory should be considered rather than making assumptions based on a demographic.

Many TAY are relying more heavily on their parents while they transition from adolescence to adulthood, by living at home, asking for financial support, or by staying on their family's health insurance plan. Although the passage of the Patient Protection and Affordable Care Act has helped increase healthcare coverage, young adults in the foster care system and unauthorized immigrants are two groups which continue to struggle to obtain reasonably priced high-quality healthcare [37]. TAY are historically the least insured of any age group, which is complicated by "aging out" of pediatric health service systems and therefore threatening continuity of care [37]. Continuing to reside in the family home during early adulthood can help with finances and can foster an ongoing connection to family at this potentially difficult time [19].

Both external support and a positive sense of personal identity increase success in navigating this period of intense growth toward achieving independence. Demographic transitions are difficult to predict and have a low impact on achieving "adulthood." Rather, accepting responsibility for one's self and making independent decisions are the most necessary steps for transitioning to adulthood [22]. Moreover, it is important to remember that different sociocultural variables set the expectations of what is expected for these youth: both in the society in which they currently live and in the heritage with which they may choose to identify [22]. Overall, youth will continue to navigate their identities as they are transitioning to adulthood. Concepts of race, gender, privilege, and other societal constructs become increasingly salient during this phase of life. Specific aspects of identity may change over this period as they contemplate what is more and less important to them.

Modern Society and Future Considerations

Current Political/Social/Cultural Perspective

The diversity of the population of the United States is estimated to continue to grow, with different ethnic and racial minority groups, multiracial groups, internationally adopted children, and immigrants [39]. There continue to be thousands of people (nearly 85,000 in 2016) with refugee status who resettle in the United States, the majority of them from Somalia, the Democratic Republic of the Congo, Burma, Syria, and Iraq [40]. This will lead to an increase in multiple languages spoken within the country and more diverse children living in settings such as foster care, migrant families, and homelessness [39].

With such a diverse population, one must consider acculturation, which is defined as "the process of social and psychological exchanges that take place when there are ongoing encounters between individuals of different cultures, with subsequent changes in either or both groups" [41] (p. 149). Indeed, Berry [42] described it as a "bidirectional and bidimensional process" which affects a person's identity within an "open/inclusive or closed/exclusive" society as well as the smaller groups within that society [43] (p. 38). When determining factors which impact a cultural identity, there have been four strategies proposed which include integration, assimilation, separation, and marginalization. Those who maintain the culture of origin while also becoming part of the new culture are believed to have employed the integration strategy. While assimilation suggests a loss of the original culture, separation prioritizes close ties to the culture of origin, and neither the new nor the former culture provides support for marginalized individuals [44].

Refugees, in addition, face logistical barriers when accessing both preventative and specialty care such as language, finances, resource availability, and stigma [40]. For this population, psychological distress can be a result of trauma involving their pre-migration experiences [3]. There is also a fear among some nonimmigrants that immigrants, refugees, and others who hold onto non-US culture and values will water down what they consider to be American-held values and/or beliefs [44]. According to Perez and Fortuna [45], undocumented immigrants endure more socioeconomic stressors as well as fear of deportation which result in greater risk for mental illness including substance use disorders and depression. In the case examples, this fear inevitably affects Lily and her family. Immigrants could be at higher risk of traumatic disorders but also less likely to seek help based on previous experiences with healthcare and uncertain immigration status [46]. Lily's family may be less likely to seek care than documented immigrants or citizens, and may be more guarded with providers, given their real concerns about deportation.

Providers should also, then, consider the potential acculturative stress on individuals, especially for TAY whose families hold tightly to a home culture, as well as how they value different elements of their identity. Specific issues these populations can face include "financial stressors and poverty, language barriers and communication difficulties, lack of access to healthcare, unsafe neighborhoods, poor housing, unemployment, underemployment, exploitation, and dangerous working conditions" [44] (p. 96). This is compounded by TAY's "heightened risk for excess emotionality, reward seeking, and poor judgment" [47] (p. 887). For example, Lily in case 3 must consider how well she fits into American culture, not only for her own identity but also for her sense of belonging, which is complicated by the added stresses of her and her family's legal status. This is a possible explanation for her nickname of "Lily," as opposed to her longer name "Lilliana." Meanwhile, Abraham in case 9 is more free to choose which parts of his Latinx, US, or Western experiences speak to him more. Alice, from case 6, has to consider her ties to her family's culture, in comparison to their desire to fit in with US culture, which is evident in her very name. Even Maaria in case 1 has to consider her name, and whether to emphasize its South Asian pronunciation or a more Western-acceptable form.

Explicit and Implicit Biases

In thinking about diversity, especially when there are externally visible distinguishing factors such as skin color, clothing or other religious identification, language proficiency and accent, and body shape and size, we must consider bias. In regard to explicit bias, there have been studies in which physicians provided lower ratings on factors including intelligence and likelihood to adhere to medical advice for African American patients and those from lower socioeconomic backgrounds compared with Caucasian Americans and patients from higher socioeconomic backgrounds [9]. There has also been negative bias against African Americans and working-class patients documented among mental healthcare professionals. When an experiment left voicemails for therapists seeking appointments, fewer working-class individuals were given appointments compared to middle-class individuals, and among the middle class, Blacks were less likely than Whites to be offered appointments [9]. Many of the patients described in the case examples have backgrounds with historical or current bias against their identified groups to highlight these considerations. In addition, attention must also be given to microaggressions, "broadly defined as behaviors that ambiguously disempower racial minorities," including microassaults, microinsults, and microinvalidations [48]. People subject to microaggressions are more likely to report mental health concerns, and microaggressions themselves can create barriers to healthcare including implicit discrimination or insensitive interactions [48].

Taking measures of implicit bias into consideration can be illuminating when addressing topics which are politically, culturally, or socially sensitive. This can include discussions on race, gender, religion, and obesity. Implicit bias involves associations and attitudes that may influence judgment and behavior which are outside an individual's conscious awareness and/or intention [49]. With regard to biases about social groups, in-group bias designates favoritism toward ones' own social group, whereas out-group bias is a negative bias toward individuals from another social group [50]. Using free, online tools such as the Implicit Association Test (IAT) can increase awareness of any biases which may exist by testing automatic associations between concepts [51].

In examining implicit associations among healthcare providers, Cooper, et al. studied associations between physician implicit bias toward Black and White people, in general, as well as physician implicit bias toward "generic" Black and White patients regarding their likely compliance with medical advice. Both measures demonstrated moderate pro-White bias [9]. Maina et al. [52] also discuss that although healthcare professionals of various training levels have implicit biases against "Black, Hispanic, American-Indian and dark-skinned individuals," Black people who are healthcare professionals are the least likely to have implicit bias when compared to other groups. There remains a lack of intervention studies with only one showing reduced implicit bias among healthcare professionals in post-intervention measures [52]. Furthermore, there is evidence that clinician bias can result in misdiagnosis of psychiatric illness in minority populations [53] and that certain minority groups (such as African American and Latinx) overall are less likely to receive accurate diagnoses [46].

Effects of Bias on Healthcare-Seeking Behaviors

According to the Institute of Medicine, disparity is defined as the lack of access to adequate healthcare or providers, communication difficulties, cultural barriers, and provider stereotyping all of which are "racial or ethnic differences in the quality of healthcare that are not due to access-related factors or clinical needs, preferences, and appropriateness of intervention" [8] (p. 3). This negatively impacts healthcare-seeking behavior in the United States as minorities experience a distrust of the healthcare system due to perceived racism [7]. In addition, the IOM reported that racial and ethnic non-minorities receive better-quality healthcare than their minority counterparts, despite controlling for access-related factors including insurance status. Having limited English proficiency (LEP) resulted in even lesser quality care [8]. Also, there are disparities in mental health outcomes for racial and ethnic minority children and adolescents, namely, that they "are at elevated risk of persistent mental disorders in adulthood," possibly due to risk factors that hinder improvement [5]. Alegria et al. posit four mechanisms: socioeconomic status (proportionately more Black and Latino children and adolescents live in poverty than Whites), childhood adversities (of which there are higher rates in people with mental disorders and they are more common in minority populations), family structure across development (there has been an increase in single-headed households in racial and ethnic minorities), and neighborhood-level factors (ethnic minorities are more likely to live in high-poverty areas with more segregation). These differences in social class, risk factors, family support, and social support could contribute to disparities [5].

TAY and Family Involvement

The parents of transitional age youth are still involved with and often advocate for their youth's medical and mental healthcare. Efforts should be made to not disempower parents or unnecessarily marginalize TAY roles. This transition is also a developmental stage for parents. Exploring the parents' individual backgrounds including where they were born and raised and how this affects the child's cultural identity is important [54]. These conversations require the TAY's permission and must be done in a way that makes the patient feel safe. Consider this in the case example of Lily, in which it would behoove a provider to make sure she fully understood the confidential nature of her relationship with a mental healthcare provider and reassure her of her and her family's safety within the encounter. Also consider the case example of Alice, whose desire for independence may make her less inclined to include family in her treatment. Awareness of parent/child differences can also help unmask intergenerational conflict caused by differing new and traditional values which Hovey [55] has identified as a specific acculturative stressor for Latinx children. Parental worries about behaviors such as sexual activity or drug use, which can be issues for all TAY, should be explored [56]. Going back to the case examples, Lily may try to avoid these discussions, and the clinician can explore her fears and provide realistic reassurance. Abraham and Becca may find that understanding their parents' perspective is helpful as they discuss current relationship and sexual identity issues with their families.

Incorporating family support systems when considering how to resolve conflicts is important. Kobus and Reyes [57] found that Mexican American adolescents identified speaking to their mothers as a useful coping skill. Familism, which is a common Latinx value, is defined as a "strong identification and attachment of individuals with their families (nuclear and extended) as well as strong feelings of loyalty, reciprocity and solidarity" [58] (p. 398). Families often choose to reside close to other family members allowing for increased engagement [59]. Similarly, collectivism allows one to form self-identity through being part of a community [60]. A loss of social support can be a particularly acute stressor for many TAY immigrants who may prioritize collectivism over individualism [55, 61–63].

In the case examples, Maaria, Sam, Becca, and Adenike all come from religious households, but not all of them identify with their family's chosen larger religious community, which may be further navigated and explored. In addition, Sam and Adenike have different backgrounds and clinical presentations, but members of both of their families express preference for prayer over standard mental healthcare – consider how a provider should engage families in conversations about evaluation and treatment. Religious involvement has been found to be protective for adolescent mental health by providing social support as well as a sense of meaning and coherence [19]. Regardless of affiliation, religious communities can provide wider family support within a group that shares norms and values. Religious involvement may reinforce more "authoritative" parenting in addition to bolstering resilience by teaching coping skills [19].

TAY with Disabilities

For youth who have disabilities, it is fundamentally important that they understand the impact of their disability on their identity. The International Classification of Functioning, Disability and Health (ICF) model states that disability is "a function of one's health, environment, and personal factors: a health condition may result in a disability through an impairment that affects one's body structure or function, an activity limitation that affects one's ability to execute a task or action, or a participation limitation that affects the individual's ability to be involved in a societal or life situation" [64] (p. 750). For Alice's and Jerome's case example situations, their medical illnesses have impacted their participation in some childhood and adolescent activities, and both struggle with wanting increased independence moving forward. In the case example of William, his anxiety and subsequent panic symptoms are affecting his ability to drive, thereby limiting his independence.

The impact of disability will likely evolve as youth transition to different work or settings where they experience a loss of services despite no change in their health condition. Socially, children with disabilities reported "social exclusion is more troublesome than the physical restrictions associated with their disability" [65] (p. 56). While experiencing discrimination negatively impacts life satisfaction, a sense of belonging has been found to be associated with improvements in a youth's life satisfaction [65]. Referring again to the case examples, Alice in particular, due to restrictions post-bone marrow transplant, is experiencing a sense of isolation from her peers, as well as feeling "stuck." When she compares herself with them, they have been able to move onto independence furthering tasks, such as secondary education and employment, whereas she feels left behind.

Cultural Formulation and Conceptualization

As the United States becomes more diverse – racially, religiously, linguistically – medical and mental health providers must consider cultural factors in diagnosis and treatment planning [53]. Specifically, they must consider how patients' cultural identities and backgrounds could affect symptom presentation and help seeking behavior [53], in addition to family understanding and involvement in treatment. Overall, providers should consider their own biases and seek to better understand that patients from different backgrounds may not present with classical symptom clusters.

The term culture "provides interpretive frameworks that shape the experience and expression of the symptoms, signs, and behaviors that are the criteria for diagnosis. Culture is transmitted, revised, and recreated within the family and other social systems and institutions" [15] (p. 14). It adds meaning to those beliefs and values within a specific social construct and can be used to create models of normative expectations [66]. These models can be used in healthcare, to help define what falls within the parameters of "healthy" and what deviates from it, and providers can then interpret cultural and social significance of symptoms and illness [53].

The *Diagnostic and Statistical Manual of Mental Disorders* (DSM-5) Outline for Cultural Formulation (OCF) was first published in 1994, helping patients create symptom and identity narratives for evaluation and treatment [67, 68]. While it was vital to begin considering patients using cultural information, there have been many changes since 1994. Specifically, the field of cultural competency education has evolved from a categorical approach (i.e., teaching facts about particular racial/ethnic groups) to the development of a framework and a set of skills [69], including ethnographic interviewing [70].

Previous approaches were less able to convey the heterogeneity of cultural groups (e.g., lumping "Asian patients" together despite there being >40 countries in Asia with very different histories, politics, languages, and culture). In the case examples, Maaria and Alice both come from "Asian" backgrounds but have inherited very different cultures and beliefs. Similarly, "Spanish speaking patients" were combined, despite there being almost 20 distinct countries in which Spanish is spoken as a primary language [71]. In addition, there are also intragroup differences, where there are some similarities, and also many cultural differences (e.g., Jewish individuals from different locales) [71]. Heterogeneity includes not only geographic, religious, dietary, and language diversity but also socioeconomic, historic, and educational diversity. In the case examples of Jerome and William, who are both African American young men, there are many differences in terms of their privilege and upbringing, which affect their identities and presentation. Similarly, Lily and Abraham are both Latinx, but their experiences are very different given their difference in citizenship status.

One concern is that broadly grouping (i.e., stereotyping) can lead to mistaken assumptions about certain cultural factors while possibly ignoring other unrelated practical issues (such as transportation and finances) in the ability or desire to seek care [68]. In addition, there is the possibility of incorrectly presuming that people who undergo similar experiences will be similarly affected; however, experiences must be considered from the specific individual's perspective. For example, certain natural disasters are traumatic for a wide net of individuals, but their effects can be felt disproportionately by people from lower socioeconomic backgrounds, due to their limited access to resources and supports, and often more dangerous environments; they might suffer more consequent symptoms [46].

Another concern is overgeneralizing based on certain cultural parameters. In the case example of Adenike, there are certainly cultural factors that make it harder for her parents and particularly her mom to understand her illness. However there are also practical difficulties, including her parent's work schedule such that they cannot visit the hospital in the daytime, when there are more healthcare providers to give explanations and space for discussion. Ideally, the clinician should have a curious inquisitiveness about the patient's cultures, backgrounds, and experiences. However, providers must also consider the agency that individuals have in choosing which identities carry personal significance. Modernization of technology and globalization have allowed for more far-reaching cultural influences [71]. Instead of assuming or assigning an identity onto a patient, the clinician must explore how youth and their families self-identify, considering the different cultural influences involved and paying attention to differences between youth and their caregivers [72]. With this inquisitiveness, the clinician gathers information that allows them to better understand the nuanced way cultural influences either build resilience or lead to symptoms and discord. In the case example, Maaria tells the provider that she's taking "a break" from religion. Alice is trying to downplay the medical identity she has been forced to take on, trying instead to be a more typical teenager. Becca and Sam both identify as religious, though they also hold fears about being rejected by their communities.

Additionally, individuals can prioritize or minimize multiple aspects of their cultural identities, "such as nationality, religion, income, age, education, sexual orientation and gender," of which these "interact and influence one another" and affect a person's subjective experiences [46]. Different individual identities should be considered from a more holistic, intersectional perspective.

An intersectional lens would posit considering how multiple identity experiences, including some longstanding patterns of discrimination which have created inequalities, impact an individual and interplay with each other in social institutions [73]. Culture is not static and is in fact very much affected by the sociopolitical climate, the economy, and narratives from religion, psychology, biology, etc. [68]. For example, from the case examples, Maaria, Sam, and Becca must all contend with their conservative religious families and communities as they explore their sexual orientation and gender identities. William's middle-class background, and having family members who have been killed by gun violence, affects him as an African American man in a different way as compared to Jerome, whose upper-middle-class upbringing has been somewhat protective for him. As Black men, they may both have similar fears of driving, but their other life experiences shape how the fear affects them, and how they are able to cope (or not) with those emotions.

The OCF pieced together medical anthropology and cultural psychiatry to outline a format for providers to discuss cultural experience across four domains [74]: cultural identity; the patient's understanding of symptoms and their etiology; patient expectations of treatment; and stressors and supports [75]. These four domains were updated in the DSM-5 [15]. The OCF was created with the goal of recognizing a variety of cultural factors that could be affecting a patient and encourages the provider to not only consider, but explicitly inquire, about them. It also encourages providers to consider similarities and differences between children and adolescents and their caregivers and to consider transgenerational strengths and differences which could lead to tension [71].

However, there have been problems in the OCF's implementation, including that it provides insufficient guidelines or can be ambiguous or repetitive. Lack of clinician buy-in has also limited its use [76]. For DSM-5, the Cultural

Formulation Interview (CFI) was developed to help clinicians gather the information needed to complete the OCF. The CFI has 16 stem questions to elicit information for the OCF and an additional 12 supplementary modules as tools to help providers. As noted in the *DSM-5 Handbook on The Cultural Formulation Interview*, "The main goal of all the components of the Cultural Formulation Interview (i.e., the core CFI, the CFI-Informant version, and the supplementary modules) is to contextualize the problem that the patient presents in a complex multidimensional way -- within the context of the person's sociocultural world, sense of identity, and ways of experiencing and understanding psychological distress. This ecological examination of the patient helps the clinician to select the appropriate treatment approach in collaboration with the patient, to enhance the patient's engagement in care...improve the therapeutic bond, …promote positive expectancy, and to accomplish other key treatment goals" [77] (p. 45).

Using a model, such as the CFI, to gather information can help a provider be more organized and thorough in assessing different cultural factors that may be relevant to a patient's care. This is especially true if the provider and patient are from different backgrounds. Even with shared cultural backgrounds, however, there can be obvious or subtle differences in experience and beliefs which could be clarified by a systematic method as groups can be heterogeneous [53]. After obtaining information guided by the CFI, the provider can conceptualize the patient on a variety of cultural parameters in a more nuanced way [71] to better understand their patient's intersectional identities, which can then help with the overall psychosocial formulation. This information can then be used in conjunction with a variety of psychiatric conceptual models to better understand a young adult's symptom expression, with the hope of forming a more accurate diagnosis to guide treatment.

Practical Guidelines and Tips

1. Utilize the tools that are available and familiarize yourself with the OCF and CFI.
2. Be aware of the normal range in appropriate development across age and cultural backgrounds, and ask patients about any issues that may impact developmental progress.
3. Encourage patients to share their expertise in their identity development, and empower them to develop their own goals and areas of concern. Ask about how youth self-identify and how supported they are in these identities. Acknowledge any struggles with these identities, and explore with the youth's family and/or friends how the different identities manifest. Incorporate general questions about the following issues into your regular histories, and explore specifics as the provider-patient relationship grows:
   (i) Gender and sexual identity
   (ii) Migration history and family migration history
   (iii) Relationship with own ethnic/cultural group
   (iv) Conflicts with familial/community identity vs. patient's individual identity
4. Encourage youth's understanding of independence including the balance between occupational goals and their post-secondary educational goals or career.
5. Strengthen youth's ability to navigate their medication regimen as well as restate physician recommendations in their own words.
6. Promote awareness of biases, and be attentive to any changes in behavior and/or communication with youth and families.

Conclusion/Summary

The population of the United States is becoming more diverse, and racial and ethnic minority groups, and those from lower socioeconomic backgrounds, bear the brunt of healthcare disparities. In addition, there are sociocultural factors delaying the transition from childhood to adulthood during this crucial time of transition, when youth explore their personal identities. In order to be more effective in symptom collection and treatment planning, mental healthcare providers must better understand identity formation. They can use guidelines such as the OCF or CFI to elicit information from patients to obtain a more complete understanding about why patients choose their specific cultural identifiers, whether those identities have affected their life experiences, and how they have interplayed with each other to help culturally conceptualize patients. Understanding these factors will allow them to provide more comprehensive care.

References

1. Colby SL, Ortman JM. Projections of the size and composition of the US population: 2014 to 2060. US Census Bur. Ed 2015;25–1143.
2. Milburn NG, Beatty L, Lopez SA. Understanding, unpacking, and eliminating health disparities: a prescription for health equity promotion through behavioral and psychological research—an introduction. Cultur Divers Ethnic Minor Psychol. 2019;25(1):1–5.
3. U.S. Department of Health and Human Services. Mental health: culture, race, and ethnicity—a supplement to mental health: a report of the surgeon general [Internet]. Rockville, MD: US Department of Health and Human Services, Substance Abuse and Mental Health Services Administration, Center for Mental Health Services; 2001 [cited 28 Jul 2019]. Available from: https://www-ncbi-nlm-nih-gov.proxy.library.vcu.edu/books/NBK44243/.
4. WHO Commission on Social Determinants of Health, World Health Organization. Closing the gap in a generation: health equity through action on the social determinants of health: commission on social determinants of health final report. Geneva, Switzerland: World Health Organization, Commission on Social Determinants of Health; 2008. 246 p
5. Alegría M, Green JG, McLaughlin KA, Loder S. Disparities in child and adolescent mental health and mental health services in the U.S. [Internet]. New York: A William T. Grant Foundation Inequality Paper; 2015 [cited 26 Dec 2019]. 26 p. Available from: https://wtgrantfoundation.org/library/uploads/2015/09/Disparities-in-Child-and-Adolescent-Mental-Health.pdf.
6. Illes RAC, Grace AJ, Niño JR, Ring JM. Culturally responsive integrated health care: key issues for medical education. Int J Psychiatry Med. 2015;50(1):92–103.
7. Smedley BD, Stith AY, Nelson AR, editors. Unequal Treatment: confronting racial and ethnic disparities in health care. Washington, D.C.: National Academies Press; 2003. p. 782.
8. Groman R, Ginsburg J. Racial and ethnic disparities in health care: a position paper of the american college of physicians. Ann Intern Med. 2004;141(3):226.
9. James SA. The strangest of all encounters: racial and ethnic discrimination in US health care. Cad Saúde Pública [Internet]. 2017 [cited 4 Jan 2020];33(suppl 1). Available from: http://www.scielo.br/scielo.php?script=sci_arttext&pid=S0102-311X2017001302001&lng=en&tlng=en.
10. Ambrose AJH, Lin SY, Chun MBJ. Cultural competency training requirements in graduate medical education. J Grad Med Educ. 2013;5(2):227–31.
11. Cross TL, Bazron BJ, Dennis KW, Isaacs MR. Towards a culturally competent system of care: a monograph on effective services for minority children who are severely emotionally disturbed. Washington, D.C.: Georgetown University Child Development Center; 1989. p. 90.
12. Schwartz SJ, Mason CA, Pantin H, Wang W, Hendricks Brown C, Campo AE, et al. Relationships of social context and identity to problem behavior among high-risk hispanic adolescents. Youth Soc. 2009;40(4):541–70.
13. Tervalon M, Murray-García J. Cultural humility versus cultural competence: a critical distinction in defining physician training outcomes in multicultural education. J Health Care Poor Underserved. 1998;9(2):117–25.
14. Kumagai AK, Lypson ML. Beyond cultural competence: critical consciousness, social justice, and multicultural education. Acad Med. 2009;84(6):782–7.
15. American Psychiatric Association. Diagnostic and statistical manual of mental disorders, DSM-5. fifth ed. Washington, D.C.: American Psychiatric Publishing; 2013.
16. Sadock B, Sadock VA, Ruiz P. Contributions of the psychosocial sciences. In: Kaplan and Sadock's synopsis of psychiatry: behavioral sciences/clinical psychiatry. 11th ed. Philadelphia: Wolters Kluwer; 2015. p. 93–130.
17. Sadock BJ, Sadock VA, Ruiz P. Theories of personality and psychopathology. In: Kaplan and Sadock's synopsis of psychiatry behavioral sciences/clinical psychiatry. 11th ed. Philadelphia: Wolters Kluwer; 2015. p. 151–91.
18. Rivas-Drake D, Stein GL. Multicultural developmental experiences. Child Adolesc Psychiatr Clin N Am. 2017;26(2):271–81.
19. Harding S, Read UM, Molaodi OR, Cassidy A, Maynard MJ, Lenguerrand E, et al. The determinants of young adult social well-being and Health (DASH) study: diversity, psychosocial determinants and health. Soc Psychiatry Psychiatr Epidemiol. 2015;50(8):1173–88.
20. Bhugra D, Gupta S, Bhui K, Craig T, Dogra N, Ingleby JD, et al. WPA guidance on mental health and mental health care in migrants. World Psychiatry. 2011;10(1):2–10.
21. Hoffman LJ, Guerry JD, Albano AM. Curr Psychiatry Rep [Internet]. 2018;20(4):Launching anxious young adults: a specialized cognitive-behavioral intervention for transitional aged youth. [cited 15 Jul 2019]. Available from: http://link.springer.com/10.1007/s11920-018-0888-9.
22. Arnett JJ. Emerging adulthood: a theory of development from the late teens through the twenties. Am Psychol. 2000;55(5):469–80.

23. de Goede M, Spruijt E, Iedema J, Meeus W. How do vocational and relationship stressors and identity formation affect adolescent mental health? J Adolesc Health. 1999 Jul;25(1):14–20.
24. Adriaanse M, Doreleijers T, van Domburgh L, Veling W. Factors associated with psychiatric symptoms and psychiatric disorders in ethnic minority youth. Eur Child Adolesc Psychiatry. 2016;25(10):1067–79.
25. Sue DW. Multidimensional facets of cultural competence. Couns Psychol. 2001;29(6):790–821.
26. Garnets LD, D'Augelli AR. Empowering lesbian and gay communities: a call for collaboration with community psychology. Am J Community Psychol. 1994;22(4):447–70.
27. Cross WE. Black families and black identity development: rediscovering the distinction between self-esteem and reference group orientation. J Comp Fam Stud. 1981;12(1):19–49.
28. Helms JE. An overview of black racial identity theory. In: Black and white racial identity: theory, research and practice. Westport, CT: Greenwood; 1990. p. 9–32.
29. Helms JE. An update of Helms's white and people of color racial identity models. In: The Handbook of multicultural counseling. Thousand Oaks, CA: Sage Publications; 1995. p. 181–98.
30. Helms JE. A race is a nice thing to have. Topeka KS: Content Communications; 1992.
31. Nadal KL. Racial and ethnic identity development for Filipino Americans. In: Filipino American psychology: a handbook of theory, research, and clinical practice [Internet]. Hoboken, NJ: John Wiley & Sons, Inc; 2011. p. 63–87. [cited 4 Jan 2020]. Available from: http://doi.wiley.com/10.1002/9781118094747.ch3.
32. Poston WSC. The biracial identity development model: a needed addition. J Couns Dev. 1990;69(2):152–5.
33. Berry JW. Immigration, acculturation and adaptation. Appl Psychol Int Rev. 1997;46(1):5–34.
34. Willsea J, Silva PC. Summary of stages of racial identity development [Internet]. Interaction Institute for Social Change; 2011. Available from: https://www.racialequitytools.org/resourcefiles/Compilation_of_Racial_Identity_Models_7_15_11.pdf.
35. Crenshaw K. Demarginalizing the intersection of race and sex: a black feminist critique of antidiscrimination doctrine, feminist theory, and antiracist politics. In: Bartlett KT, Kennedy R, editors. Feminist legal theory [Internet]. 1st ed: Routledge; 1989. p. 57–80. [cited 6 Jan 2020]. Available from: https://www.taylorfrancis.com/books/9780429969034/chapters/10.4324/9780429500480-5.
36. Bowleg L. The problem with the phrase *Women and Minorities:* intersectionality—an important theoretical framework for public health. Am J Public Health. 2012 Jul;102(7):1267–73.
37. Lui CK, Chung PJ, Wallace SP, Aneshensel CS. Social status attainment during the transition to adulthood. J Youth Adolesc. 2014 Jul;43(7):1134–50.
38. Rumbaut RG, Komaie G. Young adults in the United States: a mid-decade profile. SSRN Electron J [Internet]. 2007 [cited 17 Feb 2020]. Available from: http://www.ssrn.com/abstract=1887844.
39. Vaughn LM. Families and cultural competency: where are we? Fam Community Health. 2009;32(3):247–56.
40. Silberholz EA, Brodie N, Spector ND, Pattishall AE. Disparities in access to care in marginalized populations. Curr Opin Pediatr. 2017;29(6):718–27.
41. Redfield R, Linton R, Herskovits MJ. Memorandum for the study of acculturation. Am Anthropol. 1936;38(1):149–52.
42. Berry JW. Immigration, acculturation, and adaptation. Appl Psychol. 1997;46(1):5–34.
43. Al-Mateen CS, Rogers KM. Suicide among African-American and other African-origin youth. In: Suicide among diverse youth: a case-based guidebook. New York, NY: Springer Science+Business Media; 2017. p. 31–49.
44. Caplan S. Latinos, acculturation, and acculturative stress: a dimensional concept analysis. Policy Polit Nurs Pract. 2007;8(2):93–106.
45. Pérez MC, Fortuna L. Chapter 6. Psychosocial stressors, psychiatric diagnoses and utilization of mental health services among undocumented immigrant latinos. J Immigr Refug Serv. 2005;3(1–2):107–23.
46. Fortuna LR, Porche MV, Alegria M. A qualitative study of clinicians' use of the cultural formulation model in assessing posttraumatic stress disorder. Transcult Psychiatry. 2009;46(3):429–50.
47. Wilens TE, Rosenbaum JF. Transitional aged youth – a new frontier in child and adolescent psychiatry. Clinic Perspect. 2013;9(52):887–90.
48. Cruz D, Rodriguez Y, Mastropaolo C. Perceived microaggressions in health care: a measurement study. Zaller N, editor. PLoS One. 2019;14(2):e0211620.
49. Greenwald AG, Banaji MR. Implicit social cognition: attitudes, self-esteem, and stereotypes. Psychol Rev. 1995;102(1):4–27.
50. John-Henderson NA. Implicit Cognition. Child Adolesc Psychiatr Clin N Am. 2015;24(4):751–63.
51. Implicit Test. [Internet]. Available from: https://implicit.harvard.edu/implicit/takeatest.html.
52. Maina IW, Belton TD, Ginzberg S, Singh A, Johnson TJ. A decade of studying implicit racial/ethnic bias in healthcare providers using the implicit association test. Soc Sci Med. 2018;199:219–29.
53. Lewis-Fernández R, Díaz N. The cultural formulation: a method for assessing cultural factors affecting the clinical encounter. Psychiatry Q. 2002;73(4):271–95.
54. Rodriguez J, Umaña-Taylor A, Smith EP, Johnson DJ. Cultural processes in parenting and youth outcomes: examining a model of racial-ethnic socialization and identity in diverse populations. Cultur Divers Ethnic Minor Psychol. 2009;15(2):106–11.
55. Hovey JD. Psychosocial predictors of acculturative stress in mexican immigrants. J Psychol. 2000 Sep;134(5):490–502.
56. Dalla RL, Christensen A. Latino immigrants describe residence in rural midwestern meatpacking communities: a longitudinal assessment of social and economic change. Hisp J Behav Sci. 2005 Feb;27(1):23–42.

57. Kobus K, Reyes O. A Descriptive study of urban Mexican American adolescents' perceived stress and coping. Hisp J Behav Sci. 2000;22(2):163–78.
58. Sabogal F, Marín G, Otero-Sabogal R, Marín BV, Perez-Stable EJ. Hispanic familism and acculturation: what changes and what doesn't? Hisp J Behav Sci. 1987;9(4):397–412.
59. Cabassa LJ. Measuring acculturation: where we are and where we need to go. Hisp J Behav Sci. 2003 May;25(2):127–46.
60. Noh S, Kaspar V. Perceived discrimination and depression: moderating effects of coping, acculturation, and ethnic support. Am J Public Health. 2003 Feb;93(2):232–8.
61. Smart JF, Smart DW. Acculturative stress of hispanics: loss and challenge. J Couns Dev. 1995;73(4):390–6.
62. Sullivan MM, Rehm R. Mental health of undocumented Mexican immigrants: a review of the literature. Adv Nurs Sci. 2005;28(3):240–51.
63. Zuniga ME. Latino immigrants: patterns of survival. J Hum Behav Soc Environ. 2002;5(3–4):137–55.
64. Mann DR, Honeycutt T. Understanding the disability dynamics of youth: health condition and limitation changes for youth and their influence on longitudinal survey attrition. Demography. 2016;53(3):749–76.
65. Daley A, Phipps S, Branscombe NR. The social complexities of disability: discrimination, belonging and life satisfaction among Canadian youth. SSM Popul Health. 2018;5:55–63.
66. Arnault DS, Shimabukuro S. The clinical ethnographic interview: a user-friendly guide to the cultural formulation of distress and help seeking. Transcult Psychiatry. 2012;49(2):302–22.
67. American Psychiatric Association. Diagnostic and statistical manual of mental disorders – IV. 4th ed. Washington, D.C.: American Psychiatric Press, Inc.; 1994.
68. Kleinman A, Benson P. Anthropology in the clinic: the problem of cultural competency and how to fix it. PLoS Med. 2006;3(10):e294.
69. Mian AI, Al-Mateen CS, Cerda G. Training child and adolescent psychiatrists to be culturally competent. Child Adolesc Psychiatr Clin N Am. 2010;19(4):815–31.
70. Mezzich JE, Caracci G, Fabrega H, Kirmayer LJ. Cultural formulation guidelines. Transcult Psychiatry. 2009;46(3):383–405.
71. Aggarwal NK. Cultural formulations in child and adolescent psychiatry. Adolesc Psychiatry. 2010;49(4):4.
72. Rousseau C, Measham T, Bathiche-Suidan M. DSM IV, culture child psychiatry. J Can Acad Child Adolesc Psychiatry. 2008;17:69.
73. Eckstrand KL, Eliason J, St. Cloud T, Potter J. The priority of intersectionality in academic medicine. Acad Med. 2016;91(7):904–7.
74. Aggarwal NK. The psychiatric cultural formulation: translating medical anthropology into clinical practice. J Psychiatr Pract. 2012;18(2):73–85.
75. Lewis-Fernandez R. Editorial: the cultural formulation. Transcult Psychiatry. 2009;46(3):379–82.
76. Aggarwal NK, Nicasio AV, DeSilva R, Boiler M, Lewis-Fernández R. Barriers to implementing the DSM-5 cultural formulation interview: a qualitative study. Cult Med Psychiatry. 2013;37(3):505–33.
77. Hinton DE, Hinton L. Supplementary modules. In: Lewis-Fernandez R, Aggarwal NK, Hinton L, Hinton DE, Kirmayer LJ, editors. DSM-5 handbook on the cultural formulation interview. Washington, D.C.: American Psychiatric Publishing, Inc.; 2016. p. 45–67.

22 Supporting Connections: A Focus on the Mental Health Needs and Best Practices for Youth in Out-of-Home Care Transitioning to Adulthood

Wynne Morgan, Terry Lee, and Timothy Van Deusen

Key Points

- Youth transitioning out of the child welfare system to independence face numerous obstacles and challenges placing them at risk for poor outcomes.
- Understanding federal and state policies around transitional age youth in the child welfare system can help you as the provider advocated for appropriate services and supports to promote resilience.
- Examples of best practices for providers working with child welfare-involved young adults are outlined below.

W. Morgan (✉)
Department of Psychiatry, UMass Medical School, Worcester, MA, USA
e-mail: Wynne.Morgan@umassmemorial.org

T. Lee
Department of Clinical Services, Community Health Plan of Washington, Seattle, WA, USA
e-mail: DrTerry@uw.edu

T. Van Deusen
Department of Psychiatry, Yale University School of Medicine, New Haven, CT, USA
e-mail: Timothy.VanDeusen@yale.edu

Introduction

The transition to adulthood from adolescence is challenging for many young people but especially difficult for child welfare-involved youth. For all youth, this developmental period requires attainment of multiple developmental milestones in the areas of self-sufficiency as well as adjusting to new environments and responsibilities such as parenting, working, or continuing education [1]. In the United States, the transition from adolescence to young adulthood is an increasingly lengthy and complicated process with recent transitional age youth facing more challenges than previous generations [2]. Many transitional age youth benefit from emotional, pragmatic, and financial support from their parents and kin, but foster youth do not typically enjoy these types of family support [3]. Furthermore, many foster youth experience adverse events that increase risk for problematic emancipation, including neglect, abuse, trauma, disrupted attachments, unstable housing, multiple placements, fragmented schooling, disrupted social networks, poverty, and gestational exposures. These realities increase the risk that foster care alumni will experience negative functional outcomes, including lower education attainment, unemployment, poverty, homelessness, food insecurity, mental health and substance use chal-

V. Chan, J. Derenne (eds.), *Transition-Age Youth Mental Health Care*,
https://doi.org/10.1007/978-3-030-62113-1_22

lenges, health problems, early pregnancy and parenthood, and involvement with the justice system. The term "transitional age youth" originates from child welfare, following advocacy by stakeholders to provide developmentally appropriate services to support youth exiting foster care by "aging out" or meeting the legal age of adulthood and subsequently losing child welfare services [4]. With this focus on aging out youth, legislation, research, and grants have led to improvements to a system of care to meet the needs of this vulnerable population, but challenges continue.

Child Welfare System

The child welfare system emerged in the 1970s through advocacy from the pediatrics community following Dr. Henry Kempe's seminal article on child abuse, "The Battered Child Syndrome" [5]. Over the past 60 years, the child welfare system has evolved from a culture purely looking to ensure safety from abuse and neglect to one that considers the whole child. The federal 1997 Adoption and Safe Families Act outlined the three goals for the current national child welfare system: safety, permanency, and well-being. The term well-being assesses a child's development within four domains: cognitive functioning, physical health and development, emotional/behavioral functioning, and social functioning [6]. Permanency is a concept based on the value that youth grow up best in a family environment that is committed, long-lasting, nurturing, and stable. Permanency may be achieved by such pathways as reunification, adoption, or legal guardianship. Despite child welfare agencies' mandates and efforts to establish permanent homes for youth in foster care, some youth emancipate or "age out" from foster care when they turn 18 or 21 years old, or achieve a high school diploma. By definition, youth who age out of foster care did not achieve permanency [7].

Youth enter the child welfare system most often following concerns for child maltreatment. National data reporting of child maltreatment indicates that just under 700,000 youth are substantiated maltreatment victims each year, with a rate of 9.1 victims per 1000 children. The most common types of child maltreatment reported are neglect (74.9%) and physical abuse (18.3%), and youth may experience multiple types of abuse. In 2017, deaths from child maltreatment were estimated to be 1720 [8] (Fig. 22.1).

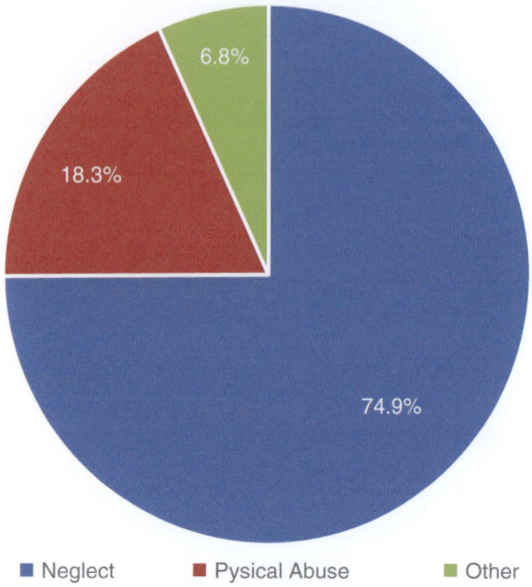

Fig. 22.1 Types of reported child maltreatment in the United States by percentage. (Adapted from US Department of Health and Human Services, Administration for Children and Families, Administration on Children, Youth, and Families, Children's Bureau. Child maltreatment 2017. https://www.acf.hss.gov/cb/research-data-technology/statistics-research/child-meltreatment 2019)

Nationally there are over 400,000 youth in foster care which is a 10% decrease over the last 10 years [9]. The average length of time for a youth in care is 19 months. Most youth are placed in a non-relative foster home (45% of youth), but efforts are made by agencies to place youth with relative foster families (32%). There is a national trend away from institutional care with just 13% of youth residing in congregate care (Fig. 22.2).

The most common path to exit out-of-home care is through reunification at 49%, with adoption as the second most common path at 24% [10]. Permanency becomes more difficult to achieve with older foster children, with rates of adoption decreasing in older adolescents to just 3% [11]. Most adolescents who are in the foster care entered as adolescents, and youth who enter the foster care system after 12 years of age are less likely to find a permanent home compared to general foster care populations [9]. While the overall numbers of youth entering the child welfare system have overall declined in the past 10 years, there has been a significant increase in the number of youth "aging out" of foster care without finding a permanent home [12]. In fact, the percentage of older youth achieving permanency has not changed in the past decade [13].

About 20,000 of foster youth age out of services annually, most at age 18 years [11]. Recent changes to federal law allow states to provide foster care to youth up to age 21 years, also known as Extended Foster Care, and claim federal reimbursement. Among all foster youth, 28% are between the ages of 12 and 17 years and 4% between 18 and 20 years old [10] (Fig. 22.3).

African American and Native American youth are disproportionately represented in the child welfare system with rates of representation in the child welfare system at 17.4 and 14.1 per 1000 youth, respectively, compared to 5.8 for Hispanic, 4.6 for White youth, and 1.3 for Asian youth [14, 15] (Fig. 22.4).

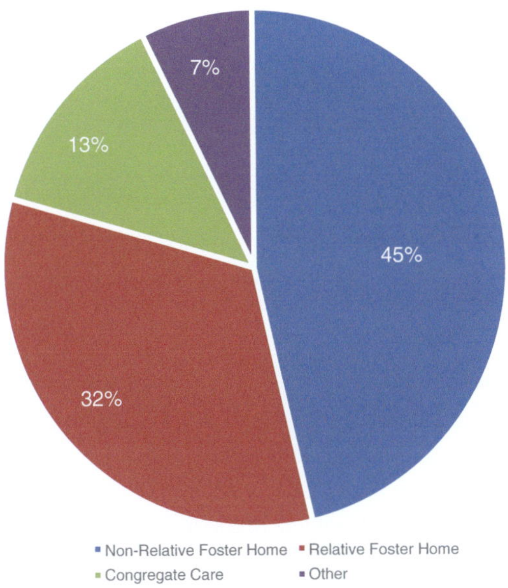

Fig. 22.2 Out-of-home placement types by percentage. (Adapted from US Department of Health and Human Services, Administration for Children and Families, Administration on Children Y, and Families, Children's Bureau. The AFCARS Report FY 2017. https://www.acf.hhs.gov/cb/resource/afcars-report-25; 2018.ge)

Legislation Impacting Transition-Age Foster Youth

Key legislation targeting older foster youth began in the late 1990s. One of the most important pieces of federal legislation supporting this population is the 1999 Foster Care Independence Act. This Act provides federal funding for independent living and transition services for older youth. The Act also created a reporting system called the National Youth in Transition Database which surveys youth between the ages of 18 and 21 years

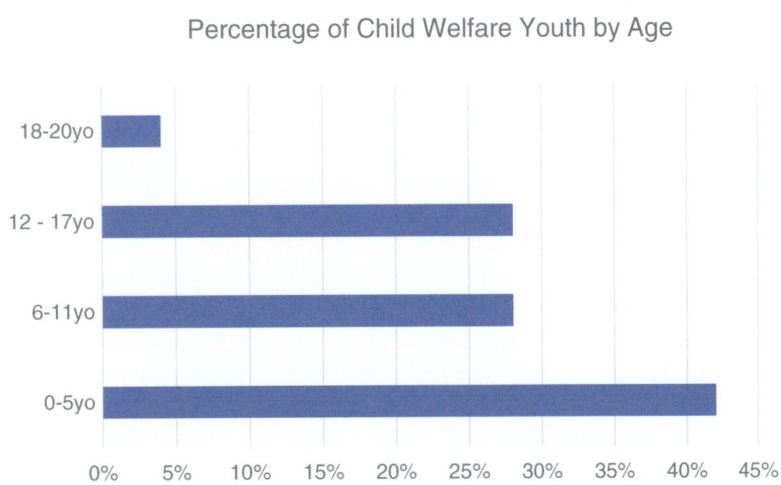

Fig. 22.3 Age of children in child welfare, by percent. (Adapted from US Department of Health and Human Services, Administration for Children and Families, Administration on Children Y, and Families, Children's Bureau. The AFCARS Report FY 2017. https://www.acf.hhs.gov/cb/resource/afcars-report-25; 2018)

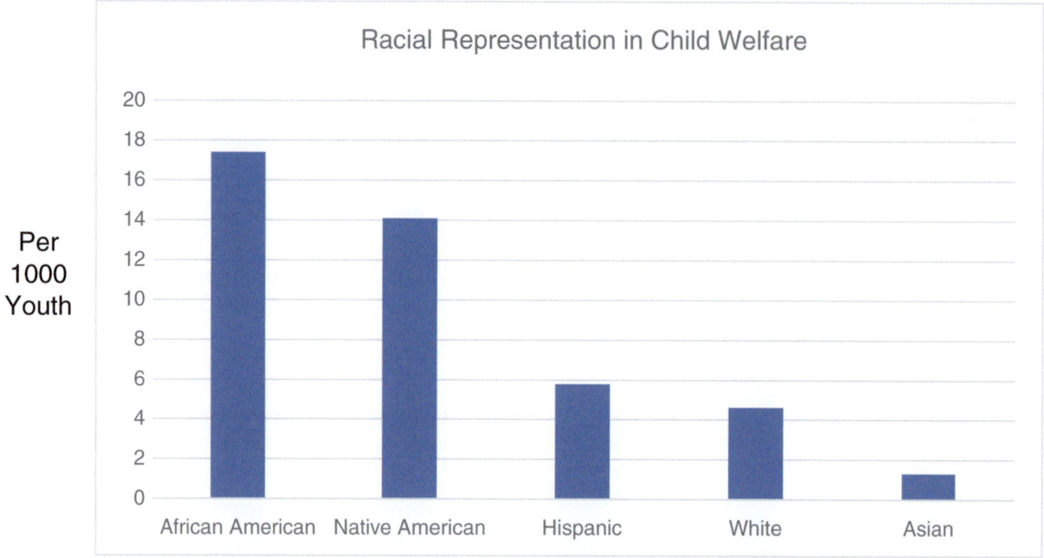

Fig. 22.4 Racial/ethnic representation in child welfare. (Adapted from US Department of Health and Human Services, Administration for Children and Families, Administration on Children, Youth, and Families, Children's Bureau. Data brief 2013-1: recent demographic trends in foster care. https://www.acf.hhs.gov/sites/default/files/cb/data_brief_foster_care_trends1.pdf; 2013)

old. This legislation was followed by the 2001 Education and Training Voucher Program which provides federal funds for postsecondary education or vocational programs for foster youth. In 2008, the Fostering Connections to Success and Increasing Adoptions Act provided voluntary Extended Foster Care (EFC) beyond age 18 years, up to age 21 years. The policy aimed to allow young people more time to prepare for adulthood with the support from the child welfare system [13]. This group of legislation establishes several services and practices to facilitate foster youth transition to adulthood.

Federal legislation outlined above sets forth requirements for youth who leave foster care due to age restrictions. A transition plan must be developed 90 days before discharge from foster care. The transition plan must be youth-directed and must address housing, health insurance, education, opportunities for mentoring and continuing support services, and workforce supports and employment services. Federal legislation requires states to develop oversight practices and coordination of health care, including behavioral health, and encourages mechanisms for ensuring continuity of care and transition to adult healthcare systems. Federal legislation offers funding to states to help with education, employment, financial literacy, housing, life skills training, transition services, emotional support, and encouraging relationships with caring adults. The federal requirement for transitioning planning at 90 days is the minimum time frame, and best practices encourage exploring and preparing for transition planning up to a year before [16].

Transition plan requirements can vary from state to state, but the Preventing Sex Trafficking and Strengthening Families Act requires specific components. When a youth is aging out of a state child welfare system, the state is federally required to provide the youth with the following: birth certificate, Social Security card, health insurance information, medical records, and a driver's license or state-issued identification card. This Act also requires case plans to offer transitional services starting at age 16 years with youth involvement in planning. The Affordable Care Act extends Medicaid eligibility to foster care alumni who aged out of care, up to age 26 years. To be eligible, the youth must have been enrolled in Medicaid while in foster care and reside in the state where either they were in foster care or have moved to 1 of the 11 states that will cover foster care alumni from other states [16]. The following website lists state Medicaid plans that will and will not cover foster alumni from another state: http://healthcareffy.org/.

The Education and Training Voucher Program is a federal program providing financial assistance (currently up to $5000/year) to foster youth and alumni enrolled in college, university, vocational, or technical training programs. Youth must enroll before their 21st birthday and remain eligible until age 23 years. Some states provide additional financial assistance for foster or former foster youth postsecondary education.

States have the option to provide developmentally modified foster care services with Extended Foster Care to foster youth up to age 21 years. To qualify for EFC, youth must be in an education or training program; working; in a program to address barriers to schooling, training, or work; or suffering a disability that prevents schooling or work. Being in Extended Foster Care has shown to help youth transition from foster care to adulthood. Youth who received Extended Foster Care are more likely at ages 19 and 21 years to be employed, enrolled in school, receive educational aid, avoid homelessness, avoid disconnection from work or school, and delay parenthood [13]. To avoid disincentives to permanency, EFC, independent living programs, and education and training supports can also be made available to youth exiting foster care through guardianship at age 16 years or older.

The 2018 Family First Prevention Services Act significantly changes the landscape of child welfare funding to support children to remain safe at home and encourage family-based placement when foster care is necessary. The other key priority of this legislation is to strengthen services for older youth. Family First allows federal funding to support older youth to live in family settings, safely care for their own children if pregnant or parenting, and expands access to independent living services. The Act also supports efforts to prevent older children from coming into care [17]. Family First also makes changes in the 1999 Chafee program to give states the flexibility to extend the Chafee program from age 21 up to age 23 years in states opting to provide EFC [16].

Overview of Foster Care Alumni Studies

The Northwest and Midwest studies are among the first series of reports that looked closely at what happens to foster care youth who age out of the child welfare system ("foster care alumni"). These reports help shed light on some of the significant challenges these youth are up against and look at ways foster services could improve their lives. These studies catalyzed change driving state and federal funding as well as program development to better serve the needs of this vulnerable population.

The Northwest Foster Care Alumni Study reviewed the cases of 659 alumni, of which 479 were interviewed, who were in the care of Casey Family Programs or in Oregon or Washington state child welfare agencies between 1988 and 1998. Youth were between the ages 20 and 33 years. The study outlined three key domains within this population: mental health, education, and employment and finances. Regarding mental health, compared to the general population, foster care alumni suffered a higher rate of mental health disorders. Within the 12 months prior to being interviewed, 54.4% of participants reported one or more mental health disorders. PTSD rates were double that of US war veterans at 25.2%, and alumni also reported major depression at 20.1% and social phobia at 17.1%. Studies in the second domain of education found alumni completed high school at a similar rate to the general population, but alumni used GED programs at six times the rate of the general population. The report also shed light on the instability in school placements with 65% of participants reported experiencing seven or more school changes in elementary through high school. The difficulty obtaining higher education was also noted with less than 3% of participants completing a bachelor's degree. The final domain of employment and finances also noted disparities compared to the general population, finding that 33% of

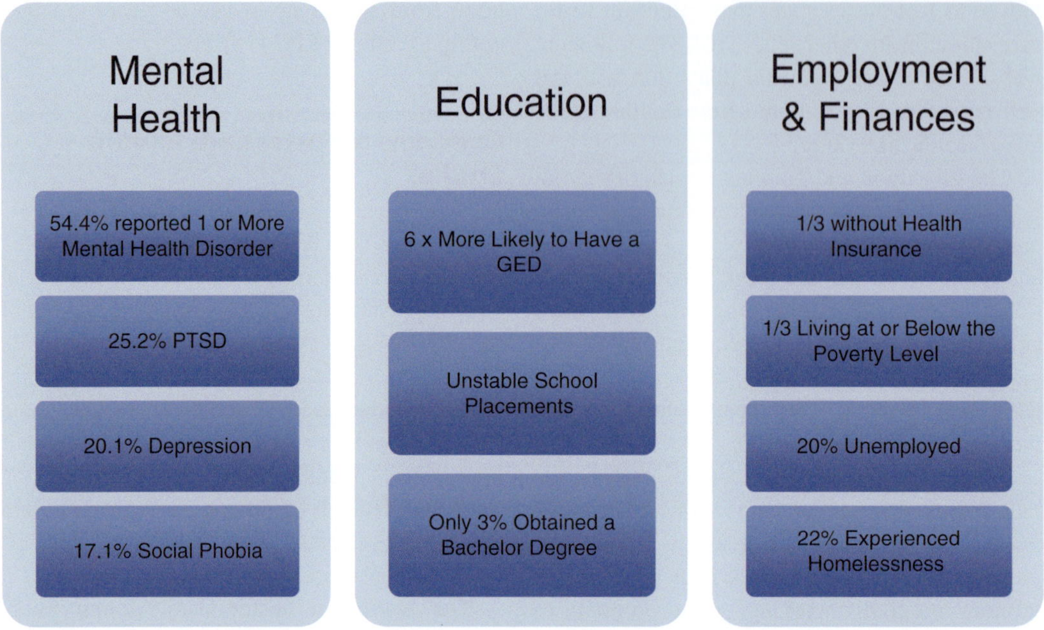

Fig. 22.5 Three outcome domains of the Northwest Foster Care Alumni Study. (Adapted from Pecora et al. [18])

alumni had no healthcare insurance, 33.2% had household incomes at or below the poverty level, and only 80.1% were employed of those eligible to work. Difficulties with stable housing were also seen with 22.2% reporting homelessness for one or more days after age 18 years [18] (Fig. 22.5).

The Midwest Study was undertaken to develop a more comprehensive view of foster youth transitioning to adulthood following a shift in federal funding (1999 Chafee Act) to support older youth in foster care. This has been the largest longitudinal study of youth aging out of foster care. Youth from Illinois, Iowa, and Wisconsin were followed from age 17 through 26 years, with five waves of data collection [3]. This study further investigated the disparities brought to light in the Northwest Study. In the domain of education, former foster youth by age 26 years were three times more likely than same peers to not have a high school diploma or GED (20% vs. 6%), while same-age peers were six times more likely to have a postsecondary degree (46% vs. 8%) and nine times more likely to have a 4-year college degree (36% vs. 4%). At age 26 years, female foster care alumni were seven to ten times more likely to have been arrested (41% vs. 5%), convicted (22% vs. 3%), and incarcerated (33% vs. 3%) since age 18 years, while male foster care alumni reported three- to eightfold increases (68% vs. 22%, 47% vs. 11%, and 64% vs. 9%, respectively). Nearly 80% of the women had at least one pregnancy by age 26 years. Financial disparities were also highlighted, with nearly 70% of women and 40% of men reporting using government assistance to access food in the last year, and of the 70% who reported earning an income, half earned $9000 or less annually, indicating concerns for poverty [3] (Fig. 22.6).

The Midwest Study also examined the effects of Extended Foster Care. At the time of the study, Illinois offered foster care up to age 21 years, while Iowa and Wisconsin terminated foster care at age 18 years. At age 19 years old, youth in Wisconsin and Iowa were 2.7 times more likely to be homeless than foster youth in Illinois, and youth remaining in foster care were at least twice as likely to complete at least 1 year of college by age 21 years [19]. Courtney et al. (2009) estimated that each dollar spent on EFC returned $2.40 in increased income, based on anticipated higher college graduation rates [20].

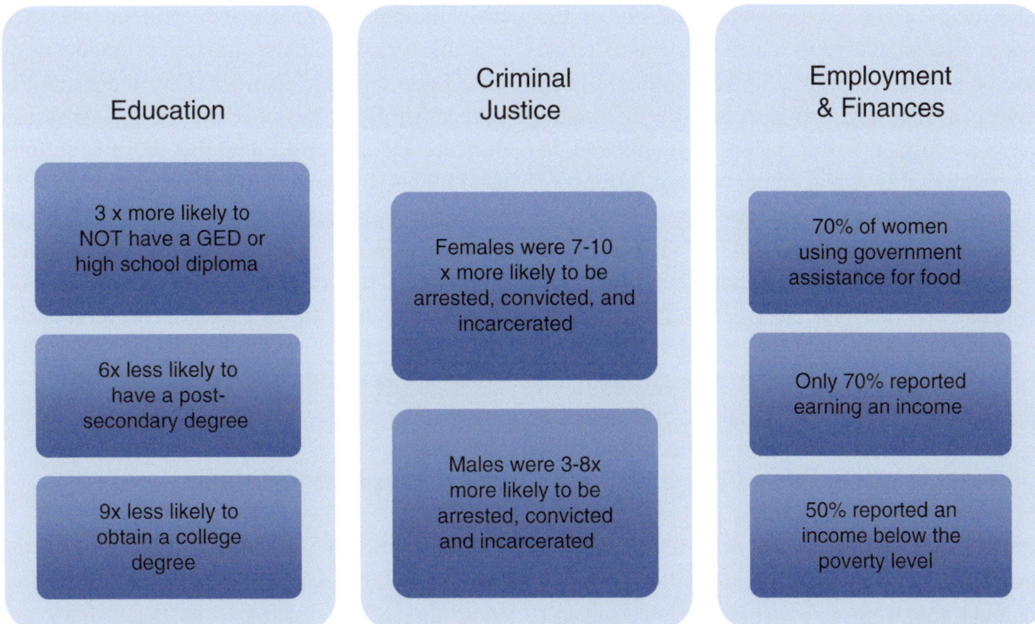

Fig. 22.6 The Midwest Study outcome domains for foster care alumni. (Adapted from Courtney et al. [3])

Transition Health Care (THC): Pediatrics to Adult Care

Reaching the age of majority, transitioning foster youth are expected to manage their own health care, and many may not be eligible to receive the number of supports that they were accustomed to while in state custody. Also, those with intellectual and/or developmental disabilities (e.g., Down's syndrome, autism) will need continued support in order to navigate transportation to appointments and assistance in understanding of the treatment that they are receiving. Many adult providers are not comfortable treating chronic childhood illnesses, and pediatricians do not have the resources to continue treating young adult patients. Pediatricians have difficulty finding adult providers who feel adequately trained in adolescent medicine, adolescent development, or adolescent behavior to take on these cases. Peter et al. (2009) surveyed internists who expressed the following identified concerns that clustered into six major themes: family involvement, patient maturity, systems issues, providers' medical competency, patient psychosocial needs, and coordination of the transition process. Health insurance is another obstacle facing young adults transitioning from foster care. Both the Midwest and Northwest studies reported that roughly 51–53%, respectively, of foster youth had no health insurance at the time of exiting foster care, which is double the rate for young adults in the general population..

Mental Health Considerations for Transition-Age Foster Youth

According to the NIMH, in 2017, young adults aged 18–25 years had the highest prevalence of serious mental illness (SMI) (7.5%) compared to adults aged 26–49 years (5.6%) and aged 50 years and older (2.7%). Former foster youth with mental illness often have past trauma histories that make it challenging for them to develop and maintain healthy adult relationships. Many will experience mistrust to new healthcare systems and providers, and their mood may easily become dysregulated as a result of insecure attachments [21]. Some researchers have shown that the more placements a child experiences, the higher the risk of attachment issues which can lead to a high risk of psychiatric morbidity in adulthood [22]. Evidence that can explain health differences between former foster youth as compared to other vulnerable young adults without foster care experience is limited. One systematic review of literature found no studies that included a sample of youth who were both homeless and had been in foster care, despite the overlapping needs of these youth in transition [23]. Supplemental studies regarding the impact of social capital on health outcomes for former foster youth as compared to non-foster peers with similar vulnerabilities, such as poverty, are warranted [24]. Also, there have been studies linking child abuse histories to mental health problems in adulthood, but not much research has looked at the effects of maltreatment while in foster care related to adult mental health [22]. Further, transitional age youth with untreated mental health disorders are at high risk for substance abuse, physical assault, and encounters with the correctional system [25]. Other studies have shown that being a victim of child abuse and neglect is commonly associated with depression, PTSD, substance use, and antisocial behaviors [26]. Entering the foster care system has been associated with a high risk of behavioral and mental health needs [27], and older youth consume more behavioral healthcare services than those of same-age peers not in foster care [28–30]. However, the use of services drops to approximately 50% when these older youth exit foster care between ages 18 and 21 years [31]. For unclear reasons, this drop may be accounted for by poor coordination between pediatric and adult providers, youth's choices in taking charge of their own care, or difficulty accessing adult services.

The Midwest Study described that the peak prevalence of alcohol abuse/dependence and other drug abuse/dependence increases from ages 19 to 26 years whereas the prevalence of non-foster youth peaks at ages 19–21 years, which decreases over time [3, 32]. Another study found that 45% of 17-year-olds in state custody, within a year of leaving care, used alcohol or illicit drugs in the last 6 months, 49% had tried one time in their lifetime, and 35% met criteria for substance use disorder [33]. Also having a diagnosis of PTSD and conduct disorder (CD) increased the chances of high rates of use and a substance use disorder. Vaughn also found that those with SUD used higher amounts than their non- foster peers and warns that those youth are at a higher risk of overdoses. White et al. (2008) found that foster alumni had higher rates of substance use and dependence than the general population, but the rates were lower in those youth who reported a constant support of a foster family [34, 35].

Psychotropic Medications

A large national probability sample of foster care children found that 14% were taking psychotropic medications: two to three times the rate of non-foster children [36]. One study reported an increased rate of antipsychotic use from 8.9% to 11.8% across 45 states over the period of 2002–2007 [37], and another found a 37.9% annual prevalence rate of psychotropic medication use for youth in foster care [38]. Among those taking medications, 72% took two or more psychotropic medications, while 41.3% received three or more medications. Data on residential care have shown substantially higher rates of psychopharmacology, with an average of 75–79% of youth in these settings taking psychotropic medications including high rates of polypharmacy [39]. Foster youth are prescribed antipsychotic medications, mainly for behavioral dyscontrol, at a higher rate than non-foster youth. Allaire et al. (2016) examined Medicaid claims from 36 states between 2000 and 2003 and found "morbid obesity" as a diagnosis at a prevalence rate of 0.5%. They also found the risk higher in females, non-White, and older adolescents and taking two or more second-generation antipsychotics increases the risk fivefold [40]. Persistently high rates of treatment with antipsychotics, particularly among foster children, gaps in metabolic monitoring, overuse of multiple concurrent antipsychotic medications, and underuse of psychosocial interventions illustrate behavioral healthcare challenges [41].

Psychosocial Treatment

Although rates of congregate care are on the decline, older youth in foster care are more likely to be placed in a congregate care, with rates approaching 60% [42, 43]. These older youth entered residential treatment facilities or group home settings instead of a family foster care home mainly for behavioral problems and required trained staff to provide care to address those issues. Unfortunately, they are less likely to be adopted, most likely emancipate from child welfare, and require support through their transition. The research base for residential group treatment effectiveness is not robust, but there is a correlation between the youth's level of functioning and their level of care in the community. Multidimensional Treatment Foster Care (MTFC) addresses the difficulty of leaving institutional care and involves a large behavior management team, including foster family involvement with treatment to support reunification. MTFC has become popular in the juvenile justice system as an alternative to youth incarceration, but it has not been widely adopted in child welfare or mental health systems [42].

There are other supports systems and approaches that help foster youth make the transition to adulthood. The Youth-Initiated Mentoring (YIM) model encourages young people to reach out and ask their potential natural supports to engage with them more and be in a relationship with them as a mentor, which could be applied among young adults with mental health conditions [21]. Another program, SPARCS (Structured Psychotherapy for Adolescents Responding to Chronic Stress), aims to enhance adolescents' abilities to cope more effectively in the moment, to cultivate consciousness, and to create connections and meaning. It draws upon mindfulness and interpersonal skills from dialectical behavior therapy for adolescents, problem-solving skills, and enhancing social support and planning for the future. Mindfulness is explained to group members as "paying attention in a particular way, on purpose, and non-judgmentally." SPARCS's focus on mindfulness, coping, and interpersonal skills makes it an ideal treatment for adolescents transitioning to independence [44]. For youth with a known history of trauma who struggle with symptoms of post-traumatic stress disorder, trauma-focused cognitive behavioral therapy (TF-CBT) has a robust evidence base for the treatment of PTSD and is recommended for first-line treatment for PTSD symptoms over medication [45].

Challenges to Address When Working with Young Adult Foster Youth

Childhood adversity is common, and the types of adversity can range from the parental separation and divorce to child abuse and neglect. But youth in the child welfare system have often undergone multiple adverse experiences which directly affect health. Research has shown a dose-response relationship between the number of adverse childhood experiences (ACEs) and increased risk of morbidity and mortality impacting health and mental health outcomes [46, 47]. Looking at the impact of ACEs on young adult foster care alumni, data from the Midwest Study show distinct subgroups related to the type and number of ACEs to which youth have been exposed. Young adults categorized as "the complex adversity group" who had high rates (average 7) of ACEs also had the highest rates of physical health and sexual health risk factors when compared to youth in the "environmental adversity group" who were only exposed to environmental adverse experiences such as a natural disaster or community violence. Not surprisingly, youth with the lower ACE scores (an average of 2.8), categorized as "the lower adversity subgroup," had the lowest risk of poor health outcomes [48].

Exposure to adversity and trauma can lead to negative physical and behavioral health outcomes. Youth in the child welfare system have often been exposed to not just one trauma but multiple traumatic events that are often chronic and cumulative. They often lack the protection and support of a parent or adult caregiver to help buffer the effects of trauma. "Toxic stress" is a phenomenon that characterizes the negative mental and physical health effects of exposure to chronic trauma, which persistently activates the body's neuroendocrine stress response system contributing to the negative health effects [49]. This activation has a direct negative effect on gene translation, immune system response, and neurodevelopment [50]. Chronic glucocorticoid exposure from the toxic stress response has a direct effect on key areas of the developing brain including the amygdala, hippocampus, and prefrontal cortex. These changes interfere with the development of emotion regulation, impulse control, concentration, and decision-making. An emerging body of research has shown that toxic stress may impact the way genes are transcribed through epigenetic changes to DNA sequences. These genetic changes may contribute to how the body responds to stress, impacting mental health [51]. Toxic stress also has a direct effect on physical health. A large body of research shows that youth in foster care, compared to non-foster peers, have increased rates of acute and chronic infections, asthma, and obesity. This is due to the physical sequelae of trauma but is also directly related to toxic stress-induced chronic immune response and inflammation [52].

Social supports can provide a buffer against the long-term effects of trauma and help youth transitioning out of care. Social supports are a central factor in well-being, impacting physical and mental health in individuals exposed to trauma. The impact of early adversity for youth aging out is linked to not only structural aspects of support such as network size but also a youth's ability to recognize and utilize available support. Efforts are needed to help build this skill set for youth aging out [53]. Foster youth transitioning out of care often lack the support network so greatly utilized by their non-foster peers as they take on more independence. Multiple moves and school settings make it difficult to form and maintain relationships [54]. Disrupted social networks are linked to higher rates of emotional distress. These frequent moves and traumas can also instill a lack of trust in people [55]. Lack of supports and social connectedness contribute to negative outcomes and increased challenges with transitioning to adulthood [56].

If not already connected, youth transitioning out of care often reconnect with their family of origin. About 64% of transition-age foster youth reported feeling very or somewhat close to their birth mothers. If they were living with relatives, nearly 95% of youth reported feeling very or somewhat close to those relatives [57]. While birth families can provide critical support during transition, reconnecting with families can also be stressful for youth. Prior to aging out, systems should be put in place to help foster youth make informed decisions around reconnecting, form realistic expectations, establish appropriate boundaries, navigate family of origin interactions, and develop skills to address possible negative interactions.

With this social vulnerability, concerns have been raised around minors in the child welfare system being at risk for child sex trafficking. On interviewing victims of sex trafficking, many of these youth were found to have histories of child welfare involvement, maltreatment, and out-of-home care [58]. The 2014 federal legislation Preventing Sex Trafficking and Strengthening Families Act shed light on this concern and aimed to provide pathways for healthy relationships to develop. Females with a history of child sexual abuse are at particular risk to engage in transactional sex for youth who recently aged out [59]. Understanding these risk factors can help drive new practices and policies which help young adults during this vulnerable developmental period.

The impact of parental incarceration in this population is also important to consider. The United States has an incarceration rate that is five to ten times higher than that in other industrialized nations and is unique in its proportion of children experiencing a parent undergo incarceration. Positive, significant associations were found between parental incarceration and health problems such as depression, post-traumatic stress disorder, anxiety, cholesterol, asthma, migraines, HIV/AIDS, and reported fair/poor health [60]. Youth in the child welfare system have increased lengths of stay when they enter due to parental incarceration when compared to other reasons for removal [61].

Best Practices: Promoting Resiliency

Child welfare systems value strengths-based approaches and resilience orientations [62]. Masten (2001) defined resilience as a class of phenomenon characterized by good outcomes in spite of serious threats to adaptation or development and emphasized that resilience is a common rather than extraordinary characteristic of individuals [63]. Ungar (2013) conceptualized resilience among maltreated youth as an interactive process between youth and their social ecology, which is influenced by youth individual characteristics (temperament and personality), the social determinants of health affecting youth and their caregivers, the quality of services provided by stakeholder agencies, and government policies addressing high-risk populations. Resilience can be promoted by ensuring the availability and accessibility of social supports and formal services and program flexibility to address individual youth specific needs [64].

A resilience orientation portends a strengths-based approach that identifies and enhances protective factors in a youth's environment. Foster youth strengths often include persistence, resourcefulness, determination, grit, and self-reliance. Latent class analysis identified four subgroups of young adults in the Midwest Study. The subgroup termed "accelerated adults" who viewed themselves as "having to grow up fast" and "take on adult responsibilities" tended to have better outcomes such as higher rates of employment and decreased involvement in criminal justice system. This group comprised about one-third of the study participants and was majority female [65]. The Midwest Study also found that foster youth with high school diplomas or GEDs were almost twice as likely to be employed as an adult [66].

Connectedness in youth who are transitioning out of care is a protective factor. Youth placed in kinship placements, compared to non-relative care, have better outcomes and more social supports [56]. Encouraging mentoring relationships can promote success, especially when working with youth in non-kinship placements. Foster youth with a positive and significant relationship with at least one adult, compared to non-mentored foster youth, fare better on general health, feelings of stress, education attainment, physical aggression, suicidality, arrests, and sexually transmitted diseases [55]. Some supportive adults enter youth's lives through interactions with the child welfare system. Important qualities of the mentoring relationship include trust, consistency, empathy, and authenticity. Transition-age foster youth value mentors who are understanding and non-judgmental, provide direct communication and advice, and have similar life experiences that they share [67].

Best Practices: Assessment of Readiness

The Casey Life Skills website contains resources for youth and coaches (providers or caregivers) to help foster youth achieve their long-term goals. The Casey Life Skills Assessment (CLSA) is a tool that helps youth self-evaluate the behaviors and competencies necessary for successful transition to adulthood (casey.org-life-skills-resources/) (Fig. 22.7).

Casey Life Skills also provides additional life skills assessments for youth with specific characteristics and circumstances. These additional assessments include assessments for healthy pregnancy, parenting of infants, and parenting young children; education assessments based on schooling level and education supports for support and assistance (Individualized Education Plan (IEP) and 504 Plan); and assessments for gay, lesbian, transgender, and questioning (GLBTQ) youth, American Indian youth, homeless youth, and younger youth with reading or developmental challenges.

After the CLS Assessment, youth and coaches can use the Resources to Inspire Guide to develop a plan for acquiring needed skills. The guide con-

Daily Living Skills

- Laundry, Home Cleanilness
- Home Safety
- Food and Nutrition

Self Care Skills

- Health Care
- Health Insurance and Benefit Eligibilities
- Peresonal Hygiene
- Adult Supports
- Medical Decision Making
- Sexuality, Sexual Health

Relationships and Communication

- Communication Skills
- Interpersonal, Relationship Skills
- Social and Family Supports
- Cultural Awareness
- Emotion Regulation Skills
- Safe Relationships & Domestic Violence

Housing and Money Management

- Budgeting and Spending Plan
- Housing, Tenancy
- (Online) Banking, Savings,
- Credit, Interest and Debt
- Emergency Funding
- Emergency Utility Support
- Home/Renter's Insurance
- Driver's License and Auto Insurance
- Vehicle ownership costs, Public Transportation

Work and Study Skills

- Resume development
- Job applications
- Job Interview skills
- Payroll and Paystub
- Employee Benefits
- Income Tax Help
- Social Security Card and Birth Certificate
- School Mental Health Services
- Viewing Child Welfare and Juvenile Justice Records
- Study Skills, Test Preparation, Tutoring help

Career and Education Planning

- Work-related Internships
- Benefits of Volunteer Work
- School Path for Deisred Work
- Finanacial Aid Knowledge
- Job training resources
- Career Mentors
- Application and Admission to Desired Post-Secondary schooling
- Adult support for Education Plans

Looking Forward

- Self-determination
- Adult Support
- Readiness for Adulthood
- Beleifs & Envisioning Successful Future
- Deslire to Heap Other Youth
- Positive Self Image
- Support System for Success

Fig. 22.7 Casey Life Skills Assessment: core competency domains. (Adapted from Casey Family Programs. Casey Life Skills [68])

tains suggestions for free or low-cost life skills training resources and encourages searching for additional resources [68].

Promising Practices

The California Evidence-Based Clearinghouse for Child Welfare (cebc4cw.org) is an online resource whose mission is to "advance the effective implementation of evidence-based practices for children and families involved with the child welfare system." The site includes a program registry and ratings of the strength of evidence for specific programs and practices. Ratings range from 1, Well-Supported by Research Evidence, to 5, Concerning Practice, and NR, Not able to be Rated on the CEBC Scientific Rating Scale. Youth Transitioning into Adulthood is one of the topic areas (cebc4cw.org-transition). At this time, in the Transitioning into Adulthood category, one program is rated 2—Supported by Research Evidence (Better Futures, described below)— and three are rated 3, Promising Research Evidence. The remaining 16 programs are rated NR—Not able to be Rated—due to a lack of available research evidence. Some of these programs target individual functional domains, such as social supports, housing, education, employment, living skills, financial literacy, health, and mental health. Other programs are more comprehensive and target multiple domains. Some are child welfare-specific, while others target general high-risk transitional age youth [69].

Education: "Better Futures" Program (Rated "Supported by Evidence" 2 Out of 5 for Strength of Evidence)

Better Futures is a program focused on improving postsecondary preparation and participation of youth in foster care with mental health concerns. The target population is youth and young adults in foster care, including youth with disabilities and/or mental health concerns, who are in their final year of high school or GED completion, open to participating in postsecondary education, and allowed to go into the community with their Better Futures Coach. Youth participate in a 4-day postsecondary school immersion experience followed by 9 months of (1) youth-directed relationship support from a coach in postsecondary education and personal experience in foster care; (2) coaching in applying achievement, partnership, and self-regulation skills to identify and attain related youth-chosen goals; (3) support for experiential activities related to career and postsecondary exploration and preparation; and (4) workshops bringing together youth, coaches, and successful near peers for learning, peer support, and networking.

A Better Futures randomized controlled trial evaluated outcomes of 67 youth involved with the Oregon child welfare system who also had some type of operationally defined mental health concern. The Better Futures intervention consisted of a 4-day 3-night Summer Institute on a university campus; individual, bimonthly peer coaching; and four mentoring workshops. At 6 months after the 10-month intervention, youth in the Better Futures group, compared to the control group, were twice as likely to participate in postsecondary education. They also scored higher in transition planning and rated themselves higher on standardized measures of self-determination, mental health empowerment, and hope. The Better Futures group trended positively in high school completion and standardized self-reports of mental health recovery and quality of life [70].

Mentoring: "Caring Adults R Everywhere" Program (Not able to be Rated)

Relationships with caring non-familial adults can enhance youth resiliency (Collins, 2010). The Caring Adults R Everywhere program is a manualized 12-week mentoring intervention designed to bolster social supports by developing and strengthening existing relationships between youth and supportive adults from the youth's natural ecology [71]. A master's-trained social worker (not the youth's child welfare worker), called an interventionist, meets with a youth aging out of foster care to identify an appropriate mentor. After screening and approval, mentors undergo training in adolescent development, the child welfare system, trauma-informed mentoring, practices of effective mentors, what to do with one's mentee, and establishing and maintaining boundaries. Youth and mentors participate in group activities and one-on-one sessions with the interventionist to strengthen and clarify expectations for the mentoring relationship.

Homelessness: "My First Place" Program (Not able to be Rated)

Foster youth experience homelessness at much higher rates than their same-age peers. The My First Place (MFP) program, located in the San Francisco Bay Area, targets transition-age foster youth at risk for homelessness [72]. The program typically lasts 18–24 months and is comprised of five core elements:

1. Ongoing case management by a youth advocate, the primary case manager, and an education and employment specialist. Foster youth work with both to achieve specific goals in the area of housing, education, employment, and healthy living.
2. MFP uses scattered site housing throughout the five-county region. The program seeks housing in safe neighborhoods near public transportation. MFP typically signs a master lease with landlords and then subleases units to program participants. Youth receive training on tenancy.
3. MFP has a property management department that maintains relationships with landlords and affordable housing partners, rents apartments, manages subleasing, oversees move-ins, and manages rent payment. The department also deals with tenant issues like property damage, maintenance, and compliance with regulations.
4. A larger organization infrastructure provides administrative and clinical support.
5. MFP collaborates with community partners, including referral sources for program youth, education and employment partners, and health and mental health provider agencies.

Financial Literacy: "MyPath Savings" (Not able to be Rated)

Limited financial knowledge and capabilities can undermine efforts to achieve financial stability. MyPath Savings is a financial knowledge and skills program for economically disadvantaged youth earning their first paychecks [73]. The program provides financial education, familiarizes youth to conventional financial products, and uses experiential teaching with peer learning and support. Topics and skills include direct deposit, checking and restricted savings accounts, and savings incentives. Youth are aided to open accounts, set up direct deposit, set a savings goal, and save a designated portion of each paycheck and provided incentives to meet savings goals.

Postsecondary Education Support

Most foster youth aspire to attend college. However, foster youth enroll in and graduate from college at much lower rates than their non-foster peers [74]. Foster youth often report that few people in their lives expect and/or encourage them to attend and succeed in college. In addition, foster youth experience a number of risk factors that negatively impact education [75]. A number of states are developing programs to support foster youth and alumni in postsecondary education, including college, community college, and vocational training. More than 30 states provide scholarships, grants, or tuition waivers to foster youth attending higher education. Casey Family Programs developed a resource report called Supporting Success that identifies and discusses 12 core program elements for improving outcomes [76] (Fig. 22.8).

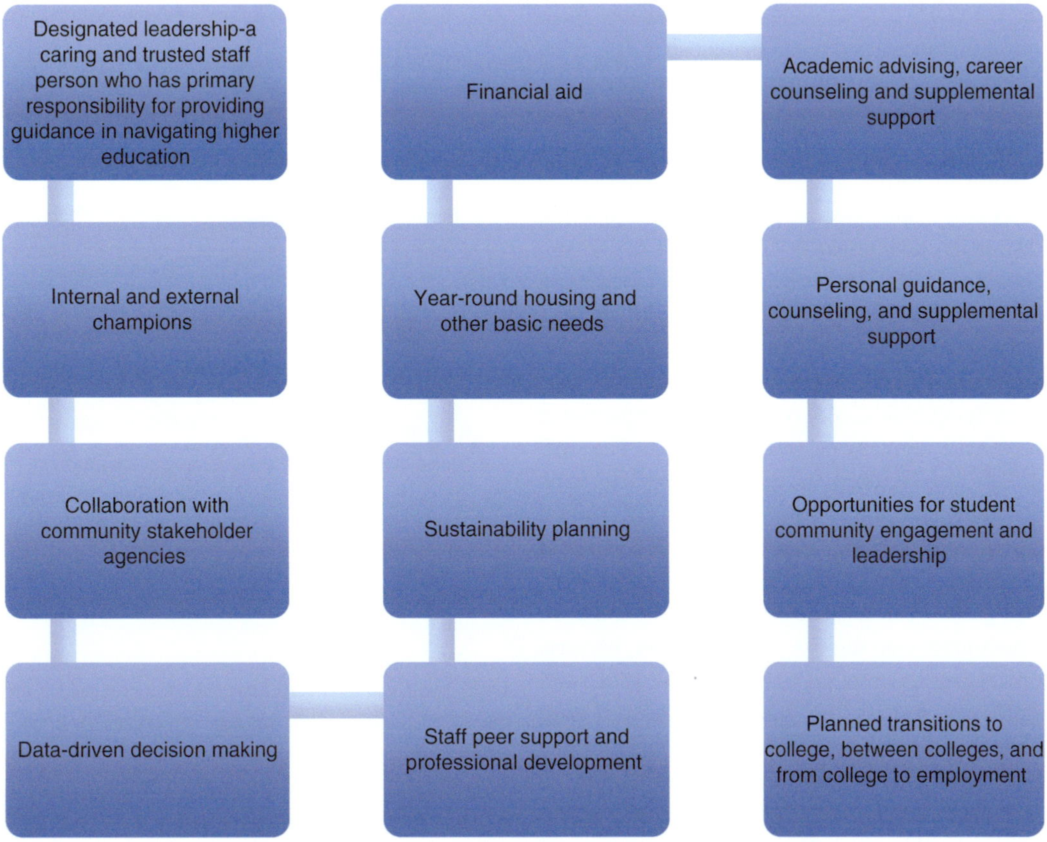

Fig. 22.8 Casey Family Programs supporting success core program elements. (Adapted from Casey Family Programs [76])

The Seita Scholars Program is a campus-based support program for foster youth and alumni attending Western Michigan University [77]. The program is named after Dr. John Seita, a graduate of the Michigan child welfare system and Western Michigan University. Coaches provide support to students in the program—Seita Scholars—with a focus on the seven lifespan development domains suggested by Casey Family Programs, academics, finances and employment, housing, physical and mental health care, social relationships and community connections, cultural and personal identity, and life skills. The program includes a scholarship at Western Michigan University. Students reside on campus and have access to 24-hour on-call support and emergency financial resources. The program uses trained master's-level campus coaches and provides training and certification for professionals working with college students who have been involved in the foster care system or other high-risk youth.

Independent Living Programs

Federal legislation provides funds to states to offer independent living programs to assist foster youth and alumni transitioning to adulthood. Program components typically involve social-emotional supports, mentoring, housing, education and training, employment, daily living skills, health and behavioral health, and financial literacy.

The Orangewood Independent Living Program (ILP) was developed by the Orangewood Foundation and provides workshops, special events, mentoring, and case management to foster youth 16–21 years old to help prepare them for the transition to independence [78]. Each month the ILP focuses on one of four key areas: education, career, relationships, and daily living, providing workshops and take-home activities. Youth can earn ILP dollars by participating in workshops and special events and completing take-home assignments. Examples of take-home activities include writing an interview thank you letter (career), completing a change of address form or getting a credit report (daily living), completing a FAFSA application (education), and identifying one's core values or completing a roommate agreement (relationships). The ILP dollars are tracked in an Orangewood bank account, and ILP youth can purchase a maximum of one $50 gift certificate per month for use at stores for groceries, clothing, and general goods. ILP dollars can also be used for bills and rent. Youth must plan the use of ILP dollars, because processing requests may take up to 2 weeks and staff may discuss the youth's requests. Foster care alumni who have successfully transitioned to independent living serve as peer mentors in the ILP. Peer mentors help establish program rapport and credibility with ILP youth, teach independent living skills, facilitate small group discussion during workshops, and serve as positive role models. Participants provide feedback at each workshop to assess interest and effectiveness (Fig. 22.9).

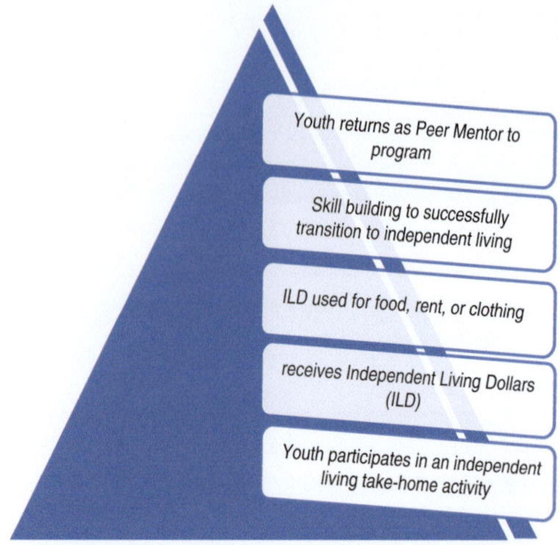

Fig. 22.9 Orangewood Independent Living Program process. (Adapted from California Evidence-Based Clearinghouse for Child Welfare. Independent Living Program Orangewood http://www.cebc4cw.org/program/independent-living-program-orangewood)

Supportive individuals are invited to participate in the youth's transition plan and attend workshops. ILP also coordinates with other programs designed to serve transition-age foster youth, such as housing, scholarships, Independent Living Specialists, and youth leadership opportunities.

Legal and Ethical Issues

Ethical, legal, and policy issues overlap because state responsibilities to foster youth should translate into policies and legislation. Given that most non-foster youth require and receive social, pragmatic, and financial support from their parents well into their 20s and beyond, one can make the case that the state and society are ethically bound to provide comparable support for a similar duration to foster youth. Vast geographic disparities in public health and behavioral health care and child welfare systems require contemplation from child and adolescent behavioral health providers and stakeholders. It is imperative to advocate for changes within local, state, and federal governments to ensure access to comprehensive services owed to this highly vulnerable population.

Behavioral health clinicians should provide and advocate for the appropriate use of psychiatric medications and trauma-informed psychosocial treatments. When working with youth who are in the care and protection of the state, providers should familiarize themselves with state laws around mental health treatment and psychotropic consent. Authority for psychotropic consent varies from state to state and may rest with the biological parents, a child welfare agency, or some other party such as a court or state-appointed consent agent. Questions about a youth's legal status, consent, release of information, and legal authority should be directed to the child welfare worker. Issues around consent and privacy have also left much of this vulnerable population out of clinical trials and other research studies, impacting the amount of evidenced-based literature on this population.

Areas of Need: Research and Policy Gaps

The Institute of Medicine and the Future of Children contemplated transition, including research and policy gaps relating to "marginalized" and "vulnerable" youth transitioning to adulthood [79, 80]. Foster youth were included in these groups, along with youth involved with the juvenile justice, mental health, and special education systems, and youth with disabilities. More research on transition-age services for foster youth is needed. A more comprehensive understanding of transition-age foster youth and outcomes will inform policy and program development. Many existing programs appear promising, but more research is required to determine the effectiveness and cost-effectiveness of programs and inform quality improvement. States are given wide latitude to develop transition programs; differences in state transition services provide opportunities to compare implementation processes and functional outcomes. Databases must be expanded, strengthened, and linked to support more rigorous evaluation and outcome tracking. Administrative data may include relevant information, including secondary and postsecondary education performance, health and behavioral healthcare utilization and outcomes, employment, justice system involvement, and participation in public assistance programs.

Legislation and policies have begun to address the myriad challenges facing transition-age foster youth, but to sufficiently support foster youth emancipation and self-sufficiency, federal legislation and policies must be strengthened to expand the availability and breadth of transition services. While recent federal legislation seeks to extend state responsibility to act as parents to foster youth beyond age 18 years, it does so mostly to age 21 years, too young given most foster youth's developmental needs. Most states provide transition services in a limited, interrupted, and piecemeal fashion, contrasted with the more comprehensive, continuous, and enduring supports many parents provide their children. Transition-age foster youth may be involved with multiple agencies because they have multiple needs, requiring integration and coordination of efforts. Moreover, federal legislation permits but does not require states to provide necessary transition services. For example, only about half the states offer Extended Foster Care, and those that do often offer more limited services than federal policies allow [81]. In addition, while states must extend Medicaid eligibility to age 26 years to foster youth from their own state, most states do not do so for foster alumni from other states [16].

Existing programs are too bureaucratic, inaccessible, idiosyncratic, fragmented, poorly responsive, and stigmatizing [80]. Transition-age foster youth will benefit from policies promoting a youth-centered, family-focused, culturally sensitive, developmentally appropriate, accessible, responsive, comprehensive, and integrated and coordinated system of transition care. This care should be continuous and seamless from adolescence to early adulthood, trauma-informed, non-stigmatizing, and socially inclusive. Accountability for outcomes must be heightened to improve the well-being of foster care alumni.

Summary

Transition-age foster youth do not typically receive the range of family supports that their non-foster peers enjoy. Foster youth often experience multiple adversities that complicate successful transition and negatively impact mental and physical health. Foster care alumni are at increased risk for negative outcomes in education, homelessness, employment, financial security, health, and behavioral health. Youth-serving public systems of care often end at age 18 or 21 years or are discontinuous with adult approximations. The federal government, states, foundations, non-government organizations, families, and current and past foster youth have begun addressing transition-age foster youth needs. Many policies and programs appear to be promising. More research is needed to assess the effectiveness and efficiency of existing programs and to inform program and policy development and quality improvement. Policies must be strengthened to increase accountability for developing youth self-sufficiency and improve transition service availability, access, responsiveness, continuity, duration, and effectiveness.

References

1. Martel A, Fuchs DC. Transitional age youth and mental illness – influences on young adult outcomes. Child Adolesc Psychiatr Clin N Am. 2017;26(2):xiii–vii.
2. Settersten RA Jr, Ray B. What's going on with young people today? The long and twisting path to adulthood. Futur Child. 2010;20(1):19–41.
3. Courtney ME, Dworsky A, Brown A, et al. Midwest evaluation of adult functioning of former foster youth: outcomes at age 26. Chicago: Chapin Hall at the University of Chicago; 2011.
4. Chan V, Moore J, Derenne J, Fuchs DC. Transitional age youth and college mental health. Child Adolesc Psychiatr Clin N Am. 2019;28(3):363–75.
5. Kempe CH, Silverman FN, Steele BF, Droegemueller W, Silver HK. The battered-child syndrome. JAMA. 1962;181:17–24.
6. Lou C, Anthony EK, Stone S, Vu CM, Austin MJ. Assessing child and youth well-being: implications for child welfare practice. J Evid Based Soc Work. 2008;5(1–2):91–133.
7. Wilson C. Integrating safety, permanency, and well-being: a view from the field. Children's Bureau, Administration for Children & Families. Health & human services; 2014. https://www.acf.hhs.gov/cb/resource/well-being-series.
8. U.S. Department of Health & Human Services, Administration for Children and Families, Administration on Children Youth and Families, Children Bureau. Child maltreatment 2017; 2019. https://www.acf.hss.gov/cb/research-data-technology/statistics-research/child-meltreatment.
9. U.S Department of Health and Human Services, Administration for Children and Families, Administration on Children Youth and Families, Children's Bureau. Child welfare outcomes 2016: report to congress; 2019. https://www.acf.hhs.gov/cb/resource/cwo-2016.
10. U.S Department of Health and Human Services, Administration for Children and Families, Administration on Children Y, and Families, Children's Bureau. The AFCARS Report FY 2017; 2018. https://www.acf.hhs.gov/cb/resource/afcars-report-25.
11. The Annie E Casey Foundation. Kids Count Data Center; 2019. https://datacenter.kidscount.org/data/tables/.
12. Johnson A, Speiglman R, Mauldon J, et al. Promoting permanency for teens; A 50 state review of law & policy. Oakland: National Center for Youth Law; 2018.
13. Rosenberg R, Abbott S. Supporting older youth beyond age 18: examining data and trends in extended foster care. Child Trend; 2019. https://www.childtrends.org/publications/supporting-older-youth-beyond-age-18-examining-data-and-trends-in-extended-foster-care.
14. U.S Department of Health and Human Services, Administration for Children and Families, Administration on Children Youth and Families, Children's Bureau. Data brief 2013–1: recent demographic trends in foster care; 2013. https://www.acf.hhs.gov/sites/default/files/cb/data_brief_foster_care_trends1.pdf.
15. Bartholet E, Wulczyn F, Barth R, et al. Race and child welfare. Chicago; 2011.
16. U.S Department of Health and Human Services, Administration for Children and Families, Administration on Children Y, and Families, Children's Bureau. Working with youth to develop a transition plan; 2018.
17. Rosenberg R, McKlindon A. The Family First Prevention Services Act can fund needed services and supports for older youth in foster care. Child trends; 2019. https://www.childtrends.org/the-family-first-prevention-services-act-fund-needed-services-supports-older-youth-foster-care.
18. Pecora P, Kessler R, Williams J, et al. Improving family foster care: findings from the northwest foster care alumni study. Washington, Casey Family Programs; 2005. https://www.casey.org/northwest-alumni-study/.
19. Dworsky A, Courtney ME. Assessing the impact of extended care beyond 18 on homelessness: emerging findings from the midwest study. Chicago: Chapin Hall at the University of Chicago; 2010.
20. Courtney ME, Dworsky A, Peters CM. California's fostering connections to success act and the costs and benefits of extending foster care to 21. Partners for Our Children Seattle; 2009.
21. Munson MBS, Spencer R, et al. Supportive relationships among former system youth with mental health challenges. J Adolesc Res. 2015;30(4):501–29.
22. Villegas S, Pecora PJ. Mental health outcomes for adults in family foster care as children: an analysis by ethnicity. Child Youth Serv Rev. 2012;34(8):1448–58.
23. Zlotnick C, Tam TW, Soman LA. Life course outcomes on mental and physical health: the impact of foster care on adulthood. Am J Public Health. 2012;102(3):534–40.
24. Collins JL, Jimenez R, Thomas LJ. Health out of foster care as young adults age out of foster care: a

phenomenological exploration of seeking healthcare services after aging out of the US foster care system. Child Abuse Negl. 2018;81:322–31.
25. Dworsky A, Napolitano L, Courtney M. Homelessness during the transition from foster care to adulthood. Am J Public Health. 2013;103(Suppl 2):S318–23.
26. Brown A, et al. Behavioral health needs and service use among those who've aged-out of foster care. Child Youth Serv Rev. 2015;58:163–9.
27. Pecora PJ, Jensen PS, Romanelli LH, Jackson LJ, Ortiz A. Mental health services for children placed in foster care: an overview of current challenges. Child Welfare. 2009;88(1):5–26.
28. Farmer EMZ, Burns BJ, Chapman MV, et al. Use of mental health services by youth in contact with social services. Soc Serv Rev. 2001;75(4):605–24.
29. Shin S. Need for and actual use of mental health service by adolescents in the child welfare system. Child Youth Serv Rev. 2005;27(10):1071–83.
30. Leslie LK, Hurlburt MS, James S, Landsverk J, Slymen DJ, Zhang J. Relationship between entry into child welfare and mental health service use. Psychiatr Serv. 2005;56(8):981–7.
31. Courtney ME, Piliavin I, Grogan-Kaylor A, et al. Foster youth transitions to adulthood: a longitudinal view of youth leaving care. Child Welfare. 2001;80(6):685–718.
32. U.S. Department of Health & Human Services, Substance Abuse and Mental Health Services Administration. National survey on drug use and health; 2014. http://www.samhsa.gov/data/release/2014-national-survey-drug-use-and-health-nsduh-releases.
33. Vaughn MG, Ollie MT, McMillen JC, Scott L Jr, Munson M. Substance use and abuse among older youth in foster care. Addict Behav. 2007;32(9):1929–35.
34. White CR, O'Brien K, White J, Pecora PJ, Phillips CM. Alcohol and drug use among alumni of foster care: decreasing dependency through improvement of foster care experiences. J Behav Health Serv Res. 2008;35(4):419–34.
35. Maliszewski G, Brown C. Familism, substance abuse, and sexual risk foster care alumni. Child Youth Serv Rev. 2014;36:206–12.
36. Raghavan R, Zima BT, Andersen RM, Leibowitz AA, Schuster MA, Landsverk J. Psychotropic medication use in a national probability sample of children in the child welfare system. J Child Adolesc Psychopharmacol. 2005;15(1):97–106.
37. Rubin D, Matone M, Muang YS, et al. Interstate variation in trends of psychotropic medication use among Medicaid-enrolled children in foster care. Child Youth Serv Rev. 2012;34:1492–9.
38. Zito JM, Safer DJ, Sai D, Gardner JF, Thomas D, Coombes P, et al. Psychotropic medication patterns among youth in foster care. Pediatrics. 2008;121(1):e157–63.
39. Brenner P, Alexanderson K, Bjorkenstam C, Hillert J, Jokinen J, Mittendorfer-Rutz E, et al. Psychiatric diagnoses, medication and risk for disability pension in multiple sclerosis patients; a population-based register study. PLoS One. 2014;9(8):e104165.
40. Allaire BT, Raghavan R, Brown DS. Morbid obesity and use of second generation antipsychotics among adolescents in foster care: evidence from medicaid. Child Youth Serv Rev. 2016;67:27–31.
41. Crystal S, Mackie T, Fenton MC, Amin S, Neese-Todd S, Olfson M, et al. Rapid growth of antipsychotic prescriptions for children who are publicly insured has ceased, but concerns remain. Health Aff (Millwood). 2016;35(6):974–82.
42. McMillen JC, Narendorf SC, Robinson D, Havlicek J, Fedoravicius N, Bertram J, et al. Development and piloting of a treatment foster care program for older youth with psychiatric problems. Child Adolesc Psychiatry Ment Health. 2015;9:23.
43. Havlicek J. Lives in motion: a review of former foster youth in the context of their experiences in the child welfare system. Child Youth Serv Rev. 2011;33(7):1090–100.
44. Weiner D, Schneider A, Lyons JS. Evidence-based treatments for trauma among culturally diverse foster care youth: treatment retention and outcomes. Child Youth Serv Rev. 2009;31:1199–205.
45. Cohen JA, Mannarino AP, Perel JM, Staron V. A pilot randomized controlled trial of combined trauma-focused CBT and sertraline for childhood PTSD symptoms. J Am Acad Child Adolesc Psychiatry. 2007;46(7):811–9.
46. Felitti VJ, Anda RF, Nordenberg D, Williamson DF, Spitz AM, Edwards V, et al. Relationship of childhood abuse and household dysfunction to many of the leading causes of death in adults. The Adverse Childhood Experiences (ACE) Study. Am J Prev Med. 1998;14(4):245–58.
47. Merrick MT, Ports KA, Ford DC, Afifi TO, Gershoff ET, Grogan-Kaylor A. Unpacking the impact of adverse childhood experiences on adult mental health. Child Abuse Negl. 2017;69:10–9.
48. Rebbe R, Nurius PS, Courtney ME, Ahrens KR. Adverse childhood experiences and young adult health outcomes among youth aging out of foster care. Acad Pediatr. 2018;18(5):502–9.
49. Shonkoff JP, Garner AS, Committee on Psychosocial Aspects of C, Family H, Committee on Early Childhood A, Dependent C, et al. The lifelong effects of early childhood adversity and toxic stress. Pediatrics. 2012;129(1):e232–46.
50. Anda RF, Felitti VJ, Bremner JD, Walker JD, Whitfield C, Perry BD, et al. The enduring effects of abuse and related adverse experiences in childhood. A convergence of evidence from neurobiology and epidemiology. Eur Arch Psychiatry Clin Neurosci. 2006;256(3):174–86.
51. Nugent NR, Goldberg A, Uddin M. Topical review: the emerging field of epigenetics: informing models of pediatric trauma and physical health. J Pediatr Psychol. 2016;41(1):55–64.

52. Forkey H, Szilagyi M. Foster care and healing from complex childhood trauma. Pediatr Clin N Am. 2014;61(5):1059–72.
53. Melkman EP. Childhood adversity, social support networks and well-being among youth aging out of care: an exploratory study of mediation. Child Abuse Negl. 2017;72:85–97.
54. Perry JC, Sigal JJ, Boucher S, Pare N. Seven institutionalized children and their adaptation in late adulthood: the children of Duplessis (Les Enfants de Duplessis). Psychiatry. 2006;69(4):283–301.
55. Collins ME, Spencer R, Ward R. Supporting youth in the transition from foster care: formal and informal connections. Child Welfare. 2010;89(1):125–43.
56. Keller TE, Cusick GR, Courtney ME. Approaching the transition to adulthood: distinctive profiles of adolescents aging out of the child welfare system. Soc Serv Rev. 2007;81(3):453–84.
57. Courtney METS, Bost N, et al. Midwest evaluation of the adult functioning of former foster youth: conditions of youth preparing to leave state care. Chicago: Chapin Hall Center for Children, University of Chicago; 2004.
58. Greeson JKP, Treglia D, Wolfe DS, Wasch S, Gelles RJ. Child welfare characteristics in a sample of youth involved in commercial sex: an exploratory study. Child Abuse Negl. 2019;94:104038.
59. Ahrens KR, Katon W, McCarty C, Richardson LP, Courtney ME. Association between childhood sexual abuse and transactional sex in youth aging out of foster care. Child Abuse Negl. 2012;36(1):75–80.
60. Lee RD, Fang X, Luo F. The impact of parental incarceration on the physical and mental health of young adults. Pediatrics. 2013;131(4):e1188–95.
61. Shaw TV, Bright CL, Sharpe TL. Child welfare outcomes for youth in care as a result of parental death or parental incarceration. Child Abuse Negl. 2015;42:112–20.
62. Lee T, Fouras G, Brown R, American Academy of C, Adolescent Psychiatry Committee on Quality I. Practice parameter for the assessment and management of youth involved with the child welfare system. J Am Acad Child Adolesc Psychiatry. 2015;54(6):502–17.
63. Masten AS. Ordinary magic. Resilience processes in development. Am Psychol. 2001;56(3):227–38.
64. Ungar M. Resilience after maltreatment: the importance of social services as facilitators of positive adaptation. Child Abuse Negl. 2013;37(2–3):110–5.
65. Courtney ME, Hook JL, Lee JS. Distinct subgroups of former foster youth during the transition to adulthood: implications for policy and practice. Chicago: Chapin Hall at the University of Chicago; 2010.
66. Hook JL, Courtney ME. Employment of former foster youth as young adults: evidence from the Midwest study. Chicago: Chapin Hall at the University of Chicago; 2011.
67. Munson MR, Smalling SE, Spencer R, Scott LD, Tracy E. A steady presence in the midst of change: non-kin natural mentors in the lives of older youth exiting foster care. Child Youth Serv Rev. 2010;32(4):527–35.
68. Casey Family Programs. Casey life skills https://www.casey.org/casey-life-skills-resources/2013. Available from: www.casey.org/casey-life-skills-resources.
69. California Evidence-Based Clearinghouse for Child Welfare. Youth transitioning into adulthood programs http://www.cebc4cw.org/topic/youth-transitioning-into-adulthood/. Available from: http://www.cebc4cw.org/topic/youth-transitioning-into-adulthood/.
70. Geenen S, Powers LE, Phillips LA, Nelson M, McKenna J, Winges-Yanez N, et al. Better futures: a randomized field test of a model for supporting young people in foster care with mental health challenges to participate in higher education. J Behav Health Serv Res. 2015;42(2):150–71.
71. Thompson AE, Greeson JKP, Brunsink A. Natural mentoring among youth in and aging out of foster care: a systematic review. Child Youth Serv Rev. 2016;61:40–50.
72. California Evidence-Based Clearing House for Child Welfare. My first place. https://www.cebc4cw.org/program/my-first-place/. Available from: https://www.cebc4cw.org/program/my-first-place/.
73. Loke V, Choi L, Libby M. Increasing youth financial capability: an evaluation of the MyPath Savings initiative. J Consum Aff. 2015;49:97–126.
74. Salazar AM, Haggerty KP, Roe SS. Fostering higher education: a postsecondary access and retention intervention for youth with foster care experience. Child Youth Serv Rev. 2016;70:46–56.
75. Salazar AM. Supporting college success in foster care alumni: salient factors related to postsecondary retention. Child Welfare. 2012;91(5):139–67.
76. Casey Family Programs. Supporting success: improving higher education outcomes for students from foster care; 2010. https://www.casey.org/supporting-success/.
77. Unrau Y. From foster care to college: the Seita scholars' program at Western Michigan University. Reclaiming Child Youth. 2011;20:17–20.
78. California Evidence-Based Clearinghouse for Child Welfare. Independent living program-orangewood. http://www.cebc4cw.org/program/independent-living-program-orangewood.
79. Osgood DW, Foster EM, Courtney ME. Vulnerable populations and the transition to adulthood. Futur Child. 2010;20(1):209–29.
80. Institute of Medicine, Council NR. Investing in the health and well-being of young adults. Washington D.C.: The National Academies Press; 2015.
81. National Conference of State Legislatures. Extending foster care beyond 18. https://www.ncsl.org/research/human-services/extending-foster-care-to-18.aspx2017.

23 Medical Leave of Absence

Parna Prajapati, Anisha Garg, and Bela Sood

Key Points

- Medical leaves of absence allow college students the opportunity to pause their education when necessary to focus on recovery from a mental health condition.
- Colleges differ in their approach to MLOA, and students, families, and providers may need to be proactive to be sure to follow the procedure and minimize disruptions or financial ramifications.
- Universities prefer not to mandate that students take LOA but reserve the right to do so when a student is refusing to withdraw and is exhibiting worrisome behavior that presents a risk to the campus community.
- Early interventions allow the student to connect to appropriate treatment and accommodations and may prevent the need for MLOA.

Case Example 1

Ron is a 19-year-old college freshman, with a history of depression and anxiety, who started his engineering undergraduate education at a reputable university. He was diagnosed with both these disorders in the preadolescent years and was stabilized on a combination of antidepressant medication and psychosocial interventions. Due to his performance during college interviews and his perceived mental health stability, his family supported a decision to stop counseling but to continue medication only with his long-standing treating psychiatrist. The mental health providers were agreeable with this plan but advised that he restart on-campus counseling if the need arose. Ron started college with excitement and energy. Although his family was well-off financially, he took up a part-time job on the weekends to have additional spending money. The stress of managing academics and his work gradually became crippling. He realized he was experiencing loss of pleasure in his hobbies; his grades were drop-

P. Prajapati (✉) · B. Sood
Virginia Commonwealth University, Department of Psychiatry, Division of Child & Adolescent Psychiatry, Richmond, VA, USA
e-mail: parna.prajapati@vcuhealth.org; bela.sood@vcuhealth.org

A. Garg
Children's Hospital of the King's Daughter, Division of Psychiatry and Psychology, Norfolk, VA, USA
e-mail: anisha.garg@chkd.org

V. Chan, J. Derenne (eds.), *Transition-Age Youth Mental Health Care*,
https://doi.org/10.1007/978-3-030-62113-1_23

ping, and he was losing hope – all familiar emotions for him from the past. In addition, the stress of perceived stigma associated with mental illness made it difficult for him to seek academic accommodations. Ron wanted desperately to appear to "fit in" with his peers. He would not discuss his unhappiness with his roommate and had no other supports in place. He missed his psychiatry appointments due to scheduling conflicts with his classes. While he was able to continue taking his antidepressant medication, he had difficulty accessing a psychotherapy appointment. The student counseling center had a 4-week wait, and he was limited to six counseling sessions. He was referred to a community provider to continue treatment, but felt increasingly isolated and unsupported. He scheduled a meeting with his advisor to discuss his options, as he wondered whether he should take some time off to focus on mental health treatment.

Case Example 2

Julia is an 18-year-old female with a history of bipolar disorder, attention-deficit/hyperactivity disorder (ADHD), and post-traumatic stress disorder (PTSD) who was stabilized on multiple medications and weekly counseling. She was accepted to a local college which was her top choice. However, she received a scholarship that allowed her to go to school in another state. Family members who lived nearby were willing to offer support, but she did not tell them about her history. Due to the severity of her symptoms and poor compliance with her medication regimen, she required three acute care inpatient hospitalizations within a month of starting college. She chose to ask the college for a "regular sick leave" and did not request a medical leave of absence. She is now wondering whether her scholarship will be affected.

Introduction

The transition to adulthood involves struggle and searching for independence, autonomy, and consolidating adult identity. Each choice, such as enrolling in an Institute of Higher Education (IHE), entering the workforce, or remaining at home, carries its own set of challenges. Often, the transition ends by entering the workforce and becoming financially independent. However, a young adult attending college can be in an "in-between" developmental stage. College youth may still be financially dependent on parents but also drift away from parental influence as they explore new relationships and experiences. Especially for youth with preexisting mental health issues, this transition phase poses a lot of challenges [1]. The freedom that comes with adulthood also carries the risk of a sense of insecurity for youth who are attempting to become socially adept, fit in with peers, and learn different skill sets [1].

Mental Health Concerns in IHEs

College mental health-related issues are on the rise, and there is a clear need to provide extensive mental health support on campus since a growing number of students with mental health needs now attend college [2]. A majority of the college counseling center directors reported having more students with greater mental health-related issues on their campuses, and the trend is moving upward. Suicide is the second leading cause of death among the young adult from age 18 to 22 years, claiming 3375 deaths just in 2018 [3]. A 2010 study found 1100 completed suicides on college campuses every year [4]. The American College Health Association survey in 2019 indicated that 17% of male students and 21% of female students in colleges surveyed felt disabling depression, with over 50% receiving both prescription medicine and psychotherapy in the last 12 months of the survey. The National Alliance on Mental Illness survey conducted in 2012 on more than 700 college students across 48 states and the District of Columbia provided alarming results of student disclosures [2]. While 73% of students experienced some form of crisis while in college, 35% did not report it to college officials due to one or more reasons. The most cited reason by students was they found a lack of mental health awareness and education in faculty, staff, and students [2]. This lack of confidence in the university's support of mental wellness and awareness of illness can have a tremendous impact on early identification, early self-disclosure, and receiving proper care.

A majority of students experience some form of stress as they enter college life, and there are services directed toward supporting students through challenging situations. Many stressors fall into the category of adjustment issues. These include incompatibility with a suite or roommate, challenges around nutrition and food, budgeting money, and acclimating to new local resources. While most of these adjustment-type problems settle down after the first few months of this transition, some students struggle with issues that rise to the level of a mental health disorder. Research shows that a mental health diagnosis is most associated with the failure to complete a college education [5]. Depending on the socioemotional maturity of the student, a lack of awareness of one's own strengths and weaknesses can have varying effects. Students may have unrealistic ideas about the adjustment to college life and poor preparation to handle challenges when they do appear. The perceived stigma of accessing on-campus mental health providers can lead students to postpone care, resulting in functional deterioration. While an IHE counseling center can serve the population who self-identify, are willing to seek assistance, and are motivated to be healthy, it does not serve that population which chooses not to seek assistance for mental health reasons. College youth are a specifically vulnerable group subject to several risk factors responsible for the emergence of mental health problems. This age group is in the midst of achieving independence in decision-making, managing finances, and staying on top of academic expectations. They are also in the midst of psychological separation and individuation from their parents. The literature suggests that roughly 50% of all lifetime mental disorders start by the mid-teens and 75% by the mid-20s [6].

Incoming freshmen who have preexisting healthcare needs may be at even greater risk of ongoing challenges. Disability-related accommodations in IHE are optimally self-requested. Treating providers should initiate conversation about this topic well in advance of the college application process. The IHE is not obliged to provide support if a student does not self-identify. Students may not know that they can receive accommodations for physical or mental health concerns. . Although the types of accommodations differ from what is available in high school, the Americans with Disabilities Act and its amendments [7] does not allow any kind of discrimination against individuals, including students (Title II for publicly funded institutions and Title III for privately funded institutions) [8]. The majority of disability-qualified students are unaware that they are entitled to these accommodations. Those who recognize their right to accommodations often do not utilize them due to perceived public or personal stigma [9]. This can be a huge risk factor for students needing a LOA in a time of crisis.

Information sharing and help-seeking behaviors can be especially challenging for those with mental health needs. These challenges include finding willing and trained providers on or near campus, complying with regular mental health provider visits, ensuring the quality of interventions (both psychosocial and psychopharmacological), and early identification of deterioration of functioning, with prompt access to services when in crisis. Adding to the challenge is the fact that students need to do these things independently while navigating academic progress in a new environment.

In the presence of environmental stressors, a biological propensity for mental and physical health challenges can [10] create a perfect storm for the appearance of health emergencies. Parents who do not live nearby may be unaware of developing crises. Even with regular communication, parents may be unable to detect regression in their child (slow to rapid decline). If the decline is rapid, the student may be unable to continue with the semester. Knowledge about what recourse they have and what the IHE offers in the way of support could prevent failure in the long term (e.g., dropping out of college permanently). When students utilize a well-designed medical leave of absence (MLOA) that has clear guidelines and procedures for reentry, the university may see a clear impact on student retention, and this may subsequently increase their college graduation rates.

What are the ways IHEs can be helpful to students who are struggling with acute or chronic health conditions that interfere with their academic progress? Other chapters discuss the university counseling center and student health services resources available on most university campuses. This chapter will discuss and provide the reader with a road map for tools available to undergraduate and graduate students in academic distress because of a health emergency. A medical leave of absence (MLOA or LOA) allows the student time to manage the crisis and return to the university when healthy and ready to re-enroll. MLOAs are generally overseen by the office of student affairs with the intention to reintegrate the student back into the academic environment once they have safely made it through the acute crisis and early recovery phases. This chapter identifies essential elements of MLOA guidelines and describes a number of college programs to provide examples of what may be available to struggling students.

Types of Withdrawals

Universities should develop a frame for an LOA that is proactive and preventative, in order to optimize utilization and reduce barriers to dealing with health emergencies which can derail education. Following the development of such a frame, the university administration should disseminate this information and available resources to staff/faculty, advisors, and the student body in regular intervals. When the information and plans are clearly defined, easy to find, and a regular part of orientation for faculty and students, the MLOA process is far easier to navigate.

More often than not, the concepts of "leave" and being "sick" inherently carry a negative connotation that one is deficient or unable to complete an academic goal in the usual manner. Negative labels, such as "academically weak," or "unable to handle college," can become secondary stressors. The internal conflict of acknowledging challenges and limitations while aspiring to become a successful, independent adult has the potential to seriously undermine self-concept and confidence. Asking for a medical leave of absence for mental health-related issues can damage self-esteem and exaggerate the youth's primary illness. Recognizing these issues, universities should create a culture wherein requesting a LOA is seen as a sign of strength. Incentives to promote help seeking can be built in to encourage proactive and timely utilization of these resources.

Withdrawals can be loosely categorized based on cause or on the manner of withdrawal.

1. *Cause of the withdrawal:*
   (a) "Primary" due to direct effect of mental health-related issues (e.g., anxiety, substance use, depression)
   (b) "Secondary" related to the psychological effects of a primary (non-mental) health-related issue (e.g., poorly controlled diabetes, mild traumatic brain injury)
   (c) "Tertiary" related to stress stemming from the psychological effects of being sick (e.g., stigma of mental health-related issues, the stress of "catching up" with school work, financial burden)
2. *Manner of the withdrawal:*
   (a) Voluntary: initiated by the student.
   (b) Involuntary withdrawal: university initiates the process due to severe aggression, substance use, violation of campus rules, etc.

Risk Factors for Voluntary LOA

Figure 23.1 depicts factors contributing to success versus failure on individual, family, and institutional levels (Fig. 23.1). Following that is a short list of risk factors for voluntary withdrawal from IHEs.

1. Individual:
   (a) Existing mental health diagnosis prior to college entry: the majority of the students who require voluntary LOA have a mental health diagnosis even before entering the IHE. Insight into one's illness and the need for additional support largely deter-

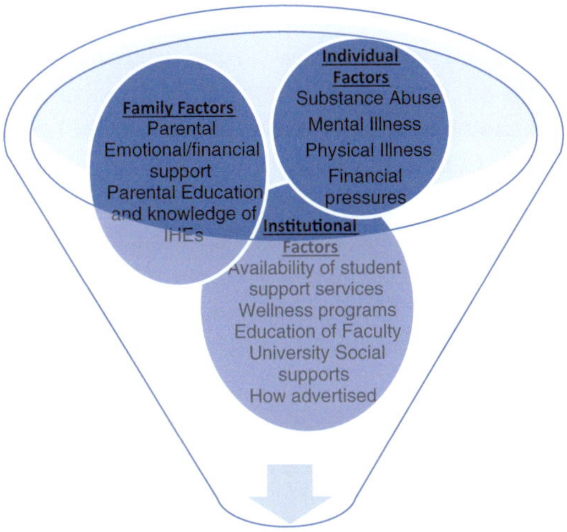

Fig. 23.1 Student success vs. failure

mine whether a student will request a LOA.

(b) Substance use: substance use among college youth is a very common problem, and it is increasing. There is evidence that leaving high school serves as a risk factor for substance use initiation as compared to entering college which may somewhat mitigate risk for SUD [11]. Treatment of substance use disorders often requires full-time engagement in a residential treatment program.

(c) Executive functioning skills: students struggling with disorganization, poor planning, and impulsive decision-making may not request or implement accommodations when indicated.

2. Family and friends:

(a) Parental/caregiver support and educational level: families with a poor level of connectedness may be inconsistent in their support for their offspring during crises. Timely help from family members who are knowledgeable about navigating the system may prevent the worsening of health problems and reduce the need to obtain an LOA.

(b) Financial stress: families with financial issues may face additional stress when students have to work to support themselves. They may have chosen to do so without an awareness that academic performance and mental health could be affected by work commitments.

(c) Local networks (friends, activities, and clubs): students who do not have local support in either family members or friends are at a greater risk of feeling isolated. Development of a network of friends, with the university providing formal and informal avenues for socialization, can meet the developmental needs of the transitional age youth.

3. Institution:

(a) Availability of on-campus mental health resources: the availability of mental health counseling resources on campus can vary by the university. Readily available on-campus providers allow students to easily access care with clinicians who are familiar with the university environment and common stressors.

(b) Availability of wellness programs: the availability of wellness programs may depend on campus leadership recognizing the importance of prevention. Institutions can offer courses in positive psychology (e.g., "How to Thrive," "Science of Happiness"), yoga, and meditation which can count toward a minor or a credit course. Outreach programs can normalize and encourage students to incorporate wellness practices into their everyday living.

(c) Training and education of faculty and staff: training of faculty and staff to recognize students struggling and triaging them appropriately without needing to be experts in mental health or wellness could be a university-wide goal to increase early identification of students who may need modifications to their schedule.

Early Identification and Interventions

Serious mental illness needs prompt attention to manage the acute event and, in turn, prevent secondary morbidities and acute health emergencies. Prompt identification and early interventions can be challenging as they are dependent not only on an individual's abilities but also awareness and accessibility to supportive people. If an individual is staying on campus, their roommate or a neighboring student can play a vital role in identifying social isolation, changes in behavior, and unsafe actions. Resident assistants (RAs) can also be an invaluable help in recognizing problems as well as serving as a resource, friend, and mentor for the struggling student. Academic professionals, such as advisors, professors, and teaching assistants, can also identify early signs and symptoms of deterioration or crisis.

Typically, students feel stigmatized and are wary of disclosing their mental health-related struggles at the college level due to several factors [9]. In turn, specific cultural norms dictate that boundaries of personal privacy are respected, and the belief that "one minds one's own business" may make it difficult for peers to determine when they should raise concerns about a peer. If education, awareness around mental health, and well-being are commonly discussed topics in the climate of an IHE, the taboo about addressing these issues can be mitigated.

The Process (Fig. 23.2)

When a situation arises that impacts a student's education secondary to health issues, the decision to prioritize one's health is paramount. A medical leave of absence provides a student with the ability to take voluntary leave from academic pressures in order to prioritize their physical and psychological health by getting appropriate treatment. LOA includes both physical and mental health concerns, in addition to other extenuating circumstances such as leave for military deployment. When considering taking a medical leave of absence, the student should first review the policy, often stated on the school website. The student should also meet with their academic advisor prior to completing any necessary forms. The advisor should be able to provide guidance and discuss the options available, depending on the needs of the student. The family may need consultation about financial impact and registration status. The withdrawal process may include completing an LOA form, writing a brief personal statement, and having documentation from their treating healthcare provider indicating the student's current diagnosis and need for treatment. Students should be aware of the time (e.g., middle of quarter, 2 weeks after midsemester) they have to voluntarily withdraw from enrollment (for nonmedical reasons) without financial penalties. Each university determines this time differently.

Ideally, medical leave of absence should be an option available at all higher levels of education institutions. A published survey of over 700 college students conducted by Gruttadaro et al. [2] found that 46% of the students felt that medical

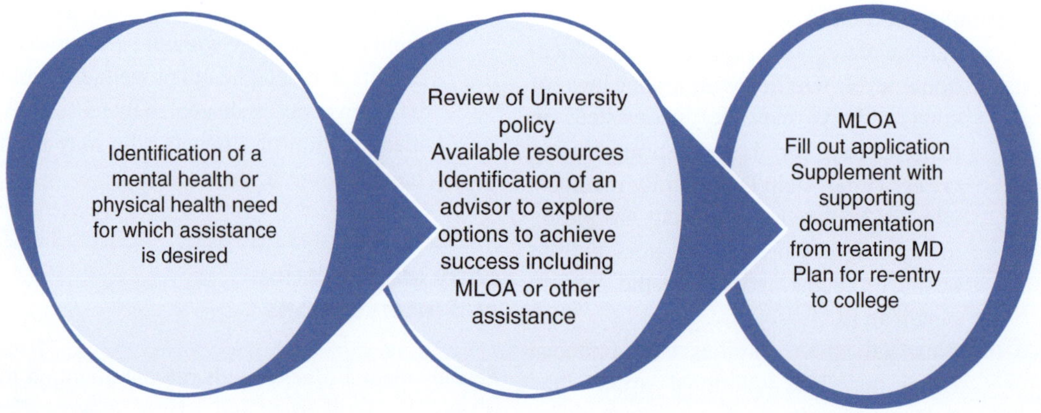

Fig. 23.2 General steps for MLOA

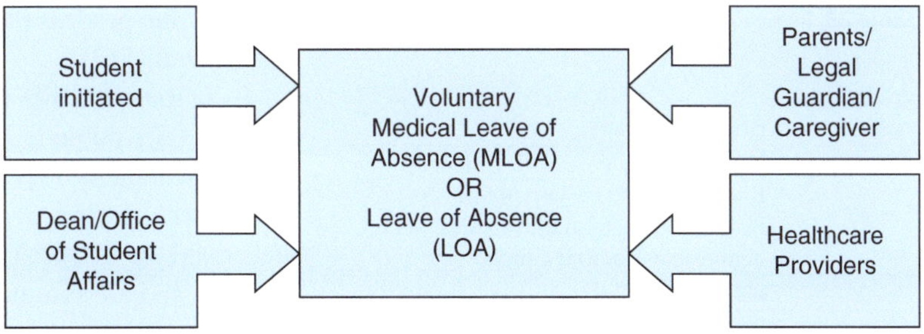

Fig. 23.3 Individual/entity commonly initiating leave of absence (LOA)

leave of absence is a critical accommodation for their success in college. Others identified help with leave of absence and returning to school after an absence being a critical support [2]. LOA should cover both mental and physical health crises that are interfering with education. Policies need to be clearly outlined and explained in an easily accessible manner. These policies need to clearly define the process of exploring LOA, seeking other options or accommodations, and, finally, the application and reinstatement process. Students in the midst of a mental health crisis are in need of support from staff, faculty, and administration. Each individual's situation is unique in its challenges and therefore requires an independent evaluation to gain understanding and intervene appropriately. Presenting various options allows the student to have autonomy, which is an important principle consistent with the ethics of making such a decision. Figure 23.3 depicts the possible involved parties contributing to LOA/MLOA decisions (Fig. 23.3).

LOA can be initiated by the student, guardian, college, or healthcare professional. By far, the students are the most common initiator, as they have the greatest experience into the academic risk their instability, albeit temporary, is posing for them. At times, a faculty member or employer-level concern can initiate a LOA request based on outlier behavior, performance, or code of conduct violations. In the latter scenario, the process would be explained by the academic advisor.

Once these requests are formally submitted, they are typically handled by the Division of Student Affairs at most universities (see Table 23.1). Often, these requests are processed with the help of the IHE's health center. According to an interview with the Associate Vice Provost at Virginia Commonwealth University, schools will sometimes use experts within the mental health field who work at the university health/counseling center to assess the student, determine if students meet the criteria for LOA, and finally provide recommendations for seeking treatment (R. Rodriguez, personal communication, November 14, 2019). Concerns often brought up when taking a LOA include falling behind in coursework, losing financial aid, losing on-campus housing, and losing scholarship support [12]. Along with consulting the academic advisor, the student should interface with the financial aid office and housing office to gain information and understand the implication of withdrawal. In many cases, when LOA is approved, the student will be refunded tuition for the current semester or quarter in which they are enrolled, with resumption of enrollment upon returning to school. This can vary depending on the IHE's refund policy [13]. The withdrawn student is not allowed to partake in school activities nor continue living in on-campus housing when disenrolled and will, therefore, require other living options. It also is important to note that once the LOA is granted, the student's transcript may often display some type of notation indicating withdrawal. However, no reasoning for the withdrawal is generally documented on the academic record, protecting the student's right to privacy [13].

Often, leadership in student affairs offices suggests that other interventions be explored before going for a LOA, e.g., accommodations in classes to meet the immediate academic needs of the student, fast-tracking a student for counseling services or mental health evaluation [13, 14]. In other words, academic leadership is keen

Table 23.1 Key of surveyed universities

University (coded by colors)	Brief description
Blue	Virginia Commonwealth University, Richmond, VA; eastern public institution, doctoral universities: very high research activity, high undergraduate, 4-year, large, primarily nonresidential
Green	Midwest public institution, doctoral universities: very high research activity, majority undergraduate, four-year, large, highly residential
Red	Eastern private institution, doctoral universities: very high research activity, majority undergraduate, four-year, large, highly residential
Orange	Southern public institution, doctoral universities: very high research activity, high undergraduate, 4-year, large, primarily nonresidential
Yellow	Western public institution, doctoral universities: very high research activity, majority undergraduate, 4-year, large, highly residential
Brown	Eastern public institution, doctoral universities: very high research activity, high undergraduate, 4-year, large, primarily residential
Purple	Eastern public institution, doctoral universities: very high research activity, high undergraduate, 4-year, large, primarily nonresidential
White	Northern public institution, doctoral universities: very high research activity, high undergraduate, 4-year, large, primarily residential
Pink	Western public institution, doctoral universities: very high research activity, majority undergraduate, 4-year, large, primarily residential
Black	Western public institution, doctoral universities: very high research activity, high undergraduate, 4-year, large, primarily residential
Indigo	Western private institution, doctoral universities: very high research activity, majority graduate, 4-year, large, highly residential

to keep the student on campus and to collaboratively work toward restabilization. Depending on university policy, safeguards for students may vary. Some public universities go to great lengths to make their policies about MLOA available to students, with a procedure in place to make the process predictable and transparent for students [13].

In preparation for this chapter, authors also viewed IHE publicly available website content about involuntary leave to gain a student/parent/consumer perspective. Two IHEs clearly described the MLOA/LOA process at the time of viewing and are summarized here.

Virginia Commonwealth University (VCU) https://dos.vcu.edu/services/medical-leave-of-absence/

The MLOA/DOA website clearly outlines the three steps for MLOA: (1) completing the MLOA Form, (2) Form Review, and (3) MLOA meeting. It also outlines a three-step MLOA reinstatement process and includes considerations, checklists, and additional resources for those considering MLOA.

VCU advises the student to review the MLOA policy, meet with an academic advisor, and to meet with a financial aid counselor prior to applying for MLOA. The process begins when the student first petitions the Dean of Students (DOS) Office in the Division of Student Affairs at VCU for a medical leave of absence from all courses. This must occur prior to the last day of classes and before a final grade has been posted. The petitioner is required to complete the MLOA form, which encompasses supporting evidence from the treating provider. Next, the form will be reviewed by a staff member to ensure it meets MLOA criteria. When the criteria are met, a meeting is scheduled with the student to discuss their planned medical leave. During this meeting, information is provided regarding MLOA, the reinstatement/re-enrollment process, and the conditions that need to be met in order to be reinstated. In order to be reinstated, evidence must be provided to prove readiness of return. This includes a completed Provider MLOA Reinstatement form, which is a letter of support from one's treating healthcare provider. After this is completed, the documentation will be reviewed by the DOS office in consultation with Student Accessibility and Educational Opportunity, Division of Academic Success, University

Student Health Services, and/or University Counseling Services. If not enrolled for three consecutive semesters, the student will have to reapply for admission. The student may be required to undergo an independent evaluation by a medical and/or psychological professional who is assigned by the university, if needed. If concerns exist that a student presents a significant risk to the safety of others within the VCU community, the DOS office may insist that the student take an administrative leave. The student may then appeal this decision.

There have been very few cases in which a student has been requested to take leave due to failure to uphold the student code of conduct (R. Rodriguez, personal communication, November 14, 2019). The counseling service opposes forced leave and encourages students to obtain assistance while remaining enrolled whenever safely possible. Each semester, VCU is expected to grant, on average, 50–70 MLOA. (Unusually, the DOS office had received less than 50 requests by the time of interview in midsemester.) It is estimated that approximately 75% of the LOA requests pertain to mental health reasons (R. Rodriguez, personal communication, November 14, 2019). The respondent was unable to provide demographic information about students requesting MLOA, as this is the first year that MLOA has been undertaken centrally by the Division of Student Affairs. Previously, MLOA was handled by each student's respective academic college (e.g., life sciences, art, business, etc.) through the Academic Regulations Appeals Committee (ARAC). This was changed to a centralized DOS review in order to expedite the process and to improve consistency with expectations and rights of students.

New York University (NYU) https://www.nyu.edu/about/policies-guidelines-compliance/policies-and-guidelines/student-leave-policy.html

On this website, NYU defines voluntary leave and procedures, and return from voluntary leave/reinstatement, and its associated procedures. It does the same for involuntary leave and also organizes other leave categories, like study abroad/study away. A search on the NYU site about personal or MLOA links users to content more specific to visa and enrollment criteria for international students.

The university recommends that the student discuss LOA with their academic advisor prior to withdrawing. A completed LOA form is submitted to NYU's Albert Student Center. The LOA request is then sent to the Department of Students (DOS) office for review and approval. The DOS office consults with the director of Counseling and Behavioral Health Services, or the medical director of the Student Health Center, depending on whether the reason is psychological or medical. An independent evaluation with the Counseling and Wellness Services may also be required, depending on the student's needs. DOS will then approve or deny the request and discuss the associated conditions. Conditions can include seeking treatment (medications and/or therapy services), leaving on-campus housing, writing a personal statement, etc. When considering reinstatement, individuals on leave must notify the DOS office 6 weeks before the start of the semester of intended return. An independent assessment interview by the Counseling and Wellness Services is required along with a completed "Certificate of Readiness to Return" from the treating provider. This independent evaluator from the Counseling and Behavioral Health Service will then provide their recommendations to the Dean regarding the student's ability to return and be successful. When requesting leave, a student is allowed a minimum of one semester (4 months) to a maximum of two semesters (8 months). Individuals who are denied a leave extension or who do not to enroll for the returned term approved by the dean are required to reapply for admission. If denied return, a petitioner has the option to appeal the decision.

In comparison, involuntary leave of absence occurs when the administration considers a student to pose a threat or is a danger to themselves or others. A student may be required to undergo an independent evaluation by the director of Counseling and Wellness Services in this case.

Administrative Considerations to LOA

Highly proactive IHEs will routinely engage the university's legal counsel in LOA/MLOA decisions to ensure an ethical and equitable approach. However, other universities may not have such safeguards. For example, private colleges may have fewer protections, and a student can be asked to leave after an involuntary LOA [15].

Lived experience can also have a major impact on university procedures. As an example, at initiation, Virginia Commonwealth University MLOAs were granted at the discretion of individual academic schools (e.g., business, engineering) within the university. This created different rules differently interpreted within each of the schools. In 2019, VCU centralized the oversight of MLOA to the Dean of Student Affairs to consolidate uniform, equitable process (R. Rodriguez, personal communication, November 14, 2019; unreferenced). The reviewing body reviews the form to evaluate appropriateness of the MLOA, or whether some other intervention is in order (such as counseling finding support within the university, to overcome challenges). The Dean of Student Affairs also ensures that the MLOA is not being requested to avoid an adverse outcome such as expulsion from the university for other reasons. As of the time of publication, the university will assess the first centralized cohort and will evaluate if the standardized approach has changed reinstatement outcomes, as well improved faculty and student satisfaction with the process.

Involuntary leave generally occurs when faculty or peers raise an alarm regarding behavior that is inconsistent with student code of conduct, or behavior that is bizarre or threatening [16]. Generally, well-informed faculty know to contact the Student Affairs Office or the school's behavioral intervention team to raise their concerns, while a peer might speak to a resident assistant (RA) who may escalate the concern up to the Dean of Student Affairs. For some universities, the Dean of Student Affairs Office will have a behavioral intervention team or threat assessment team that includes representation from the university communication team, campus law enforcement, university counseling services, legal counsel, faculty from the office of student conduct office, a human resources representative, and, sometimes, even the president of the university [16]. The unifying characteristic of these teams is the multiple departments that are represented for consensus decision-making. These threat assessment teams often meet regularly. Threat assessment is a topic that has garnered national interest after the Virginia Tech massacre, and universities across the nation have developed teams to prevent sentinel events from occurring on campus. At best, threat assessment teams are well connected locally and nationally to agencies such as the FBI and state police who can provide them with more information about possible threats that those agencies pick up through social media [17]. In addition to threat assessment teams, universities have also begun to develop care teams which oversee students who are referred for mental health concerns or aberrant behaviors. The care team often meets regularly and may flag certain students for review by the threat assessment team [16].

Reinstatement

If the student is seeking to return to the same IHE, the reinstatement process can be similar to the withdrawal process in reverse. As in the case of applying for leave, a student may need to complete a reinstatement form and provide documentation from the treating provider indicating readiness of return and recommendations (if any) for continued treatment. Sometimes, reentrants are asked to write a brief statement explaining the completion of any university expectations during their leave. In addition, the student may need to notify the Dean of Students Office prior to the planned semester or quarter of returning. In some IHE's this is required as early as 8 weeks beforehand. The Student Affairs Office will then review the student's request, often involving the campus mental health/counseling center or other services if indicated and determine whether or not they have completed all expectations for reinstatement. Some institutions may also require a psychological evaluation completed independently by a professional of the university's choosing to assess the readiness of return [18]. Generally, the letter from the provider regarding fitness to re-enroll must speak to the resolution of the specific issues in the MLOA and what would be helpful for the student when they return [18].

Leave of Absence and the Legal System

From time to time, the legal system weighs in on what are considered the "rights" of college students. Lawsuits against universities have helped other institutions revamp their MLOA policies. It is clear that leaves of absence for mental health needs are sometimes necessary. However, it must be considered to be the last resort when reasonable accommodations cannot help stabilize the medical or mental health crisis.

In 2018, a class action lawsuit was brought against Stanford University for perceived violations of anti-discrimination toward students who suffered from mental health issues [19]. Students claimed they were being forced to leave the campus, sometimes under threat of expulsion. Students also expressed concerns that the university would often not provide additional support or resources, but, rather, exclusively encourage a leave of absence. Students additionally alleged that favorable guidance or opinions made by their off-campus treating providers, mental health professionals, were not followed nor taken into consideration by the university. Upon return, plaintiffs charged that they were required to write personal statements "accepting blame" regarding their behaviors leading to the forced LOA [12]. A confidential settlement was reached in October 2019 which resulted in negotiated revisions to the leave of absence policy and procedures. This case is considered a landmark win for those with mental health concerns, according to the Disability Rights Advocates (DRA) [19]. The DRA is hopeful that this case will bring about change and implement progress for other colleges and universities across the country to help advocate for those who suffer from mental health disabilities. In addition, the university has partnered with The Jed Foundation to help build and develop programs addressing mental health needs. According to The Jed Foundation (JED) website, one of the foundation's missions is "to guide schools through a collaborative process of comprehensive systems, program and policy development with customized support to build upon existing student mental health, substance use and suicide prevention efforts." Designated "JED Campuses" embark on a 4-year strategic partnership that not only assesses and enhances the work that is already being done but helps to create positive, systemic change in the "campus community" (JED). This program is affiliated with over 200+ colleges and universities nationwide, spreading mental health awareness.

Until the 1960s, higher institutions adopted a law of in loco parentis, a Latin phrase meaning "in place of the parent," generally describing the legal relationship of a temporary legal guardian, including an entity, and a minor. This in turn meant the university would act with parental prerogative (rights, duties, and responsibilities) toward students. Following a series of several court cases, this concept evolved and ultimately dissolved in the 1990s, so that the relationship has changed between universities and students, allowing students their constitutional rights and protections. Despite the demise of in loco parentis for IHEs, legal cases have since occurred where universities have been found negligent in providing protections for students. An example of this is *Mullins v Pine Manor College (1983)*, after a female student was raped on campus. The student sued the college for failing to protect her from the incident, and the courts ruled in her favor [20]. IHE sometimes continue to struggle to find a balance between the duty to protect and allowing individual rights.

Results from a Survey Conducted by Authors

The authors conducted a convenience survey with several universities in the USA to gain more understanding about the medical leave of absence process and how teaching institutions implement policies for LOA. Authors reached out to 11 universities/colleges with an attempt to be geographically diverse by contacting IHE in four regions (i.e., North, West, South, East USA) with the results presented below. Authors included information available publicly on university websites. In cases where information was either restricted for public use or was not available, the authors attempted to obtain this information via telephone. A convenience survey was used due to accessibility, efficiency, and limited financial resources. Although the information obtained was enlightening and educational, our findings are limited due to a small sample size and inability for clear generalization. See Tables 23.1 and 23.2.

Authors found that about three-fourths of LOA requests are mental health related. In two of the universities (Blue and Green), they occurred most commonly in students in the freshman and sophomore years. However, Orange University described the majority of LOA requests being from students in their senior year (R. Rodriguez, personal communication, November 14, 2019; Green University, personal communication, November 11, 2019; and Orange University, personal communication, December 17, 2019).

Authors noticed that universities used different terms for leaves of absence and varied in policies for accommodations and reinstatement. After reviewing LOA from different universities, some areas of concern were noted from students' personal experiences. For example, student status and eligibility for campus services were cut off when TAY were no longer an "active" student (Yellow University, personal communication, December 9, 2019).This introduces barriers such as loss of school health insurance, campus housing, and school services including access to the campus mental health counseling center (Hartocollis, 2019; Yellow University, personal communication, December 9, 2019). This could ultimately cause further disruption and distress to the student who is already suffering from a mental health crisis.

One university presented the option to purchase extended school health insurance out of pocket, therefore, maintaining the ability to continue counseling services through the university. It was noted that out-of-pocket costs for insurance were often high and therefore unlikely to be a viable option (Yellow University, personal communication, December 9, 2019). At other universities, this parallel of employee offered continuation of health coverage (COBRA)-type benefit would continue health insurance but not permit disenrolled student to access on campus care (V. Chan, personal communication, June 19, 2020). Housing loss for freshmen and sophomores can be more problematic than for juniors and seniors who usually establish off-campus apartment living. Students who take MLOA generally lose student housing eligibility. Some sites even suggest that after LOA is granted, students may have 24–48 h and not more than 5 days to move out. This can intensify stress, making it

Table 23.2 Survey of a university sample chosen based upon geographic location

US regions	University	Responded to request	Allows LOA?	Information available on website?
North	White	☒	☒	☒
	Green	☐	☐ "medical withdrawal"	☐
West	Pink	☒	☐ "hardship withdrawal"	☐
	Yellow	☐	☒	☐
	Black	☒	☒	☒
	Indigo	☐	☐	☐
South	Orange	☐	☐ "medical withdrawal"	☐
East	Brown	☐	☒	☒
	Blue	☐	☐	☐
	Purple	☒	☐ "excused withdrawal"	☐
	Red	☒	☐	☐

Information obtained from respective school websites [Refs. 2, 4, 5, 11, 17, 18, 20–23]

more difficult for the student to prioritize their mental health needs. In some situations, unstable home situations complicate the students' recovery. With loss of campus-based housing, these students may have to return to an environment that could be triggering and cause further exacerbation of their symptoms. A student may speak with the housing office to explore options, which are often limited.

Case Example 1: Continued

Ron met with his advisor, who offered to help him get connected more quickly to a local psychotherapist. He also discussed the procedure for taking a MLOA. Ron reviewed his options with his family and his outpatient psychiatrist, and they all agreed that he would take the rest of the semester off and move back home with his family. He completed an application in which he proposed a plan to complete one community college course and volunteer at the humane society for 10 h per week in addition to attending psychotherapy sessions twice per week. With regular therapy sessions and close follow-up by the psychiatrist, Ron achieved stability once again. He contacted the university weeks in advance of the new semester, submitted an application for reinstatement in which he reported on his experience, and had his psychiatrist and therapist write letters attesting to his participation in treatment, current status, and future recommendations. He continued to see his therapist twice per week via telehealth (to minimize need for travel) and was able to cut down to once-weekly sessions later in the semester as he continued to demonstrate improvement.

Case Example 2: Continued

Being in another state, at a new university, with new adult responsibilities, including newly acquired independence, was becoming a stressor for Julia. Her mental health worsened, causing a crisis and leading her to return home for family support. She subsequently lost her scholarship, and she had to enroll locally in a community college. While her list of regrets clearly included her medication non-compliance, she also described the feeling of being "lost" while pursuing an education in an unfamiliar state where she did not know insurance work-arounds, struggled to connect with local mental health providers, and had no knowledge of college mental health resources. She left college without exploring any of the campus resources that were available. Again, stigma played a big role in Julia not feeling comfortable disclosing her mental health needs to her college. She described several attempts to locate mental health services by either searching the college website or reaching out to friends for help, both with no success.

Julia needed tremendous support in navigating resources. She was a scholarship recipient, and her fear of losing it was completely reasonable. Lack of knowledge about leave of absence, the "unknowns" about what happens to scholarships during LOA, stigma associated with disclosures, and difficulty navigating healthcare resources all contributed to her suboptimal transition to college. It was very critical for someone like Julia to get connected with services locally with additional information about what can happen while she is on LOA. College website clarity around these issues would have helped. A lack of institutional climate and culture that supported conversations around mental health and wellness contributed to her academic and mental health challenges.

Conclusions

Mental health problems that require professional intervention are common (one in five people). That applies to students entering college as well. After the Virginia Tech massacre, IHEs have recognized the importance of mental wellness on campus. Mental wellness is an essential part of optimal academic performance, and efforts need to be directed toward developing supportive structures for students. The expansion of university counseling centers and attention to institutional climate improvements that support not only the students' academic progress but their whole body wellness are examples. Of these services, mental health is an increasingly important focus in many IHEs. Despite these expansions, primary and secondary prevention efforts may not avert student regression. Sometimes, students decompensate to the point where temporary or even permanent leave of absence is necessary. LOA policies are not standard in all universities, but authors recommend that it should be an available strategy for all students who may need extra support to complete their education. For IHEs, the investment in making such procedures clear and relatively straightforward can provide guidance through many crises and sentinel events and minimize loss of talented students. The administrative structure within an IHE should provide clear policies that students can easily access. Delineating the roles and responsibilities of the Dean of Student Affairs, appointing committees with a mandate to fairly and equitably assess leave requests, and convening a team to deal with threat assessment are good initiatives for IHEs. The medical leave of absence is an excellent tool to provide an opportunity for students to focus on recovery and return back to the IHE to complete their degree in a healthy and happy manner.

References

1. Davis M. Addressing the needs of youth in transition to adulthood. Adm Policy Ment Health Ment Health Serv Res. 2003;30(6):495–509.
2. Gruttadaro D, Crudo D. College students speak: a survey report on mental health. Retrieved from National Alliance on Mental Illness website: https://www.nami.org/About-NAMI/Publications-Reports/Survey-Reports/College-Students-Speak_A-Survey-Report-on-Mental-H.pdf. 2012.
3. Centers for Disease Control and Prevention. Web based injury statistics query and reporting system. 2018.
4. Wilcox HC, Arria AM, Caldeira KM, Vincent KB, Pinchevsky GM, O'Grady KE. Prevalence and predictors of persistent suicide ideation, plans, and attempts during college. J Affect Disord. 2010;127(1–3):287–94.
5. Hunt J, Eisenberg D, Kilbourne AM. Consequences of receipt of a psychiatric diagnosis for completion of college. Psychiatr Serv. 2010;61(4):399–404.
6. Kessler RC, Amminger GP, Aguilar-Gaxiola S, Alonso J, Lee S, Ustun TB. Age of onset of mental disorders: a review of recent literature. Curr Opin Psychiatry. 2007;20(4):359.
7. Feldblum CR, Barry K, Benfer EA. The ADA Amendments Act of 2008. Tex. J. on CL & CR. 2007;13:187.
8. Hawke CS. Accommodating students with disabilities. New Dir Comm Coll. 2004;2004(125):17–27.
9. Eisenberg D, Downs MF, Golberstein E, Zivin K. Stigma and help seeking for mental health among college students. Med Care Res Rev. 2009;66(5):522–41.
10. Arain M, Haque M, Johal L, Mathur P, Nel W, Rais A, Sandhu R, Sharma S. Maturation of the adolescent brain. Neuropsychiatr Dis Treat. 2013;9:449–61. https://doi.org/10.2147/NDT.S39776.
11. White HR, Labouvie EW, Papadaratsakis V. Changes in substance use during the transition to adulthood: a comparison of college students and their noncollege age peers. J Drug Issues. 2005;35(2):281–306.
12. Hartocollis A. Feeling suicidal, students turned to their college. They were told to go home. [Internet]. 2018 [cited 2019 Dec]. Available from: https://www.nytimes.com/2018/08/28/us/college-suicide-stanford-leaves.html.
13. Medical leave of absence [Internet]. 2019 [cited 2019]. Available from: http://bulletin.vcu.edu/academic-regs/ugrad/medical-leave-absence/.
14. Involuntary Leave of Absence and Return Policy [Internet]. 2019 [cited 2019Dec2]. Available from: https://stanford.app.box.com/v/involuntary-leave-of-absence.
15. Bingham T. Discrimination in education: public versus private universities. J Law Educ. 2007;36:273.
16. Eels GT, Rockland-Miller HS. Addressing and responding to disturbed and disturbing students: understanding the role of administrative teams in institutions of higher education. J Coll Stud Psychother. 2011;25(1):8–23.
17. National Threat Assessment Center. Enhancing school safety using a threat assessment model: An operational guide for preventing targeted school violence. US Secret Service, Department of Homeland Security; 2018. pp. 1–32.
18. NYU. Student leave policy [Internet]. 2018 [cited 2019]. Available from: https://www.nyu.edu/about/policies-guidelines-compliance/policies-and-guidelines/student-leave-policy.html.
19. Anderson G. Stanford changes leave policies on mental illness [Internet]. 2019 [cited 2019 Dec]. Available from: https://www.insidehighered.com/news/2019/10/08/stanford-changes-leave-policies-mental-illness.
20. Lee P. The curious life of in loco parentis at American Universities [Internet]. Scholar.harvard.edu. 2011 [cited 17 June 2020]. Available from: https://scholar.harvard.edu/files/philip_lee/files/vol8lee.pdf.
21. Leaves of Absence [Internet]. Handbook.fas.harvard.edu. 2019 [cited 2019 Dec 20]. Available from:

https://handbook.fas.harvard.edu/book/leaves-absence#four.
22. Long AB. Introducing the new and improved Americans with disabilities act: assessing the ADA amendments act of 2008. Northwest Univ Law Rev Colloquy. 2008;103:217.
23. Medical Withdrawal [Internet]. [cited 2019 Nov 19]. Available from: https://odos.illinois.edu/community-of-care/resources/medical-withdrawal/.
24. FIRE's Guide to due process and campus justice — Full Text - FIRE [Internet]. FIRE. 2019 [cited 20 Dec 2019]. Available from: https://www.thefire.org/research/publications/fire-guides/fires-guide-to-due-process-and-campus-justice/fires-guide-to-due-process-and-fair-procedure-on-campus-full-text/#__RefHeading__2512_2127946742.
25. Hardship Withdrawal Petition for Courses [Internet]. Office of the University Registrar. [cited 5 Dec 2019]. Available from: https://registrar.washington.edu/students/hardship-withdrawal-petition-for-courses/.
26. Hunt J, Eisenberg D. Mental health problems and help-seeking behavior among college students. J Adolesc Health. 2010;46(1):3–10.
27. Learn About JED Campus [Internet]. [cited 2019 Dec]. Available from: https://www.jedcampus.org/about/.
28. Leave of Absence Request [Internet]. UCLA graduate programs. [cited 2019 Nov]. Available from: https://grad.ucla.edu/academics/graduate-study/leave-of-absence-request/.
29. Undergraduate Degrees and Programs [Internet]. [cited 2019 Dec]. Available from: https://exploredegrees.stanford.edu/undergraduatedegreesandprograms/#leavesandreinstatementtext.
30. Virginia Tech Academic Relief [Internet]. [cited 2019 Nov]. Available from: https://www.healthcenter.vt.edu/medical_records/academic_relief.html.
31. Watkins DC, Hunt JB, Eisenberg D. Increased demand for mental health services on college campuses: perspectives from administrators. Qual Soc Work. 2012;11(3):319–37.
32. Withdrawal [Internet]. [cited 2019 Dec]. Available from: https://catalog.utexas.edu/general-information/academic-policies-and-procedures/withdrawal/.
33. Withdrawal from Classes [Internet]. 2019 [cited 2019 Dec 1]. Available from: https://secretary.temple.edu/sites/secretary/files/policies/02.10.14.pdf.

Index

V. Chan, J. Derenne (eds.), *Transition-Age Youth Mental Health Care*,
https://doi.org/10.1007/978-3-030-62113-1

B

C

MIX
Papier aus verantwortungsvollen Quellen
Paper from responsible sources
FSC® C105338

If you have any concerns about our products,
you can contact us on
ProductSafety@springernature.com

In case Publisher is established outside the EU,
the EU authorized representative is:
Springer Nature Customer Service Center GmbH
Europaplatz 3, 69115 Heidelberg, Germany

Printed by Libri Plureos GmbH
in Hamburg, Germany